Myelodysplasias and Exstrophies:
Significance, Prevention, and Treatment

Edited By
David B. Shurtleff, M.D.

Professor
Department of Pediatrics
University of Washington
Seattle, Washington

Illustrated by
Cathy Herndon

G&S

Grune & Stratton, Inc.
Harcourt Brace Jovanovich, Publishers
Orlando New York San Diego Boston London
San Francisco Tokyo Sydney Toronto

Grune & Stratton, Inc.
Orlando, Florida 32887

Distributed in the United Kingdom by
Grune & Stratton, Ltd.
24/28 Oval Road, London NW 1

Library of Congress Catalog Number 86-80920
International Standard Book Number 0-8089-1816-8
Printed in the United States of America
86 87 88 89 10 9 8 7 6 5 4 3 2 1

Dedication

Dedicated to all patients, their families, and affected friends who have contributed their lives and feelings to this work; and to all my own family, students, colleagues, and co-workers. And especially to J. Timothy Stuntz, M.D., physician and neurosurgeon, who was a living author, colleague and friend, who died during publication of this text. No truer friend to the mentally impaired ever existed. All to whom this text is dedicated above will understand the addition of his name. Without him, this work would have been impossible.

Contents

Section I: History and Philosophy

Section II: Initial Medical Treatment

Section III: Management of the Neurogenic Bowel and Bladder

Foreword

This book has been written to provide both the general reader and the specialist with a comprehensive understanding of the complex issues involved in the growth and development of children kept alive by our modern technology, despite being born with major malformations. It describes our clinical experiences drawn from a computerized data file that has evolved over a period of 28 years. This work is an incomplete study that is being used as a model by which we measure the progress of our regional demonstration, clinical research, teaching, and patient care program. The disorders described in this text were medical curiosities, most of whom died, until only one quarter of a century ago. Little has been written about the exstrophies and the tail bud anomalies. They and the other forms of myelodysplasia, mostly meningomyeloceles, share the three problems of (1) impaired mobility, (2) impaired sphincters, and (3) central nervous system disabilities that until the social changes of the last decade rendered individuals with these malformations handicapped. Because we have such large numbers of patients with meningomyelocele, they have served as a model for analysis of our treatments and hypotheses. When appropriate, we have referred to studies that include lipomeningoceles, myelocystoceles, and other lower spinal cord lesions as myelodysplasia. When studies are applicable to all impaired, disabled, or handicapped children, we have attempted to use the most appropriate term, as defined in Chapters 1 and 2. Although the literature has been carefully reviewed and cited, this text is unique in that most of the data about our patients has been computer generated. I hope each reader will find at least a portion of this text both of interest and a guide to help at least one patient.

Acknowledgments

This text would not have been possible without the support and input of many organizations and individuals. The longest and largest support was provided over 25 years by the March of Dimes-Birth Defects Foundation through a series of different grants that both started the project and provided long-term support, a critical need for those of us who study chronic disease. Many March of Dimes volunteers not only provided financial support, but also worked in the clinic on research projects and provided guidance and counsel. They include: Felix Montes, Mort Bobrow, Bob Perry, Charles Massey, Charles Russell, Talley Goiney, Carla Freeman, Torchy Torrence, and many others. I regret there is not sufficent space to name them all.

The four people most responsible for the production of this text include a March of Dimes Volunteer, a volunteer investigator who spent many hours over many years helping me develop and maintain the computerized data file, a collaborator as a graduate student, a contributor in her own right as a professional educator, Cynthia Shurtleff, M.Ed., my wife. The statistical analyses and the computer drawn charts and graphs would not have been possible without the assistance of Jan Lamers, B.S., a colleague for 14 years. The actual reduction of ideas to print would have never occurred without tireless effort under the stress of criticism by both the typist-editor, Betsy Brown, B.A., and the technical editor and my daughter, Hillary Shurtleff, M.A.

Intellectual contributions to this text have been recognized formally in each chapter by listing the author or coauthors, researchers, and reviewers. This documentation, however, does not include recognition of many past and current students and colleagues whose ideas have been incorporated. Whether each of the primary authors' opinions are original or learned from others, can no longer be distinguished. In an attempt to place their contributions in some order of perspective, we have identified the person who wrote the original draft first with coauthors in order of their contribution (except Chapter 17 that was written in segments and then rewritten for constancy of editorial style). Researchers provided original unpublished data included in Chapter 15. Reviewers provided criticism and offered suggestions. Not all of the original authors', coauthors', researchers', and reviewers' suggestions have been incorporated. Unacceptable, inaccurate, and inappropriate statements are, therefore, the responsibility of the principal author.

Although all chapters are a composite of the ideas of numerous individuals, several warrant special mention. The first two chapters are, undoubtedly, the most controversial and were the most difficult to write. Their multiple revisions by the technical editor attempted to synthesize a diverse literature with the primary author's beliefs and practice. The criticisms and encouragement of the reviewers are particularly appreciated since the existing format reflects our own views. We hope they will be of value to the reader. Chapters 9 through 11 have been written by our clinic nurses and urologists with the intent to reflect our practice and dialogue with patients. Hopefully, this section will be of value to both laymen and professionals. Chapter 15 reflects more original observations and incorporates more controversial concepts than any other. We are appreciative of the considerable effort expended by the large number of reviewers and contributors. As mentioned above for Section 3, the primary author only supplemented Sections 5 and 6 primarily written by educators, psychologists, and therapists.

Not listed among contributors to this text are a number of persons I would like to acknowledge. Students not listed except in the bibliography include Robert Goiney, M.D., Larry Kuhns, M.D., Paul Montes, M.D., Gary Okamoto, M.D., M.P.H., Sandra Davenport, M.D., Lowell Sever, Ph.D., Charlene Butler, Ed.D., Jan Carr Sousa, RPT, MS, Colleen Sheehan Van Ness, OTR, MPT, Margaret Bartlett, MPT, and Kathy Hinderer, RPT. Colleagues not recognized elsewhere include Sterling Clarren, M.D., E. Franklin Stone, M.D., Warren Chapman, M.D., David McLone, M.D., Robert Jones, FRACS, Sigvard Hansen, M.D., Howard King, M.D., Theodore Wagner, M.D., John Sharrard, FRCS, Laurence Gordon, M.D., Margaret Hill, R.N., P.H.N., Maurine Swanson, R.N., Deborah Gregory, M.S.W., Arline Broy, M.S.W., and Kenneth Vanderhof, Esq. The fundamental scientific philosophy that is the basis for the data collection and analysis presented in this text has been derived from the early teachings of my undergraduate advisor Professor Hooten and residency program director Allan Butler, M.D., and his staff. This philosophy is simple: if you can observe a difference, you can measure it; if you can measure a difference, you can quantitate, compare, and analyze it. Both the academic career of the primary author and his interest in the subject of this test were created by Robert A. Aldrich, M.D., Philip Dodge, M.D., Douglas McKay, M.D., Josef Warkany, M.D., Julian Ansell, M.D., Professor Michael Laurence, FRCP, and Malcolm Menelaus, FRACS. A few of the parents and patients who have provided insight into many of the problems discussed in this text include Kent Smith, Executive Director of SBAA, Betty Pieper, SBAA, Nan Gingher, Adult Network SBAA, Joulian Joubert, Septogenarian (deceased), Janice Tasker, her mother Mary Shandorf and foster brother Michael Eakin (deceased), Doynell Martin and her adopted daughter Lori Ann (deceased), Barbara Stanton (deceased) and family, Gary Kettles, MBA, Leon McCleerey, Ph.D., Fred Gross, Frank Prewoznick and family, Joanne Keyser Armstrong, Charolette Hotelling, Francis and Jerry Rinder, and Adam, Blanche, and "Doctor Doc" Pallister

Other financial support required to complete this work included early support by the institutional Clinical Research Center NIH Grant Number RR-37 and Children's Orthopedic Hospital and Medical Center study R-24-3; recent support from NIHR Grant #G008436-05, Shriner's Unit of Honolulu, and a quarter century of support from gifts and bequests to the Division of Congenital Defects.

I apologize to the many other students, colleagues, friends, patients, and their families who have contributed in many ways to this work but have not been mentioned.

Contributors

Authors

Julian Ansell, M.D.
Professor and Chairman, Department of Urology, University of Washington, Seattle, Washington

Kevin Dunne, M.B., B.S., F.R.A.C.P.
Fellow, Division of Congenital Defects, Department of Pediatrics, University of Washington, Children's Orthopedic Hospital and Medical Center, Seattle, Washington

Gayle Fay, Ph.D.
Director, Neurodiagnostic Clinic, Children's Orthopedic Hospital and Medical Center, Seattle, Washington

William Friedrich, Ph.D.
Assistant Professor, Department of Psychology, University of Washington, Seattle, Washington

Patricia Hayden, M.D.
Professor, Department of Pediatrics, Chief of Birth Defects Clinic, University of Washington, Children's Orthopedic Hospital and Medical Center, Seattle, Washington

D. Kiko Kimura, R.N.
Nurse Clinician, Children's Orthopedic Hospital and Medical Center, Seattle, Washington

Kay Wicks, R.N.
Tertiary Care Nurse Supervisor, Children's Orthopedic Hospital and Medical Center, Seattle, Washington

Lynn Wolf, M.O.T., O.T.R.
Research Associate, Department of Pediatrics, University of Washington, Children's Orthopedic Hospital and Medical Center, Seattle, Washington

Researchers

Brian Dudgeon, M.S., O.T.R.
Clinical Head, Division of Occupational Therapy, Children's Orthopedic Hospital and Medical Center, Seattle, Washington

William Friedrich, Ph.D.
Assistant Professor, Department of Psychology, University of Washington, Seattle, Washington

Ken Jaffe, M.D.
Assistant Professor, Rehabilitation Medicine, Adjunct Assistant Professor, Department of Pediatrics, University of Washington, Children's Orthopedic Hospital and Medical Center, Seattle, Washington

Craig McDonald, B.A.
Research Associate, Department of Rehabilitation Medicine, University of Washington School of Medicine, Children's Orthopedic Hospital and Medical Center, Seattle, Washington

Joyce Shaffer, Ph.D.
Consultant Psychologist, Division of Congenital Defects, Children's Orthopedic Hospital and Medical Center, Seattle, Washington

Jan Carr Sousa, R. P. T., M.S.
Former Research Associate, Division of Congenital Defects, Department of Pediatrics, University of Washington, Seattle, Washington

Ronald Lemire, M.D.
Professor, Department of Pediatrics, Director, Inpatient Services, University of Washington, Children's Orthopedic Hospital and Medical Center, Seattle, Washington

Michael Mayo, M.D.
Associate Professor, Department of Urology, University of Washington, Seattle, Washington

John McLaughlin, M.D.
Associate Professor, Department of Pediatrics, Chief, Neuromuscular Clinic, University of Washington, Children's Orthopedic Hospital and Medical Center, Seattle, Washington

Joyce Shaffer, Ph.D.
Consultant Psychologist, Division of Congenital Defects, Children's Orthopedic Hospital and Medical Center, Seattle, Washington

David Shurtleff, M.D.
Professor, Department of Pediatrics, Head, Division of Congenital Defects, University of Washington, Children's Orthopedic Hospital and Medical Center, Seattle, Washington

Hillary Shurtleff, M.A.
Technical Editor, Division of Congenital Defects, Children's Orthopedic Hospital and Medical Center, Seattle, Washington

J. Timothy Stuntz, M.D.
Clinical Associate Professor, Neurological Surgery, University of Washington, Head, Division of Neurosurgery, Children's Orthopedic Hospital and Medical Center, Seattle, Washington

Josef Warkany, M.D.
Professor of Research, Department of Pediatrics, University of Cincinnati, Children's Hospital Research Foundation, Cincinnati, Ohio

Reviewers

Michael Bayles, Ph.D.
Professor, Department of Philosophy, University of Florida, Gainesville, Florida

Luciano Dias, M.D.
Assistant Professor, Department of Orthopedics, Northwestern University, Chicago, Illinois

John Freeman, M.D.
Professor and Head, Division of Pediatric Neurology Johns Hopkins Hospital, Baltimore, Maryland

Richard Marshall, M.D.
Professor and Head, Division of Neonatology, Department of Pediatrics, Washington University, St. Louis Children's Hospital, St. Louis, Missouri

Malcolm Menelaus, F.R.C.S., F.R.A.C.S.
Chief Orthopaedic Surgeon, Royal Children's Hospital, Melbourne, Australia

Douglas McKay, M.D.
Professor, Department of Orthopedics, George Washington University, Chairman, Pediatric Orthopedic Surgery Department, National Children's Medical Center, Washington, D.C.

Philip Pallister, M.D., D.Sci. hc.
Adjunct Professor of Medicine, Montana State University, Bozeman, Montana, Clinical Professor, Department of Pediatrics, University of Washington, Seattle, Washington

Lynn Staheli, M.D.
Professor and Director, Department of Orthopedics, University of Washington Children's Orthopedic Hospital and Medical Center, Seattle, Washington

Lynn Wolf, M.O.T., O.T.R.
Research Associate, Pediatrics, University of Washington, Children's Orthopedic Hospital and Medical Center, Seattle, Washington

SECTION I

History and Philosophy

Hillary Shurtleff
David Shurtleff

1

Decision Making for the Treatment or Nontreatment of Congenitally Malformed Individuals

This chapter examines the influences affecting the decision-making process involved in caring for congenitally malformed individuals. Before examining the techniques of care, it is necessary to understand the various influences that affect the decision for treatment or nontreatment and that impact long-term care.

The decision for or against providing care for congenitally malformed individuals is not simple. It involves a complex of interacting influences, including (1) cultural beliefs concerning the significance and treatment of birth defects; (2) current treatment technology; (3) available resources; and (4) public policy. In monocultural societies, the first three components are usually synthesized into a clearly understood public policy, but in our polycultural society in the United States, the interaction of these components is more complex. Health care providers should attempt to identify all four components since participants in a care decision for an impaired child may be dissimilarly affected by these influences and, therefore, may approach each treatment decision differently.

Each component must be considered because the participants in such a decision usually have different experiences and beliefs, which can directly influence their understanding of and, therefore, choice of, treatment. Three potential types of differences between participants exist: (1)

MYELODYSPLASIAS AND EXSTROPHIES: SIGNIFICANCE, PREVENTION, AND TREATMENT
 ISBN 0-8089-1816-8

family members disagree among themselves and with others in society; (2) the family's beliefs differ from medical recommendations; and (3) health care providers disagree among themselves.

To better understand these differences that are important to the process of making a treatment decision, it is helpful to understand how they evolved throughout history. This discussion will lead to a better understanding of current prenatal and postnatal decision-making processes involving severely congenitally malformed fetuses and infants who will always bear impairments because their original defects cannot be cured.

CULTURAL BELIEFS

Historical Background

The following anthropological data indicate birth defects have existed for a long time: the neolithic skeleton of a child with hydrocephaly, found in Seeburg, Germany;[134] the 10,000–12,000-yr-old skeletons of persons with spina bifida excavated in Morocco;[330] the 5,000-yr-old skull of an anencephalic located in a holy burial ground in ancient Egypt;[301,962] the late Saxon skull of a person with Down syndrome (with microcephaly and excessive brachycephaly), found in Leichestershire;[134] the high percentage, 7.3 percent, of skeletons with first sacral spinal clefts (spina bifida) from Romano-Britain;[134] and the protohistoric skeletons of persons with lumbosacral neural arch defects found in Modoc tribe burial grounds in Arizona (this tribe had the highest known incidence of this defect).[87,431]

Societal attitudes toward these malformations are indicated by where these remains were found. For example, since the skull of an anencephalic was buried in a holy burial ground for apes and ibis, the person with this defect must have been considered holy. Moroccan and Modoc remains were buried with similar findings from other members of the group, suggesting their acceptance as equals. More substantial records of attitudes can be found in written material. The oldest written record of reactions to congenital malformations may be the Babylonian tablets,[599,630] dating back to 1,700 B.C. These tablets reveal 62 prophesies, both positive and negative, derived from congenital defects.[599,630]

The long history of attitudes toward congenital malformations includes a changing spectrum of social attitudes as well as differences between cultures at a given time. Attitudes toward the initial treatment or nontreatment of the congenitally malformed are briefly discussed in this chapter, and attitudes as they affect the rights and socialization of the same group are discussed in the next chapter.

Attitudes Toward Treatment or Nontreatment

Historically, in monocultural societies, public policy concerning the congenitally malformed almost directly reflected the relationship of a society to its resources. Although, as Alland[23] has pointed out, environment was not an active force, it was a selecting agent; that is, it influenced societal change or adaptation. Monocultural responses form the basis for the development of current cultural beliefs within polycultural societies.

Some societies with abundant food resources were able to preserve all individuals. Kwakiutl native Americans of the Pacific Northwest coast had such abundant resources they were able to care for their disabled.[498] The masks made by this tribe indicate some congenital malformations may have even been respected. For example, Noolthmal masks represented Treacher-Collins syndrome,[498] and owning this type of mask was considered a powerful privilege.[743] Today, Kwakiutl Indian behavior reflects this heritage: most members of this group preserve their congenitally malformed infants.

In nomadic societies, mobility required crippled members be left behind or eliminated. The north central native American, Athabaskan and central plains Indians, survived by tracking and hunting moose, caribou, and buffalo; thus, they did not preserve their defective or old individuals (for example, the old arrowhead maker in Hiawatha was left behind to care for himself[659]). Today, the Athabaskan and plains Indians are affected by their heritage in that some still do not accept congenitally malformed infants.

Overpopulated societies, such as China and Hawaii, eliminated defective infants as a means of population control. Today, in both China and Hawaii (as in the other American states), abortion is a method of birth control accepted by some. In China, where girls are being "suppressed," there is an increased risk of cot death for female infants; Emery[304] not only points to this increase, but suggests that as many as one in ten cot deaths may be due to filicide.

Today, the spectrum of reactions to congenitally malformed individuals, as exemplified by responses to infants with meningomyelocele, reflects similar relationships between public policy and societal resources. On one extreme, Gross and associates[427] in Oklahoma as well as Lorber[666] in England recommend treating only the most promising cases of meningomyelocele. As Gross and associates stated, the poor quality of some survivors of modern surgical treatment has led to an alarming number of dependents on the state and a resulting drain on limited social resources.[426] In addition, in Great Britain, houses with steep stairways inaccessible to individuals with wheelchairs and fewer societal resources make it more difficult for paralyzed individuals to develop productive adult life-styles[318] than in the United States.[729,736,901]

At the other extreme, McLone and associates[740] in Chicago as well as Reigel[901] in Pittsburg advocate treating all infants with meningomyelocele referred to them. These authors participate in active parents' groups and assist families in obtaining appropriate societal resources such as social services, education, and vocational training services. In the United States, public laws mandate education, vocational training, and access to public places, advantages not available in Great Britain, but unfortunately, implementation of these laws is not uniform in all areas of our United States. Oklahoma apparently has less to offer, according to Gross and associates,[427] than Pittsburg and Chicago. Variations in the availability of local resources may reflect differences in local beliefs and in turn result in the availability of fewer resources regulated by state agencies. McLone and Riegel offer one alternative to depriving the impaired of life, as recommended by Gross and associates.

Although these varied reactions to the congenitally malformed exist, we in the polycultural society of the United States share to different degrees the influence of one main cultural group: the Anglo-Saxons.

Development of Anglo-Saxon Beliefs

Preventing child abuse and treating congenitally malformed infants are both influenced by how much human life is valued and are, therefore, clearly linked. If, for example, a culture does not value normal infants, it is even less likely to value defective infants.[59] In the 1700s, the pressure of overpopulation affected attitudes toward children. Swift's "A Modest Proposal" satirized the growing lack of concern for the value of human life found in the overpopulated slums of Ireland.[59,1139] In 1798, Malthus[59,690] predicted the inability of society to support its ever-larger number of children (both normal and abnormal). This reaction foreshadowed attitudes brought by the planned increase in number of children in the middle 1800s stimulated by the Industrial Revolution and described by Charles Dickens in such works as *Oliver Twist*.[270] At this time, children were kept alive as cheap labor, but often were treated so poorly that they died early. They were even deliberately maimed so they could make money begging or in circuses.[59]

Almost a century after Malthus's prediction, Darwin pointed out that not only were abortion and infanticide a form of population control used around the world, but that only "savages" practiced them.[59,246] This greater concern for the value of human life reflected a reaction against earlier inhumane attitudes. During the second half of the century, attitudes toward congenitally malformed individuals, both adults and children, generally followed the trends of prevention of cruelty to children coincident with the rapidly expanding industrialization of Europe and the resultant availability of goods and services. This more humanistic movement was reflected in England by the new child abuse laws and the conversion of foundling homes to hospitals. For example, infants were no longer sent to Great Orman Street to die in what had been a foundling home, but were sent there to get cured in what is now a famous children's hospital in London.[59] In the United States, development of a society for the protection of children led to the passage of legislation creating maternal and child health services.[59]

Later in the early 20th century, large numbers of surviving, unproductive children were perceived as a burden, and the simultaneous social preoccupation with eugenics reintroduced an attitude favoring the elimination of defective children. This movement justified life according to its utility, that is, its usefulness to the state. During this time, Justice Oliver Wendell Holmes, representing the United States Supreme Court, ruled that sterilization of a microcephalic, mentally retarded woman was legal and appropriate, claiming that "three generations of idiots is enough."[141,403] In 1941, a group of Americans recommended compulsory euthanasia for the mentally retarded and congenitally deformed.[1210] These views prevailed at the same time as the actual starving to death of mentally and physically handicapped children by Pfannmueller and other physicians in Nazi Germany.[1210]

Recently, Lejeune,[631] the geneticist who first identified trisomy 21, considered disposing of fetuses and newborns who did not reach minimal specifications of normalcy. He came to the following conclusion:

> For millennia, medicine has striven to fight for life and health and against disease and death. Any reversal of these terms of reference would entirely change medicine itself. It happens that nature does condemn. Our duty has always been not to inflict the sentence but to try to commute the pain. In any forseeable genetical trial I do not know enough to judge, but I feel enough to advocate.[631]

Current, positive attitudes toward the value of the lives of the congenitally malformed are reflected in legislation described in Chapter 2, in the designation of this decade as the International Decade of the Disabled, and in the appointment of 1984 as the International Year of the Disabled. The public is becoming more aware of children with physical defects.[205] For example, the following four advertisements show how disabled persons are entering life-style advertising: a man with elbow canes, used because of paralysis due to polio, advertises the Voyager, A Chrysler-Plymouth van; a young man doing wheelies in a wheelchair on a boardwalk alongside a pretty girl shows off his Levis; a Vietnam veteran sitting in a wheelchair shaking hands with a man in a motorcycle praises

Kodak;[685] and a woman in a wheelchair playing basketball illustrates a Safeway bag and promotes fitness with the following caption: "Being disabled doesn't mean being unable." It is important for health care professionals to keep abreast of changes in social attitudes such as these in order to better inform parents of the potential for their impaired infant.

Reactions Affect Severity and Prevalence

Not only can a society react to "defective" individuals, but, through its reactions, it can also influence the severity and prevalence of a disease. As Moore and associates[773] have illustrated in *The Biocultural Basis of Health*, a certain group's reaction to a particular disease can "increase or decrease the severity" as well as the prevalence of that disease. The authors used the example of measles. The disease is usually not fatal in Western cultures,[773,799] but it is in a South American Indian tribe. Moore and associates[773] and Neel[799] attribute this high fatality rate to the tribe's social rejection of individuals with measles.

In a similar manner, the severity and prevalence of children with severe meningomyelocele are different where they (1) are all treated aggressively, as in Atlanta, Chicago, Pittsburg, and the Pacific Northwest[737,819,905,1058] (see Chapter 5); (2) are not all treated early but are kept alive with antibiotics, as in Ohio;[325] or (3) are managed so that many or all die, as in Sheffield, England,[671] and Oklahoma.[427] The prevalence is highest and the morbidity lowest in the first group. the prevalence is high, but the morbidity is also high in the second; and the prevalence is the lowest, but the morbidity the highest in the third. These results are examples of medical interreactions within different social contexts, but social contexts also affect prevalence at birth.

Elwood and Elwood[301] noted an inverse relationship between social class and prevalence at birth of meningomyelocele, but it is difficult to determine whether the relatively lower prevalence for individuals from higher social classes is due to better nutrition, a higher use of prenatal diagnosis and improved pregnancy outcome, better medical care, or some other factor or combination of factors, as discussed in Chapter 3.

Fuchs[380] has noted the effect of different life-styles on infant death rates in Utah and Nevada. Since the populations he studied are similar in most respects except for their religious preference, Fuchs attributed the difference between death rates in the two states to life-styles based on religion. Unlike most people in Nevada, most people from Utah are Mormons and, therefore, do not smoke, drink alcohol, or divorce. Fuchs attributes the low infant death rate in Utah to this "healthy" Mormon life-style and the high infant mortality rate in Nevada to the less healthy life-style of many people in that area. This trend is also remarkable in that

Mormons do not accept abortion even for defective fetuses, whereas many people in Nevada use abortion for both social and eugenic reasons. It is important for health care professionals to realize that these different cultural life-styles and beliefs exist and influence group as well as individual health. At the same time, we must recognize the possibility of dissimilar genetic stocks contributing to the differences in health.

Within our patient population, we have seen the dramatic effects of cultural beliefs on the severity and prevalence of congenital defects. Athabaskans and Kwakiutls (described above) now have similar resources and technology. Both are similarly influenced by public policy. But most of our Athabaskan patients with myelomeningocele have died, whereas all of our Kwakiutl patients with the same defect have lived. Since all of the other variables involved in the care of these native Americans are similar, cultural beliefs based on historical background (described earlier) must be an important determining factor.[498] Athabaskans historically have not accepted infants with meningomyelocele, whereas Kwakiutl native Americans have. Different mortality rates may be due to dissimilar parenting, as it is affected by cultural influences. We have described the influence of good parenting on the survival and well being of severely impaired children with meningomyelocele.[729]

Practitioners aware of these "biases" can affect the outcome of treatment. For example, by careful examination of beliefs and by encouraging parents from a social group that does not accept impaired infants to give up their congenitally malformed infant for adoption if they are prone to agree with their heritage, we can be relatively certain the infant has a better chance for survival. However, we cannot rightfully insist on removal of an impaired child from all parents from certain social groups since some may not agree with their heritage and may want their child regardless of the severity of the malformation.

Two families with whom we have worked, both from mountain tribes in Vietnam, exhibited opposing extreme reactions to their children's defects. We believe these different responses were due to the dissimilar beliefs of their tribal cultures. In one family, a trisomy 21 infant was taken home from the hospital only to be killed by the father, who then attempted suicide. We found out later that, according to this family's culture, death is more acceptable than living with a congenitally malformed child. Had we been aware of this cultural bias, we would have been able to suggest adoption or some other alternative. The other Vietnamese family had a child with a congenital defect of the blood. Instead of being disgraced when they found out the infant needed a transfusion, the family expressed joy since, in their culture, receiving blood is considered holy. Knowing this cultural belief prior to our discussion with the family would have alleviated our concern about informing them.

We have also observed variation within cultural groups, best exemplified by exceptions within a group of nonreligious, unwed mothers and within more religious groups consisting of Mormons and Spanish American Catholics. Generally, the nonreligious, unwed mothers tend to abort their fetuses and give up their deformed babies for adoption, whereas Mormons and Catholics tend to avoid abortion and opt to care for their children. However, exceptions always occur within groups. We have dealt with a number of unwed mothers without religious affiliation who have given birth to severely congenitally malformed infants and have taken excellent care of them. In addition, we have observed antiabortion Catholics opt for abortion of fetuses suspected of being abnormal. Black and Furlong[101] also discovered variations within groups. While most Protestants, Jews, and people with no religious preference planned to terminate their pregnancies if serious defects were detected and most Catholics did not, these trends were not without exceptions.

We have to be prepared, therefore, not only for parents' reactions as members of their culture but also for their reactions as individuals. For these reasons, we always discuss an affected fetus' or child's condition with the parents after ascertaining their personal feelings, family attitudes, and cultural beliefs. Some of the most unhappy parents we have known have been seen by health care providers who have not asked parents about their attitudes toward termination, relinquishment, or treatment versus nontreatment before providing the parents with recommendations contrary to firmly held beliefs (see Chapters 4 and 5).

In addition to affecting initial care decisions, sociocultural beliefs will subtly affect aspects of daily care, particularly since congenitally malformed infants often require comprehensive home care as well as modification of the home. Social attitudes, particularly when the parents have rejected their subculture or family norms, may lead later not only to complete rejection of the child and family, but to any number of reactions, including conflict, parental depression, neglect and overprotection. If health care providers are aware of the disparity between different parents and among general societal, local, cultural, family, and parental attitudes toward the congenitally malformed and how these beliefs may differ, they can anticipate problems and more easily help patients and families make informed decisions that will be most acceptable in the long-term. For further discussion of family adjustments to impaired children, see Chapter 18.

Parental Reactions to Health Care Providers

Parental beliefs affect not only their reactions to their congenitally malformed child but also their encounters with health care providers. Misunderstanding caused by discrepancies between family beliefs and medical recommendations can hinder the decision-making process.[362] Snow[1081] defines *disease* as a "malfunctioning maladaptation of biologic and psychophysiologic processes in the individual" and *illness* as "personal, interpersonal and cultural reactions to disease and discomfort," and points out that a patient's illness must be revealed before effective treatment can be undertaken.

The most outstanding example of cultural influence on health care practice was presented by Meleis and Jonsen.[746] They described a number of physician errors in dealing with the family of a man with Hodgkin's disease. Because the practitioners knew little about Arab customs, they violated many of the family's cultural beliefs. By the time they made the prognosis of death, the family was extremely hostile, particularly since, according to the Arabs' belief, the mention of death destroys all hope. The man's family would have been much happier had the physicians simply said they had done all they could and that it was up to Allah. We have had two such experiences with families of congenitally impaired infants but have been fortunate enough to known of the families' deep-rooted cultural beliefs and have, thereby, avoided any errors by adhering to the recommendations of Meleis and Jonsen.[746] In one case, a Moslem leader, and in the other, Gypsy leaders willingly described the patients' and families' expectations and worked closely with us to arrive at a treatment plan acceptable to all.

We had another experience similar to the one described by Meleis and Jonsen[746] but with one of our Catholic patients who became extremely upset when another physician suggested abortion. "He wants to kill my child," she said. We know that practitioner well, and he does not use the term killing for termination of a pregnancy. Although *killing a fetus* is usually not used interchangeably with *therapeutic abortion* or *termination*, we are aware that some of our patients find both phrases equal to the term *killing*. We suspect, too, that most health care providers take offense if the phrase *killing the fetus* is used instead of *therapeutic abortion* or *termination of pregnancy*, although all three expressions refer to the end of life for the fetus. Abortion and whether or not to treat an infant or an older child or adult are personal and emotional issues. It is difficult to discuss them because, although we can use the most medically accurate terms possible, we cannot always appreciate their effects on specific listeners whose feelings about these issues vary enormously.

In a physician–parent conference, on the other hand, health care providers can ask questions about beliefs and can carefully observe parental reactions to these emotion-laden topics. We have observed many parents accept with relief a 50-percent chance for retardation because they had believed the prognosis to be a hopeless 100-percent. Others have expressed horror at the mention of a 15-percent chance for mental retardation or at the mention of a mild impairment. Even more subtle facial expressions and body attitudes, such as a smile or a drooping face and shoulders, can be interpreted as hopeful acceptance or depressed rejection; these indicators are of paramount importance in parent interviews. We believe health care providers should also ask parents directly whether or not they wish to even discuss certain alternatives such as abortion or treatment versus nontreatment before suggesting such options.

Health Care Provider Biases

In order to be able to more accurately assess parental beliefs, we need to be aware of our own biases. Practitioners' beliefs affect both treatment and treatment outcome, as suggested in Chapters 4 and 5. Todres and associates[1167] discovered physicians who perceived themselves as religiously active were likely to recommend surgery for an infant with Down syndrome and a duodenal atresia or for an infant with severe meningomyelocele. Religious activity, religious affiliation, and physician age, sex, and job type define groups of practitioners with different biases. In order to offer the best advice possible, we should make ourselves aware of frequently unacknowledged influences such as recent experiences and personal beliefs.

The same actions and statements have been labeled both as "preservation" by a representative of one group and as "murder" by another. It is much easier to write about personal bias than to determine its existence. Personal opinions are biased only relative to the bias of others. Regardless, all practitioners should attempt to understand their own as well as their patients' families' biases and recognize that any decision must conform to individual, cultural, and group biases of all involved.[368,1209] The best protection against having one's bias become isolated and different from general and local society bias is to cooperate with nonmedical review boards as recommended by the President's Commission, the American Academy of Pediatrics, and parent organizations (see Chapters 2 and 5).

We are not suggesting health care providers know all cultural beliefs about health, but sociocultural beliefs are such a significant influence on the health–disease continuum that they can't be ignored. Medical education should help health care providers to see the moral nature of medical decisions and to counsel the "real decision makers"—the parents.[1183] We have learned that families are openly willing to share their beliefs before discussing treatment options. Trying to be more aware of the influence of beliefs and of individual deviations from societal or cultural norms will enable the practitioner to provide better care. While many different cultural beliefs coexist in a polycultural society like ours, general trends can be identified and can, thereby, inform us of potentially important attitudes. The health care provider's understanding can be expanded through careful questioning and listening, increased clincial experience, and reading.

TECHNOLOGY

Attitudes toward congenitally malformed individuals and treatment decisions are directly affected by technological advances. Particularly in the last several hundred years, the rapid development of technology has, as Alland[23] has described it, "provided the impetus for change." More recently, attitudes toward children with meningomyelocele, in particular, have coincided with the technical ability to treat back lesions and hydrocephalus, as reviewed in Chapter 5.

Before the 1950s, when the technology was first available to implant artificial devices and treat infections, severely congenitally malformed children either died or, rarely, lived with grossly deformed bodies and severe mental retardation (see Chapter 7). Technological advances of the past three decades allow many children with congenital deformities to live and to appear relatively normal (see Chapters 5–15). (Although modern technology has allowed more severely malformed infants to survive, it has also allowed many survivors to appear more normal; see Chapters 20 and 21.) As a result, societal attitudes toward these children are changing from rejection of a few suffering "monsters" to acceptance of many relatively normal-appearing and functioning but impaired or disabled children.

Currently, various reactions to congenitally impaired infants exist. This may, in part, be because the effect of more advanced technology of the past two decades has not yet had a full effect on the adult population, nor has it been fully realized by some authors (see Chapters 4–15, 20, and 21). In addition, differences between opinions of authors quoted in Chapters 4–15 may be due to variable acceptance or knowledge of advances in technology as well as variations in availability. For example, when physicians attended medical school 25 years ago, little was known about the care of many congenital defects. As an example of evolving technology, this text describes two malformations with more favorable outcomes than indicated in previous publications (see Chapters 4 and 8). Health care professionals who have graduated in the last 5 years, moreover, are very likely to have studied only the university-hospitalized, poor-prognosis patients with congenital malformations. Most medical students and resident physicians are not exposed to the outpatient care and socialization experience of the disabled. If health care providers do not know all of the technological treatment alternatives and current improved oucomes, then it is realistically and practically the same as if the alternatives did not exist. Thus, health care professionals should be encouraged to obtain consultation or to refer infants with rare and severe congenital malformations to special care centers such as those centers reporting better results. In turn, if local physicians and regional centers are to offer medical care, they must be responsible for remaining current in the rapidly advancing field of care of the severely impaired infant and child.

AVAILABLE RESOURCES

If a society is able and willing to care for congenitally malformed individuals, then those individuals will have better outcomes and will be more acceptable to society. In turn, society, having experienced a profitable and pleasant experience with the disabled, will be more willing to allocate funds to enable the congenitally impaired infant or child to become a functional adult. Thus, treatment for congenitally impaired individuals can progress in a positive spiral rather than regress in a negative spiral of death and preventable handicaps.

Availability as well as allocation of resources must be considered. In a small country with limited resources, governments may not feel they can afford the luxury of caring for malformed individuals. Countries with greater resources may be better able to offer such care. However, in most countries, allocation of resources presents a problem. A society as a whole may be well-off, but individual parents of congenitally malformed infants may not be able to access those resources. For example, many pregnant women or parents of congenitally impaired children in the United States cannot gain access to diagnosis and treatment because of the high cost, regardless of ethical or moral considerations.

Haynes and associates[477] found that socioeconomic status influenced treatment outcome. The mortality rates for indigent versus nonindigent infants with meningomyelocele were 50% versus 22%, and the shunt infection rates for the same two respective groups were 45% versus 15%. The authors attributed these differences not only to the less healthy life-styles and inadequate transportation of the poor, but also to the differences in the health care available. House staff in a public hospital cared for indigent infants, whereas attending staff in a private hospital cared for nonindigent infants. Thus, the patients with money, unlike the poor patients, benefitted from more skilled physicians and more sophisticated techniques.

Although in the United States federal laws mandate care for malformed infants and provide adoption, medical, educational, and rehabilitation services, these laws are not implemented with equal opportunity in all parts of the country. However, we have found that it is possible to alter the allocation of public resources when they are inadequate to provide for the needs of the handicapped. For example, health care professionals interested in the care of congenitally malformed children worked with government and voluntary agencies to ensure passage of the humanities legislation noted above and discussed more thoroughly in Chapter 2. These professionals should continue to advocate change in order to favorably affect public policy.

PUBLIC POLICY

Cultural beliefs, current treatment technology, and available resources all influence public policy concerning the treatment of congenitally malformed individuals. Public policy in turn affects those variables if policy is expressed as legislation that provides for technological development and resources.

In the United States, we must abide by laws that document public policy. In other words, although one subgroup in our country (for example, the National Organization of Women) may believe that life begins at birth and another subgroup (for example, devout Catholics) that life begins at conception, legally we must abide by our abortion laws that imply life begins at approximately 24 weeks' gestation. During the first 24 weeks, health care professionals must allow the mother to choose whether she will abort or arrange treatment for her embryo or fetus. After 24 weeks, however, unless the pregnancy is a threat to the mother's life, abortion is illegal. The infant's rights may begin at 24 weeks of age, but medically indicated treatment is not legally mandated under recent child abuse prevention laws until after birth.[190] If a child aborted with prostaglandin or sodium chloride remains viable, legally that child must be treated. *Logically*, we see no difference between aborting a 24-week-old fetus and killing the surviving abortus or defective but viable infant. However, *legally*, there is a difference.

What is most important is that we as health care providers, despite our personal beliefs, must abide by public policy expressed in laws and court decisions. One alternative is to withdraw from providing the type of care we find morally unacceptable and refer the patient to another health care professional. If, however, we feel these public policies are inappropriate, we can also work within the system to change them. As mentioned earlier, legislation for subsidized adoption rights for the handicapped[16] and education for all[297] have been passed as a result of strong advocacy movements (see Chapter 2).

DECISION MAKING: PRENATAL VERSUS POSTNATAL

Prenatal and postnatal decision making must be differentiated for three reasons: (1) as discussed above, public policy concerning the treatment or nontreatment of embryos or fetuses in the first two trimesters differs from that in the last trimester and postnatally; (2) the accuracy and understanding of prenatal and postnatal diagnoses differ dramatically for most conditions; and (3) prenatal diagnosis, before 24 weeks gestation age, unlike later diagnosis, is often confused with an implied consequence: abortion.

The Accuracy and Understanding of Prenatal and Postnatal Prognosis

The health care profession's experience with prenatal diagnosis is so limited, due to its newness, that in many cases we cannot use information from these procedures to make accurate prognoses. Some diagnoses such as trisomy 13 or 18 and anencephaly have well-known outcomes. Others, like trisomy 21, are more variable.[631] We have not yet obtained enough information about the natural progress of many disorders, including hydrocephalus and meningomyelocele (see Chapter 4). Prenatal diagnosis in the first trimester is frequently less accurate for some conditions than in the last trimester and much less accurate then than postnatally. Adding to the above problem is the disagreement in our society about termination of any life in the first trimester. Abortions of malformed fetuses limit our ability to learn how these fetuses would have developed in utero, whether the pregnancy would have been carried to a viable termination, and what the quality of postnatal life would have been.

When counseling parents, health care providers must keep these problems in mind. Because prenatal diagnosis, unlike postnatal diagnosis, is clouded by a large number of unknowns, we msut be careful not to be overly optimistic or overly pessimistic.

Prenatal Diagnosis and Its Implied Consequences

Whereas postnatal diagnosis does not necessarily have an implied moral consequence, prenatal diagnosis does. Marion and associates[693] found that 21 out of the 62 (33 percent) patients who declined amniocentesis (95 accepted) did so due to moral issues. Thirteen declined because they would not consider abortion as an alternative, and five declined because they wanted babies regardless of any defect. These data agree with our own experiences. As few as 5 percent of all pregnancies at risk that were referred to our prenatal clinics were found to be abnormal and led to consideration of abortion. Only 75 percent of these affected pregnancies were aborted; some parents elected to continue the pregnancy despite knowing the fetus had trisomy 21 or such severe defects as ienencephaly. This high-risk prenatal clinic population is different from our parents of congenitally malformed children, only 22 percent of whom indicate they would opt for abortion if they were found to have impaired fetuses. The high-risk prenatal clinic population was actually pregnant, and a high proportion had sought prenatal diagnosis with intent to terminate abnormal pregnancies. The parents of our patients were not pregnant and had had experience with some badly impaired infants who had become well-adjusted, disabled children and adults.

Use of Prenatal Diagnosis

Parents at risk generally fall into three basic groups: (1) those who want prenatal diagnosis and termination if the fetus is defective, (2) those who want prenatal diagnosis in conjunction with improved pregnancy outcome, and (3) those who do not want any children.

We have found that individuals who opt for prenatal diagnosis are generally a preselected group. We believe this is because the general public perceives genetic counselors as able to offer only termination or delivery of a congenitally malformed child as alternatives. With the exception of Harrison and associates,[461] most of the genetic literature does not discuss the full range of expression of deformities and the possibility for improving pregnancy outcome.[48,156,228,387,444,623,761] The potential for improving pregnancy outcome, using open neural tube defects as an example, is discussed in further detail in Chapter 4.

Health Care Provider Bias and Prenatal Diagnosis

As we have noted above, health care provider bias should be recognized when dealing with sensitive issues. Most people involved with prenatal diagnostic procedures state they recommend a full range of options to parents when a malformed fetus is diagnosed, but often their messages may be contradictory. On the one hand, these health care professionals justify genetic counseling by the utilitarian argument that they will effect a reduction in the occurrence of congenital malformations. This implies abortion is the consequence if an impaired fetus is detected.

On the other hand, most of these professionals recommend allowing patients to make decisions in the absence of any persuasion. This double message is implied by the two passages taken from the same article and quoted below:

> Since Down's syndrome is the most commonly identified cause of severe mental retardation, the amount of future reduction of severe mental retardation will depend, partly, upon the proportion of older gravitas who use prenatal chromosomal diagnosis.[15]

> Decisions concerning the use of prenatal chromosomal diagnosis and abortion of affected fetuses are personal decisions. It is imperative that they be reached on the basis of available information and in the absence of coercion[15]

However, Lejeune[631] describes, as our experience shows, that the variation of trisomy 21 is great, with few very severely retarded among the natural survivors. Can counselors making the statements above really be unbiased? Will they refrain from even subtle influence by innuendo and body language?

We have observed a so-called unbiased health care professional give what we consider biased genetic-prenatal counseling. He informed a defective fetus's parents of their options in the following manner:

> We detected positive alpha-fetoprotein levels. That means your baby is affected with spina bifida and will be mentally retarded, paralyzed, and incontinent. Most families prefer to have an abortion rather than have a baby with this defect. Do you want termination, or do you want to have a handicapped baby?

Not only did this health care provider not present the full spectrum of possibilities, but he recommended termination in the manner in which he presented options for pregnancy management.

The Accuracy and Understanding of Prenatal Diagnosis Counseling

In addition to presenting information in a biased manner, counselors may present inaccurate data, as described earlier in this chapter. In addition, we have seen counselors quote grossly out-of-date material. One example, a book published in 1983, reads as follows:

> Where active treatment (for myelomeningocele) is given, including several operations shortly after birth, most survive, but of that number virtually all are totally paralyzed from the waist down and incontinent with no present hope for improvement[496]

Data from centers caring for these children reveal this statement to be grossly inaccurate. Not "virtually all" are hopelessly handicapped patients, but 70–80 percent are effective and competitive[737,819,901,1045] (see also Chapters 4–15). In addition, health care providers or counselors seeing patients prior to the need for prenatal diagnosis may have difficulty conveying the information so that it is easily understood,[362,877] and parents may not fully understand the real causes, despite explanations given by these providers or counselors.[877]

Availability of Resources

In addition to genetic counseling possibly being biased and associated with inaccuracies, it is provided much less frequently than it should be.[877] Adams and associates[15] found 6–28 percent "use ratios" (amniotic fluid specimens divided by live births) by women at risk in Alabama, California, Manhattan, and Nebraska. Marion and associates[693] initially found that only 41 percent of patients in Atlanta, Georgia, who were offered amniocentesis accepted the procedure. This ratio increased to 69 percent between 1976 and 1978, probably because "peer support' was introduced into genetic counseling sessions. Overall, 61 percent of their patients counseled opted for prenatal diagnosis. In general, low use ratios for prenatal testing exist in poor and minority groups.[15,101,348,693] Individuals in rural settings tend to use prenatal testing less than those in urban environments, and blacks tend to use this testing less than whites.

Individuals who use the prenatal diagnosis represent a preselected segment of our society for two main reasons. The first reason is socioculture beliefs such as religion, discussed earlier in this chapter. Another type of belief, interracial prejudice, might explain lower prenatal diagnosis rates in black Americans:

> These white folks don' care nothin' 'bout you and me and they don' want to see us flerishin'. That's why so much of that medicine they always after us 'bout takin' is agains' us. These doctors ain' nothin' but white folks, too.[1081]

Convincing health care providers to educate black Americans that prenatal diagnosis is not synonymous with racial discrimination and abortion may help to increase the rates or prenatal diagnosis in this population. Also, individuals in rural populations may not have access to or may not know about prenatal diagnostic test centers. Marion and associates[693] suggest that accessibility and publicity would increase use ratios in the lower socioeconomic, predominantly black population they studied in Atlanta.

Reassurance Through Prenatal Diagnosis

The chances of even a couple at risk having a congenitally malformed child are still relatively small, as noted previously. Thus, not only is prenatal diagnosis more likely to inform a couple of a normal pregnancy, but as Father Williams[1216] has pointed out, it allows parents at high risk to overcome fears that prevent them from having more children. Because prenatal diagnosis allows the removal of this fear, more women at risk will get pregnant when they know prenatal diagnosis is available and can allow them to avoid having another impaired child (either through improved pregnancy outcome or abortion). We have found Father William's prediction to be true. With the introduction of each new prenatal diagnostic test, many of our patients' mothers who were at risk of having another malformed child conceived.

Not only does prenatal diagnosis usually result in the detection of a normal fetus and in reassurance to high-risk mothers, but even if a malformed fetus is identified, alternatives besides abortion are chosen by some of our patients.

Decision Making When a Malformed Fetus is Detected

Public policy in the United States mandates that health care providers provide up-to-date, modern information. Most authors generally accept parents' legal and moral rights to the most accurate information about the chances for having a congenitally malformed child and, once a defective child is discovered, for treatment alternatives.[295,609,760,781,880] (For specific prognoses, see Chapters 4–15). In the United States, health care providers have a contract with parents to give the most informed advice possible (as opposed to giving them biased advise). As Fletcher[347] points out, we have a moral obligation to tell the "truth."

It is not always easy to define the "truth," however, since the exact outcome of a fetus or infant with a particular diagnosis is usually unpredictable, as noted above in the discussion about accuracy of prenatal diagnosis. We can offer only probabilities for outcomes (see Chapter 5). In addition, a given prognosis changes as new treatment techniques, illustrated in Chapters 4–15, evolve.

When a congenitally malformed child is detected in utero before 24 weeks, three basic parental positions usually exist: (1) the parents choose to have the baby because they do not believe in abortion and/or they believe a congenitally malformed infant is equal to a normal one; (2) the fetus is any place in the spectrum from normal to severely malformed, and the parents opt for an abortion; and (3) the parents are undecided.

In the first two cases, we believe the parents should be allowed to carry out their decision since it is their legal right. In the third case, we present the probabilities as we know them and advise the parents only if they indicate they want our professional opinion. It is particularly important for health care providers to take responsibility for at least recommending a course of action since parents cannot appreciate the stress of long-term care of a congenitally malformed child[754] and may not be able to carry the burden of guilt that often accompanies the decision to abort even the most severely malformed fetus. We have observed that, when approached with treatment alternatives, most parents (approximately 65%) ask us as health care providers to do what we believe is most appropriate to improve the outcome of their pregnancies and treat their children regardless of prognosis. The other 35% ask that we do what they believe is the best choice based on their own beliefs and the information we have provided them.

Decision Making After Week 24 and Postnatally

After 24 weeks of gestation, we believe the physician is legally bound to act as the advocate for the fetus or for the child.[936] Although consideration of pregnancy management for improved outcome for the fetus is new, we explain our recommendations in Chapter 4 and will limit this discussion to the infant born alive. The generalities in this part of the chapter will be expanded in Chapter 5. Some have argued that reaching a decision for or against treatment based on a physician's recommendation with parental approval is inappropriate because of parental coercion. The process of providing a definite recommendation, however, has worked well in our clinic, possibly because we explain our own biases and all options for management with anticipated outcomes and attempt to be sensitive to the parents' beliefs.[730] Our process has several safeguards.

First, if the physician does not feel the parents are acting in the best interests of the infant, then relinquishment or referral to Children's Protective Services may be appropriate, as discussed in Chapter 5.

Second, if the parents do not feel the physician is acting in their best interests or in the best interests of their child, and if our recommendations conflict with legally sanctioned parental desires, we encourage referral to another health care provider.

Third, we use peer review to assure that nontreatment decisions are not only legally sanctioned but technically and morally appropriate. As practitioners, we work within societal contexts; we are judged by our peer groups. The President's Commission on Ethics in Medicine and Medical Research, the United States House of Representatives, and the United States Senate have established the moral and legal right for treatment of malformed infants and children.[190] The Federal regulations recommend a formal review by a committee of peers. For more than a decade, we have used both peer review and concurrence by advocacy groups for the disabled and handicapped. We require that at least three physicians with expertise in the care of the patient's problem agree to a nontreatment plan in writing in the patient's record. We have also regularly reviewed our decisions with our federally mandated state Developmental Disabilties

Planning Council and Protection and Advocacy Agency for the Handicapped. Our process, as described more fully in Chapter 5, is socially and legally sanctioned according to three court decisions, two for withholding treatment[172,1010] and one for withdrawal of treatment.[521,522]

Individualization

Recent United States public policy described above is part of a new approach to the congenitally malformed: these individuals are increasingly perceived not as magical or monstrous but simply as human.[403,599] In this approach, the importance of the individual is stressed. The provision of health care is viewed in terms of its effect on each patient. Essentially, it involves managing congenital malformations by treating individuals within a context.

McCormick's philosophy[712] is basic to this approach. He argues that infants should be treated (1) when a life of only suffering is not simply prolonged, (2) when there is any chance of error, and (3) when the infant has potential for human relationships.

First, it is important to differentiate between morbidly versus chronically ill patients. For each particular procedure, the health care provider must determine (and inform the parents) how the infant might benefit from the procedure. On the two extremes of the continuum, the infant may either live a happier life as a result of certain procedures or may simply have inevitable death forestalled. If the infant is morbid and the procedures in question will merely prolong his or her life, the procedures should be foregone and the infant be allowed to die. If, on the other hand, the infant is impaired but not morbid, procedures that will in any way benefit the child should be undertaken.

Second, when there is any doubt, treatment should be undertaken since mistakes in predicting oucome can be made.

Third, the potential for human relationships must be considered. Hufeland clamins that "if the physician presumes to take into consideration in his work whether a life has value or not, the consequences are boundless and the physician becomes the most dangerous man in the state."[1210] Uncontrolled medical technology may be detrimental to individuals and families, according to Duff and Campbell.[291] They use this rationale to argue that parents should make the final treatment decisions (since parents bear the consequences). We agree that medical technology must be controlled and that physicians alone should not determine the value of patients' lives. However, we disagree with Duff and Campbell[291] in that physicians should provide parents with their experience and knowledge about treatment and outcome probabilities as well as provide them with a clear recommendation as to the most appropriate course of action.

Quality-of-life decisions should not be made by health care providers alone. We do need, however, to determine whether or not each particular child should or should not receive a specific treatment. Treatment decisions become difficult unless we take into consideration human value. How do we determine value or quality? Where does pain and consequent suffering fit into all of this? Basing the decision on Aristotle's criteria, "the capacity for happiness," is difficult since happiness is a nebulous concept. We have found McCormick's criteria[712] of "potential for human relationships" to be more understandable and applicable despite the difficulty, identified by Speer,[1097] of determining the value or quality of life. If there is no possibility for the malformed infant to develop a human relationship with the biologic parents, we seek relinquishment and treatment under state auspices, as discussed in Chapter 5.

If a decision to withhold treatment for a severely congenitally malformed child is reached with the biological parents, we recommend appointment of a legal guardian to represent the child's interests.[1045] We warn the parents that such action will protect them, as in Shane Lemmell's case,[1010] in which representatives of the right to life stimulated a wrongful death action against the State of Washington and the primary author because we were not surgically treating a multiply malformed infant. Relinquishment protects the biologic parents and allows the advocates of the right to life an opportunity to adopt a severely congenitally malformed infant. There is, therefore, no justification for withholding treatment from a child because of potential stress on the biologic family. Both family and child can be served.

SUMMARY

The home and family situation should reflect the macroculture, that is, society as a whole, not just the microculture of the single family involved. In other words, the current approach of our society (our macroculture) is to preserve the life of many congenitally malformed infants who would have been allowed to die 10–20 years ago. Some of these infants, despite significant congenital malformations, can now live relatively normal lives in the mainstream of life.

Today, if parents want their physically malformed, normal-intellect or mild-to-moderately retarded infant to be allowed to die, other parents may be willing to adopt and care for that child. Thus, despite the biological parents' personal and cultural beliefs, a child is now able to live and experience human relationships due to recent changes in social attitudes, treatment technology, societal resources, and public policy.

Hillary Shurtleff
David Shurtleff

2

The Rights and Socialization of the Unexpected Minority[403]

The previous chapter dealt with influences on initial decisions to treat or not treat congenitally malformed fetuses and infants. This chapter will deal in more depth with the rights of the disabled as reflected in public policy and general societal expectations. Health care providers must understand these rights and expectations, not just the technicalities of medical care since understanding them can have profound effects on initial as well as long-term management.

Current attitudes toward the rights and socialization of the congenitally malformed are changing for three main reasons. First, these individuals are becoming more accepted by society.[205,754] More positive attitudes toward children with meningomyelocele in particular may be due to greater numbers surviving with more normal appearance. Second, large numbers of spinal cord–injured civilian accident victims and veterans of the Vietnam war currently are joining with the congenitally disabled to make a powerful lobby for the impaired, disabled, and handicapped.[1174] Third, legislation protecting the disabled and handicapped and assuring equal opportunities has been passed within the last decade. These laws have resulted from the disabled advocating for themselves and have allowed congenitally malformed children to grow up to become effective advocates for their own interests.

MYELODYSPLASIAS AND EXSTROPHIES: SIGNIFICANCE, PREVENTION, AND TREATMENT
 ISBN 0-8089-1816-8

SOCIETAL ACCEPTANCE

The term *unexpected minority* most accurately describes the congenitally malformed, who are not acknowledged as a minority, but are discriminated against for appearing abnormal.[205,754] The congenitally malformed are perceived as inferior. This perception interferes with normal socialization and reduces a disabling condition to a handicap.[870]

As discussed in Chapter 1, current positive attitudes in the United States have changed from the negative ones of the first half of the 20th century when negative labels were accepted. For example, Justice Oliver Wendell Holmes described mentally retarded microcephalics as "idiots,"[141,403] and a group of Americans used the words "monsters and imbeciles" to describe the congenitally malformed and mentally retarded.[1210] Despite the current, more humane attitudes, negative labeling still occurs. For example, one author[496] in a 1983 text on medical ethics used the word "vegetable" to describe severely mentally retarded children with meningomyelocele and hydrocephalus. We agree with Sondra Diamond's response to this negative labeling. She is a woman with cerebral palsy, who reacted in the following manner to the term "vegetable," used in a *Newsweek* article to describe the handicapped:

> I'll wager my entire root system and as much fertilizer as it would take to fill Yale University that you have never received a letter from a vegetable before this one, but, much as I resent the term, I must confess that I fit the description of a "vegetable" as defined in the article. . . .
>
> Due to severe brain damage incurred at birth, I am unable to dress myself, toilet myself, or write; my secretary is typing this letter. Many thousands of dollars had to be spent on my rehabilitation and education in order for me to reach my present professional status as a Counseling Psychologist. My parents were also told, 35 years ago, that there was "little or no hope of achieving meaningful 'humanhood' " for their daughter [afflicted with cerebral palsy].
>
> Have I reached "humanhood"? Compared with Doctors Duff and Campbell, I believe I have surpassed it!
>
> Instead of changing the law to make it legal to weed out us "vegetables," let us change the laws so that we may receive quality medical care, education, and freedom to live as full and productive lives as our potentials allow.[481]

Often, negative labeling occurs because individuals, health care providers included, do not use accepted terms—such as *impairment*, *disability*, and *handicap*—in the same manner. Therefore, we will repeat the definition of these three terms and will use them as defined throughout this text. The World Health Organization defines *impairment* as "any loss or abnormality of psychological, physiological, or anatomical structure or function"; *disability* as "any restriction or lack of ability to perform an activity in a manner or within the range which is considered normal"; and *handicap* as a "disadvantage for a given individual, resulting from an impairment or a disability, that limits or prevents the fulfillment of a role that is normal (depending on age, sex, social, and cultural factors) for that individual."[1182,1236] Basically, an *impairment* is an abnormality that cannot be seen; a *disability* is a restriction that can be seen; and a *handicap* is a restriction that can be seen and that is a social disadvantage. Given these definitions, it is easy to understand why many of our patients prefer not to be labeled handicapped.

Physical Appearance

The interaction between an individual child and others is just as important as labeling. The effect of facial appearance on normal socialization is first identified through interactions between both mothers and nurses with premature infants. Nurses tend to give higher intelligence prognoses to infants they perceive as physically attractive,[7,224] and mothers tend to have more negative feelings for children with craniofacial anomalies than for normal children.[572] In addition, an infant's physical attractiveness may be predictive of the quality of the relationship with the parent.[7] We believe that, once these reactions are recognized, they can be overcome by properly counseling parents and educating nurses of these infants. According to some authors, people will interact more with a child if he or she appears normal.[561,923] This theory affects initial as well as long-term management, including decisions of when to close an infant's meningomyelocele lesion (see Chapters 5 and 6) and whether to recommend a wheelchair or braces for a paralyzed child (see Chapter 15).

Physical attractiveness plays a role in the socialization of any individual. As Berscheid[94] points out, there may be some validity to Freud's claim that "anatomy is destiny," particularly in a society like ours that stresses youth and beauty. Physically attractive individuals often receive preferential treatment.[10,94,95,1084] Because of these prejudices, health care providers may be better able to serve congenitally malformed individuals if they help to make their patients as physically attractive as possible. In addition, health care professionals can assist in changing societal prejudices against individuals with physical malformations.[770,892]

Physical appearance is an important determinant of group membership.[1129] For example, mainstream society in the United States in the era of 1933 to 1945 tended to reject people in wheelchairs but accept the sight-impaired person who wore pince-nez spectacles, somewhat a reversal of our current social mores.[93] As documented in Chapter 1, persons in wheelchairs are entering into the modern mainstream of life, including Madison Avenue advertising, but the person with the pince-nez has been replaced by the sight-impaired person with contact lenses.

This social code of accepting only persons with certain appearances can be deadly. Reid[897] and Lightowler[648] recommend euthanasia or nontreatment of severely paralyzed *infants*. The utilitarian criteria for euthanasia or nontreatment suggested by these two authors apply also to accident victims and Vietnam War veterans.[1044] Is the paraplegic meningomyelocele person more or less likely to be productive compared with a traumatic quadraplegic? If Reid and Lightowler extended their age criteria to include adults as well as infants, would they not also include themselves? We believe the mainstream of our culture accepts the impaired or disabled victims of war, accidents, and congenital malformation, but will accept neither euthanasia nor nontreatment for them. To do otherwise is to allow prejudice to rule.

Although prejudice is group-defined to a large extent, it is possible to partially overcome the effects of physical appearance with "interpersonal warmth, kindness and responsiveness."[7] No better example can be found than Franklin D. Roosevelt, who led this country despite being disabled during an era when the disabled were not accepted. He claimed that public funds would be repaid "many times" by the increased productivity of handicapped individuals, considering what he saw as a vast economic waste caused by prejudice.[93] In addition, it is possible to identify reactions to physical appearance as Richardson and associates[924] have done and either modify physical appearance to suit those prejudices when possible or attempt to change existing attitudes among the able-bodied.

Richardson and associates[924] found that, regardless of cultural background or individual characteristics, children in the United States preferred to have as a friend, in decreaseing order, a child with no handicap, a child with crutches and a brace on the left leg, a child in a wheelchair with a blanket covering the legs, a child with the left hand missing, a child with a facial disfigurement near the left side of the mouth, and finally, an obese child. As discussed in Chapter 13, obesity can be avoided, whereas the other disabilities need education of peer groups. Reactions to physical appearance have been further defined by other authors, as is discussed below.

Physical appearance is particularly important during early education experiences. Adams and Crane[9] have found that, although preschool children can identify attractive versus unattractive children, they do not attribute good or bad personality characteristics based on attractiveness until they are older.[7] However, Jones and Sisk[561] have found that children as young as 4 and 5 discriminate against the disabled, and Dion[278] discovered that 3-year-old children distinguish between "pretty" and "homely" people just as much as their 6½-year-old peers. Regardless of when this phenomenon begins, physical appearance affects interactions with peers.[7,9,204,278,279,505,607] Because of peer prejudice, we have boys and girls wear polypropylene braces, as opposed to obvious metal braces, beneath socks and contemporary clothing, as discussed in more detail in Chapter 15. In addition, we stress appropriate body fat stores and socially acceptable self-toileting, discussed in more depth in Chapters 9–13 and 17.

If stigmatization begins with the education process, as Goffman[407] suggests, it may be influenced by teacher attitudes. Teacher expectations reflect student attractiveness,[7,204] whether the children are in preschool[7,9] or elementary school.[8,12–14,620] Langlois and Downs[606] explain this by stating that not only do teachers prefer nonaggressive children, but negative evaluations of unattractive children reflect an actual tendency for these children to be aggressive. In addition, the authors found that different expectations for unattractive versus attractive children may actually influence behavior. These prejudices must be overcome before new education opportunities can be fully realized.

Not only do parents and teachers respond to individuals, but they may teach children to respond to others in a similar manner. Through subtle reinforcement,[606] parents' and teachers' expectations of whether a child will use a stereotype is associated with whether the child will actually use that stereotype.[7] We have witnessed school staff and peers reinforce dependent life-styles for visibly disabled children despite medical prescriptions to foster independence. Professionals who wish to change attitudes should attempt to influence not only children, but also their teachers, mothers, and health care providers to recognize and deal with these socialization behaviors.[1167]

Paradoxical Reactions to Physical Appearance

Two traditional, paradoxical approaches to physical malformations currently exist in our society.

First, according to the beauty-is-good hypothesis, physical appearance is associated with innate worth. For example, Hogarth's paintings of inmates of mental institutions with ugly, deformed faces clearly show the historical link between facial deformity and mental deficiency.[7] The story of Cinderella also reflects this beauty-is-good and ugly-is-evil paradigm: the main character is beautiful, good, and kind whereas her stepsisters are ugly, wicked, and cruel.[606] Other characters reflect this beauty-is-good and ugly-is-evil paradigm: Captain Hook, Long John Silver, Pinocchio, Rumpelstiltskin, The Ugly Duckling, and numerous witches.[7] The ugly-is-evil paradigm has been incorporated into the belief system of lower-class black Americans who believe someone may curse a pregnant woman and, thus, cause her infant to "bark like a dog"[363,1081,1082] and that a woman's actions can cause her fetus to be "marked" by God. Mary

Shelley's novel, *Frankenstein*,[1026] perhaps best depicts the beauty-is-good hypothesis, but with an additional theme: the monster, though not evil at first, becomes evil; negative societal reactions to his ugliness actually *cause* him to become evil.[94] Shelley's story may reflect actual behavior, as indicated by Langlois and Downs's findings[606] mentioned above.

In conflict with the beauty-is-good hypothesis is the beauty-is-only-skin-deep theory. The beast in "Beauty and the Beast"[96,136] fits this paradigm; however, this fairy tale character becomes beautiful when his innate goodness is realized. Part of this physical reflection of innate quality may be due to the nature of fairy tales: they are, to a large extent, based on physical symbols. More recently, films such as *Mask*, *Elephant Man*, and *Just the Way You Are*[93] reflect the beauty-is-only-skin-deep theory.

As Kapp-Simon[572] points out, these two hypotheses put children with congenital malformations in a conflict situation: on the one hand, they are told their inner selves, not their physical appearances, matter; and on the other hand, they are encouraged to become as beautiful (or normal) as possible, which implies their physical appearances really do make a difference. If parents and health care providers understand this paradox, they will be better able to help congenitally malformed individuals understand the situation. Part of the solution lies in a realistic understanding of these two paradoxical paradigms and part of it lies in normalization.

Normalization

The principle of normalization, "making the lives of mentally retarded persons as normal as possible,"[495] is currently popular. We believe this concept is helping the congenitally disabled to integrate into society. Normalization is a prime motivating force and should be achieved during early childhood.[244b] Mainstreaming, placing children with learning and physical disabilities into regular classrooms rather than self-contained classrooms, arose from the principle of normalization, and for the most part, we have found our congenitally malformed patients to have benefitted from mainstreaming and from other general normalization concepts, despite the several drawbacks discussed by Hoffmaster.[495]

Hoffmaster[495] claims the normalization principle leads to "moral absolutism" wherein normalizing measures are "imposed,"[1230] and individuals are not allowed the 'freedom to choose" between different alternatives.[944] However, we believe it is important to allow individuals a choice. For instance, although it may be more normal and/or acceptable to move around on two legs than in a wheelchair, children with congenital malformations may want the freedom to use the latter instead of walk with the aid of cumbersome braces, as discussed in Chapter 15.

Socially Acceptable Behavior

In order to be able to act and behave as much like their siblings and peers as possible but, at the same time, be allowed the freedom to be individuals, congenitally disabled people must first learn independence in daily activities, particularly in self-toileting skills. Others will neither tolerate nor comment on malodor. Bad breath is the most readily seen example on public television. Several years ago, a popular commercial for mouthwash showed friends and business associates turning away from someone with bad breath; only the person's lover said something about the bad breath—and that was done indirectly, by offering the mouthwash. In our society in the United States, the mainstream concept is that cleanliness and sexiness are paramount. Multiple subliminal and overt messages reinforcing these beliefs reach us through advertising. Because of these beliefs, we teach our patients independence in daily activities, particularly socially acceptable hygiene, as early as possible, as discussed in Chapters 9–15 and 17.

Shoeing and Iversen[1032] suggest that, when an adult paraplegic patient is "physically ready and [has] an intact mind," he or she will relearn dressing and locomotor activities quickly. The injured adult learned early in childhood that malodors and improper hygiene are not acceptable. This is markedly different from a congenital paraplegic who does not learn the social necessity for independence in self-care skills during childhood. A congenitally malformed child does not relearn skills. Instead, despite physical and social impediments, an impaired child frequently must acquire new skills after a childhood of tolerance and dependence on care providers.

Primarily, therefore, the achievement of independence and socialization begins with the family and family expectations. Congenitally malformed individuals who may be perceived as cute and pitied at first become tiresome as they continue to demand care while they get older. The problems posed by the perception of what the older impaired child should do and actually does do may be avoided if children are encouraged from the beginning to learn age-appropriate independent skills. Performance is clearly influenced by expectations.

In addition to learning independent activities of daily living, congenitally malformed individuals may be taught to overcome prejudice by using particular socialization techniques. Cobb and Hancock[205] suggest entering social events through able-bodied siblings, keeping abreast of topics of interest to peers, and explaining disabilities in a way that minimizes stigma. These techniques may help individuals to avoid what the authors have identified as a "'Catch-22' bind": congenitally malformed children need 'superior personal qualities," but they can't develop these since they're isolated.

Finally, able-bodied children and adults involved in school with the impaired must be taught to see the child behind the physical defect. An annotated bibliography for helping the able-bodied learn more positive attitudes is available.[1036] Some of the better sources are also listed in the bibliography of this text.[5,149,323,560,1087,1111,1228] More reasearch on the long-term effectiveness of programs to change attitudes needs to be obtained.[205]

Demographic Changes

Demographic changes have contributed to attitude changes in this country. While the number of children born with congenital malformations has decreased with the decline in the birth rate (as the birth rate incidence has remained constant), the number of children with congenital malformations living (prevalence) has increased since more of these infants now survive as the result of improved care. Thus, the percentage of children with "limitations of activities" has dramatically increased; since 1960, the percentage of these children has more than doubled.[804] Individuals with any level of limitation have increased 111 percent, and individuals with severe limitations have increased 122 percent.

As the birth rate decreases and the population size remains relatively stable, society becomes more interested not only in the well-being of the individual, but in the individual's ability to contribute to the whole.[963,964] Healthier children lead to healthier adults, who, in turn, create a healthier society.[21] As the number of disabled individuals increases and the demographics change so that we have an older population, each person capable of contributing is valued more. Thus, disabled persons are becoming more accepted by society and are being offered more opportunities to contribute.

Legislation and Advocacy

Adequate legislation for protecting the disabled did not occur in the United States until the 20th century and then probably as an extension of the civil rights movements. In the 20th century, changes in the family in America toward a more democratic orientation[649] put more emphasis on the importance of the individual. This trend accompanied social changes toward acceptance of the disabled (as discussed in Chapter 1 and previously in this chapter) that have led to legislation for the establishment and protection of minority rights.

Newman[805] summarizes the important rights movement dates: in 1912, the United States Child's Bureau formed; after World War I, in 1918, legislation for vocational rehabilitation for soldiers passed; in 1920, legislation for the vocational rehabilitation of handicapped civilians passed; in the 1930s social security began; and in the 1940s, services were provided for the nonphysically handicapped. For the past 10 years, legal mandates for all disabled individuals have dramatically improved in the United states. This change is most exemplified by the Rehabilitation Act of 1973. This law deinstitutionalizes individuals with mental retardation and provides all types of disabled and handicapped individuals with access to work, socialization, and enjoyment of life. In addition, the 1975 Education for All Handicapped Children Law, Public Law 94-142, provides children with equal opportunities for education.[297] Most recently, Section 405 of the Rehabilition Law was unsuccessfully applied to the rights of disabled infants and to treatment at birth. As a result of this failure, the United States government reauthorized funding for prevention of child abuse and included "withholding medically indicated treatment" in the Child Abuse Amendments, Public Law 98-457.[190] In particular, these last three laws will profoundly and favorably alter the outlook and opportunities for the congenitally malformed for whom medical treatment is described in this text.

The Revolution in Education

Recent legislation for the normalization of education for the handicapped has been called a "quiet revolution."[403,463] The Education for All Handicapped Children Act of 1975, Public Law 94-142, legislates education for all impaired, disabled, and handicapped children, with emphasis on the individual child's needs through Individual Education Plans (IEPs).[297] Learning environments must include the child's able-bodied peers and take into consideration a number of factors that were mentioned above and are more fully discussed in Chapter 17.

Several judicial decisions have been important in providing the educational opportunities for the disabled provided by Public Law 94-142. The "Brown Decision" set the precedent for this law.[137] Another case, the "Pennsylvania Association of Retarded Children (PARC) Versus the State of Pennsylvania" furthered the cause of education for all since the court required the state to provide access to a free public education for every retarded child.[857,858] In addition, in the "Peter Mills Versus the Board of Education of the District of Columbia" case, the court ruled that money is no excuse to exclude children from an education and that the law authorizes funds for excess costs.[863] Finally, the United States Supreme Court ruling in the "Tatro" case assured that children at school should be provided with assistance for clean intermittent catheterization (CIC) and that such needs are not adequate reasons to exclude children from equal education.[528]

The revolutionary quality of Public Law 94-142 is far from being implemented universally, however. In order to be a complete revolution, its intent must be implemented by parents and professionals—medical and educational as well as social—and the impaired and disabled themselves. Often, professionals do not back this law because they are unaware of its provisions or disagree with its intent. In order to provide health care providers with an insight into what educational programs are indicated, we have described them extensively in Chapter 17. Some administrators state that they are against implementation of these programs because the extra costs involved have not been provided. We believe advocates working with educators and lobbying for funds will make the revolution in education even more successful than it has been.

Despite the advantages of Public Law 94-142 and the problem with funding, the following additional problems exist. First, there is ambiguity in the specifications of the law.[534,1034,1130] Second, children are often placed in inappropriate programs and are trapped by labels such as *learning disabled* and *retarded*.[18,244b,557,870] Third, coordination among educational services is lacking,[244b,831] and fourth, schools may be inadequately or inappropriately staffed.[823,1173] Many regular classroom teachers without appropriate training may be forced to help disabled children take care of their physical needs. Fifth, these teachers may not want to or have the time to help with self-care. Sixth, care may not be available at schools located near certain students' homes. Seventh, architectural barriers are still a problem.[823,1173] Eighth, many children miss school for therapy and surgery. Ninth, peer teasing interferes with the education process.[823,1173] Tenth, as Miezio[754] points out, there can be disagreements between the parents and the school. These ten problems will be further discussed in Chapter 17.

Despite the problems listed above, we believe Public Law 94-142 provides for better education of many impaired or disabled individuals than was available prior to its passage. Most parents report being satisfied with schools.[517,1130]

Parents and Professionals: View of the Congenitally Malformed

Traditionally, one of the problems in the socialization of congenitally malformed children was the lack of mutual understanding between parents and both medical and educational professionals.[244b] The world views of parents differ from those of medical and educational professionals[244b,843,950] and understanding how these perspectives differ will help to reduce potential conflicts between different groups as well as facilitate the best possible care.

The medical professional may want the parents to adopt a treatment regimen that interferes with other areas of the family's life that the family views as more important than the problem being addressed by the professional. Primarily because of their training, physicians and therapists tend to treat parents of the congenitally malformed according to the social pathology paradigm in which parents become patients and, as such, are only allowed to accept the professional's decisions. If parents attempt to actively participate by attempting to explain that a particular treatment is causing more harm than good, they are treated as if they are maladjusted or acting inappropriately.[403,870] Many health care professionals trained in the care of acute disease are accustomed to total control by prescription and resent parental resistance to their suggestions, particularly when they are dealing with chronic disorders. Patience and understanding of the child and of the family's complicated life may help avoid this conflict.

The parents, on the other hand, may not be capable of negotiating with medical professionals and, thus, may be judged as noncompliant because they are just not able to carry out the prescriptions.[1130] Even worse, we have witnessed school or independent center therapists give professional advice to a family that conflicts with the advice of other health care professionals. As a result of this type of conflict, young patients are left to develop their own loyalities. They either follow the daily care suggestions of their therapists and report noncompliance to their physicians or lose the good will of their therapists and follow the recommendations of their physicians. Such conflicts can be prevented by interprofessional communications that take into consideration a particular family's life-style and the needs of the patient.

More effective communication may also help parents and educators to work together. Parents and educators may disagree concerning (1) whether the child is exceptional, (2) what problems, if any, the child does have, and (3) where the child should be placed. One of the main causes of disagreement is misleading verbal performance, common in children with hydrocephalus, as discussed in Chapter 16.

According to Darling,[243b] parents may be relluctant to challenge health care providers and educators for fear their child will be adversely affected or for fear they are too socially or educationally inferior to become involved. Parents may experience ambiguous feelings: they do not want to cause disturbances and create negative attitudes toward their children, but they feel society should accept their children and provide appropriate programs.[710,869] Other parents may not know or understand what exactly the law mandates.[142,517,1130,1176] Poor, minority families may be especially unlikely to benefit from the law due to language and cultural barriers.[142,1130] Parents may be at a disadvantage with schools because they lack the money and resources of the school systems when a controversy develops as to the most appropriate educational program for their children.[403,1130] "Professional parents"[324] may be overinvested in their child's handicap; that is, fighting the school system may be their role in life, and any improvement in their child's condition may represent a threat to that role. Finally, many parents *are* able to get appropriately involved with their children's schooling.

Advocates for parents and their children can be parents, health care providers, or teachers, but those employed by the schools have the most difficulty in helping with problems because they are in conflict with their source of salary. In order to take full advantage of educational opportunities, we refer educational problems to private educational consultants who provide parents with another opinion in regard to their child's educational needs. With recalcitrant schools, we refer our patients to our Washington State Protection and Advocacy Program, a federally mandated program available in all of the United States.[896] As health care professionals, we meet with families and educators and write appropriate nursing, occupational therapy, and physical therapy orders for inclusion in the individual education plan.

Fortunately, parents and professionals are rarely in conflict. They are most often able to work together for the benefit of individual children, and, in general, where conflict does exist, the relationship between parents and professionals is improving. Health care professionals are learning more about disabled children and their parents through new curricula,[434,879] new techniques of instruction,[915,1123] and textbooks.[106,245b] Most studies show that health care providers exposed to developmental disabilities in their training have more positive attitudes toward disabled children.[915,1101,1232] Educational professionals are learning more about congenitally disabled children and their parents and about how to teach positive attitudes and acceptance to their able-bodied peers.[247a,770,892] Parents are becoming more active advocates as part of the general consumerism movement.[245a] Partially because of support from parent groups, parents now have a better awareness of involvement strategies and recent legislation.[244a] We agree with the many authors[225,244b,245a,557,870,1078,1093,1130] who have recommended that parents should participate actively in monitoring laws, challenging authority, and, most importantly, advocating for disabled children.

Finally, parents must teach their congenitally malformed children to advocate for themselves. Adolescents and parents alike must be taught that protection and pity foster attitudes and behaviors of helplessness and, thus, hinder independence. Teenagers and young adults, if they have been in good medical, educational, and social management programs, should have arrived at a point where they can take care of themselves (see Chapters 19–21).

SECTION II

Initial Medical Treatment

David Shurtleff
Ronald Lemire
Josef Warkany

3

Embryology, Etiology, and Epidemiology

Embryology, etiology, and epidemiology are among the most important matters to be discussed with parents of a newborn with major malformations. First, embryology tells us something about when the congenital malformation originated and rules out suspected causes that may needlessly worry parents; many events can be definitely excluded because they occurred later in the pregnancy, after the embryopathologic event. Second, etiology, if it can be established, assists in defining prognosis. Third, epidemiology, in addition to etiology, helps allay unspoken parental concerns by correctly defining recurrence risks.

EMBRYOLOGY

Embryology of the Neural Tube

The nervous system develops by neurulation, the formation of a tubular structure.[635] At gestational age 18 days, the embryo consists of three layers of cells (the ectoderm, mesoderm, and endoderm) making up the embryonic disk. At approximately this time, ridges build up on either side of the midline on the dorsal surface of the embryonic disk. These neural folds begin to fuse at about day 22. At this time, six or seven mesodermal somites have formed. Fusion of the neural folds begins at the level of the third to fourth somite; this area later develops into the

MYELODYSPLASIAS AND EXSTROPHIES: SIGNIFICANCE, PREVENTION, AND TREATMENT
 ISBN 0-8089-1816-8

occipital bone. At the head end (rostral), the neural cells multiply rapidly. This area later folds and grows laterad, forward and backward, to form the brain and its related parts. At about 24 days, the most rostral opening of the neural tube, the anterior neuropore, closes at the level of the lamina terminalis, a thin, flat plate.[635] Precisely where the posterior neuropore closes is not definite, but closure occurs at approximately day 28. Thereafter, the tail (caudal) end of the spinal cord develops by canalization and then retrogressive differentiation of a caudal cell mass.[635]

During canalization, the caudal end of the neural tube, the caudal cell mass, develops when some cells orient themselves around vacuoles, which coalesce and enlarge in a somewhat irregular manner. The vacuoles later connect with the central canal of the spinal cord that was previously established rostral to the posterior neuropore by neurulation. The largest and most caudal area of the central canal is known as the ventriculus terminalis, found within the conus medullaris. Later differential growth rates make the conus medullaris "ascend" to the level of the second lumbar vertebra. From the conus medullaris, a slender terminal filament (the filum terminale) extends to the tip of the coccyx.

Embryology of the Hindgut

This topic is important because of the association of myelocystocele with exstrophy of the cloaca (see below). Simultaneous with neural development, the anterior abdominal wall forms with development of the hindgut and cloacal membrane.[1198] The hindgut is first recognizable at about 32 days of age as a tube located in the midline with a dilated, terminal, blind sac (the cloaca) and with a membrane on the inner (ventral) curve of the tube (the cloacal membrane) (Fig. 3-1). Ventral to the hindgut is the allantoic diverticulum, which extends rostrally and ventrally in the umbilical cord. Shortly thereafter, the urorectal septum develops between the allantois and the hindgut; this mesodermal septum extends caudally, dividing the allantois and the cloaca into, respectively, the urogenital sinus on the ventral side and the rectum on the dorsal side. The urorectal septum continues to grow, medially and caudally, toward the cloacal membrane and then fuses with it to form the primitive perineum at about age 49 days. The anterior section of the cloacal membrane becomes the urogenital membrane and the dorsal section, the anal membrane. Both of these membranes perforate into the amniotic space to form the urethral opening anteriorly and the anus posteriorly. Mesoderm thickens the walls of these primitive structures to form the abdominal and perineal musculature, the bony pelvis and musculature of the gut, and the urinary bladder and sphincters. The urogenital septum develops parallel and anterior to the urorectal septum to separate the

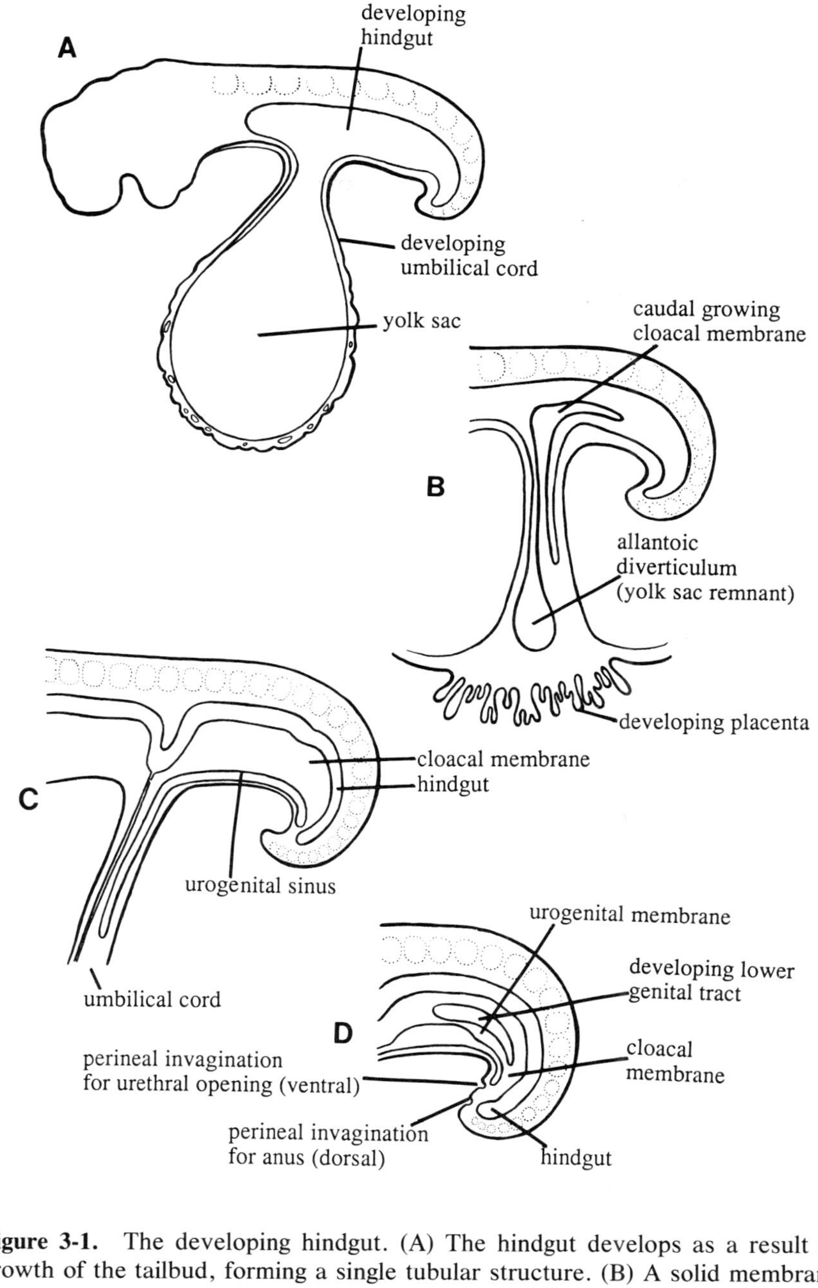

Figure 3-1. The developing hindgut. (A) The hindgut develops as a result of growth of the tailbud, forming a single tubular structure. (B) A solid membrane separates the developing hindgut into an anterior and posterior tube that will develop into the hindgut and urogenital sinus. (C) A second membrane forms between the anterior urinary system and the medially placed genital tract. (D) These structures perforate the perineum at the sites of perineal invagination for the urethra and the anus and, in the female developing genital tract, the vagina.

urinary tract (on the anterior side) from the primitive reproductive organs (on the dorsal side) between the urinary tract and the rectum.[1198] Two ridges, the genital ridges, migrate caudad and mediad to form the genital tubercle from which the external genitals develop.[846,1098]

EMBRYOPATHOLOGY: ABERRANT NEURULATION AND POSTNEURULATION

The above brief review of the embryology of the areas in which major malformations discussed in this text develop serves as a framework for discussions of embryopathology and the clinical relevance of myelodysplasias.

Encephalocele, Craniomeningocele, and Anencephaly

Errors in neurulation (failures of fusion) cause many malformations of the nervous system such as anencephaly and meningomyelocele.[635] Postneurulation neural tube defects consist of encephaloceles and skin-covered lumbosacral lesions. Most rostral neurulation defects appear along the closure line to the anterior neuropore and are lethal conditions. These range from anencephaly to craniorachischisis.[633]

Malformations that develop in the head after neurulation are, essentially, hernias of the brain coverings and are called encephaloceles. In the United States, most of these occur in the occipital region. These herniations were, until recently, thought to have the same consequences as true neurulation malformations, that is, death or severe mental retardation. The severe morbidity from simple herniations, however, is due essentially to secondary complications of trauma during vaginal delivery or to infection and can be prevented with modern treatment methods, discussed in later chapters.

Myelodysplasia

True meningomyelocele (myelomeningocele) is believed by most doctors to be the result of a failure of fusion of the neural folds during neurulation. Failure to fuse can be associated with neural tissue overgrowth[845] or with disorientation of the neural cells.[249a,635] It is not currently known whether these changes of cellular disorientation and overgrowth are sequential, causal, or simply related to failure of the neural tube to close.

A hypothesis recently proposed by Jennings and associates[551] involves a more cephalad closure of the neural folds, entrapping posterior fossa contents to create the Arnold-Chiara malformation.[189] This displacement creates serial somite closures more rostral to the nervous system than normal. When the site of final closure is reached at the posterior neuropore, too much nervous tissue remains within the forming neural canal, inhibiting or preventing closure.[551] Although this embryopathologic process may explain the most common meningomyelocele with a placode (defined below) that involves the high and midlumbar spine, it does not explain the less common cervical or thoracic lesions not involving the lumbar area.

Regardless of the mechanism of formation, two clinically important features about meningomyelocele remain. First, the neural tube is open with what was meant to be the central canal lying exposed on the dorsal surface of the sac, the so-called zona medullovasculosa[635] or the placode[739] (Fig. 3-2 A and B). This placode is surrounded by a rim of membranes, variable in thickness and inconsistently covered with epithelialization. Second, the posterior neuropore closes at about 28 days postconception; only events prior to that time can possibly be etiologic, if the most popular nonclosure theory is accepted. Other, less widely held theories suggest the tube closes and then "ruptures"[385,833] or claim that the blood supply fails to develop.[1190] At present, these latter theories are less accepted for lack of supportive documentation.

Open sacral and lumbosacral lesions could conceivably develop because the canalization process opens into a previously formed open defect. Essentially, little is known about the differences between causes and mechanisms accounting for the formation of meningomyelocele variants, including a range of malformations from open lesions with the nervous system contained within an open neural canal (Fig. 2A and B) to huge cystic meningomyelocele lesions with the neural plaque either on the dorsal surface (Fig. 3-2C) or with the cord connections lying in a definite neural canal with nerves traversing the sac, adhering to the dorsal (back) surface, and then reentering the neural canal before exiting the foramina (Fig. 3-2D).

Meningocele

Meningoceles are clinical entities comparable with the cranial and frontonasal meningoceles that are hernias of membranes involving little or no dysgenesis of the underlying nervous system. They might result from pathoembryogenesis of the meninx primitiva or the dura mater as it develops from the mesoderm at 25–52 days gestational age. Meningoceles may appear as in Figure 3-2D, with fully functioning nerves entering the sac and adhering to the dome before returning to their exit foramina.

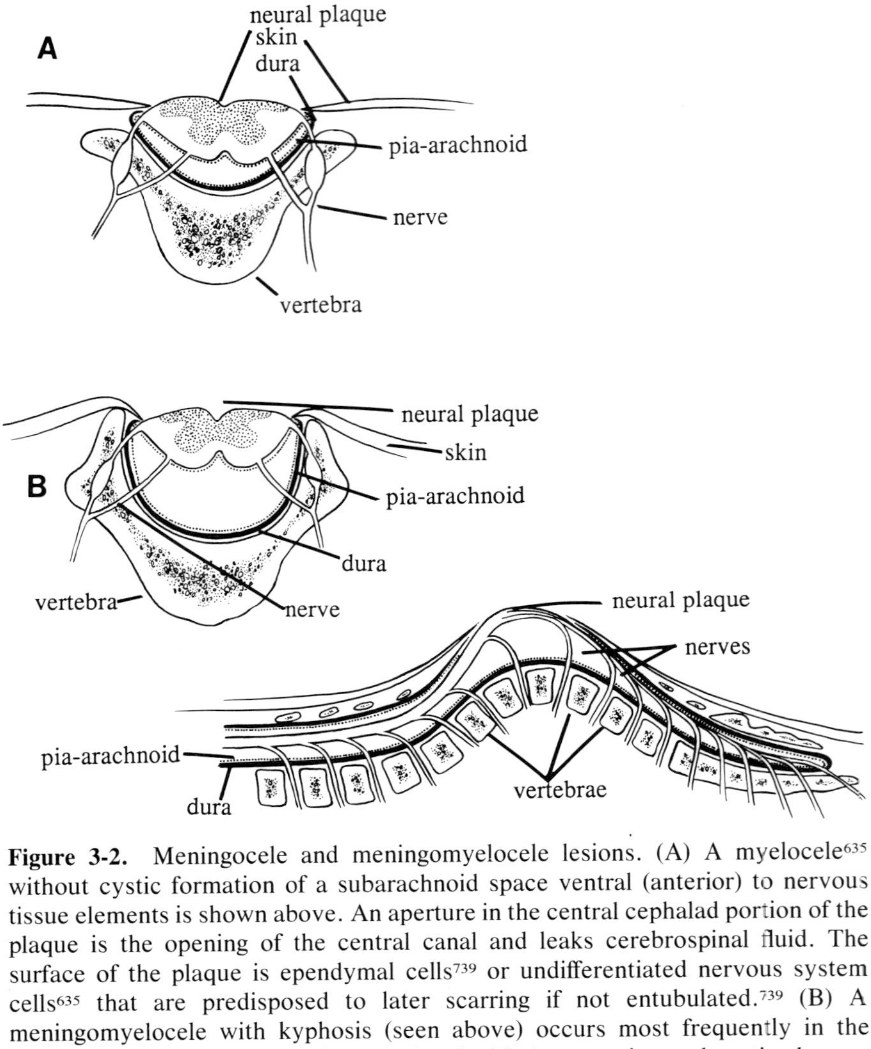

Figure 3-2. Meningocele and meningomyelocele lesions. (A) A myelocele[635] without cystic formation of a subarachnoid space ventral (anterior) to nervous tissue elements is shown above. An aperture in the central cephalad portion of the plaque is the opening of the central canal and leaks cerebrospinal fluid. The surface of the plaque is ependymal cells[739] or undifferentiated nervous system cells[635] that are predisposed to later scarring if not entubulated.[739] (B) A meningomyelocele with kyphosis (seen above) occurs most frequently in the thoracolumbar area and may be associated with degeneration and cystic changes as well as chronic inflammation in the plaque. Our only case of this type was delivered early (see Chapter 4) and was associated with high-level paralysis, as is seen with most of these cases delivered after labor via either cesarean section or vagina. (C) The most commonly seen meningomyelocele may be barely protruding or may assume a sessile large protrusion (shown). This lesion has been most frequently described as having no epithelial covering, but, invariably, affected infants have been delivered after labor via vagina or cesarean section. As with type A, the placques are covered by inflammatory and undifferentiated nervous system cells. All variations are associated with varying degrees of paralysis (see also Chapter 4, Case 3, Fig. 4-2).

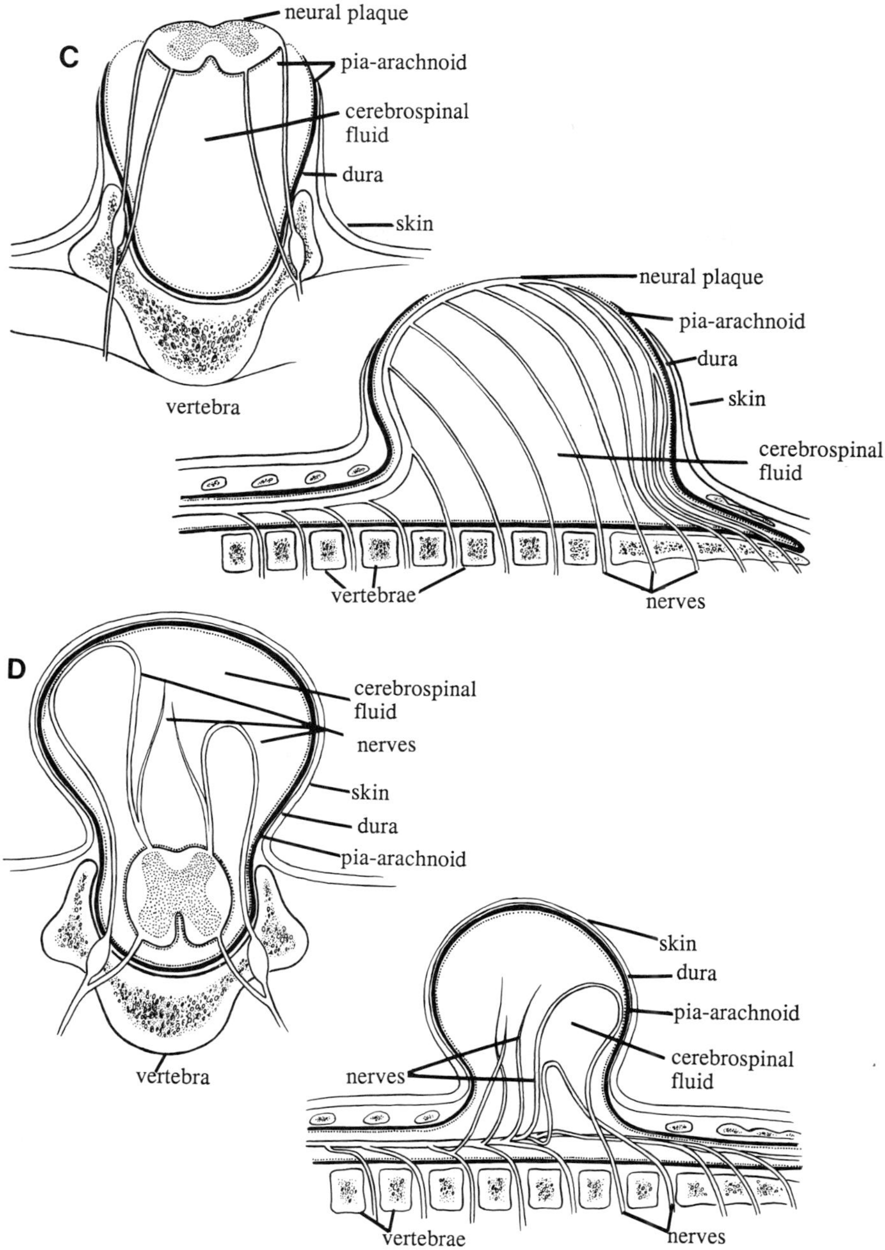

Figure 3-2. *(continued)* (D) This type of lesion can be associated with incomplete covering, as illustrated in the photograph in Chapter 4 (Fig. 4-2), or it can have a full-thickness skin covering, as illustrated here. If completely covered with skin and associated with paralysis, the lesion is classified clinically as a meningocele. Meningoceles have only a few or no nerves attached to the dome of the sac. The illustrated meningomyelocele has a clear membrane with nerves imbedded in the dome of the sac and occasionally returning to their exit foramina in the neural canal.

Some nerves may end in the dome of the sac but without apparent loss of function. The most commonly recognized form of meningocele has all nervous system elements within the neural canal, with only the meninges forming the sac. The meningoceles have skin coverings, with no evident paralysis.

Meningoceles are included in this text because they represent abnormal development in an area that involves mesoderm, epithelium, and nervous tissue. Progressive loss of nervous system function occurs in some children and adults with previously resected meningoceles because of tethered cord, scarring at the site of repair and growth of lipomas, or dermoids, as discussed in Chapter 6. Furthermore, there is a clinical gradation between patients with asymptomatic meningoceles and patients with meningomyeloceles covered with varying degrees of epithelialization that is not a true skin covering and with different degrees of nerve involvement in the sac and of resultant paralysis (see case 5, Chapter 4). For the above reasons, patients with meningoceles and meningomyeloceles deserve the same careful follow-up to assure normal function.

Lipomeningomyelocele, Lipomeningocele, and Lipomyelocele

All of the neural tube lesions of the lower spine may be associated with abnormal growth of epidermal or mesodermal tissue later in life. Fat is the most common tissue presenting by itself in association with open lesions of the spinal canal, as in a lumbosacral lipoma.[632] Lipomas of the neural tube most frequently present with some degree of meningocele formation, and most have no nerve function impairment initially. They can be associated with both split spinal cord (diastematomyelia) and with tethering of the cord by an enlarged, thickened filum terminale. The most common lipomas present at birth with connections to the filum terminale, the conus medullaris, or the lower spinal cord itself. Most of these lipomyelomeningoceles or lipomeningoceles extend in the rostral direction up the spinal canal and have a firm, thick transverse band at the most caudal level of the intact spinal column.[793] This band kinks and tethers the spinal cord.

Lipomas of all sorts in the lumbosacral area are thought to arise from either lipid cells of the zona epithelioserosa enclosed during surgical repair or from aberrant differentiation of primitive caudal mass cells into lipomas during the stage of canalization.[632] The latter origin accounts for most sacral lipomas apparent at birth and, therefore, like meningoceles, the lipomas are covered with a full thickness of skin and subcutaneous tissue. Sacral lipomas theoretically develop between gestational age 28 and 34 days or later, but no embryologic data have been published about these lesions. Most of them will progressively increase in size, pressing on contiguous nerves, and cause loss of function.

Diastematomyelia (Diplomyelia)

Like lipomas of the sacral area, duplication of the lower spinal cord or diplomyelia is thought to develop during the postneurulation period of cord development. It occurs alone or with mesodermal elements such as fibrous bands or bone and cartilagenous spurs that pass from the ventral to the dorsal wall of the spinal canal. These lesions can be seen in association with the various types of meningomyelocele. They can both account for progressive loss of neural function and be detected by contrast roentgenography (Fig. 3-3). Diastematomyelias can be resected; however, associated spasticity cannot be neurosurgically corrected, only arrested if it is progressive.

Myelocystocele

Myelocystoceles develop from within the neural tube and can have more than one cyst, one of which communicates with the central canal of the spinal cord. They are covered with skin and can be barely noticeable or as large as an infant's body. Most grow in size after birth and require neurosurgical resection. Many are associated with open defects of the ventral surface such as exstrophy of the cloaca.

Exstrophy of the Urinary Bladder and Cloaca

The pathogenesis of exstrophy of the cloaca and bladder is poorly understood.[1198] The exstrophies develop between 32 gestational days, when the hindgut is first identifiable as a tube, and 49 days, when the hindgut meets the primitive perineum by perforation of the anal membrane to form the anus. In complete exstrophy of the cloaca, the original cloacal membrane creating the anterior wall of the rectum and colon as well as the posterior wall of the urogenital sinus does not form, but develops only partially with various structures such as rectovesical, uterine, vaginal, and urethral or perineal fistulae. The original cloacal membrane does, however, form completely in urinary bladder exstrophy. The most common cited theory for the development of exstrophy is Patten and Barry's contention[846] that the genital tubercles migrate more caudally than normal, leaving insufficient mesoderm anteriorly, which later perforates. Rickham[928] extended this hypothesis to include the most extreme degree of caudal displacement to account for perforation of the primitive cloaca anteriorly, producing exstrophy. Three other theories

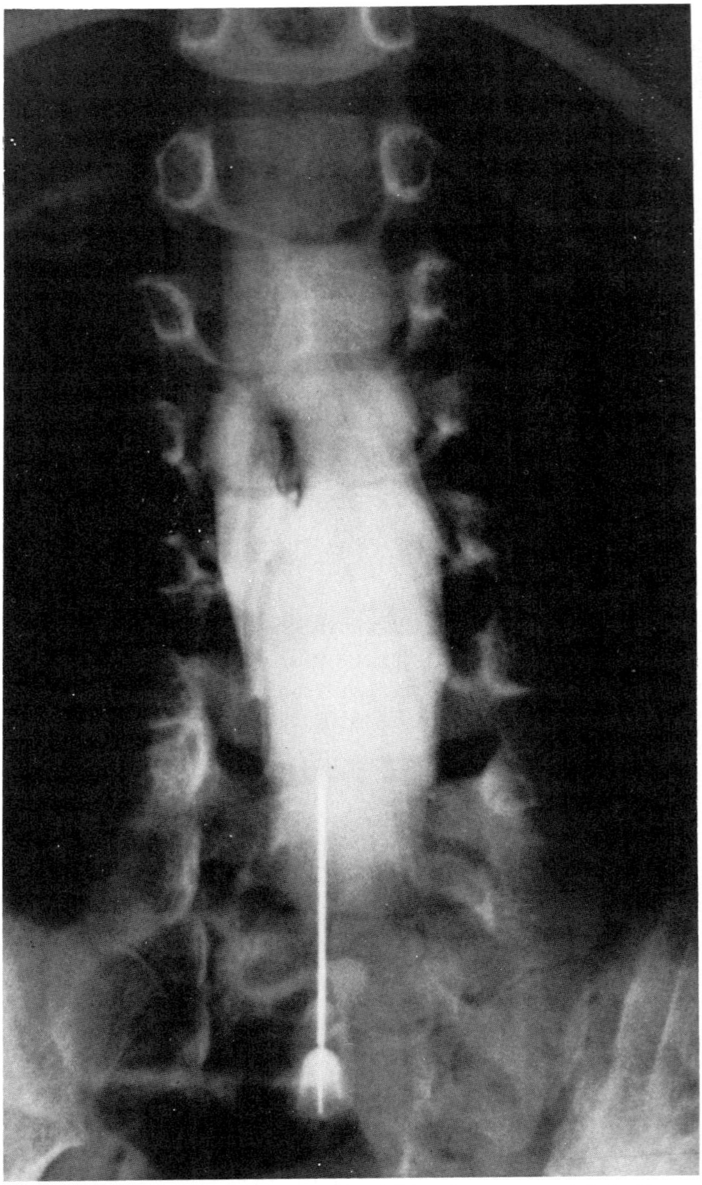

Figure 3-3. Diastematomyelia. This shows a metrizimide myelogram of a child with increasing spasticity in the lower legs. The radioluscent defect in the lumbar area is a diastematomyelia that was surgically removed with cessation of the progressive spasticity, and resulting in some modest recovery.

include partial formation of the anterior wall of the hindgut by incomplete ventral-rostral folding of the tail fold,[1098] persistence of an abnormally large cloacal membrane that prevents mesodermal closure,[696] and failure of fusion of the mesoderm anteriorly.[1083] A number of partial exstrophies and abnormal urethral and anal openings occur with various types of myelodysplasia. As mentioned above, cloacal exstrophy is associated with myelocystocele. In our series of 621 myelodysplasia patients, 43 (7%) had exstrophy of the cloaca, and 21 (4%) of the 578 remaining had epi- or hypospadias or rectal fistulae.

ETIOLOGY

Embryology and embryopathology, wherever possible, should be supplemented with a knowledge of etiology in order to assist prognosis. Nothing is known about the etiologies for most of the lesions mentioned in this chapter, with the exception of those few causes of open neural tube defects listed in Tables 3-1–3-4. Epidemiological studies suggest that neural tube defects constitute a spectrum resulting from similar causes acting at slightly different times during embryogenesis.[301] Most reports consider the hydrocephalus-anencephaly-meningomyelocele spectrum to be a continuum.

Familial Recurrence

In almost all reports from the eastern United States and the United Kingdom, there are descriptions of families with both anencephaly and meningomyelocele. In the Pacific Northwest, we have families with meningocele, meningomyelocele, and hydrocephalus in siblings; only one known family with meningomyelocele and ienencephaly; and none with meningomyelocele and anencephaly. In other families, more than one anencephalic child occurred. We have observed concordance in identical twins for exstrophy of the cloaca[727] and for meningomyelocele (one set of a total of five pairs of twins and 621 cases of meningomyelocele; see the section on Trends of Occurrence later in this chapter for a more in-depth discussion of epidemiologic studies of twinning as they relate to etiology). A multiple center study we participated in reported a slight increase in bifid vertebrae among siblings of children with meningomyelocele.[614]

In one family with three children with meningomyelocele, two female siblings and both parents had spina bifida occulta of the L5-S1 and L3,4-S2 vertebrae. These two female siblings were advised to have prenatal diagnoses, and each has had a normal child. Another family has been reported by Sever[1002] as having meningomyelocele with a three-

Table 3-1
Suspected Environmental Causes[a]

Etiology or Association	Probability Rating	Defects	Studies
Alcohol	5	Intrauterine growth retardation, myelomeningocele, short palpebral fissures, thin philtrum, thinned upper vermillion, microcephaly	Clarren and Smith, 1978[198]; Goldstein and Arulanantham, 1978[410]
Aminopterin (methotrexate)	5	Anencephaly, hydrocephaly, meningomyelocele, encephalocele, multiple skull anomalies	Milunsky et al., 1968[763]; Warkany et al., 1959[1199]
Amphetamine	0	Meningomyelocele (1 child)	Erikson et al., 1978[315]
Clomiphene	3	Anencephaly, microcephaly, meningomyelocele, skeletal deformities of chest and limbs, microcephaly, sacral dysgenesis	Singh and Singh, 1978[1070]; Nevin and Harley, 1976[802]; Dyson and Kohler, 1973[294]
Defects of midline developmental fields	1	Meningomyelocele, exstrophy of the urinary bladder, gastroschisis	Hunter, 1984[515]; Opitz and Gilbert, 1982[829]
Diabetes (maternal)	5	Caudal regression; other multiple defects including anencephaly, meningomyelocele	Soler et al., 1976[1090]; Stewart and Stoll, 1979[1120]
Fever	4	Anencephaly	Chance and Smith, 1978[175]; Clarren et al., 1979[197]; Smith et al., 1978[1074]; Miller et al., 1978[759]; Shiota, 1982[1020]; Hunter, 1984[515]

Folate deficiency	4	Neural tube defects	Smithells et al., 1983[1079]; Laurence et al., 1981[617]; Seller and Nevin, 1984[998]
LSD (multiple drug ingestions)	2	Multiple neural tube defects: meningomyelocele, meningocele, anencephaly, hydrocephaly, congenital heart disease (CHD)	Jacobsen and Berlin, 1972[535]
Miscarriage (association, not etiology)	5	Meningomyelocele	Elwood and Elwood, 1980[301]; Hunter 1984[515]; Leck, 1966[625]; Nishimura et al., 1968[813]; Record, 1950[894]
Nitrate excess	1	Meningomyelocele, anencephaly, encephalocele	Knox, 1972[590]; Scragg et al., 1982[994]
Nutritional deficiency	3	Neural tube defects	Knox, 1972[590]; Leck, 1983[629]
Rubella	2	Meningocele, microcephaly, mental retardation (MR), cataract, CHD, etc.	Lundstrom, 1962[678]
Thalidomide	3	Meningomyelocele, anencephaly, reduction malformation of limbs	Taussig, 1962[1146]
Tissue bands	2	Anencephaly, facial clefts, constriction bands on limbs	Jones et al., 1974[559]
Trichlorophenoxybenzamine	0	Neural tube defects	"2,4,5-T," 1977[1172]
Trimethadione	1	Meningomyelocele, cleft lip and palate, CHD, omphalocele	Nichols, 1973[807]
Twinning	1	Meningomyelocele, Arnold-Chiari malformation, encephalocele	Hindse-Nielson, 1938[488]; Knox, 1974[592]; Layde et al., 1980[622]

Continues

Table 3-1 *Continued*

Etiology or Association	Probability Rating	Defects	Studies
Valproic acid	4	Meningomyelocele	Dalens et al., 1980[240]; Hurd et al., 1983[516]; Robert et al., 1983[933]
Zinc deficiency	2	Meningomyelocele	Leck, 1983[629]; Sever, 1973[1007], 1957[1005]

[a] Reviewers of large series of neural tube defects (spina bifida aperta, meningomyelocele, and anencephaly) came to the conclusion that genetic predisposition to these anomalies is polygenic and that additional intrauterine environmental factors play a part in causation. This was suggested by observations in areas of high frequency[168] and in areas of low frequency.[169] Findings suggested a multifactorial etiology dependent on genetic predispostion and environmental triggers. Such explanations are general, and searches for specific factors, environmental as well as genetic, have been made and should be continued.

We believe neural tube defects can be caused by a number of etiologic factors and, therefore, should be considered polyetiologic. In these tables, some cases of neural tube defects and their putative etiologies are listed. In many instances, the suspicions of causation are more justified than in others. Added to the suspected causes are numbers (1–5) that indicate a subjective evaluation of the probable validity of the suspicion of causal connections.

Table 3-2
Suspected Chromosomal Anomalies[a]

Etiology	Probability Rating	Defects	Studies
Triploidy (69 XXX)	4	Encephalus, meningomyelocele, cleft palate	Creasy and Alberman, 1976[230]; Simpson et al., 1972[1067]
Trisomy 13	5	Encephalocele, meningomyelocele	Warkany et al., 1966[1200]
Pseudotrisomy 13–15	5	Arhinencephaly with encephalocele	Marshall et al., 1964[695]; Miller and Selden, 1967[758]
Trisomy 18	5	Meningomyelocele, encephalocele, prominent occiput, low-set malformed ears, micrognathia, CHD, short sternum, prominent calcaneus, dermatoglyphics, excess arches	Menashi et al., 1977[747]; Passarge et al., 1966[844]; Taylor, 1968[1147]; Warkany et al., 1966[1200]
Trisomy 8 (46 XY, 47 XY)	3	Spina bifida occulta	Theilgard et al., 1977[1161]
Partial trisomy 11 (T-6P+; 11 q−)	3	Anencephaly, craniorachisch	Wright et al., 1974[1240]
Trisomy D XX	3	Encephalocele, cleft palate	Creasy and Alberman, 1976[230]
45 X	3	Encephalocele	Creasy and Alberman, 1976[230]; Haddad and Wilkins, 1959[443]

Continues

Table 3-2 *Continued*

Etiology	Probability Rating	Defects	Studies
46 XXY q+	3	Exencephaly	Creasy and Alberman, 1976[230]
Ring chromosome	3	Anencephaly	Schmid et al., 1975[983]
Unbalanced translocation	3	Craniorachischisis and meningomyelocele, anencephaly	Wright et al., 1974[1240]
Cytoplasmic inheritance gonadal mutation (mothers have several affected children with different fathers)	1	Meningomyelocele, meningocele, microcephaly	Nance, 1974[794a]

[a] See footnote to Table 3-1.

Table 3-3
Suspected Gene-Determined Anomalies[a]

Etiology or Association	Probability Rating	Defects	Studies
Dominant	1	Meningomyelocele	Wilner, 1949[1223]
Dominant	1	Meningomyelocele in family with spondylolisthesis; spina bifida occulta	Sever, 1974[1002]
Dominant (with large environmental influence)	1	Spina bifida, sacral agenesis	Demenais et al., 1982[255]
Dominant	1	Spina bifida, spondylolisthesis	Amuso and Mankin, 1967[37]
Dominant	1	Cranium bifidum occultum	DeMyer, 1967[258]
Dominant	3	Anterior spina bifida, meningoceles, neurofibromatosis	Borberg, 1951[115]; Campbell, 1951[155]; LaVielle and Campbell, 1958[619]
Dominant or recessive	1	Anterior sacral meningomyelocele, anal stenosis	Say and Coldwell, 1975[974]

Continues

Table 3-3 *Continued*

Etiology or Association	Probability Rating	Defects	Studies
Recessive and X-linked	1	Meningomyelocele, MR, arthrogryposis, limb reduction malformations	Pallister and Opitz, 1985[836]
Recessive	1	Meningomyelocele, hydrocephaly, anencephaly	Lorber, 1965[667]
Recessive	5	Anencephaly, occipital encephalocele, cleft palate, polycystic kidneys, genital anomalies, polydactyly, Meckel syndrome	Fried et al., 1971[371]; Hsia et al., 1971[510]; Meckel, 1822[745]
Recessive	4	Encephalocele (rare), cleft lip and palate, tetraphocomelia, clitoral or penile enlargement, Roberts syndrome	Freeman et al., 1974[369]; Roberts, 1919[935]
Recessive	5	Encephalocele, hydrocephalus, retinal detachment, Hydrocephalus Agyrio Dysplasia and Encephalocele, HARD syndrome	Chemke et al., 1975[184]; Pagon et al., 1978[834]
Polygenic recessive	3	Meningomyelocele	Carter et al., 1976[170]; Timson, 1972[1165]

[a]See footnote to Table 3-1.

Table 3-4
Syndromes of Unknown Origin[a]

Probability Ratings	Defects	Studies
2	Meningomyelocele, ankyloblepharon filiform	Kazarin and Goldstein, 1977[576]
5	Myelocystocele, cloacal exstrophy, "meningocele"	Beckwith, 1966[81]; Marshall and Muecke, 1962[696]; Warkany, 1971[1198]
2	Meningomyelocele, sacrococcygeal teratoma	Fraumeni et al., 1973[365]
2	Hydrocephalus with occipital encephalocele, micrognathia, short limb dwarfism	Dinno et al., 1976[275]
4	Meningomyelocele, anencephalus, absent spleen, cardiac defects, Ivemark syndrome	Ivemark, 1958[530]; Van Went et al., 1977[1179]
2	Spinal defects Omphalocele Exstrophy Imperorate anus and Spinal defects, OEIS complex (hemivertebrae, sacral meningocele)	Carey et al.; 1978[161]

[a] See footnote to Table 3-1.

generational history of spondylolisthesis and spina bifida occulta. Not only are family histories important when evaluating the significance of spina bifida occulta, but the clinician should be concerned with the age of the patient: the fifth lumbar vertebra has been reported as bifid by roentgenographic studies in 16 percent of all normal 7–8-year-olds and 2.2 percent of all normal adults; the first sacral vertebra is bifid in 51.6 percent and 26.4 percent of the same two respective groups.[1137] In both groups of 7–8-year-olds, the bifid roentgenographic appearance decreases with age as the posterior laminae calcify.

Familial recurrence must also be interpreted with caution because of possible nongenetic causes for meningomyelocele. One mother with three affected male children was known to be a severe alcoholic; all three children were microcephalic and had facial features of the fetal alcohol syndrome.[198]

The occurrence of known syndromes that include meningomyelocele indicates the heterogeneous nature of this defect[499,582,713,1045] (Tables 3-1–3-4). Some patients with multiple anomalies in addition to a meningomyelocele have chromosome disorders (Fig. 3-4, Table 3-2). Taylor[1147] reports three of 27 patients with trisomy 13 had meningomyeloceles. We have one patient with the same 46,T (8′11)(q21P14) balanced chromosome translocation in a normal mother and normal sibling. Therefore, the presence of a chromosome abnormality may be associated with a congenital malformation, but not causally related. Careful family history, physical examination, and special studies may reveal one of the known types of inheritance, listed in Tables 3-1–3-4.

Etiologic Heterogeneity

Heterogeneity was found in our series of 621 cases of meningomyelocele. We have been able to identify malformations as potentially caused by chromosome abnormalities, folate deficiencies, recessive inheritance, and maternal alcoholism. Only two types of chromosome-related cases occurred in our sample in addition to the family mentioned above under familial recurrence: one trisomy 13 and one trisomy 18. One family with dominantly inherited nerve palsies included a mild form of meningomyelocele; and two families had severe, recurrent fetal alcohol syndrome. Six of 123 women attempting a second pregnancy after having given birth to children with open neural tube defects had low red blood cell folates while on adequate diets and taking multiple vitamin capsules containing 40 mg of folic acid.[1238] These women were provided adequate supplementation to raise their red blood cell folate and subsequently conceived normal children. Within the near future, several large studies will, we hope, answer the question raised by Smithells and associates[1079] as to whether folic acid deficiency is a cause for some open neural tube defects. To date in a local study, 69 pregnant women with prior meningomyelocele children were given preconceptual supplements and had normal children. In addition, we have observed two cases with hydrocephalus, severe brain malformation, meningomyelocele, arthrogryposis of all four extremities, and radial digital ray reduction malformations; all of these malformations are complex anomalies, possibly recessively inherited.[835] Finally, a woman has given birth to seven children, three of whom had hydrocephalus, small meningomyeloceles or meningoceles, and severe retardation despite early adequate treatment. All three were by different fathers. Two were girls and one a boy. This family history and the two mentioned above raise the question of maternal cytoplasmic inheritance,[91] a field defect as an expression of dominant inheritance,[829,1223] or maternal gonadal mutation.[1198] The above 13 cases have suspected etiologies, leaving 608, or 98 percent, of the cases with an unknown etiology. Our percentage of diagnosed causes of meningomyelocele, lower than those reported by Holmes and associates' 12 percent,[499] may be accounted for by their inclusion of encephaloceles.

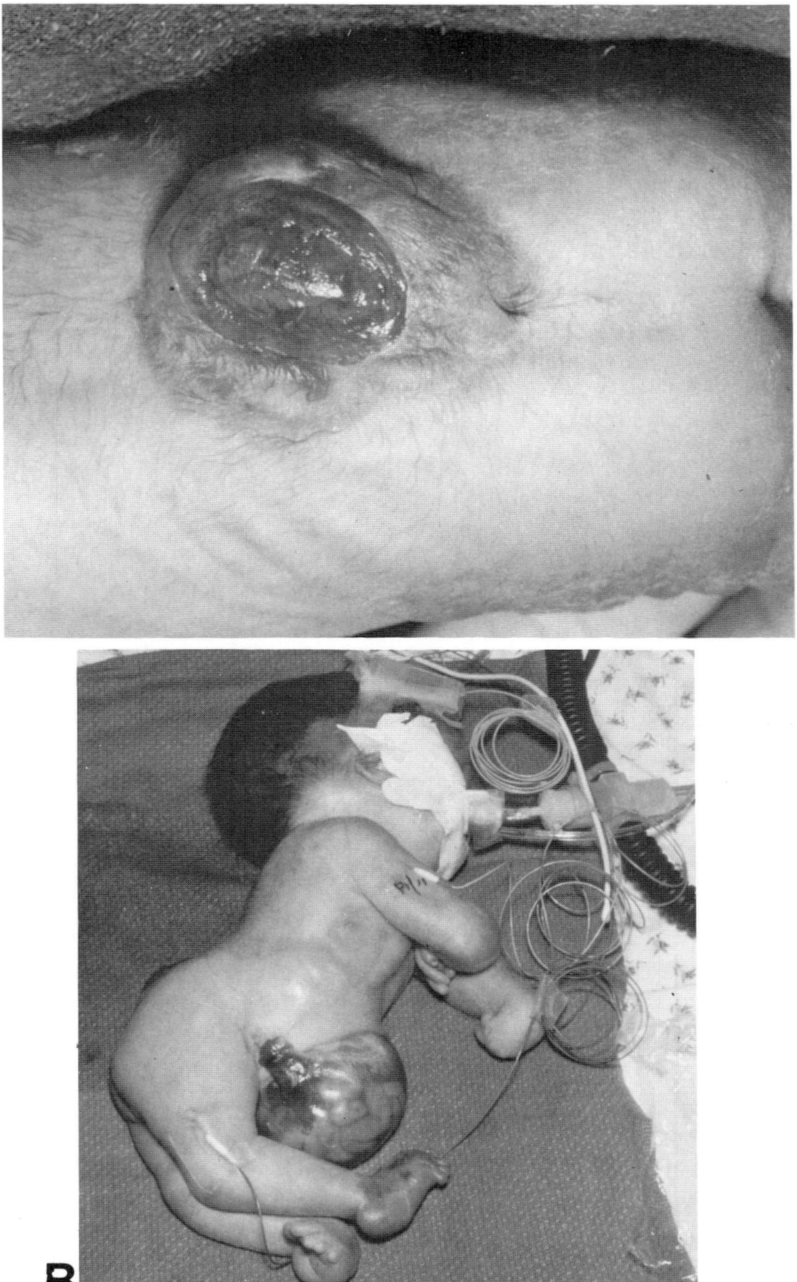

A

B

Figure 3-4. Multiple defects. This shows a child born with multiple defects and a small, relatively easily repairable meningomyelocele (A), as well as microcephaly, advanced hydrocephalus, cardiac malformation, omphalocele, and rigid deformities of all four extremities (B). The nonmeningomyelocele defects caused death on day 2. The chromosome analysis revealed Trisomy 13.

EPIDEMIOLOGY

Epidemiologic contributions to the understanding of etiology are of less importance to the clinician than their contribution to the understanding of treatment outcome, to be discussed later in this text. However, a brief review of the historical and ancestral background of these diseases, as it relates to our Seattle data, allows a greater understanding of the malformations discussed.

Ancestry and Historical Background

It is interesting that almost all of our Pacific Northwest families with meningomyelocele children trace their ancestry to Ireland, Scotland, or Wales or are of Mexican or Spanish descent. There seems to be little question that meningomyelocele is more common among the Celts and northern Indians, but rare among blacks.[301,626] Curiously, the parents' concerns are allayed by learning racial propensities and evidence for a long history of open neural tube defects in prehistoric, Roman, Anglo-Saxon, and medieval burials excavated in the United Kingdom.[134] By joining our knowledge of the history of this part of the world with these findings among human remains, we can presume the early Celtic people were the original racial stock to bring open neural tube defects to the area.

These Copper Age invaders of the northwestern land mass came at a time when there was a contiguous Ireland, Scotland, and Wales (during the melting of the last Ice Age before the English Channel separated Ireland) and have occupied these three countries continuously since their earliest appearance at about 1500 B.C. Their continued survival has been in part because of the mountainous, easily defended terrain; sporadic but temporary invasions resulted only in the capture of towns at the outlets of valleys since Hadrian, the Roman conqueror, built his wall south of this difficult country in an effort to keep the barbarians out of England. This relatively pure racial strain created Stonehenge and the Barrows as well as a stone architecture complete with a rich archeological history that only incidently traces the origin of open neural tube defects of the spine. The Celts were, however, not the only prehistoric people to have open neural tube defects, as we pointed out in Chapter 1. The oldest spinal defect, discovered in Morocco and believed to be over 12,000 years old,[330] may be the ancestor of the current Spanish-Mexicans noted to have a higher prevalence at birth (our series)[1128,1178] than other non-Celtic races.

Two mothers of offspring in our series with meningomyelocele associated with fetal alcohol syndrome are both North American Indians. Their racial propensity toward the birth of children with open neural tube defects of the spine as well as their alcoholism may be a dual influence. Further evidence to support the frequent occurrence of open neural tube defects among indigenous American populations is provided by Strassburg and associates,[1128] who noted that the Mexican-American population in the Los Angeles area has the highest prevalence at birth of open neural tube defects.

Incidence and Prevalence

Definitions of incidence and prevalence, concepts presented by Hook[503] and Sever,[1003] underlie studies of treatment as well as causation. The definition of incidence as prevalence (the number of births per unit of population at a given time) at birth, offered by Sever,[1003] is the same as that used by Elwood and Elwood.[301] Prevalence at birth provides three basic types of information. First, it is descriptive of the frequency of new cases added to a population. Second, it considers the loss of new cases of neural tube defects due to spontaneous abortion and stillbirth by miscarriage. Thus, Nishimura and associates[812] found that meningomyelocele occurred ten times more often in embryos 3–10 weeks of gestational age, obtained by induced abortion, than in children born at or near term. Creasy and Alberman[230] also noted high prevalences of central nervous system (CNS) defects in spontaneous abortions, with meningomyelocele common among later abortuses. In the future, induced abortion secondary to population screening by serum alpha-fetoprotein, ultrasound, and both amniotic alpha-fetoprotein and acetylcholinesterase will further increase the difference between incidence in early pregnancy and prevalence at birth. Third, prevalence at birth includes both stillbirths and live births with death in the next few hours or days, as reported by Laurence and Tew.[618] This concept of prevalence at birth is of particular interest to the clinician caring for open neural tube defects of the spine and possibly seeing only children referred to a tertiary medical center. What, indeed, are the types and degrees of severity and potential survival of children with meningomyelocele who arrive at different children's hospitals throughout the world? These characteristics are not known.

In the state of Washington, our Health Department claims that 87–96 percent of children born with open neural tube defects of the spine were reported by treating hospitals, 45–48 percent by birth certificates, and only 4–13 percent by viral statistics reporting forms (birth or death certificates) between 1981 and 1983.[850] Of these, 71–82 percent were reported by our Seattle-based tertiary treatment center. Since 71–82 percent of all patients in our area are referred to us, any comparison of effectiveness of treatment in other centers should consider what percentage of the total population is being referred to them. Prevalence at birth may not be reflected in prevalence at referral, particularly in densely populated areas where there are several centers with different selection for treatment policies. In addition to the possible effects prenatal diagnosis and abortion may have on referral patterns to treatment centers, changes occur due to selection for treatment processes documented by Feetham and associates[325] (see also Chapter 5). It will be increasingly important for clinicians to understand treatment outcome as measured by what percentage of patients detected in early gestation (early gestation prevalence) and what percentage of patients born (prevalence at birth) they are treating. Are they treating only survivors of an alpha-fetoprotein screening program with a high percentage of skin-covered meningoceles? Are they treating mostly infants referred with low-level meningomyelocele lesions preselected by the referring physician? What is the death rate of fetuses detected in the first trimester?

Trends of Occurrence

In addition to giving us an understanding of the spectrum of severity of open neural tube defects of the spine presented for treatment, epidemiology has provided valuable information concerning trends of occurrence of neural tube defects; these data may allow insight into etiology and development of resources for the care of children born with meningomyelocele. Long-term trends since the 1940s have demonstrated a decreasing prevalence at birth of meningomyelocele in the United Kingdom and Canada[301] and the United States.[1226] Within these long-term movements occur shorter term "epidemics" and yearly variations with a higher prevalence at birth reported in winter months.[241a] During the latter part of the 1970s, prevalence in the United States at birth has been relatively stable, at 0.6–0.9/1000 in Atlanta and at 0.4–0.6/1000 in 1200 hospitals across the United States, as reported by the National Birth Defects Monitoring Program.[1226] This program includes surveillance by hospital discharge diagnoses according to the Center for Disease Control's Birth Monitoring Program (CDC-BDMP) classification for approximately one third of the births in the eastern geographic two thirds of the United States (the reporting source furthest west is Nebraska).[1176] Recently, we have noted an insignificant rise in the prevalence at birth of meningomyelocele, suggesting, perhaps, that our low levels represent a stabilized rate.[850]

Throughout the last decade, the prevalence at birth of meningomyelocele in Washington state has been approximately 0.3–0.5/1000 births.[850] Van den Berg[1178] reported 0.5/1000 live births from northern California, and Strassburg and associates[1128] reported 0.38/1000 live births for whites (not Spanish) from Los Angeles. They reported the Spanish-

American prevalence at birth to be 0.47/1000, confirming the higher rate for Mexican-Americans suggested by Van den Berg's much more limited data[1178] and our own information. These western United States data confirm Hewitt's east-to-west decreasing gradient,[483] also observed in Canada.[301] The North American continent east-to-west decreasing gradient is similar to the increasing gradient observed from the southeast to the northwest British Isles.[301] These gradients occur within racial groups and suggest a geographic, environmental influence.

Geographic gradients that may reflect environmental causes for open neural tube defects are no more understood than the vague implications of environmental influences suggested by the inverse relationship between social class and prevalence at birth of meningomyelocele,[301] mentioned in Chapter 1. Since it was first described by Naggan and MacMahon,[791] the influence of poverty has been confirmed by most studies. Unfortunately, with the exception of folic acid deficiency,[1079] studies of infections, poor nutrition, and other given causal factors within the broad category of socioeconomic circumstances provide no more precise etiologic clues.[301] Specifically, described clusters of the incidence of meningomyelocele are etiologically unlike classic infections and can only be explained as occurring by chance, according to Elwood and Elwood.[301] Leck[626] reports seasonal and geographic variations that led him to believe there are environmental influences of considerable importance that may include nutrition.

Epidemiologic studies among twins suggest that open neural tube defects are to some degree genetically determined (they are more frequently concorded among like-sexed twins). But Elwood and Elwood[301] point out that conclusions from twin observations are difficult because of uncertainties about estimates of sibling risks and sex influences. The lack of concordance in both identical and fraternal twins suggests subtle environmental influences.

Recurrence Risks

Regardless of the interpretations of twinning and the occurrence of open neural tube defects, the sibling recurrence rate is of great interest to the clinician. Early studies suggested the recurrence risk to be 5 percent. More recent studies suggest the recurrence risk is 4–5 percent in the United Kingdom and 2–3 percent in the United States.[301] Other recent recurrence risk data[545,707] suggest recurrence among siblings to be near 2 percent. An apparent decrease in recurrence risks with lower general population incidence provides further evidence of an environmental influence.[515]

SUMMARY

In general, epidemiological data have included diverse clinical entities as a group in order to identify clues or trends. We agree with Khoury and associates[582] and Holmes and associates[499]: open neural tube defects are caused by a variety of mechanisms and agents. More specific studies of identical etiology groups need to be undertaken. Information to date from a variety of sources has provided insight into some causes and mechanisms of open neural tube defect formation, but much work remains to be done in the areas of (1) embryogenesis and its derivations, (2) case and family histories, (3) maternal age and parity, (4) social class and migration, (5) secular trends, (6) multiple, potentially additive, environmental factors, and (7) differences between single neural tube defects and those associated with other major malformations.

David Shurtleff

4

Prenatal Diagnosis: Prevention and Management for Improved Pregnancy Outcome

Advances in intrauterine diagnosis as well as in the treatment of children born with major congenital malformations have had a profound effect on the type of counseling that can be offered to parents of such fetuses and children. Intrauterine diagnosis and the subsequent management of the pregnancy are the subjects of this chapter. We will limit our discussion to meningomyelocele because a group managed after prenatal diagnosis is large enough to allow statistical analysis and comparison with our larger series of patients managed following full-term pregnancy and labor.

Prenatal diagnosis includes genetic screening by family history as well as biochemical or enzyme and roentgenographic or ultrasound examination of pregnant women.[228,760] We will mention briefly only those prenatal diagnostic techniques used in the diagnosis of neural tube and cloacal malformations (Table 4-1). The least invasive is maternal serum alpha-fetoprotein screening. As a single test, it should be relied on only for general population screening since its accuracy in detecting a fetus with a neural tube defect is 60–70 percent compared with 90–95 percent for examination of amniotic fluid for alpha-fetoprotein. Approximately 5 percent of open spine lesions will be epithelial or true-skin-covered and will be associated with normal serum and amniotic fluid alpha-fetoprotein levels. Other malformations, placental (fetal) bleeding into the amniotic fluid, fetal compromise and death, or an error in gestational age can raise

MYELODYSPLASIAS AND EXSTROPHIES: SIGNIFICANCE, PREVENTION, AND TREATMENT
 ISBN 0-8089-1816-8

Table 4-1
Methods of Prenatal Diagnosis

	14–16 Weeks Gestational Age			14–40 Weeks Gestational Age			
	Serum	Maternal Amniotic Fluid					
Clinical Entity	Alpha-Fetoprotein	Alpha-Fetoprotein	Acetyl-cholinesterase	Ultra-sound	Routine X-ray	Amino-graphy[a]	Fetoscopy**[b]
Anencephaly	+	+	+	+	+	+	+
Caudal regression syndrome	−	−	−	±	±	−	−
Craniobifida, not skin-covered, all types	+	+	+	±	±	±	±
Skin-covered cranial meningocele	±	±	−	±	±	±	±
Diasematomyelia	−	−	−	−	−	−	−
Exstrophy of the urinary bladder	+	+	−	+	−	±	±
Exstrophy of the cloaca	+	+	−	+	−	±	±
Lipoma (sacrococcygeal and all types)	−	−	−	−	−	−	−
Meningocele	−	−	−	±	−	±	±
Meningomyelocele, not skin-covered	+	+	+	±	−	±	±
Skin-covered meningomyelocele	−	−	−	±	−	±	±
Myelocystocele	−	−	−	+	−	±	±
Neuroenteric fistulae	−	−	−	−	−	−	−

Key: +, majority of lesions can be detected; ±, accuracy limited or insufficient data to evaluate; small lesions may be missed; −, method usually will not detect the clinical entity.
[a] Limited use with modern refined ultrasonography.
[b] Limited applicability because of risk of bleeding or leakage of amniotic fluid.

alpha-fetoprotein levels in amniotic fluid and lead to incorrect diagnosis of a neural tube defect.[228,387] Elevated amniotic fluid acetylcholinesterase, a central nervous system (CNS) enzyme, is specific in the 99–100 percent range for open neural tube defects without epithelial or skin covering and can be used to differentiate other abnormalities from open CNS conditions associated with elevations of alpha-fetoprotein.[129] Amniotic fluid acetylcholinesterase can also be used to diagnose open neural tube defects after the 20th week of gestation. Alpha-fetoprotein levels rise in the presence of normal fetuses by 20 weeks to the same levels reached as early as 14–16 weeks gestation in the presence of an open neural tube defect or one of the other abnormalities listed above.

Campbell[157] added ultrasound as a potent prenatal diagnostic tool and reported detecting 25 of 28 fetuses with open neural tube defects of the spine. The three cases detected by alpha-fetoprotein but not ultrasound were small low-lumbar or sacral-level lesions associated usually with less paralysis and a higher incidence of normal intellect.[1045] Roberts and associates[934] report, in addition, 100 percent accuracy with ultrasound in diagnosis of anencephaly in utero, an experience we have shared. They[934] reported an improvement in accuracy of detecting meningomyelocele from 36 percent in an early study to 80 percent in a later study with more experienced ultrasonographers and more accurate machines. They also reported missing only 1-cm-diameter sacral-level lesions. These studies discuss only elimination by termination or carrying a severely defective fetus to term.

Simultaneously with the development of techniques for intrauterine diagnosis of meningomyelocele, others described damage to nerves exposed in large defects due to compression of labor and confinement in late pregnancy,[1107] trauma to peripheral nerves during breech delivery,[890] or trauma and infection.[1104,1105]

Harrison and associates[462] first recommended cesarean section delivery of fetuses with large meningomyelocele lesions but presented no supportive data. They described this recommendation for "innovative" care as so obviously beneficial as to not need an investigation to prove its efficacy. Chervenak and associates[188] recently reported both a technique for cesarean section to avoid trauma to a large meningomyelocele sac, with a 75 percent good result. The obvious benefits include avoidance of trauma to the exposed spinal cord and delivery into a sterile environment with scheduled neurosurgery to follow immediately. In areas like the Pacific Northwest, where neurosurgical units are distant from isolated, small obstetrical units, transportation of the mother and baby in the protected, sterile, in utero environment to a treatment center that can handle both the delivery and neurosurgical care will also eliminate postnatal hazards associated with travel. In addition, parents can be counseled over a number of weeks so that they will be able to select the most appropriate treatment after they have overcome their initial shock.

In utero diagnosis of meningomyelocele has been most common, in our experience, after the last legal age to terminate, 24 weeks of gestational age. We offer various methods of delivery to provide either maximum safety for the mother or reduced risk of further damage to the fetus's exposed nerves.

MANAGEMENT OPTIONS

As mentioned above and in Chapter 1, genetic counseling literature usually offers termination as the only alternative when an unborn baby is diagnosed as severely congenitally malformed.[48,281,444,623,761] However, other options are available to parents who would not desire abortion or who have a diagnosis established after the pregnancy is beyond the allowable age for termination. These options are as follows: (1) natural birth with its attendant risks to the mother and child, (2) cephalocentesis or puncture of the ventricles of the fetal head to drain cerebrospinal fluid (CSF) and relieve cephalopelvic disproportion, followed by vaginal delivery with attendant risk to the baby[281,402,1221]; (3) cesarean section after a trial of labor with potential trauma to unprotected, exposed tissue involved in open defects; (4) cesarean section before onset of labor to protect congenitally exposed organs from trauma and infection[187,206,462]; and (5) intrauterine, fetal surgery.[203,402,1221] Delivery by cesarean section prior to labor in order to avoid trauma to the fragile hydrocephalic head; to the exposed nervous system with myelodysplasia; or to the intestines with exstrophy or omphalocele should improve pregnancy outcome by avoiding trauma to the exposed organs.[187,188,727,889,890,1104,1107]

SEATTLE EXPERIENCE

Recently, the Departments of Obstetrics and Gynecology at the Swedish Hospital Medical Center and the University of Washington have developed a system that allows a pediatrician, familiar with the treatment of and the prognosis for severe multiple congenital defects, to participate in prenatal counseling and pregnancy outcome planning. The following eight case reports illustrate the recommendations and potential options, including treatment for minimizing damage to the fetus's CNS.

Case 1

The managing physician examined case 1 in the uterus of a gravida 1, aborta 0, mother by ultrasound at 26 weeks of gestation because of a failure of the cranial size to develop according to the obstetrician's expectations. The examination revealed the diagnosis of microcephaly and an occipital encephalocele. We advised the physician that severe microcephaly associated with an encephalocele causes either death in early childhood or mental retardation of a marked degree. The family immediately requested termination. But since the pregnancy was beyond 24 weeks, the obstetrician advised the parents to let the pregnancy go to term as legally required and use vaginal delivery as the safest course for the mother. In addition, the parents were informed that labor and vaginal delivery could possibly further damage the exposed nervous system in the encephalocele and worsen the mental retardation. Such trauma could be avoided by cesarean section before the onset of labor. Although the parents initially desired termination and accepted vaginal delivery, they later changed their minds and requested elective cesarean section to give their child the best chance for survival. The baby was delivered by cesarean section with severe microcephaly, had the occipital encephalocele removed at the request of the parents, and is severely developmentally delayed at 30 months of age. This case illustrates how parents can bond to a fetus, despite an extremely poor prognosis.

Case 2

Because the head did not engage due to suspected cephalopelvic disproportion, the managing physician performed ultrasound and diagnosed case 2 in utero at 39 weeks gestation of a woman with no prior pregnancies. She and her husband were counseled that the infant would, without doubt, be mentally retarded because of the lack of brain tissue secondary to far-advanced in utero hydrocephalus. Delivery occurred by vagina after transvaginal cephalocentesis. The infant died after 18 days with an essentially absent brain and such an advanced degree of hydrocephalus as to be hydranencephalic. A high thoracolumbar meningomyelocele accompanied atrophied legs and fixed severe hip flexion contractures and equinovarus.

Case 3

The managing physician first used ultrasound to see case 3 at 21 weeks postconception because of sudden weight gain and suspected polyhydramnios in a mother of three children. At that time, the fetus had a head of normal proportion for gestational age with increased cerebral ventricle size and a lesion in the thoracolumbar spine diagnosed as an open neural tube defect (Fig. 4-1). At this time, the alpha-fetoprotein in the amniotic fluid (AFAFP) remained within the expected high-normal range. At that time, acetylcholinesterase was not available as a diagnostic

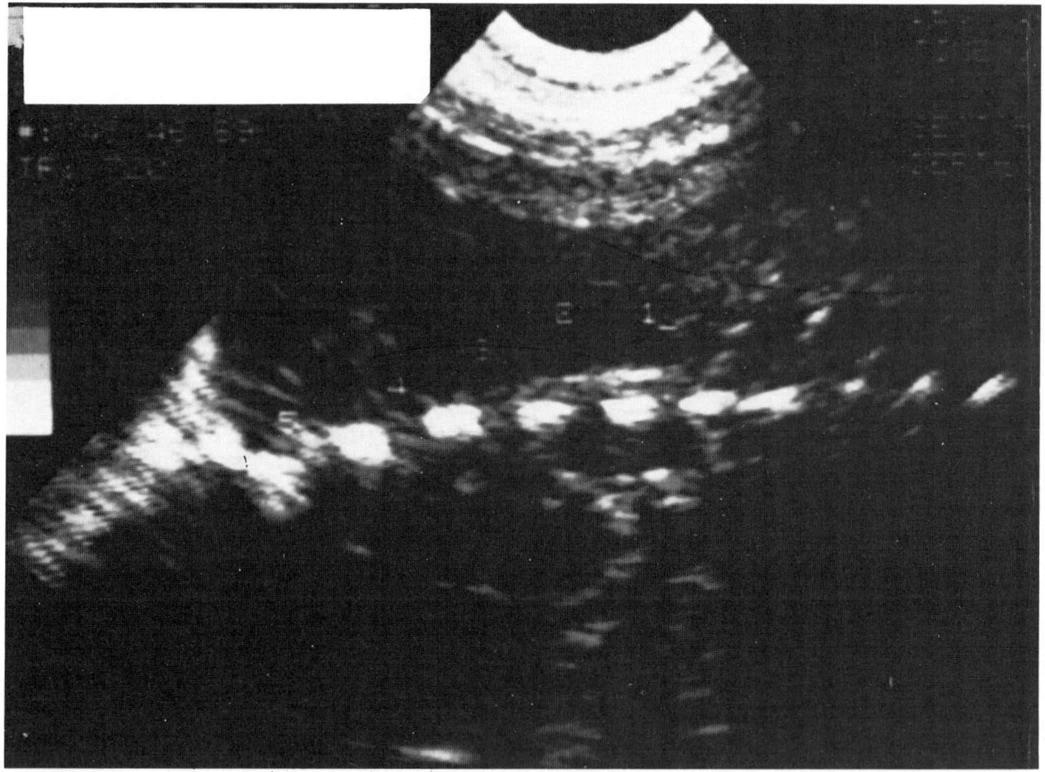

Figure 4-1. Case 3 with a head of normal proportion with increased cerebral ventricle size and a lesion in the thoracolumbar spine. Sagittal view of fetus at 21 weeks gestational age. Pelvis is to the left. The dark black area with numbers 1–5 represents the meningomyelocele sac posterior to lumbar vertebrae that show up as white. Cephalad to the sac the posterior vertebral arches can be seen.

test. Immediate counseling offered the family the options of termination or the birth of a severely disabled child but not the possibility of either in utero treatment or elective cesarean section. Despite the care with which the physician presented the two choices during the original counseling session, the family became distressed because abortion was mentioned as a possibility. Opposed to exposing the fetus to greater risk, they sought alternative medical management to continue the pregnancy with hope for the best possible pregnancy outcome. After learning that the ultrasound examination demonstrated both flexion and extension of the fetal hips and knees and also that the brain mass appeared to be adequate, we offered the following prognosis.

The degree of hydrocephalus was consistent with normal intellect; that is, we estimated 1 cm of frontal cortex by the time of delivery if the fetal brain continued to develop, and if progressive hydrocephalus did not develop. However, a malformation of the brain could cause the anatomically adequate mass of brain to malfunction, resulting in retardation.[741,819,1045,1053] With neuromotor lesions at or distal to the level of L_3, such as this child was thought to have, mental retardation is moderate to mild in 15 percent of cases; the remainder have normal intellectual capabilities.[1045]

With full extension and flexion of the hip and knee, the child would probably have a neural tube defect with neuromuscular function distal to the third lumbar vertebra (L_3) level. The child would have the ability to walk with braces and crutches unless further loss of neural function occurred. Greater loss of function could occur due to degeneration of the neural plaque exposed to amniotic fluid or as a result of surgery to close the back. The baby would most likely have paralysis of the urinary and anal sphincters.[1045]

We stressed that these prognoses were based on our experiences with a select population: children born throughout the Pacific Northwest with open neural tube defects of the spine and referred to our program in Seattle.[729] We also warned the parents that we were projecting from birth back into the first trimester and that we had no experience with meningomyelocele diagnosed early in utero; therefore, we could not predict whether the legs would become paralyzed or the brain distorted from hydrocephalus before we could initiate treatment.

Pregnancy management included the following options mentioned above: (1) serial follow-up by ultrasound with consideration of an intrauterine CSF shunt if the hydrocephalus progressed too rapidly, although it has been documented that very few children with open neural tube defects develop massive hydrocephalus[741,671]; (2) elective cesarean section prior to labor; (3) routine labor and delivery; (4) if labor fails to progress properly, ventricular puncture via cephalocentesis; or (5) labor, with a cesarean section if labor does not progress properly. If cesarean section prior to onset of labor was chosen, serial amniotic fluid examinations during the last trimester would allow the obstetrician to determine maturity of the fetal lungs by lethicine/sphyngomyelin (L/S) ratio before performing the cesarean section; this would be necessary to avoid infant lung disease due to prematurity. In addition, if elective cesarean were chosen, the section could possibly provide the following three benefits for the baby: (1) protection from potential trauma to an open neural tube defect from tight confinement in the uterus during the last stage of full-term pregnancy and from labor and passage through the vagina; (2) sterile delivery would preclude bacterial contamination of the open lesion during passage through the vaginal tract; and (3) neurosurgical repair of the infant's spine could be scheduled to immediately follow the cesarean birth, thereby lessening exposure to airborne bacteria. Options 3, 4, and 5, above, would run the risk of trauma from labor and potential infection arising through the punctured membranes and damage to the CNS from cephalocentesis or labor.

The family wished to give the child the maximum potential at birth—that is, follow-up by ultrasound and consideration for either intrauterine CSF shunt and/or delivery by cesarean section at the time of lung maturity.

The infant was born after 35 weeks gestation. A thin, intact epitheleal membrane covered an otherwise classic meningomyelocele lesion with protruding neural plaquė and nerves (Fig. 4-2). The CSF contained no cells. No paralysis was evident. Our surgeons immediately closed the infant's lesion without incident, and no infection occurred. Repeat ultrasound examination of the brain following delivery showed a stable ventricular cerebrospinal space.

Because of slowly progressive hydrocephalus at the age of one year, a CSF shunt was placed; it has been revised twice. By Bayley's infant developmental scale, the child's developmental quotient was normal at age 3 years. He has no evident motor paralysis in his legs and ambulates without a limp. This case illustrates that not all parents accept termination and that high thoracolumbar anatomic level lesions can have minimal or no paralysis.

Case 4

An ultrasound was performed because the mother of case 4 described a sudden decrease in fetal movements at 38 weeks gestation; she had no prior pregnancies. Case 4 was diagnosed in utero as having a lumbosacral sac and a minimally enlarged ventricular system of the brain, with a normal biparietal diameter of the fetal skull. We informed the mother the

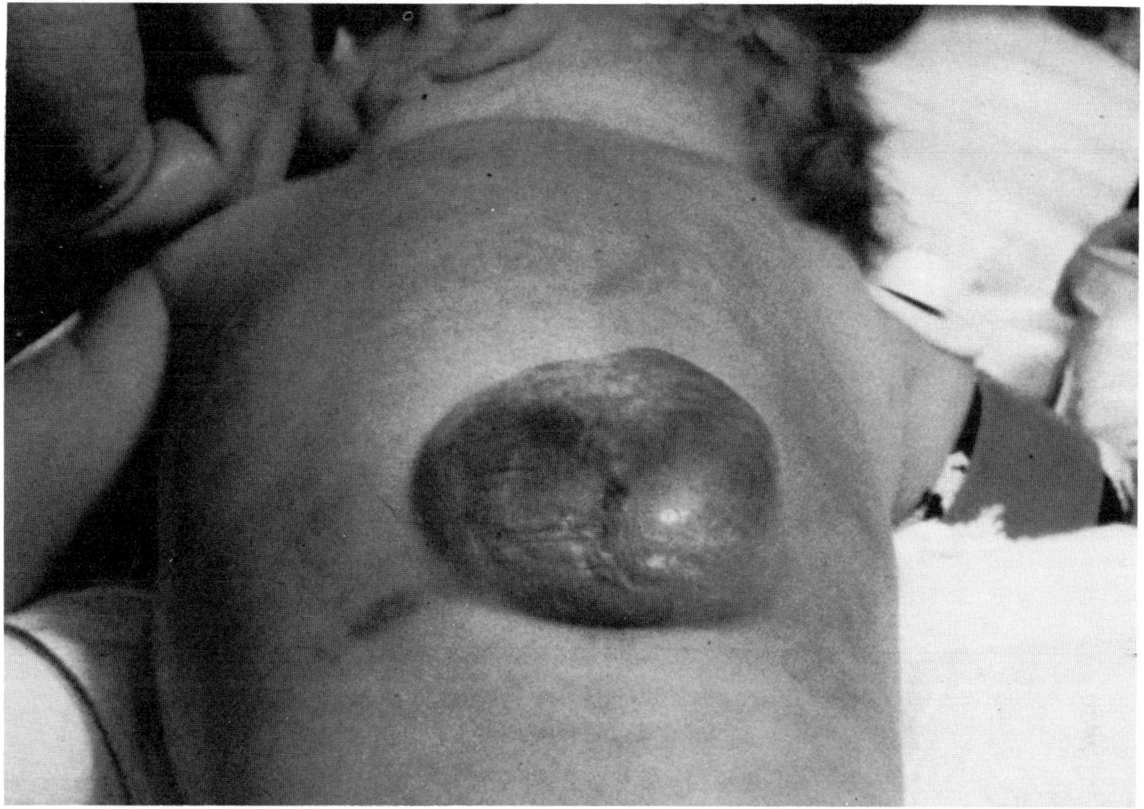

Figure 4-2. A thin, intact epitheleal membrane covering an otherwise classic meningomyelocele lesion in the same region of the back as suspected by in utero ultrasound and demonstrated in Figure 4-1. Except for the epithelial cover, this is a typical meningomyelocele with the neural plaque in the cephalad-dorsal portion of the sac wall (Fig. 3-2A). Spinal fluid was clear. No paralysis evident.

meningomyelocele sac had most likely ruptured and either pressure on the nerves or a myelitis from the vernix caseosa and amniotic fluid had caused the cessation of movement. We had no precedent upon which to offer advice as to possible recovery. We did mention Stark's theory[1104] theory of in utero confinement as an explanation for the loss of muscle function. We further explained that postnatal myelitis from trauma and infections can show recovery for 6 months post insult, despite a long-existing argument in the literature about whether infants born with open meningomyelocele lesions recover muscle function if operated on soon after birth (see Chapters 5 and 6). Despite the tentative theories, the parents opted for cesarean section to avoid further damage and to allow possible healing of the lesion. The surgeons repaired the back within 4 hours and described considerable arachnoiditis. The baby's legs appeared normal, with what appeared to be adequate muscle mass, but were never observed to move spontaneously. What was palpated as muscle mass at birth atrophied. The joints, mobile at birth except for the fixed flexion posture of infancy (see Chapter 15), gradually became contracted at the knees and ankles.

This case suggests Stark's theory[1104] that late intrauterine compression of a rapidly growing fetus can cause pressure on the neural plate and rupture the meningomyelocele sac, resulting in irreversible loss of neural function.

Case 5

The managing physician palpated a mass in addition to the fetus and subsequently diagnosed case 5 by ultrasound in a woman at 38 weeks gestation. She had had one uneventful prior pregnancy. Ultrasonography demonstrated a large thoracolumbrosacral mass filled with fluid and a small spinal defect (Fig. 4-3). After being presented with the same options as the parents of case 3, but without the alternative of abortion because of fetal age, the parents requested elective cesarean section. A nonparalyzed boy with a 32-cm head circumference and an intact 31-cm-circumference meningomyelocele containing fluid and nerves was delivered via an unusually large uterine incision (Fig. 4-4). There was one monocyte in the otherwise normal CSF. At 2 years of age, he has no need for a CSF shunt and has no evident paralysis. His development is normal, and he has walked without a limp since 19 months of age.

This case illustrates a lesion that would have had to rupture to allow delivery. The absence of paralysis has never before been observed by us in the presence of such a large lesion.

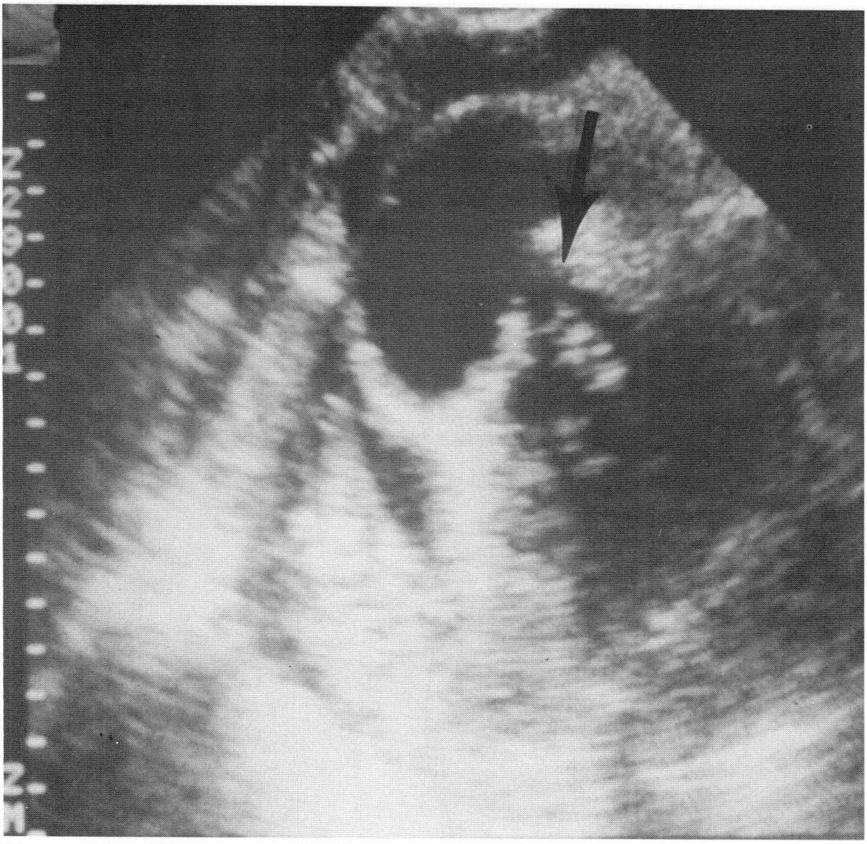

Figure 4-3. Ultrasonography demonstrating a large thoracolumbrosacral mass filled with fluid and an arrow pointing to a small spinal defect.

Case 6

Due to advanced maternal age, a 38-year-old Roman Catholic woman underwent amniocentesis at 16 weeks of her first gestation. An unconfirmed report of normal chromosome analysis and "an elevated alpha-fetoprotein" combined with a suspected "open spine" seen by ultrasound led her genetic counselor to describe the options of abortion or birth of a severely congenitally malformed child with meningomyelocele. When we saw her in our center 1 week later, she was informed that the alpha-fetoprotein level in the amniotic fluid was high but within normal limits and that there was no evidence for either a spinal defect or hydrocephalus by repeat ultrasonographic examination. She opted for abortion. The fetus was normal.

This case illustrates that some parents cannot consider even a very

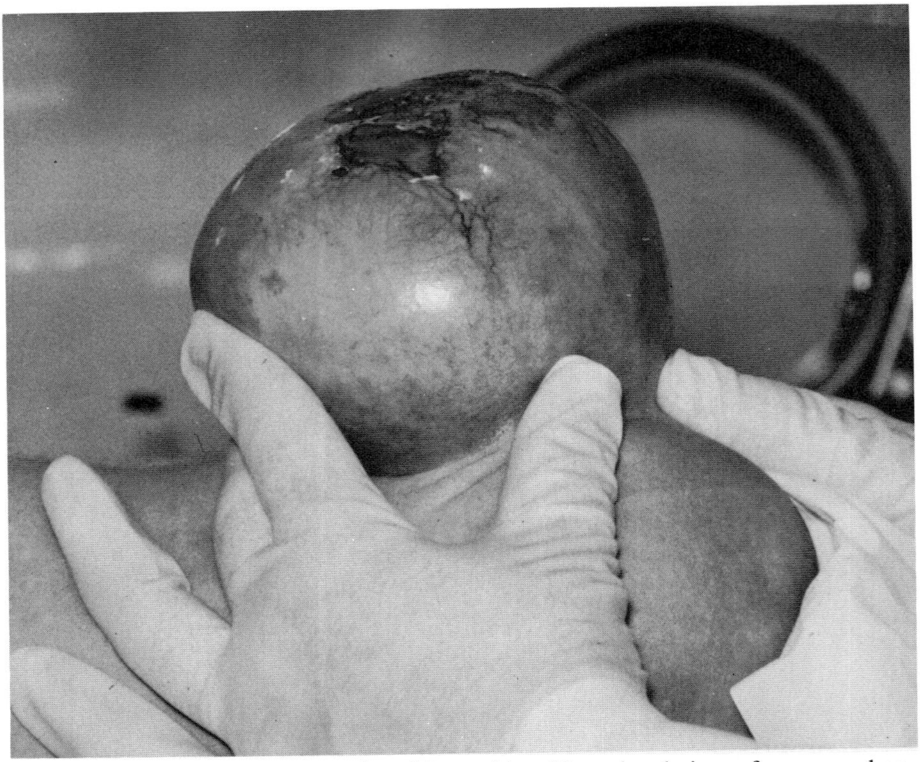

Figure 4-4. Case 5: A nonparalyzed boy with a 32-cm head circumference and an intact 31-cm-diameter meningomyelocele demonstrated in utero by ultrasonography in Figure 4-3. The zona vasculosa is evident with an incomplete epithelial covering. Nerves exited the spine defect, some attached to the dome of the sac, and most reentered the spinal canal (see Fig. 3-20, which is similar but with an incomplete epithelial covering).

small risk of having a deformed child and that religious or cultural background may not predetermine a personal response, as was discussed in Chapter 1.

Case 7

Case 7 presented in utero at 23 weeks gestation of a mother with two previous, normal pregnancies. The physician performed ultrasound for biparietal measurement to estimate fetal age and noted moderate hydrocephalus. This finding was not reported to the parents until 27 weeks gestation. The parents wished to terminate the pregnancy and were upset at the delay. Because we initially counseled them at 28 weeks of gestational age, we gave them the same pregnancy management options as for in utero hydrocephalus but ordered an amniotic fluid acetylcholinesterase determination. Detailed examination of the spine on four occasions between 28 and 32 weeks gestation revealed no lesions. Alpha-fetoprotein was normally high, as expected for gestational age, but acetylcholinesterase was elevated to diagnostic levels. Before learning the acetylcholinesterase level was elevated, we informed the family that 85 percent or more of congenitally hydrocephalic infants without meningomyelocele detected in utero were severely mentally retarded or die in the perinatal period.[186,206,402,744,1221] Finally, at 36 weeks gestational age a small L5-S3 meningomyelocele was detected. With evidence of a low lumbrosacral meningomyelocele, we reduced the risk for retardation to a minimal or moderate degree of only 15 percent.[741,1045] Subsequent delivery was by cesarean section. The infant had no evident motor paralysis in the legs but did retain urine postnatally, suggesting neurogenic incontinence will develop. Her neurological examination is normal, but she is too young to test for development. CSF remained culture negative despite growth of pseudomonas from the surface of the meningomyelocele sac. The infant developed a 4 × 6 cm superficial skin necrosis and slough that required split-thickness grafting. At 2 weeks of age, she had a shunt revision because of persistent subcutaneous collections of CSF around a first shunt system.

This case illustrates both the value of using acetylcholinesterase as a prenatal diagnostic test after alpha-fetoprotein has risen at 20 weeks of gestation and the difficulty of detecting small lumbrosacral meningomyelocele sacs. Also, parents must be warned of poor tissue response in the premature infant as well as the possibility for intrauterine infections.

Case 8

Because the mother of case 8 described decreased fetal movements at 32 weeks gestational age in her first pregnancy, the managing physician performed ultrasound and interpreted it as demonstrating cebocephaly with massive hydrocephalus and a single ventricle, paralyzed legs, large thoracolumbosacral meningomyelocele, omphalocele, and partial absence of the right abdominal wall and chest. We advised the family of a hopeless prognosis with death in early infancy. If the fetus survived to term, we recommended cephalocentesis to correct cephalopelvic disproportion and a low vaginal delivery. The mother presented 2 weeks later in labor and delivered a stillborn infant with atrophy of the legs, far-advanced hydrocephalus, and a massive meningomyelocele but no body wall defects.

This case is one of two infants with meningomyelocele in this series who died in utero prior to a planned delivery. These cases, along with the fetus we subjected to cephalocentesis, suggest that multiply malformed and hydranencephalic, nonviable infants can be recognized in utero. They will affect the prevalence-at-birth data reported from referral centers treating infants with meningomyelocele detected after birth and alter series' outcomes, as discussed in Chapters 3–7.

Case Reports: Summary

These eight cases range in severity from a fetus with microcephaly and encephalocele, and another fetus with large meningomyelocele with multiple anomalies and a prognosis of severe impairment, to a very good prognosis for a fetus with hydrocephalus and a small, lumbosacral meningomyelocele, and even a normal fetus. All but two of the eight pairs of parents, when informed of the potential for improving their babies' impairments, eventually chose elective cesarean section. One mother was so frightened by initial genetic counseling and the remote possibility of a congenitally malformed child she requested termination. Another mother delivered a stillborn infant. The initial shock and fear was resolved by two sets of parents who initially requested termination but later opted for elective cesarean section despite a poor prognosis. Two of the four with very limited prognoses opted for delivery via cesarean section; one has fulfilled that prognosis, and the other is as able as his normal siblings. The third died after vaginal delivery and transvaginal cephalocentesis, and the fourth was stillborn.

TOTAL SEATTLE EXPERIENCE

To date we have counseled 19 pairs of parents with fetuses with neural tube defects diagnosed in utero (Table 4-2). Three of the six (50 percent) diagnosed at 23 weeks gestational age or younger chose termination. One mother given a prognosis of stillbirth or neonatal death for a fetus with ienencephaly carried to term; the others had meningomyelocele and hydrocephalus and a more hopeful prognosis.

Five of the remaining 13 diagnosed after 24 weeks gestational age demonstrated severe paralysis (two), multiple anomalies (one), and advanced hydrocephalus (two). Three sets of parents chose cephalocentesis and vaginal delivery for fetuses with far-advanced hydrocephalus (less than 1 cm of frontal cerebral mantle) in a full-term infant with meningomyelocele,[1053] another with advanced hydrocephalus only, and a third with multiple anomalies. The last two delivered spontaneously as premature stillbirths. The two infants diagnosed in the third trimester with

Table 4-2
Prognosis, Method of Delivery, and Outcome

Gestational Age at Time of Diagnosis	Prognosis: Poor	Prognosis: Guarded[a]	Prognosis: Terminate	Method of Delivery: Stillborn	Method of Delivery: Cephalocentesis	Method of Delivery: Cesarean Section	Outcome
24 Weeks		3	3	—	—	—	Death
		2	—	—	—	2	One normal DQ[b]; no paralysis (case 3); 1 neonate
	1			One immediate death			
24 Weeks	5			2	1	—	Three deaths
						2	One death; 1 normal DQ in wheelchair
	—	8	—	—	—	8	No loss, 4[c]; low lumbar, 2; sacral, 2; 6 normal DQ; 2 too young
At delivery of elective cesarean	—	—	—	—	—	Total: 10[d]; breech, 3; routine repeat, 2; both, 1; twins, 2; maternal ITP,[e] 1; fetal distress, 1	Low-lumbar, 3; lumbo-sacral, 2; sacral, 4; all normal DQ
Total	6	13	3	3	1	22	29

[a] See text, case 3; legs move in utero, stable hydrocephalus.
[b] Developmental quotient.
[c] Motor level at last examination; age 6 months to 4 years of age.
[d] Indications for cesarean section.
[e] Mother noted to have idiopathic thrombocytopenic purpura; cesarean section was timed to coincide with platelet transfusion.

severe paralysis were delivered by cesarean section; one has since died despite treatment, and the other, at age 4 years, is intellectually normal and wheelchair mobile with totally paralyzed legs.

An additional eight patients with meningomyelocele diagnosed in utero in the latter part of pregnancy but before onset of labor, as well as the two diagnosed before 24 weeks gestational age, were delivered by cesarean section. Seven have low-lumbar or sacral-level paralysis or no paralysis; all of these patients should develop biped ambulation (Table 4-2).

In all, parents of 12 of 18 patients diagnosed in utero chose elective cesarean section; three chose early abortion of their fetuses; one selected cephalocentesis; and two gave birth to stillborn infants prior to anticipated delivery by cephalocentesis.

Because this group represents too small a series to analyze, we added ten cases of elective cesarean section with minimal (four cases) or no (six) labor from our general population of newborn referrals from 1979 onward (the same time interval that we cared for the infants with intrauterine diagnoses; Table 4-2). None of these mothers described a decrease in fetal movements as did the mother reported in case 4 above, suggesting that confinement without labor is not a frequent cause of paralysis. Three (one before death) of the 22 patients born after elective cesarean section had high-level lesions (17 percent), and 20 had low-lumbar or sacral-level lesions or motor loss (83 percent; Table 4-3). Of the patients born during the same time period but after labor and either cesarean section or vaginal delivery, 18 (62 percent) patients had high-lumbar or thoracic-level lesions, and 11 (38 percent) had low-lumbar or sacral-level lesions or no motor loss (Fisher's exact, $p = .009$; Table 4-3). These data suggest that cesarean section before the onset of labor may reduce the extent of paralysis, as suggested by Stark and Drummond,[1107] Ralis,[889-890] and Chervenak and associates.[188]

In addition, most of these infants born by early cesarean section had few or no white blood cells in the CSF aspirated from their intact meningocele sacs, suggesting the absence of inflammatory processes. Our surgeons have described a lack of arachnoiditis in all but one of their patients born by elective cesarean section; that child's mother noted a decrease in fetal movement prior to delivery, thought to be due to sac rupture (case 4). The lack of arachnoiditis has made back repair easier. Late gestational confinement with rupture of the meningomyelocele sac may cause a sterile meningitis and trauma to the exposed neural plaque and nerves; this situation accounts for late gestational loss of fetal movement and permanent paralysis in some children born with meningomyelocele.

The child with arachnoiditis and high-level paralysis demonstrated

Table 4-3
Lesion Level, Method of Delivery, and Motor Loss for Meningomyelocele Lesions Diagnosed in Utero and Carried to Term

Lesion Level	Labor and Cesaraen Section or Delivery		Cesaraen Section Without Labor		
	Percentage	Number of Patients	Percentage	Number of Patients	
T12	16.87	14	10	3	
L1-2	4.82	4	0	0	
L3	18.07	15	5	1	
L4-5	46.99	39	35	7	
Sacral	13.25	11	30	7	
No motor loss	0	0	20	4	
Total[a]		83		22	
Fisher's Exact Comparisons					Fisher's Exact Comparisons
T12,L1-2	62	18	17	2	$p = 0.009$
Sacral, no loss	38	11	83	10	
T12, L1-2, L3	40	33	15	3	$p = 0.029$
L4-5, Sacral no loss	60	50	85	17	
T12, L1-2, L3, L4-5	87	72	50	10	$p = 0.0008$
Sacral, no loss	13	11	50	10	
T12, L1-2	22	18	10	2	$p = 0.1950$
L3, L4-5, Sacral no loss	78	65	90	18	

[a] X^2, 14.02; degrees of freedom, 2; $p < 0.01$.

very limited mental development and died in the second year of life. Two others born after elective cesarean section were discharged home and developed severe bulbar palsies secondary to the Arnold-Chiari malformation. One of these two also developed progressive loss of neural function in the lower extremities, but contrast study revealed no evidence for scarring, tethering, or an intraluminal mass. Both are now stable following tracheostomy, gastrostomy, and tracheal separation from the larynx. Although both are improving and can now swallow more effectively, time will determine whether they will completely outgrow their bulbar palsies and associated velopharyngeal and pharyngolaryngeal incompetencies. We could not distinguish prenatally any more than we could at birth the three who developed postnatal neurologic sequelae from those who did not.

Other infants have loss of function due to early abnormal embryogenesis, leading to atrophy of the paralyzed muscles and fixed joint contractures, such as equinovarus, by the time of delivery. Infants with these deformed, nonmobile joints have been accurately differentiated from those with functioning muscles and mobile joints of the lower extremities.

WHY PREGNANCY MANAGEMENT OPTIONS SHOULD BE OFFERED

We believe many parents will choose management of pregnancy that may offer improved outcome rather than abortion, particularly when the diagnosis is made after 24 weeks gestational age. Even theoretical advantages have led most parents (9/12; 75 percent) in the absence of a definitely poor prognosis to choose cesarean section rather than abortion, cephalocentesis, or possible further nerve damage from confinement, labor, and vaginal delivery. Even a significant number of parents (2/5; 40 percent) of fetuses with very poor prognoses diagnosed after 24 weeks gestation chose cesarean section. Only two of five also chose improved pregnancy outcome with diagnosis of uncomplicated meningomyelocele before 24 weeks gestational age. Only three of six with serious defects diagnosed in this early period chose termination.

In addition, a recent survey of parents of congenitally malformed children in our clinic and of young adults born with meningomyelocele indicate most would not accept abortion (Table 4-4). These data are suspect since they represent opinions of people not actually pregnant with congenitally malformed fetuses. When appropriate, physician counselors should discuss with parents the full range of pregnancy management options, from termination to intrauterine treatment and elective cesarean

Table 4-4
Seattle Survey Results: Acceptance of Abortion

Parents of Children with Meningomyelocele
1. Would choose abortion, 23%
   Would not abort an affected fetus, 56%
   Undecided, 21%
2. Would use prenatal diagnosis
   - With abortion as only alternative, 5%
   - With abortion and improved pregnancy outcome as alternatives, 57%
   - Would not use prenatal diagnosis, 23%
   - Undecided, 15%
3. Reasons against abortion
   - Personal, 64%
   - Religious, 23%
   - Both, 13%
4. Knew of increased recurrence risk
   - Yes, 85%
   - No, 15%
5. Knew of possible preventive value of folic acid
   - Yes, 10%
   - No, 90%
   - Wished more information, 46%

Young Adults with Meningomyelocele
1. Would choose to abort a fetus with meningomyelocele, 10%
   Would not choose to abort, 90%
2. Would use prenatal diagnosis, 90%
   Undecided, 10%
3. Knew of increased recurrence risk, 100%

section, for four reasons, listed and explained below: (1) prenatal screening programs will be more accepted by the general public; (2) parents' beliefs and subsequent treatment requests vary; (3) the expression of open neural tube defects is variable; and (4) prenatal diagnosis with improved pregnancy outcome is a cost-effective adjunct to screening programs.

Public Acceptance of Prenatal Screening Programs

Cultural and religious beliefs influence some parents to reject prenatal diagnostic programs that offer pregnancy termination as the only alternative to delivering a congenitally malformed child (see Chapter 1). Offering alternative methods of pregnancy management as opposed to termination alone invalidates arguments that human life advocates use to describe prenatal diagnosis and elective abortion as synonymous. The wider the pregnancy management options, the greater the number of people who can be effectively served.

Parental Beliefs

Depending on their personal beliefs, parents accept or reject prenatal screening accompanied by termination. One pair of parents, described earlier, could not accept termination because of their cultural and ethical values. Another accepted termination despite an avowed religious belief.

Parents may also reject prenatal screening based on the "treatment" alternatives available, as mentioned in Chapter 1. Current reports show only 6–38 percent of parents participate in prenatal screening programs when termination is the only alternative to delivery of a congenitally malformed child.[15,64,504,653,1089] These programs offered amniocentesis screening for chromosomal defects in pregnancies of women over the age of 35 years. The authors suggest that low-use percentages were due to lack of knowledge and do not mention antiabortion attitudes as a deterrent to participation in their programs. We believe that some members of general society, particularly antiabortion cultural and religious groups, are likely to reject both prenatal diagnosis and its associated single option, termination, on moral and ethical grounds (see Chapter 1). In our racially and culturally heterogeneous nation, caution should be exercised in initiating maternal serum alpha-fetoprotein screening (MSAFS) to detect open neural tube defects when termination is the only alternative to delivery of a congenitally malformed child.[28,29]

However, prenatal screening can be separated from an implied consequence of abortion (see also Chapter 1); it can lead to options for improving pregnancy outcome, discussed throughout this chapter. We believe even families with antiabortion ethics would use prenatal screening if they were informed of the possible alternatives to improve pregnancy outcome as well as abortion of the fetus.

Variability of Expression of Open Neural Tube Defects

Open neural tube defects can be identified in utero by chemical tests,[48,129,228,761] described above. As we mentioned, these tests, unfortunately, cannot distinguish the bad-prognosis cases, including hydranencephaly, encephalocele, microcephaly, anencephaly, and high-level thoracolumbar lesions, from those neural tube defects with relatively better prognoses, such as meningomyelocele with minimal degrees of, or no, paralysis. Ultrasound can distinguish anencephaly from microcephaly with encephalocele and from hydranencephaly or meningomyelocele.[157,934] It would appear from our series that the ultrasound findings of hydrocephalus with meningomyelocele in midtrimester can be associated with a higher proportion of better prognosis cases (13/18 cases; 71 percent; Table 4-2) than suggested by others who have carried out termination or cephalocentesis in most of their cases.[402] Delivery by cephalocentesis contributes to the poor prognosis. Others recommending elective cesarean section have not indicated the quality of the infants' lives.[187,1221]

Extrapolating data from meningomyelocele children who have been treated and transferred to regional centers after birth to make predictions for the meningomyelocele fetus detected by in utero diagnosis may be misleading. We currently cannot be sure what percentage of early fetuses with meningomyelocele and aequate leg movement and mild hydrocephalus will (1) be prematurely stillborn, (2) lose muscle function, (3) develop severe hydrocephalus before lung maturity allows safe delivery by cesarean section, or (4) develop more severe degrees of mental retardation or bulbar palsy. The two of 22 cases (9 percent) with severe bulbar palsy approximates in frequency the rate among our cases of meningomyelocele seen over the past 27 years (approximately 5 percent).[563] Moreover, our preliminary data reported herein are limited, and therefore, additional descriptions of the natural history of prenatally diagnosed meningomyelocele are needed.

Complications associated with open neural tube defects may be further reduced by improved postnatal care, as discussed in Chapters 5–7. Prenatal diagnosis and delivery by cesarean section may contribute to even more reduction in the degree of mental retardation and paralysis, as suggested by McCullough and Balzier-Martin[716] as well as others.[187,203,1221]

Cost-Effectiveness

Discussions about screening programs using intrauterine diagnosis and abortion as the only alternative to delivery of an impaired infant emphasize cost-effectiveness.[444,623,960] Costs for the care of the congenitally malformed child have been compared with the cost of screening, confirmation of diagnosis, and abortion of affected fetuses. However, these theoretical models do not take into consideration the degree of compliance with prenatal screening programs offering abortion as the only alternative.[64,504,653,1089] Nor do they consider the cost-effectiveness of more modern medical care, delivery techniques, and education that will enhance the ultimate outcome by reducing acquired morbidity and its associated handicaps. We have demonstrated the lower cost of care of the early surgically treated child compared with the more severely paralyzed and retarded patient with a neglected open neural tube defect.[1062] Furthermore, we have documented the lower cost of care for the minimally impaired compared with the more severely paralyzed.[1058] As indicated by our series and case reports in this chapter, further potential cost savings can be realized by using cesarean section to reduce the percentage of wheelchair-dependent patients with open neural tube defects from 41 percent to 10 percent. Money would also be saved by the shorter hospitalizations of 9–27 (average, 16) days for infants postcesarean section compared with 13–49 (average, 22.5) days for our other meningomyelocele patients seen during the same time period; these shorter initial hospitalizations significantly reduce the cost from an average of $11,088 to $7,979 (a 29 percent reduction). These low-level lesion patients not only cost society less to care for, but a higher proportion will become contributing adults.

From a purely utilitarian viewpoint, a prenatal diagnosis program that offers both abortion and options for improved pregnancy outcome with in utero treatment and elective cesarean section delivery prior to the onset of labor is the most economical of the following three possible programs: (1) termination, (2) both termination and improved pregnancy outcome options, and (3) no screening at all. Because some parents cannot accept abortion (Table 4-4), a prenatal diagnosis program offering termination as the only other option to the birth of a congenitally malformed child will be underused, and therefore, some pregnancies with meningomyelocele will go undetected and be delivered after labor. These affected pregnancies will result in a higher proportion of more severely paralyzed children. The third option, not to use prenatal diagnosis at all, is obviously the most expensive social option.

By adding elective cesarean section to options available to those in society participating in screening programs, we can expect less severely paralyzed infants among those who are detected either too late for legal abortion or whose parents cannot, for whatever reasons, accept abortion. Because increased numbers of people will participate without organized opposition from prolife groups, we can also expect fewer affected children to be born. The extension of utilitarianism to include improved pregnancy outcome as an alternative is coincident with the "preservationist" concepts of those who believe in the ultimate value of life. Such a spectrum of options, from abortion to reduction in the degree of impairment, is more consistent with a true choice for parents than is the choice between natural birth with its attendant causes for increased impairment or abortion.

SUMMARY

We propose that prenatal diagnostic and screening programs for open neural tube defects take into consideration the heterogenity[499,582,1045] and variability of open neural tube defects[1045] as well as clarify intrauterine diagnosis by careful ultrasound[157] and chemical examinations.[48,129,229,387,444,623,761] The range of possible impairments and management options (including termination, cephalocentesis, intrauterine treatment, and cesarean section delivery without labor) should be provided to the parents. Such counseling will allow adherents to an antiabortion ethic to use chemical and ultrasound screening to provide for improved pregnancy outcome and, at the same time, will allow freedom of self-determination for those accepting abortion when a fetus is diagnosed as severely congenitally malformed.

David Shurtleff

5

Selection Process for the Care of Congenitally Malformed Infants

In a book about the care of congenitally malformed individuals, a chapter should be devoted to a discussion of selection of the best method or methods of treatment. Medical technology, considered in this type of a discussion, must be applied within the context of those cultural and social influences presented in Chapters 1 and 2. Criteria for selection of treatment should be based on past experiences and should be appropriately altered according to new technology as it is integrated with current cultural and social influences.[57] The main goal of this chapter is to describe our recommended process for selection of treatment for individuals with congenital malformation, a process in constant need of modifications.

THE HISTORY OF MYELODYSPLASIA

To describe such a process of selection, we will begin by reviewing suggestions from the past. Although congenital malformations have been described as existing for thousands of years, as noted in Chapter 1, the process of understanding medical care for individuals with severe types of caudal and neural tube defects did not begin until 1632, when Nicholas Tulpius first described a meningomyelocele lesion; he called it spina bifida operta. In 1691, Ruysch[957] first made the distinction between two forms of

MYELODYSPLASIAS AND EXSTROPHIES: SIGNIFICANCE, PREVENTION, AND TREATMENT
 ISBN 0-8089-1816-8

this congenital malformation: paralytic meningomyelocele and nonparalytic meningocele. Morgagni[776] first linked the meningomyelocele sac with hydrocephalus in 1769. In 1806, Ferris related the paralysis of the legs to the sac, warned against ligature from the meningocele without paralysis, and distinguished paralysis of the meningomyelocele type of lesion.[332] Despite the early description of nerves in the sac and a warning against ligature by Tulpuris and later confirmations, 196 years later Trowbridge[1169] recommended ligation although his patients died. In addition, in 1883, Newbigging advocated puncture or ligation of the sac although almost all of his patients also died—but due to poor nursing care, according to the writer.[1105] In 1858, Jackson[532] first lamented and clearly delineated the complications of surgical treatment for meningomyelocele. Morton[778] recommended iodide sclerosing solution, a practice reported by a commission in 1885 as being more hazardous than leaving the patient alone or providing minimal closure surgery.[694]

Until Lister applied Pasteur's basic observation—that bacteria cause infectious disease—to surgery, selection of treatment for infants with various forms of myelodysplasia appeared to be no problem since operations caused putrefaction and demise.[654] Lister showed how aseptic precautions improved surgical results by decreasing the most dreaded complication, infection, at that time a hazard for both patient and surgeon.

In 1892, Bayer[71] recorded the first well-described surgical experience with major malformations. He recommended aggressive treatment for all infants with meningomyelocele; this suggestion coincided with the more humanistic movement of the 19th century mentioned in Chapter 1 and was later recommended by Sharrard and associates[1022] in 1963. Bayer initially described good results of surgical repair of 14 unselected patients with "spina bifida operta," only to write 5 years[72] later of his "sad experiences." A 59 percent mortality rate developed sooner or later, despite his meticulous procedure. He described three contraindications for operating on patients with spina bifida operta: (1) hydrocephalus of a "decided" degree, (2) paralysis, and (3) complications in the sac. These are, to the author's knowledge, the first published selection criteria. However, it is more appropriate to consider them contraindications to surgery since Bayer attempted to protect patients from surgery that would do more harm than good. It took Bayer 5 years and a few dozen cases to modify his aggressive approach,[72] a change that took Lorber 8 years and 270 cases some 80 years later.[666] In their 1963 and 1971 papers, the Sheffield group, Sharrard and associates,[1022] and Lorber[666] did not review the literature.

Shortly after Bayer, in 1905, Moore[772] reviewed the literature and suggested that one not operate at a "tender age" and that operation would not cure paralysis nor be effective in the presence of a large growing sac or overt hydrocephalus. He suggested that one should operate only after the age of 5 years and only to remove an unsightly tumor. One of his seven patients died immediately postoperatively, but 86 percent had skin-covered meningoceles and did not die. During this period, he described death as predominantly due to two causes: (1) infection and (2) hydrocephalus. Both of these causes remain concerns for modern authors discussing selection of treatment for newborns with meningomyelocele.[180,729,741]

Despite the possibility of fatal infection common in 1918, Frazier[366] suggested the surgeon wait until 1 year of age to operate in order to allow the sac to epithelialize and the strong to declare themselves. He was in agreement with most writers of his era.[594]

In 1932, Penfield and Cone[856] described their own studies of cerebrospinal fluid (CSF) absorption by the arachnoid-dural sac. These studies were based on fundamental studies of CSF production and absorption by Dandy.[241b] Penfield and Cone[856] demonstrated that similar absorption took place in the membranes of the meningomyelocele sac. They suggested that exacerbation of an existing hydrocephalus or onset of progressive hydrocephalus follows excision of this absorptive surface. Since that time, both confirmatory and contradictory reports have suggested, respectively, that hydrocephalus is and is not related to sac excision that removes absorptive surface and stops leakage of CSF.[a]

By 1933, Kolodny[594] urged "early" closure to avoid infection and stated that sac excision did not worsen or precipitate hydrocephalus in most of his patients. He operated on 60 patients, 32 (54 percent) before 1 month of age and four (7 percent) after age 1 year. He carefully dissected the filum terminale and nerves free from the dura to prevent further neurologic loss and added improvement of neurologic function as well as the prevention of infection to the list of indications; Sharrard and associates[1022] confirmed these two observations 30 years later, as did McLone and associates[741] 50 years later. Others agreed,[282,357,701,1076,1105] but still others demonstrated neither improvement in function with early closure nor loss of function with delayed closure.[118,132,180,433,1080] Some of these authors reported no difference in infection rates with early versus delayed closure.[180,1080]

Kolodny[594] reported an immediate mortality of 5 percent, but this figure increased an additional 19 percent with follow-up immediately after discharge from the hospital. Forty-four (59 percent) of the group of 79 operated and nonoperated patients had meningoceles. Three years later,

[a] See references 282, 357, 433, 479, 524, 525, 594, 621, 666, 671, 700, 741, 1020, 1071, 1077, and 1105.

in 1936, Siris[1071] reported an immediate 32 percent mortality among 37 operated patients. He operated on only 45 percent of a total of 84 referred to his service, 23 (62 percent) during the first month of life and five (14 percent) over 1 year of age. He recommended treating infected sacs with an open cradle and heat lamp. Some cases developed huge cystic sacs with progressive hydrocephalus. On several occasions the sac would rupture, and subsequently the hydrocephalus would temporarily arrest before the sac refilled. After several such episodes, the process would abate, and he recommended operation at that time.

Siris agreed with Kolodny about two operative results: (1) it was harmful to operate on infected cases, and (2) surgery would not help those with severe paralysis or other deformities. Most authors since that time have recorded severe and life-threatening deformities of the brain or other organs and presence of infection as contraindications to surgery.[b] Like Kolodny,[594] Siris[1071] noted that most of his unoperated children died of ascending ventriculomeningitis, the same cause for death of seven (54 percent) of the 13 who died following surgery. Siris noted that his 35 percent mortality rate (13/37) was not as good as Kolodny's 5 percent, but failed to note Kolodny's 19 percent who died shortly after hospital discharge (24 percent total mortality, an insignificant difference: (χ^2 = 1.38, degrees of freedom = 1). In addition, Kolodny reported 44 of 79 (56 percent) cases as meningoceles, while Siris reported 20 of 84 (24 percent), a significantly larger proportion of mildly involved cases than in Kolodny's series ($\chi^2 = 17.2$, df = 1, $p < 0.01$). We mention these differences and similarities in these two early studies to emphasize the need for careful evaluation of the types of cases in each series subjected to various treatments. Outcomes of series will depend to some extent on the severity of involvement of cases referred. Outcomes today are compared among series with little detail as to the types of cases being evaluated. McLone and associates[741] in Chicago recently compared their outcomes with those of Lorber and Salfield[671] in Sheffield. The Chicago group had 35 percent high-level lesions and the Sheffield group had 70 percent ($\chi^2 = 26$; df = 1, $p < .001$). Was the Sheffield group much more severely involved at the time of referral? If the authors had recorded the condition of their cases by comparable definitions at the time patients entered their studies, we could better appraise the difference in approach.

Despite the introduction of antimicrobial agents and a general decline in infant mortality during the early 20th century,[380] few changes were recommended for selecting treatment modalities for infants born with meningomyelocele. By 1943, Ingraham and Swan[525] still recommended

---

[b] See references 132, 180, 282, 357, 666, 671, 1021, 1058, 1077, 1105, and 1115.

surgery at 12–18 months unless there was a thin, uninfected sac that threatened to rupture. Another 20 years later, Doran and Guthkelch[282] still recommended delay of surgery for 3–18 months, despite observing both that infection was likely to cause death and that neural function was lost in the first 24 hours of life. They warned against operating on grossly hydrocephalic and severely paralyzed infants or those with other fatal anomalies. Doran and Guthkelch added "encephalocranial disproportion" as a contraindication to surgery. As described, this entity is probably the clinical manifestation of a brain malformation detailed by Cleland[202] and now known as the Arnold-Chiari type II malformation[131] that remains a highly fatal complication of meningomyelocele.[563,741] Doran and Guthkelch[282] stated that early closure prevented meningitis and reported a 30 percent mortality, strikingly similar to the earlier mortality rates of Kolodny[594] and Siris.[1071] Doran and Guthkelch[282] also reported that 13 percent of their severely physically malformed survivors were confined to wheelchairs, but experienced "survival not without enjoyment." They also suggested that medical, social, and family resources available for the care of the congenitally malformed child should be taken into account when considering surgery; this general recommendation is still applicable in some areas today.[357,380,428,729,927,1058] Later that same decade, Matson[700] listed similar indications and contraindications to surgical treatment in an editorial written in response to a number of inquiries concerning the increased survival of infants born with nonepithelialized myelochisis and meningomyelocele. He thought antimicrobials and improved neonatal care allowed all impaired neonates to live in larger proportions and, thus, caused the increase in referral to regional treatment centers of infants born with open neural tube defects of the spine.

Doran and Guthkelch[282] also mentioned that eight of 107 (7 percent) infants not operated on survived to $2\frac{1}{2}$ years of age. This selected group's survival is remarkably similar to both the natural survival of that era described by Laurence[612] and the 12 percent rate of survival of an initially "untreated" group recently reported by Gross and associates.[428]

From the reports of Bayer[71,72] until the editorial by Matson,[700] authors have described their indications for surgical treatment and their contraindications. These recommendations were derived solely for the benefit of their child patients. The mid-20th century witnessed the evolution of two different types of medical care criteria for infants born with meningomyelocele. One approach, treatment for the benefit of the infant, was similar to the approaches developed in the 19th and early 20th century. The other, new approach, fundamentally quite different, was publicized by Lorber[666] and is discussed below.

SELECTION VERSUS NONSELECTION

Lorber[666] listed the same contraindications to surgery that have been discussed in the first part of this chapter: (1) severe or "decided" hydrocephalus, (2) severe paralysis, and (3) other congenital deformities. He added kyphosis and level of lesion and defined the degree of hydrocephalus to include moderate degrees, although he also reported much more severe hydrocephalus as compatible with normal intellect[670] (see Chapter 7). The difference in his approach is the utilitarian assumption that these infants are of negative value and, therefore, society and families are better off not treating them. In fact, he uses the high death rate as justification for use of his criteria for selection for nontreatment, but he still claims to recommend the criteria for humanitarian reasons.[665] Unlike Doran and Guthkelch,[282] Lorber and Salfield[671] describe the more severe forms of meningomyelocele as causing nothing but suffering and life "without enjoyment." They primarily justify not operating on or providing any medical treatment for these children by claiming they are a burden to their families and society.[671] Lorber and Salfield[671] have been joined by others who recommend not only withholding surgery and antibiotics, but also keeping the infants away from parents to assure death for those selected into the nontreatment group.[210,428,433,486,1106] These authors recommend hospitalization or care in a nursing home to assure compliance with the nontreatment protocol, claiming discharge home may cause the family to bond with the infant and subsequently insist on treatment.

Discharge into foster and nursing homes after the use of criteria similar to Lorber's but without adherence to a complete nontreatment protocol led to the use of antibiotics, good nutrition, and a 70 percent survival rate reported in one study.[325] This study apparently confirms Matson's opinion[700] in the previous decade; general improvement in care, not surgery, can account for the improved survival of infants born with major congenital defects. Perhaps the positive effects of mothering and parental advocacy led Guiney and MacCarthy[433] to recommend keeping an untreated baby in the hospital until the infant dies because "fundamental to its [selection policy] implementation is the belief that infants selected for nonoperative management will die in infancy." They claim that "measures to facilitate death of those not actively treated" are not a necessary sequel. However, when the infant thrived, they did perform surgery before discharge home and transferred 33 of 132 (25 percent initially nonoperated patients to the treatment group,[433] a practice in agreement with our recommendations.[729,1058] These data describe failure of a selection process in the hands of "compassionate" physicians. Guiney and MacCarthy[433] and McLaughlin and associates[729] did not insist on death for their patients "selected" for nonoperative management. Lorber, during discussion of a paper given in 1974, suggested that phenobarbital should be provided to quiet hungry infants to accelerate the dying process, a comment not included in recordings of the proceedings but noted in the press.[248b]

To recommend no surgical procedures and then provide inadequate nutrition and no other forms of treatment as well as to confine the patient to a hospital or nursing home for protection against parental bonding and advocacy is nothing more than prescribing a program that assures the prognosis; this approach equals euthanasia.[73,349,557,897,937,1045] Such behavior suggests that the method of management is more a determinant to survival than any inherent aspect of the selection criteria. Indeed, authors who prescribe this type of program have succumbed to what Veatch[1184] has described as the "technical criteria fallacy," which illustrates how bias can affect outcome of treatment and prevalence, as discussed in Chapter 1. Physicians who prescribe programs sure of producing death have become so infatuated with their technical abilities to accumulate data and tally scores that they misunderstand the nature of the difficult decisions they are making.[1184] As useful as these criteria for a poor prognosis may be in looking at populations and advising parents, they still lack sufficient accuracy in the individual case. In a given case, we are incapable of predicting with sufficient accuracy either the ultimate outcome of a "good candidate" or the quality of survival of a "severely affected" infant and should offer parents the full range of possibilities with and without treatment[c].

For the many reasons reviewed above and in Chapter 1, we believe that the utilitarian ethic, an emphasis on benefits for the family and society at the child's expense, is not acceptable. Neglected infants, deprived of succor, will die. Studies that support selection for nontreatment by reporting the high mortality rate for those not treated as justification for their policy of selection of nontreatment are unethical, inhumane, and illegal.[73,349,367,639,712,937] Freeman[367] has most appropriately summarized criticism of selection of meningomyelocele infants to die and their placement in nursing homes without subsequent reassignment to the treatment group if they overcome complications, as described by Gross and associates in 1983:[427]

> What they have done, they have done well. We would argue that what they have done well should not have been done at all.[362]

The anger and grief caused by lack of communication and lack of treatment for those few who survive have been described by Pieper.[870]

---

[c] See references 144, 251, 282, 357, 700, 927, 1045, 1105, 1115, and 1252.

The suffering created by those who select for death has been best described by an anonymous parent under the pseudonym of Roger Pell[854] after he and his wife agreed with their physician's decision not to treat their son Peter, born with meningomyelocele. After the birth of a normal child, the Pells were ecstatic and experienced great joy. There were, however, other thoughts and feelings about their first born child.

> ". . . Then she ticked his feet and the little legs didn't respond. . . . She began sobbing again. . . . Peter James Pell died of meningitis . . . but there is grief, too—grief for Peter. . . . Did we do the right thing? Is taking a life, no matter how incomplete or deformed, an act of murder?"[854]

Joanne and Roger Pell's "Agonizing Decision" describes a complaint of many parents whose requests for treatment of their afflicted child are rebuffed.[870] Many of our patients' parents have written about their appreciation for having done all that was possible before their infant or older child died despite our therapeutic efforts. To add the grief of self-blame for "taking a life, no matter how incomplete or deformed," by asking parents to allow their child to die without treatment is, indeed, inhumane.[854] This opinion is diametrically opposed to the recommendation of others that parents should condemn their baby to die.[291]

INDICATIONS AND CONTRAINDICATIONS FOR TREATMENT

As the alternative to selection for utilitarian reasons, others have continued their predecessors' search for improved treatments and emphasize the need to consider the individuality of each patient and the need to continue to care for each patient regardless of whether early surgery is advised or not.[d] Treatment may have to cease in the presence of a complication when it will only prolong dying. Treatment should also be initiated if an unoperated patient either overcomes a complication that precluded surgery or is developing an increasing degree of disability.[35,433,881] Whenever a nontreatment decision is reached, we adhere to the process of open public and peer review described in Chapter 1.

At the opposite extreme from those who would withhold all forms of treatment for many or a majority of infants born with meningomyelocele, others advocate immediate surgical closure of all of them.[368,741,792,819,901,1022,1252] Their reasons for immediate closure are to preserve neural function,[741,1022] prevent ventriculomeningitis, increase survival, and decrease morbidity.[741,792,819,901,1021,1252] Several cite their inability to allow these children to suffer a lingering death or, worse, to

[d] See references 118, 131, 144, 180, 251, 368, 433, 700, 730, 741, 792, 901, 927, 932, 1045, 1077, 1115, and 1231.

see a rare child grow up more deformed than if treatment had been offered.[368,1022,1252] Others cite social insistence on treatment[819] or results of treating all of these infants as having potentially the same results as treating only those selected.[741,792,901] The authors that state that all patients should be treated without selection do not usually mean immediate surgery for all. Sharrard and associates[1021] exempted 10 out of 630 (2 percent) because they were moribund or in the processes of dying from birth trauma, cardiac malformations, failure of their lungs to expand, or other concomitant anomalies. McLone and associates[741] state that they usually do not operate to decompress the posterior fossa with hindbrain or midbrain symptoms because of a lack of success claimed by Park and associates.[838] McLone and associates[741] also state that "*nearly all* children born with myelomeningocele[s] should have their lesion[s] repaired surgically within 24 hours of birth." These exceptions to surgical treatment are consistent with the social and ethical concepts discussed above and in Chapters 1 and 2. Both the President's Commission for the Study of Ethical Problems in Medicine[881] and the American Academy of Pediatrics with seven other groups have produced statements[34] saying that treatment that either will not affect or will only prolong the process of dying should not be provided.

We believe, also, that all children born with meningomyelocele should be treated, but some will benefit more from nonsurgical treatment or surgery delayed until resolution of infection or central nervous system (CNS) trauma.[729,1058] Medical treatment prior to surgery may improve the success of back repair and CSF shunt procedures in some complicated cases.

THE PROCESS OF CARE SELECTION

Initial Evaluation and Care of the Neonate

The three basic reasons for careful initial evaluation are (1) to inform and counsel the parents and family, (2) to help them to decide whether or not to refer the baby for further evaluation and care, and (3) to prepare the person(s) to whom the referral is made so proper action can be initiated without delay. The guardian, parent(s), and family will initially want to know what the problem is, whether anything can be done to "cure" the baby, and, frequently, why the problem occurred. It is important to carry out as complete an evaluation as facilities permit and to quickly initiate an appropriate management plan.[1105] Indecision, delay, misinformation (overly optimistic or overly pessimistic prognoses), or insufficient information increases the family's distress. Proper information should be tempered with cautious optimism if any doubt exists. Otherwise, the parent–infant bonding process may be inalterably disturbed, as with the case of the incorrect in utero diagnosis that led to the abortion of a normal fetus (case 5, Chapter 4).

If the infant is an obvious candidate for surgical therapy, he or she should be referred for consultation with an experienced pediatric neurosurgeon. If doubt exists, a thorough medical evaluation is in order. Transfer to a regional center with a pediatric service capable of complete evaluation, coordination of therapies, and proper discharge planning is in the patient's best interest. Finally, referral or consultation should be arranged with an appropriate indication of the parents' desires and patient's status. For instance, do the parents desire aggressive surgical therapy regardless of prognosis? Can they accept nonsurgical, compassionate ameliorative and supportive care? Or are they undecided? In order to insure initiation of a realistic management plan without falsely optimistic or pessimistic expectations, the evaluation described below should be conducted.

Evaluating clinical status of the infant's brain and lower extremity muscle function is the first step. The low-level neuromotor patient with functioning quadriceps and hamstring muscles (or palpably existent, fleshy muscles) and intact neonatal neurological examination should be urgently referred to preserve existing muscle function or maximize return of muscles temporarily nonfunctioning due to cord shock.[741] We agree with Charney and associates[180] that delay in making a decision for surgery is appropriate with high-level lesions associated with paralysis and atrophy of the thigh muscles.

History: Assessing Brain Damage and Malformation

The long-term outcome of any program will depend to a significant degree on the severity of involvement of the patient admitted. Brain damage, malformation, and trauma as well as the type of infection, if any, are major determinants in the long-term outcome of infants entering a treatment program with any form of myelodysplasia. Therefore, these complications should be identified.[180,513,1053,1058,1059,1105,1248] As much information as possible should be obtained from the obstetrician and parents about the type of delivery and labor, early signs of birth trauma, and exposure to infection and teratogenic agents, such as anticonvulsants (listed in Tables 3-1–3-4). Care must be exercised to relieve anxiety and guilt about wrongly suspected causes. Both parents should be reassured that events occurring after the first month of pregnancy can be unequivocably denied as causative. Feelings of guilt and self-blame are commonly mentioned by parents but not expressed to authority figures and to persons not well known to the family. Reassurance as to the insignificance of imagined causes is therapeutic for parents. Even with obvious clinical features of a teratogen-produced malformation, such as fetal alcohol syndrome, questions about such relationships should be discussed only after unequivocal confirmation and at a later, more appropriate time. This early history should elicit only information that is of value in treating the infant. In particular, the types of bacteria and their patterns of sensitivity to antibacterials that are common in the hospital in which the baby was born should be learned from the hospital epidemiologist or bacteriologist.

MANAGEMENT

Observation

The infant should be placed in a warm isolette or covered incubator. Clothing, diapers, and linens should be sterile, and the infant should be handled only with sterile gloves. The plexiglass shield of the isolette will allow observation that, in turn, will yield a significant amount of information; at the same time, temperature can be stabilized, and open lesions can be protected from airborne infections. There are six important observations: (1) the general body tone, color, and movements; (2) the nature of the meningomyelocele or meningocele lesion, the exstrophy lesion, or the imperforate anus; (3) the deformities of the head; (4) the lower extremity motion, range of motion of the joints, and positional deformities; (5) the passage of stool and urine; and (6) the clinical features that may suggest a particular syndrome or other, complicating anomalies.

General Body Tone, Color, and Movements

General color and body movements can indicate whether the infant is vigorous and healthy or pale, immobile, and brain-damaged. Hemiparesis may be expressed in an upper extremity and should be differentiated from Erb's palsy. Triplegias are incompatible with any satisfactory form of biped ambulation and make manual propulsion of a wheelchair and self-hygiene difficult. Spontaneous movements of the lower extremities may be reflex or may be coordinated and purposeful. Stark[1105] has described lower extremity movements as being (1) flail, due to lower motor neuron damage, (2) reflex only, due to absence of upper motor neuron connections with a group of flail muscles between the isolated reflex activity and the higher normally innervated muscles, (3) no flail muscles, but just uncontrolled reflex movement, and (4) reflex with partial upper motor neuron control. A protuberant anus can easily be seen in the presence of a lax perineal floor and atrophy of the buttocks. Tightly flexed hips and knees suggest absent extensors of those joints. Extended knees suggest strong, unopposed quadriceps muscles, sometimes with a medial hamstring that has ridden over the medial condyle of the femur and is functioning as a knee extensor.[749,1077,1105] Rigid feet in equinovarus and fixed hip or knee deformities suggest long-standing paralysis that probably reflects congenital paralysis from the first trimester or loss of function early in utero. Mobile joints with palpable but nonfunctional muscles suggest cord shock or recent paralysis from the trauma of labor and delivery (see Chapter 4).

The Meningomyelocele or Meningocele Lesion

Direct observation of the lesion will reveal epithelialization, CSF leakage, presence of putrefaction or hemorrhage, anatomical vertebral levels involved, and surface area of the lesion relative to the baby's back. The presence and extent of kyphosis and of dorsolateral protuberance of vertebral alae can be determined through observation and palpation. Complete examination of the lesion should include aspiration of CSF, as described in Chapter 6. Presence of blood or infection, kyphosis and deformed vertebrae, and the size of the lesion will all alter the prognosis, as outlined in Table 5-1 and explained in later chapters of this book.[1043,1105]

After the physical examination, presence of brain mass and of intracranial bleeding, the status of the heart and urinary tract, and the type of myelodysplasia should be further defined by ultrasonography or computerized axial tomography (CT scan).[54,199,718,1053,1105] Since closure of the back is followed by evidence of progressive hydrocephalus in a majority of infants with meningomyelocele and since CNS infection and bloody CSF are contraindications to CSF shunt procedures, we recommend they be identified and treated prior to back closure.

Exstrophy Lesions

In general, exstrophies of the urinary bladder or cloacal exstrophy necessitate particular considerations; they are discussed separately in Chapter 8.

Deformities of the Head

The presence of hydrocephalus at birth (which causes cephalomegaly, sunset sign, craniotabes, a bulging forehead, prominent veins, and a bulging fontanelle) may be associated with other brain malforma-

Table 5-1
Prognosis

	Infancy	Childhood	Adolescence	Adulthood
CNS abnormality	85% require a CSF shunt	Average, one shunt revision; at any point in time; 20% may not be needed	Same as for child; rare occurrence of hydromyelia or onset of hydrocephalus or two-compartment hydrocephalus	Same as for teenage but shunt dependency not known
	NOTE: A higher intellectual performance may be possible (see Chapters 4 and 7)			
Bleeding	Contraindication to CSF shunt and back closure	Expect CNS damage with increased risk for mental retardation and cerebral palsy		
Infection	Same as for bleeding			
Late onset of loss of neural function	Rare	5%–10% may have tethered cord or dysplastic mass in the spinal canal	10%–15% may have tethered cord or dysplastic mass in the spinal canal	Rare
Mental Retardation				
L2 and above	50% mentally retarded			
L3	35% mentally retarded			
L4 and below	15% mentally retarded			
Open neural tube defects	—	—	—	—
Infection	1%–2% (see Chapter 6)			
	Other malformations: dependent on type (see Tables 3-1–3-4)			

Continues

Table 5-1 *Continued*

	Infancy	Childhood	Adolescence	Adulthood
Exstrophy lesions				
		Only rare CNS involvement		
Urologic abnormalities	Need to maintain infection-free, unobstructed flow of urine	Delayed acquisition of urine control; 70%–80% sexually acceptable, but majority dependent (see Chapter 12)	L4-5 and sacral 30%–40% independent and 30%–40% dependent but socially acceptable; only 10%–15% of thoracic and L1-2. Onset of uremia: percentage not known.	L4-5 and sacral 50%–60% socially acceptable; only 30%–40% of thoracic and L1-2. Renal failure percentage not known.
Bowel abnormalities	Need to avoid constipation and obstipation	Same as for urine control (see Chapter 12)	—	—
NOTE: Early age of self-toileting skills is possible but, in our experience, these skills are not maintained (see Chapter 12)				
Musculoskeletal abnormalities				
Spine				
T	Usually no problems	Kyphoscoliosis 20%–30%	Increasing to 80%–90%	50% symptomatic
L1-2	Usually no problems	Same as for T	—	—
L3-5	Usually no problems	Kyphoscoliosis 10%–20%	Increasing to 40%	50% symptomatic
Sacral	Usually no problems	Kyphoscoliosis 1%–3% (see Chapter 15)	10%	50% symptomatic

Hips				
T12	40% contractures dislocate	Both become less common through age 3 years, then increase in frequency; see Chapter 15	—	—
L1-2	45% contractures dislocate	— —	—	—
L3	25% contractures dislocate		—	—
L4-5	20% contractures dislocate		—	—
Sacral	5% contractures		—	—
Knees				
T12 an L1-2	25% contractured	70%	65–70%	65–70%
L3	30% contractured at birth but only 15% by age 3 years	increase to 40% by age 12 years	45%	40–45%
L4-5	15% contractured at birth to 5% by age	increase to 20% by age 12 years	20%	25–30%
Sacral	15 contractured at birth to 24 months of age	1–2% by age 6–12 years of age	3–5%	1–2%
Feet				
T12&L1-2	18% at birth with fixed deformities	deformities increase to 45% by age 5 years	30–80%	35%
L3	10% at birth with fixed deformities increase to 25% by age 3 years	20%–30%	30%–35%	50–55%
L4-5	20–25% at birth with fixed deformities	25–35%	20–25%	30%

Continues

Table 5-1 *Continued*

	Infancy	Childhood	Adolescence	Adulthood
Sacral	0% at birth have fixed deformities	5–15%	2–5%	0%
	For more detailed description of musculo skeletal deformities see Chapter 15			
Ambulate				
T12	Standing frame	20%–25% ambulate with extensive aids	15%	Few ambulate
L1-2	Standing frame	45%–50% ambulate with extensive aids	15%–20%	A few more ambulate
L3	Stand only	75%–85% ambulate with long leg braces	60%–75%	50% ambulate
L4-5	Rarely walk	85%–95% ambulate with short leg braces	90%	90%
Sacral	Rarely walk	95% ambulate without aids	100%	100%
NOTE: Ambulation in patients with midlumbar lesions is dependent on CNS impairment (cerebral palsy) and status of quadriceps and gluteal muscles; the latter is difficult to evaluate in neonates (see Chapter 15)				
Skin care	Preventable but all levels are 90%–100% at some time in life due to loss of sensation, poor perineal hygiene, and ill-fitting shoes or braces (see Chapter 14)			
Obesity	All levels are at risk, but the more paralyzed are at higher risk. Preventable but still too frequently a complication (see Chapter 13)			
Sexual function	Potential as an adult should be discussed	Potential as an adult should be discussed	Possible in all females with fertility; problems with pregnancy. All males capable of orgasm, erection (perhaps with surgical implants), and potency; fertility must be evaluated after puberty (see Chapter 21)	

Laryngeal and pharyngeal palsies	20%, with half needing tracheostomy, gastrostomy, and tracheal separation	Rare	Rare	Rare
Seizures	10%	15%	15%	15%
Ocular palsies and poor vision	58%	35%	35%	35%
Visual Perception and ocular motor incoordination; poor type motor control	95%	95%	95%	95%
NOTE: Important education and vocational problem. Should be properly evaluated. See Chapter 16.				

See also Shurtleff.[1045] Prognosis should be varied to include capabilities of local health, education, and social resources and changing (hopefully improving) technology.

tions.[341,646,662,1116] The fontanelle is usually soft at birth; sutures may be widely spread, but lax despite markedly advanced hydrocephalus. Tension rarely increases until after age 2–7 days, even if the back has been closed shortly after birth; this is due to factors discussed in Chapter 7.

Rarely, myelodysplasia is associated with the Dandy-Walker syndrome,[354] a diagnosis indicated by the presence of a large posterior fossa and transillumination. Most frequently, a small posterior fossa with a sharply cut-off inferior portion of the occiput and a ''scrawny'' neck are indications of the Arnold-Chiari type II malformation, by far the most common brain anomaly associated with meningomyelocele.[131] The more severe clinical forms of this malformation (e.g., the ''peach syndrome'') cause weakness and atrophy of neck and arm muscles and paralysis of cranial nerves. They are related to more serious cerebral dysfunction, including mental retardation, occulomotor incoordination, and laryngopharyngeal palsies.[851] Examination of cranial nerves often reveals optic muscle palsies[688] as well as poor gag and swallow reflexes and a croupy, hoarse cry resulting from paresis of the ninth and tenth nerves.[342,479,1042,1045] Careful examination of the eyes, palate, and ears will lead to detection of other anomalies associated with chromosomal or other syndromes (see Tables 3-1–3-4).

Lower Extremity Movement and Range of Motion of the Joints

Pulling, tickling, and pinching or holding the baby up from the mattress by placing the hands under the abdomen will allow a rough estimate of useful, coordinated movement as opposed to useless cord reflexes in the lower extremities. Absence of movement despite the visible and palpable presence of a muscle may mean infant noncompliance or temporary cord shock after the trauma of labor and delivery.[331,889,890,932,1105] We have observed good lower extremity function disappear temporarily even without labor and after the utmost care in handling an open meningomyelocele. Just exposure to air and temperature changes may produce temporary cord shock. McLone and associates[741] have observed that 37 percent of their patients develop improved muscle function across at least one major joint. Those who delay treatment either do not witness or do not mention such a return.[180,427,671] Stimulation for lower extremity movements should be above the waist to avoid reflex reactions. Pin pricks or touching the lower leg or foot may lead to isolated contralateral or ipsilateral reflex activity. A child with muscle power that allows only hip flexion and adduction will usually be unable to walk effectively as an adult. (For more on the relationships of functional ambulation to the levels of paralysis, see Chapter 15.) Because of the importance of knee flexion and extension for ambulation, a good examination for knee flexion and extension is important for counseling the family. Response to sensory stimulation is too variable to be of value. However, we have found motor function to be of great importance in predicting the infant's ambulation potential as well as intellect (Table 5-1).[616,666,1045,1060] Motor level is not well correlated with the roentgenographic definition of the level of abnormal vertebra, the level of sensory loss, or the anatomic site of the open skin lesion.

Anorectal Pathophysiology

Anal wink is a frequently recorded finding, but it has little significance. An anal wink is usually present, but it does not indicate cortical reception of pain on stimulation. The muscle contraction is usually an isolated sensory-motor arc reflex.[1105] Anal tone may be weak or absent at birth, and a rectal prolapse may, rarely, be present or develop. These signs are not indications for colostomy. Even most infants with a patulous anus gain anal tone. Almost all patients have at birth, or develop, a tight, spastic reflex sphincter with the useful function of assisting in stool retention, but as a clinical finding in an infant, this type of sphincter cannot be used as a prognostic sign for normal anal function (see Chapters 10 and 12). The child with a patulous anal sphincter will have more prolapse, stool staining, and accidents, but he or she can be taught to be socially acceptable. Toilet training for appropriate stool elimination is dependent on sensation as well as voluntary motor control and, therefore, cannot be tested until later in childhood.

As with lower urinary tract anomalies, a high incidence of imperforate anus or perineal fistulae anterior to the anal sphincter occurs with various types of myelodysplasias. These malformations are also amenable to conservative management without recourse to colostomy.

Urinary Pathophysiology

Absence of a palpable urinary bladder suggests a weak or nonexistent urethral spasm or resistance and is sometimes found in association with a flail or weak anal sphincter. The urinary sphincter mechanism can be tested only indirectly. The examiner can identify the capacity to retain urine with abdominal palpatation. If urine leaks or spurts with pressure, a weak sphincter or active detrusor is present, and bladder capacity will be small or vary. The presence of a large, distended urinary bladder implies a spastic sphincter and weaker detrusor with urine retention. A compensated urinary bladder will empty by reflex contraction if the intravesical pressure is suddenly increased by the Crede method. A distended bladder with outlet spasm will either be large and turgid (frequently with positive transillumination) or will manifest by a ureterovesical incompetence, bilateral hydronephrosis, and hydroureter visible by ultrasonography. We usually perform both cranial and abdominal ultrasonography prior to our initial counseling with parents of a meningomyelocele child because of the rare child who has, in addition, renal agenesis or hydronephrosis of such a degree as to be incompatible with life.

We have seen edema from the midabdomen distally present with iliac vein obstruction secondary to an enlarged, otherwise asymptomatic urinary bladder in the neonate with meningomyelocele. Management of urinary tract obstruction in the neonate is now only rarely surgical, as discussed in Chapter 11.

Other Anomalies

Other significant anomalies are polydactyly, radial ray hypoplasia, arthrogryposis, fused or anomalous ribs, and cardiac or renal anomalies.[e] (see Table 3-1). Palm- and fingerprints, hair pattern, facial features, and ear formation should be carefully observed in consideration of fetal alcohol syndrome, chromosomal errors, or field defects typical of the syndromes; the presence of syndromes or other malformations can alter the prognosis. An otherwise uncomplicated, low-level meningomyelocele may appear as part of a syndrome that is, in itself, incompatible with life (see Figs. 3-4A and 3-4B). Whereas the authors noted above include these subtypes in the overall group of children with meningomyelocele,[f] others eliminate them from consideration and discuss only uncomplicated meningomyelocele.[741,901] We include all types of myelodysplasia because of the need for primary care physicians, pediatricians, and surgeons to be aware of the differential diagnoses associated with meningomyelocele lesions. Otherwise, unnecessary operative procedures will be performed on children with meningomyeloceles and other fatal anomalies.

If superficial or hidden anomalies suggest a chromosome disorder or if preliminary examination indicates other organ anomalies, definitive studies should be carried out to confirm diagnosis before conferring with the parents about a decision for the most appropriate form of treatment.

Decision for Management

After completion of the initial evaluation, the parents should be fully informed of the contents of Tables 3-1–3-4 and this chapter, as modified for their child. During this discussion, we write down a summary for the

[e] See references 131, 180, 282, 325, 357, 666, 669, 671, 701, 1021, 1058, 1077, and 1105.
[f] See references 131, 180, 282, 325, 357, 666, 669, 671, 701, 1021, 1058, 1077, and 1105.

parents (and keep a carbon copy) containing pertinent points listed in these tables. We have learned that most parents are not able to remember all of the complex issues discussed at our counseling sessions. A written list allows them to review and later question us about subjects pertinent to their child. General booklets do not provide adequate specificity and only confuse or frighten new parents. This list is supplemented by a personal care loose-leaf notebook provided the parents by our nurse. As each problem is addressed, the family is given current recommendations to include in their child's care book. The parents' wishes should be carefully considered by the physician in charge so that treatment (i.e., surgical closure, deferment of surgery, or relinquishing custody and establishing guardianship) can be clearly prescribed for the reasons discussed in Chapter 1. The parents' wishes should be followed unless the physician recognizes that the parents' decision is based on the parents' own interests at the expense of the child.

Also as discussed in Chapter 1, we believe *communication* among the parents, primary health care providers, and specialists to be an essential component of care for the child with a severe congenital malformation.[243a] Repeat, detailed, and careful discussions between the family and concerned professionals are necessary because of the complex and dynamic nature of congenital malformations and because of the development of new treatment modalities. With the passage of time, the competence of the family to assimilate information about these complex disorders increases.

In our discussions, we quote recent data that suggest better survival potential for children with congenital malformations.[741,729,819,901] In our experience, the percentage of patients with myelodysplasia who are referred to us have fewer contraindications to treatment (23 percent) compared with 10–20 years ago (52 percent) (Fig. 5-1). In addition, complications after initial treatment have dramatically decreased from 12.5 percent before 1965 to 3.4 percent after 1973 (most of the latter 3.4 percent were severe Arnold-Chiari malformations) (Fig. 5-2). The better condition of infants as a result of early referral and fewer complications as a result of improved treatment have allowed an increasing percentage of children at risk to survive. Now, over 90 percent of infants operated on early in our program survive to at least 10 years of age (Fig. 5-3).

We discuss with our parents the results of treatment described in Chapters 6–8, 12, and 15 and Table 5-1; being confronted with this large number of problems presented by their congenitally malformed infant is an apparently horrendous experience for the parents. Parents so informed, however, express appreciation, in contrast to complaints about lack of information recorded by others.[370,459,882] Several of our group of physicians and nurse coordinators review the list, described above, with

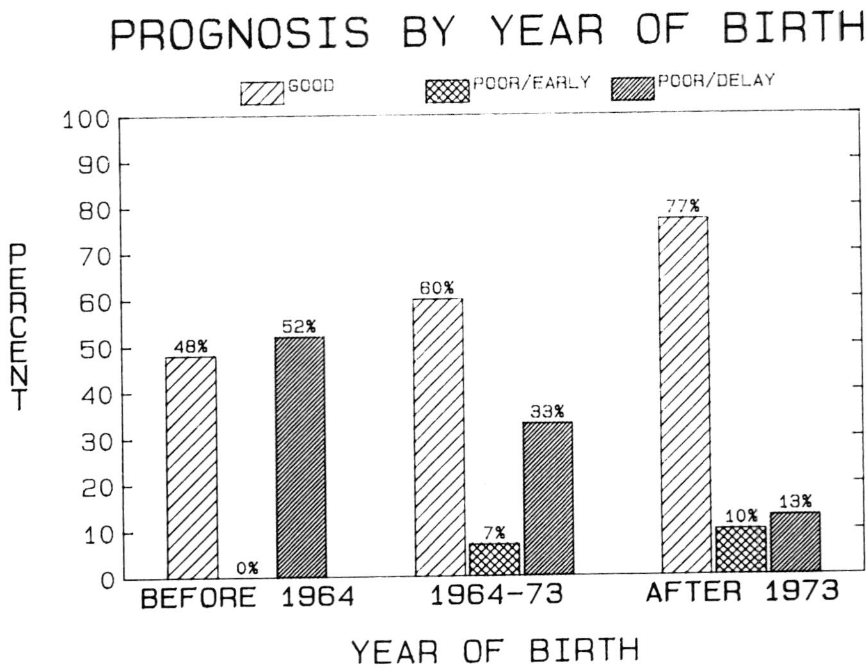

Figure 5-1. Prognosis by year of birth prior to initial treatment. All 275 infants seen at or before 1 week of age and prior to any treatment from 1957 through September 1985 are included. Complications leading to a poor prognosis include primary birth trauma to the central nervous system and infection. Prior to 1964, the majority of the 44 cases were referred after considerable delay. After 1974, improved neonatal care and transport as well as obstetrical care (discussed in Chapter 4) have further improved prognosis for the 88 cases referred. Those patients with poor prognoses but operated on early had high-level lesions with higher risk for mental retardation but neither infection or blood in the cerebrospinal fluid. The differences in proportion between the patients in the good and poor categories of the three eras is significant ($\chi^2 = 15.6$; df $= 2$; $p < 0.01$).

the parents during the initial hospitalization, and we explain possible complications, medical treatment, and how to operate equipment.

For each child, one pediatrician and one nurse are assigned as advocates responsible for helping the family care for their child and to assure parental understanding (see Chapter 22).

Initial plans to defer back closure and CSF shunt surgery are altered if the infant overcomes the complications that caused deferral of early operation and if the back is not epithelialized. Initial decisions for aggressive surgical treatment may be altered if untreatable complications arise as a result of brain destruction from a high-pressure shunt obstruc-

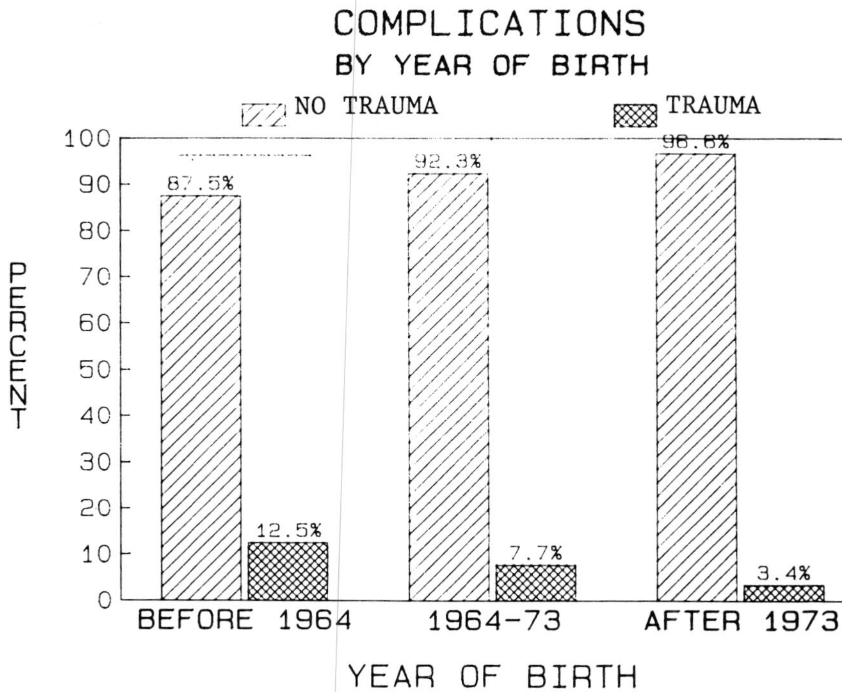

Figure 5-2. Complications following treatment of myelodysplasia by year of birth. The 185 patients in this figure are some of the same as those in Figure 5-1. The three eras reflect, in addition to the comments in Figure 5-1, time periods during which there were considerable differences in quality of care. Up until 1964, we were comparing the effectiveness of back closure or cerebrospinal fluid shunt as the primary procedure on the 16 patients in this era. Since 1974, we have had a number of technical improvements in care (discussed in Chapters 6 and 7). The majority of complications of the 117 patients seen in this last era are now shunt infections and bulbar palsy from the Arnold-Chiari malformation. The differences in proportions among those without postoperative complications in the three eras are insignificant (Fisher's exact for before 1964 and 1964–1973, $p = 0.4$; before 1964 and after 1973, $p = 0.15$; and 1964–1973 and after 1973, $p = 0.20$).

tion or CNS infection. We assure the parents from the beginning that we will review openly and frequently the progress and prognosis of their child, and that we will not recommend treatment for treatment's sake or research purposes; we recommend treatment only if the child will possibly benefit from the procedures. We will not withhold treatment against the family's wishes even if there is only a slight chance of success, and we will recommend treatments that will decrease morbidity and relieve suffering, even if life prolongation is not a goal. More frequent

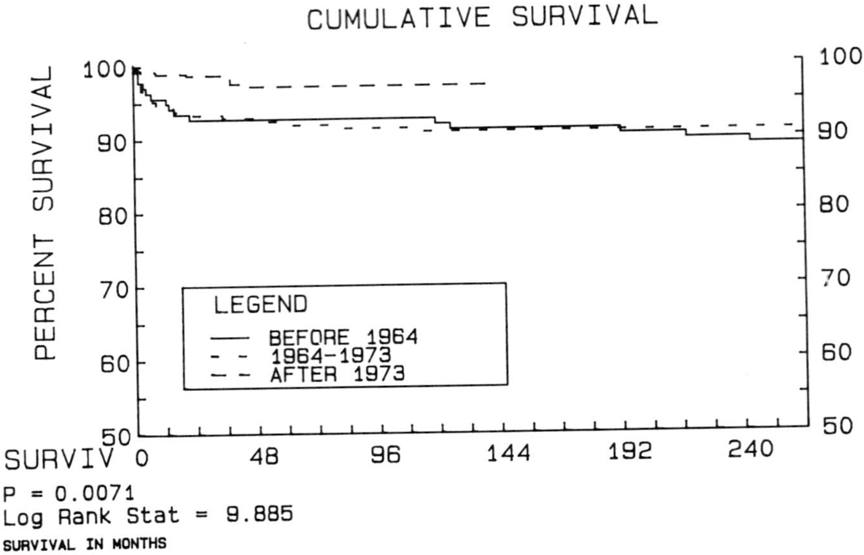

Figure 5-3. Cumulative survival. All 711 infants seen at or before 1 week of age and prior to treatment from 1957 through August 1985 have been divided into the same groups by year of birth as in Figures 5-1 and 5-2. The age is on the abscissa in months. Percentage of survival is calculated by standard actuarial methods. The improved survival for the most recent group is significant (log sub statistic = 9.885; $p = 0.0071$). Improved survival is probably due to the better condition of infants at the time of referral, as demonstrated in Figure 5-1, and lower complication rates (discussed in Chapters 5 and 6). The last cell with five observations for the 136 patients seen before 1964 was 480 months; age, 252 months for the 209 patients born between 1964 and 1973; and age, 132 months for patients seen since 1973.

review, at least weekly, is planned for infants with conditions for which we have deferred surgical or medical treatment.

Most parents accepting a nonsurgical treatment program for their infants are emotionally and technically incapable of providing nursing care, and when a nonsurgical treatment program is chosen, most parents readily relinquish custody. When we recommend placement in a nursing or foster home, we emphasize the need for skilled nursing care rather than for mothering in order to prevent increasing the guilt parents already feel about the placement of their child outside the home.[244a,370,459,470,697,882] Care should be exercised to protect mothers from being required to care for infants at the insistence of a nonsupportive spouse, family, or society.

On the other hand, some mothers can nurse an infant with an untreatable and fatal defect, sometimes contrary to their family's beliefs, as discussed in Chapter 1. A mother wishing to care for her child regardless of the degree of deformity should be allowed to do so. If a mother is to take a child with an open defect home, we close the lesion for ease of care. Repetitive surgical procedures can be justified even in a severely malformed infant or child if loving parents care for the baby between hospitalizations and realistically foresee future possibilities. A surprising number of these severely malformed children do well,[741,819,901] even despite a delay in surgical care.[180,729] Lack of full information and denial of the opportunity to care for their child breeds severe resentment among parents who have the capacity to "mother" a severely malformed child.[870]

Adoption Possibilities

Preconceptual parental disharmony, impending parental separation or divorce, and out-of-wedlock conception are some of the problems of parents who refuse treatment for relatively mildly malformed children. We have encouraged relinquishment and even initiated deprivation hearings in these kinds of situations. The children have subsequently been adopted under the Washington State–subsidized adoption plan, also available in some other states. These plans pay for medical care, education, and extra costs of daily living expenses. We have not witnessed the increased marital stress[470] noted by others[697,1158] (see Chapter 18). For the above reasons, we agree with DeLange[251] that the child should be provided other social accommodations if the impairment is going to be too heavy a burden for a particular family. There are national adoption programs for congenitally malformed infants and children, such as the program provided by the Spina Bifida Association of America. One family in our clinic has adopted one child with meningomyelocele and three with trisomy 21 in addition to foster parenting two other children with meningomyelocele and a child with severe cerebral palsy.

We cannot stress in this text either too strongly or too frequently the need for health care professionals to recognize the dual responsibilities: to the infant and to the parents. Relinquishment can serve both.

On the other hand, we have noted that some of the least congenitally malformed children have been placed for adoption and some of those most severely affected remain in their natural homes. Health care professionals should support each family's need to care for its physically malformed infant, and when that option is not feasible because of family structure, resources, or beliefs, professionals should support the child by providing both medical care and referral for surrogate "mothering." Indeed, in our clinic we now care for one profoundly, two moderately, and one mildly retarded adopted children with meninogmyelocele whose parents relinquished them at birth. The two with moderate retardation are in wheelchairs and are unable to perform transfers at 6 and 12 years of age. The profoundly retarded child is confined to bed.

Monetary Costs

For details of monetary costs of treatment and the effect of early, delayed, and supportive treatment for infants and children with high-level lesions, we refer the reader to two recent publications describing higher total costs (medical care, education, and custodial care) for those who receive delayed or no surgical therapy.[1058,1061] Higher costs to the states were primarily due to abandonment,[470,1061] resulting in higher custodial costs. Increased intellectual and physical impairment among the groups provided delayed or no surgical treatment probably account for the higher rate of abandonment and resultant higher custodial costs[1061] (Table 5-2). Other authors[180,427,671] disagree but have not presented financial data to support their opinions (see Chapter 4 for a discussion of the cost-effectiveness of prenatal diagnosis with improved pregnancy outcome).

SUMMARY

It should be noted that our clinic provides consultative care for local residents, many of whom live hundreds or thousands of miles from our tertiary referral center. We must, therefore, communicate with primary care providers in writing, by telephone, and through local conferences and seminars. We believe communication among the specialists, parents, and primary health providers to be an essential component of care for a child with a chronic physical malformation. We recommend that establishment of a supportive home, natural or surrogate, is just as important a goal as surgical correction.

In conjunction with the dual responsibilities mentioned above is the most important concept of the decision-making process: to choose the most beneficial and humane treatment for the child. That decision should include assurance of a supportive family and of surgical procedures that will lessen morbidity and relieve suffering and not just prolong life without hope. We have had successful judicial review of our decisions, when they have led to nonsurgical treatment and death, and when they have led to withdrawal of treatment and death in a child who was initially operated (see Chapter 1).

Relinquishment not only provides some infants the opportunity for treatment and supportive adoptive homes, but helps families in the following ways: (1) it relieves parents incapable of caring for a congeni-

Table 5-2
Costs of Care of Meningomyelocele During Childhood[a]

	1977[b]	1985[c]
Medical costs		
Shunt plus revisions	$9,114 (Shunt plus 1.7 revisions)	$5,285 (Shunt plus 0.77 revisions)
Back closure with shunt	$8,786	$11,088
Back closure without shunt	$4,320	$6,412
Spine fusion	$4,844	$16,925
Hip operation	$1,280[d]	$3,245
Ankle or foot operation	$1,280[d]	$2,266
Decubitus	$4,333	$12,619
General surgical	$1,003	$1,852
Total medical	$34,960	$59,692
Social costs[b]		
Special education for all 18 years (in excess of regular education costs)		$66,608
Institutional or foster care for 18 years		$106,634

[a] Costs for care of a population can be calculated from tables and graphs of frequency for each complication. Reduced infection rates are associated with lower cost of cerebrospinal fluid shunts relative to greater increase in costs for other types of care. The decreased number of shunt revisions in the 1980's accounts for the lower cost. Spine fusion ranged from $1,494 to $68,174 so that a single expensive and complicated case increased the average cost. Several prolonged hospitalizations for decubiti caused the greater than average increase.

[b] Calculated from Bricker and associates[126] × 1.16 inflation from consumer price index, US Bureau of Economic Analysis, 1984, and Bricker and associates.[126]

[c] Actual costs of 20 average cases for each procedure.

[d] Average cost of nonspine orthopedic procedures.

tally malformed child (for whatever reasons) from bearing the guilt of allowing their child to die untreated; (2) it protects the family of the untreatable child from harassment with inappropriate legal action by "right-to-life" groups, as most poignantly illustrated by the "Baby Jane Doe" case of Stonybrook, New York[1117]; and (3) it provides for a family in want of a child.

David Shurtleff
J. Timothy Stuntz

6

Back Closure

Previous chapters have discussed the selection of various treatment methods. This chapter addresses the advantages, disadvantages, and outcomes associated with different types of modern operative procedures to close an open meningomyelocele, reconstruct a meningocele, or repair a lipoma of the conus medularis. We will discuss the closure of the lesions associated with exstrophy in a separate chapter (Chapter 8).

OPEN MENINGOMYELOCELE CLOSURE

Infection

As discussed in Chapter 5, most authors state that the two most important reasons for closing an open meningomyelocele are to prevent infection and to preserve existing or potential nerve function.[a] To prevent infection, early closure, before colonization of bacteria occurs on the newborn's skin, has been advocated.[442,1020,1021] Others state that there is no increase in infection or loss of muscle function with delayed closure.[180,671] Prevention of postoperative cerebrospinal fluid (CSF) fistulae and of the resultant potential entry for infection has been stressed as a reason for watertight closure of the outer membrane of the meninges, the

[a] See references 183, 438, 442, 524, 621, 700, 732, 739, 1021, and 1052.

MYELODYSPLASIAS AND EXSTROPHIES: SIGNIFICANCE, PREVENTION, AND TREATMENT
 ISBN 0-8089-1816-8

dura mater.[183,442,600,700,739,1227] To control CSF leakage further, some authors have advocated an additional closure of myofascia over the dura mater.[58,103,195,246b,261,600,785] Sealing off CSF leakage and removing the portion of the surface of the sac that may have been absorbing CSF can cause acute hydrocephalus, wound breakdown, and infections.[435,524,621,700,856]

We have noted the relationship between closure and the acute onset of hydrocephalus. We attempted to relieve the hydrocephalus in some cases by initial insertion of a CSF shunt prior to back closure and, in other cases, by insertion of a shunt with the onset of hydrocephalus after back closure, only to discover infection was equally likely to compound treatment.[1052] More recently, we have used early closure and temporary control of hydrocephalus with 1,4:3,6 dianhydro-D-glucitol until infection could be eradicated and the CSF cleared of cells.[1059] A CSF shunt was then inserted when there was little or no evidence for a central nervous system (CNS) inflammatory process.

Preservation of Neural Function

Preservation of neural function has led most authors to advocate careful protection of the neural plaque and careful closure of the arachnoid-dura.[435,524,600,621,700,739] McLone[739] and others have described the need for meticulous care of the exposed neural elements prior to surgery. They should not be allowed to become dry or traumatized by scrubbing, tight bandages, clothing, or allowing the infant to lie on his or her back. Only sterile saline or Ringer's lactate should be applied to sterile, nonadhesive dressings held loosely in place by an elastic stockinette. If the infant is to be transported, a protective bandage with a doughnut of sufficient size to prevent touching the neural plaque should be applied in a manner that will prevent slippage. As indicated in Chapter 4, we also recommend avoidance of late pregnancy fetal confinement and avoidance of trauma from labor and vaginal delivery because of potential trauma to, or infection of, the exposed neural elements. Reconstruction of the neural tube by invaginating the plaque, as recommended by McLone[739] and Nash,[796] and simple replacement of the plaque into the neural canal will be discussed in more detail below under "*Neural Element*."

Restructure of Myofascial Planes

A third general objective of open meningomyelocele lesion closure is prevention of orthopedic deformities. One of the more important and frequent late complications of large lesions involving the thoracolumbar area is kyphoscoliosis.[62,239,684,1055,1125] Two types of closures have been effective: one involving bone and myofascial procedures and the other involving only myofasica. Mustarde[785] has recommended myo-osseus flaps, and Edgerton[296] has used bone grafts during initial closure. Sharrard and Drennan[1019] as well as Reigel[900] have recommended resection of parts of vertebrae to correct kyphosis at the time of initial closure. Details of myofascial closures (including flaps and grafts) will be discussed later in this chapter.

The following three therapeutic objectives are incorporated to varying degrees in descriptions of many different techniques for closing open neural tube defects of the spine: (1) prevention of CNS infection, (2) preservation of neural function, including prevention of tethering at a future date, and (3) restoration of myo-osseous deficits of the spine. Essentially, most discussions of how to close open neural tube defects concentrate on closure of the neural elements, osseous and myofascial planes, or subcutaneous tissues and skin. Rather than discuss different authors' types of closure, we will incorporate their concepts into the following three aspects of open meningomyelocele closure: (1) neural elements, (2) myofascial planes, and (3) subcutaneous tissue and skin.

Neural Elements

McLone[739] first emphasized the importance of the junction between the lateral edges of the neural plaque and the sac. The edges of the neural plaque, with proper formation, would have rolled up from a ventral and lateral position to fuse in the midline and form the dorsal aspect of the spinal cord. The junction of the neural plaque and the sac, created by failure of entubulation, is formed by the continuation of the pia-arachnoid that covers the ventral surface of the neural plaque and extends laterally and ventrally along the sides of the plaque to line the inner surface of the sac (Fig. 6-1A). They meet the dura mater along the lateral and caudal aspects of the lesion and extend ventrally to form a continuous covering on the dorsal surface of the neural canal. Thus, the neural plaque floats on a fluid space created by a continuum (Fig. 6-1A). The essence of McLone's technique can be understood as closing two tubes, one within the other, by enfolding the inner tube, the neural plaque (Fig. 6-1B).[739]

The exposed surface of the plaque is ependyma that would have developed into the lining of the central canal of the cord. This ependymal surface is continuous with the central canal cephalad to the defect. The medial portions of the neural plaque, on each side of the median raphe, represent the ventral or basal (motor) portion of the cord, whereas the lateral parts of the plate correspond to the dorsal or alar (sensory) plates.[733] The neural plaque (including the dorsal layer, comprised of

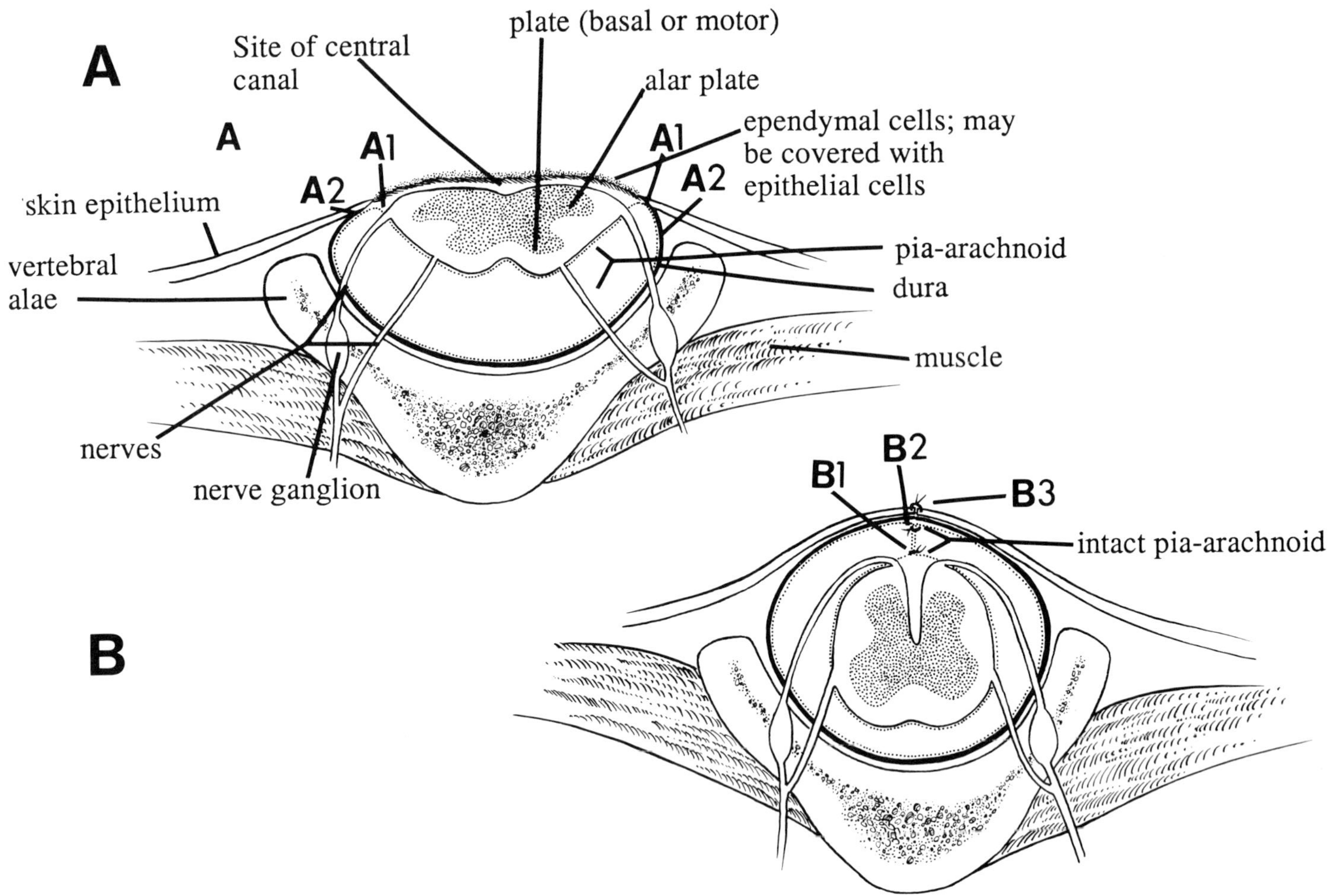
A
Site of central
canal
plate (basal or motor)
alar plate
A
A1
A2
A1
A2
ependymal cells; may
be covered with
epithelial cells
skin epithelium
vertebral
alae
pia-arachnoid
dura
muscle
nerves
nerve ganglion
B
B1
B2
B3
intact pia-arachnoid

ependymal cells) is rolled into a tube by folding together and suturing the edges of the neural plaque and pia-arachnoid. Care is taken to dissect away any epithelium or non-nervous system tissue since it can develop into dermoids or scarring that cause cord tethering.[742,903,1188] Then, without interrupting the arachnoid, the dura mater is brought to the midline and the arachnoid-dura sutured to form a second tube (Fig. 6-1B). McLone's method of closure necessitates no separation of the arachnoid, invaginates and entubulates the neural plaque, and provides enclosure of both the ependymal dorsal surface of the neural plaque and a double layer of arachnoid, one around the entubulated plaque and another lining the dura mater (Fig. 6-1B).[739] Microneurosurgical techniques are necessary when operating in this area because this pia-arachnoid junction was to have been the dorsal surface of the cord, and both significant blood vessels and nerves enter the neural plaque along this border (Fig. 6-1B). McLone's technique is more refined than the method originally described by Nash,[796] and it avoids damage to the plaque, nerves, and blood vessels. His objectives are to preserve neural function and, hopefully, avert future scarring that will lead to progressive nerve damage. Closure of the central canal of the spinal cord and suspension of neural tissue in a pia-arachnoid–lined CSF compartment is performed to prevent adhesions of the neural elements to dura or myofascia at the closure site. It is hoped such a closure will reduce or eliminate cord tethering later in the child's life.[739]

Guthkelch and associates[438] compared the use of an entubulation technique (not explained in sufficient detail to enable one to judge its comparability with McLone's method) with simple replacement of the neural plaque, used by us[600] (Fig. 6-2) and others.[183,442,1227] Our method of closure also includes myofascial flaps, as illustrated in Fig. 6-2 and

---

Figure 6-1. Surgical closure. (A) The abnormal covering of plaque and pia-arachnoid may be ependymal cells or ependymal cells covered by a thin layer of epithelial cells without skin appendages or subcutaneous tissue. This corresponds to Figure 3-2C and figure 4-2. the space between the neural plaque and the open spinal cord may be pia-arachnoid and dura mater, or pia-arachnoid and a thin layer of epithelium (see Figure 3-2D and Figure 4-4). The junction of the epithelial layer, pai-arachnoid, and the dura mater, or a combination of all three, occurs along the lateral edge of theneural plaque. The true skin joins with arachnoid-dura and the beginning of abnormal epithelium or may completely cover the plaque. (B) McLone's closure.[739] Each edge of the neural plaque, shown in A (A1 and A2), is folded to the midline (B1, then B2). All epithelial elements are carefully removed, and the edges of neural plaque are sewn together via sutures in the pia-arachnoid (A1) to form a tube closure in the midline (B1). The pia-arachnoid is kept intact.[739] The skin is then approximated, tension free, in the midline (B3).

discussed in the next section. The ependyma is left exposed to arachnoid as opposed to McLone's method. McLaurin states he has rarely been able to preserve the integrity of the arachnoid membrane so that the subarachnoid space is not violated.[733] Guthkelch and associates[438] reported no differences in loss or recovery of neural function, but follow-up was too short to assess the potential for McLone's procedure to prevent tethering from scarring. We have observed one of two entubulated plaques closed by others develop tethering.

Detailed studies of preoperative muscle strength and sensory levels will need to be compared with postoperative and long-term repeat evaluations in a sufficiently large population to finally answer the question as to the value of reconstituting the microenvironment of the neural plaque, as suggested by McLone.[739] Other potential causes for loss of nervous system function due to leaking of CSF, infection, and compression of nervous tissue by myofascial flaps also need to be assessed.

Most authors would agree with us that excision of the neural plaque, as proposed by Guthkelch and associates,[438] should be avoided and a watertight arachnoid-dural closure should be accomplished with fascial grafts, if possible.[183,442,739,903,1188,1227] Cord shock in the neonate as well as a relatively poor predictive value of muscle strength in the neonatal period for later neuromotor function is discussed further in Chapter 15. McLone and associates[741] report that 37 percent of infants improve motor function across at least one major joint between initial exam and later follow-up. This degree of inability to accurately predict future muscle function suggests caution. Excision of a functionless plaque and lower cord may be considered later when surgically correcting a spinal curvature or to eliminate deforming spasticity of the lower extremities.

Osseous and Myofascial Layer

Despite descriptions of bank[296] and autologous[111] bone grafts and use of myo-osseous flaps[785] and kyphectomy,[900,1019] there have been no long-term evaluations of these recommendations. Failure of bone growth, high blood loss, and mortality seem to have dissuaded most surgeons from pursuing kyphectomy repairs on infants. Many, however, still perform minimal osteotomies of protruding malformed alae, modified after Mustarde,[785] to assist in closure and to lower the profile of dorsally protruding bony masses that threaten flap graft survival and later cause decubiti. In addition, the theoretical use of bone paste for in utero repair remains under study.[751]

Others, however, have recommended myofascial layers be placed over the dural closure to add protection and to help prevent formation of CSF fistulae. Ingraham and Hamlin[523] were of the opinion that neither repair of the vertebral arch deformity nor replacement of muscle was of critical value. They and others believe skin and subcutaneous tissue to be adequate closure over the dura mater, and myofascial flaps or grafts to be only optional or useful as patches when there is insufficient dura mater.[58,739,801,1227]

Other groups have recommended the use of lattissimus dorsi with or without overlying skin as rotational flaps across the midline[103,195] and to the midline.[261] Habal and Vries[442] criticize these grafts as associated with high blood loss. We have observed that cross-midline grafts containing skin pose problems of approach when later spine surgery is indicated for correction of kyphoscoliosis. Skin swung across the midline in myocutaneous grafts has blood supply that compromises subsequent incisions for spinal surgery. McLaurin[733] states theoretically that progressive gibbus deformity will be prevented by the pull of these posteriorly placed muscles.

A final group has recommended lumbodorsal myofascial flap graft or free graft closure.[438,442,600] When a *flap graft* or pedicle is made, a piece of myofascia is cut on three sides, lifted up, and folded over the lesion, leaving blood supply to the flap graft intact via the uncut, folded side. A *graft*, on the other hand, involves removing a section of myofascia by incising all four sides, undermining the graft to separate the tissue and attaching it over the lesion. We believe spine stability has been improved in our patients by lumbodorsal myofascial *imbrication* (bilateral flap grafts or pedicles folded across the midline and attached to the myofascia of the opposite side of the open spine defect; Fig. 6-2).[600] When insufficient tissue is available laterally, free myofascial grafts or partial lattissimus dorsi flaps supplement closure, most commonly in the sacral area (see "Myofascial Closure"). Free myofascial grafts supplement closure in the sacral area.

Skin and Subcutaneous Tissue

The final stage of open meningomyelocele closure has received the most attention in the literature. Skin closures fall into one of three types: (1) rotational skin flaps, (2) delayed closures, and (3) midline closures with relaxing incisions for bipedicle grafts when necessary. We will discuss all three closures below. Most discussions accept the primary midline, tension-free closure as optimal. Generally, longitudinal closure is preferable because of possible later surgical procedures for orthopedic correction of spinal problems.[733] Preservation of blood supply can also be accomplished by horizontal, oblique, *T*, and *V-Y* closure. The exact dimensions of the lesion are not as important as its magnitude relative to the infant's size and the corresponding availability of skin. As a rule,

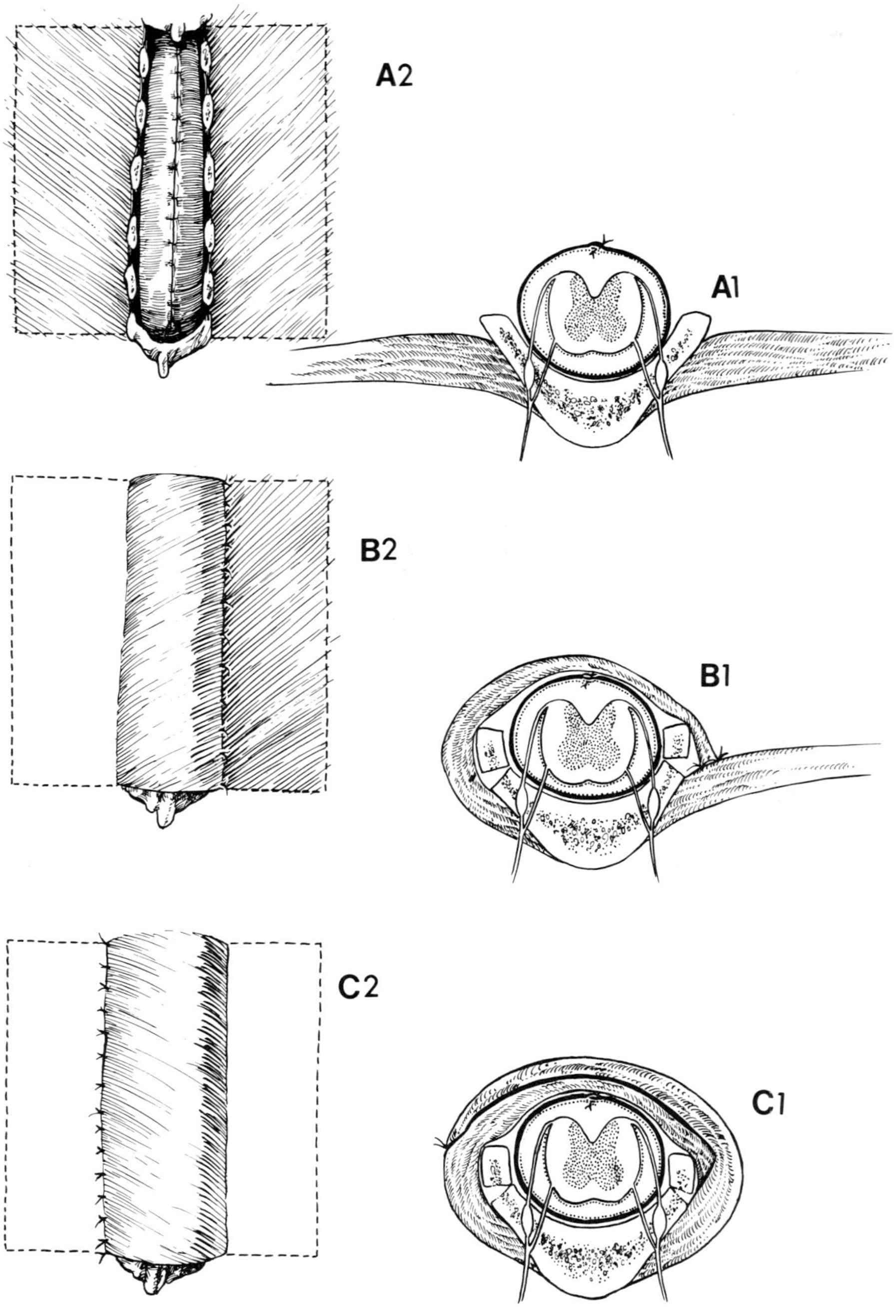

Figure 6-2. Imbrication. After removal of epithelium and excess pia-arachnoid and dura mater, the neural plaque is dropped back into the neural canal with nerves, and the margins of the neural placque are folded (A1). The ependymal surface of the plaque is open and facing dorsally. After excess pia-arachnoid and

lesions resulting in a skin defect less than half the width of the back can be closed directly.[733] Only the so-called large lesions (in relationship to the size of the infant) require consideration of one of the following three types of grafting techniques.

Rotational Skin Flaps

A rotational skin flap graft is a single pedicle graft swung across the midline. Patterson and Till noted in 1959 that relieving incisions were needed in approximately one fourth of their cases, and they advocated rotational flaps for large lesions.[848] Later, Davies and Adendorff[246b] described single rotational flaps across the midline performed on five infants with an average size lesion of 7.5 × 6 cm. Bajaj and associates[58] described the use of bilateral rotation flaps, one lateral cephalad and the other lateral caudad, swung across the midline with a transverse closure; essentially, one flap is cut out on each side, and then both flaps are layed, one below the other, side-by-side over the lesion, and sewn together. The ten patients had lesions measuring from 5.5 × 4.5 cm to 7.5 × 12.5 cm. They mentioned "ten patients who survived," but did not clarify their mortality rate.[58] They also mentioned hematoma formation and swelling due to CSF leakage, but did not discuss the management or outcome of these complications.

Delayed Closure

Two types of delayed closure have been recently described. Nelson and associates[801] have described three cases closed by delayed pedicle grafts. They undermined the graft from the medial and lateral borders on one or two occasions before bringing both grafts together in the midline for a vertical closure on day 7–10. One developed an abscess. In another small series, Winston and associates[1227] described the use of Teflon (Codman and Shurtleff, Billerica, MA) mesh to repeatedly snug up skin margins of three open meningomyeloceles measuring 7 × 5.5 cm, 10.5 × 7 cm, and 6 × 6.5 cm. Teflon® mesh was placed in the space between

---

all epithelium have been excised, pia arachnoid and dura are closed over the open neural plaque to form a single nervous system membrane: tube A.[(600)] The paraspinous muscles and, if necessary, protruding vertebral alae are then cut to free up superficial myofascia.[(A2)] One muscle flap is then folded over to be sutured to the base of the opposite side at B1 and B2. The opposite side is then freed up and folded over the top of the other flap graft and sutured over the top of the first muscle flap (C1 and C2). If the deformed vertebral alae protrude, they are cut with an osteotome and included in the muscle flap, as shown in B and C.

both edges of the skin so that the subcutaneous tissue would grow into the Teflon®; mattress sutures also held the Teflon® to the skin several centimeters from the skin margins. Every 2–3 days, the Teflon® pieces were firmly resutured together, putting maximum tension on the skin margins toward the midline. This technique achieved full-thickness closure in 7–10 days without skin grafts, relaxing incisions, or rotation flaps. Although closure time was more rapid than with Nosik's use of Tantalum mesh,[815] concern about infection requires further evaluation of a larger series.

Bipedicle Grafts: Immediate Closure

A bipedicle graft is created by incisions made on each side of the defect, parallel to the midline near the midaxillary line (Fig. 6-3). These incisions create bipedicle grafts. The width of each graft should be at least one half the width of the defect, and the length of the graft should be no greater than twice its width.[58,801,1255] Immediate closure by bipedicle grafts (Fig. 6-3), with natural healing or application of split-thickness grafts to the sites left open by the relaxing incisions, would appear to be the most popular and effective technique to close large meningomyeloceles.[442,600,733,739,848,1255] At the time of initial closure, we routinely apply split-thickness grafts to any open sites left by relaxing incisions. We can usually discharge patients after a total of 10–14 days, a week or more before those subjected to delayed skin-to-skin or split-thickness graft closure of donor sites, as described by Habal and Vries.[442]

MENINGOMYELOCELE CLOSURE: SEATTLE METHOD AND RESULTS

Up until this point, we have described separate layer components of our closure techniques in relation to those aspects discussed by others. In reality, the entire process of handling the open meningomyelocele lesion—from birth through closure and stabilization of CSF dynamics with complete healing of all wounds—is one continuum. We recommend that referring physicians handle the open lesion, as discussed in an earlier section of this chapter, by protecting the lesion against trauma and drying with the use of sterile, nonadhesive, loosely held bandages kept moist with sterile saline or Ringer's lactate solution. In addition, we recommend immediate referral to a center experienced with meningomyelocele repairs, with the infant prone or side-lying and handled by sterile technique in an isolette. If the sac is intact and full of fluid, it should be protected so as to avoid rupture.

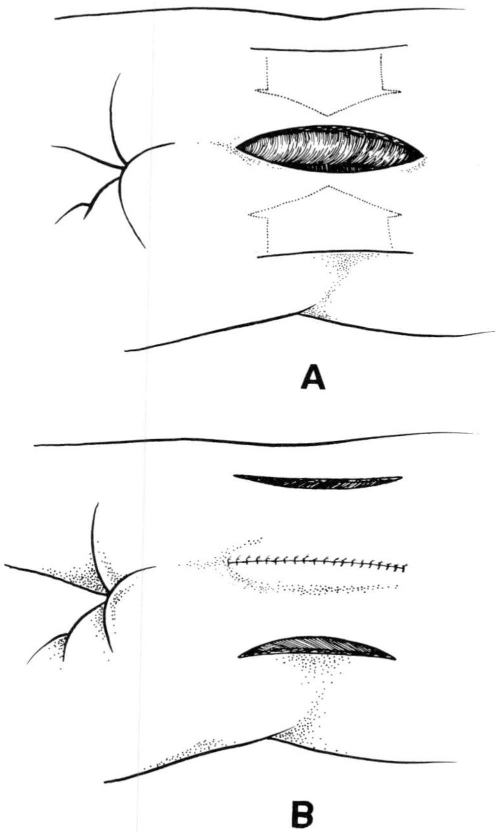

Figure 6-3. Bipedicle, full-thickness grafts. If the lesion cannot be closed tension free by a midline straight *T*, *Y*, or horizontal closure, an area at least one-half as wide as its length is undermined, and longitudinal incisions are made on each side of the defect (A). The medial borders of these full-thickness grafts are then closed in the midline. Split-thickness grafts from the posterior thighs are then placed over the skin defects left on each side (B).

When the infant arrives, we culture the plaque surface and CSF aspirated from the subarachnoid space ventral to the plaque, as illustrated in Figure 6-1.

The needle should enter lateral to the sac via normal skin and pass medially between veretebral alae and thus into the enlarged ventral subarachnoid space. The needle should not enter via the midline above the lesion or in the cisterna magna because malformation of cord and the Arnold-Chiari malformations obliterate the dorsal subarachnoid spaces in these areas. We begin intravenous antibiotics as if we are treating bacterial meningitis. Antibiotics are chosen on the basis of epidemiologic studies at the hospital where the baby was born or at our own hospital or, in the cases that present with infected CSF, sensitivity studies of the organism. Unless indicated otherwise by these studies, we use gentamycin 5–7 mg/kg/day and Staphcillin (meticillin, Bristol Laboratories, Syracuse, NY) 100 mg/kg/day. Back repair is scheduled to immediately follow assessment and discussion with the family as outlined in Chapters 3 and 5. Only in children with thoracic and high-lumbar lesions associated with atrophy of muscles ennervated at levels distal to L2 (maximum of hip flexor and adductor function) do we delay closure and discuss potential outcome with parents as recommended by Charney and associates[180] (see Chapter 5). We believe the increase in risk for CNS infection, permanent loss of neuromotor function in exposed nerves, and local infection with subsequent arachnoiditis and later cord tethering to be too great to delay closure.[741] All parents, even those who do not wish to care for their children, are relieved by early surgical intervention. In the event they cannot, for whatever reasons, care for a child with meningomyelocele, they can relinquish, and adoptive parents can be found as discussed in Chapter 5. The less an infant is handicapped, the easier will be adoption.

During the surgical procedure, CSF is sent for analysis of cell, protein, and sugar content as well as culture. The wound is irrigated liberally with $\frac{1}{4}$% Neomycin solution or a 1:1000 solution of Bacitracin. Intravenous antibiotics begun preoperatively are continued until pre- and intraoperative cultures demonstrate no growth after 48 hours. With the aid of magnification during dissection, we preserve the neural elements at the subarachnoid junction with the neural plaque. We have not used the somatosensory-evoked potentials recommended by McLone and associates[742] and Reigel[903] or electromyographic recordings of the anal sphincter.[538] Nor have we used somatic nerve stimulation and urinary or rectal pressure sensors as suggested by Pang and Casey[837] and Shapiro and Fried.[1012]

Regardless of the surgeon's technical preferences, three layers of closure should be accomplished. Because of the unique anatomical features, the repair must be individualized.[733] Our closure methods are described below.

Closure of Neural Elements

During the past ten years, we have used five methods to close the neural tube. The plaque was removed from a 4-year-old child with lower extremity spasticity and no useful motor function or sensation in the lower extremities, and a watertight arachnoid-dura closure was accomplished prior to kyphectomy and spinal fusion. The difficult-to-manage spastic diplegia that existed preoperatively was converted to a relatively easily managed flail diplegia. The four other types of closure performed on our Seattle patients were as follows: (1) in two cases, the plaque was invaginated and entubulated with both a pia-arachnoid and watertight, arachnoid-dural closure as described by McLone[739]; (2) on 107 occasions, the plaque was replaced into the spinal canal without entubulation but with a watertight, arachnoid-dura closure; (3) the plaque was replaced into the spinal canal with a myofascial duraplasty in two cases; and (4) only dura was used to close over an open plaque in one case because of insufficient arachnoid (Table 6-1).

Myofascial Closure

Three of the lesions in our Seattle group were covered directly by only full-thickness skin and subcutaneous tissue with only partial myofascia coverage (Table 6-1). On 24 occasions, paraspinous myofascia was turned caudally to provide adequate coverage. These flap grafts were folded over low-sacral fascial defects. When inadequate myofascia was present, free patch grafts were created for three patients to supplement this type of closure. Four lesions were covered by patch grafts only. On 79 occasions, bilateral flap grafts were imbricated; 74 were paraspinous myofascia (Fig. 6-2), and five cases with insufficient tissue needed partial gluteus maximus or lattissimus dorsi. These flap grafts were turned caudally and medially to complete the two-layer closure. Lattissimus dorsi flap grafts are created by freeing superficial layers of muscle and fascia from just below the scapula. If there is also insufficient myofascial tissue in the lumbosacral area, partial lattissimus dorsi flaps can be turned caudally and medially. The latter are folded caudally towards the coccyx after incisions that free up superficial layers of lattissimus dorsi. We have observed that both lumbosacral myofascial flaps imbricated across the midline and latissimus dorsi grafts function as spinal extensor muscles, essentially replacing the erector spinous muscles. We have also observed stabilization of kyphotic lesions when adequate muscle has been trans-

Table 6-1
Surgical Closure

Surgical Method	Number of Cases	Number[a] With Lipo
Neural tube		
Arachnoid/Dura	107	12
Excision of cord	1	
Dura only	1	
Myofascial duraplasty	2	
Entublated cord, two-layer arachnoid	2	
Total	113	12
Myofascia		
Imbricated lumbodorsal myofascial flap grafts	74	5
Midline grafts cephalad to caudad to midline	24	6
Myofascial (lattissimus dorsi or gluteal) imbricated flap grafts	5	
Patch grafts (free myofascia) plus myofascial flap grafts	7	
No myofascial closure (or incomplete)	3	1
Total	113	12
Skin		
Vertical	65	12
Horizontal	5	
Oblique	1	
*Y-V**	14	
*T**	3	
Bipedicle, double	21	
Bipedicle, single	4	
Total	113	12

* Y, V and T = shape of closure after trimming away excess skin.
[a] Lipomyelomeningocele.

planted across open spine defects, which agrees with McLaurin's hypothesis.[733]

Lesions in the low-sacral area were closed by myofascial layers using one of three techniques where no myofascial layers were available locally.[733] Those techniques were (1) medially imbricated myofascia from superficial gluteus maximus on one occasion, (2) caudally folded lattissiums dorsi flap grafts on four occasions, and (3) the only four completely covered by free myofascial grafts. None of the myofascial grafts or flaps broke down, became infected, allowed a CSF fistula to form, or needed reclosure.

Skin Closure

Our approach to skin closure has incorporated three basic principles: (1) approximate only good full-thickness skin, (2) provide closure that is tension free, and (3) approximately in the midline so as to preserve blood supply to all portions of grafts that will allow later midline vertical incisions for skeletal surgery. Partial skin layers from the edge of the lesion break down easily and do not take well as grafts. Tension-free approximation of skin closure is necessary to prevent skin slough, the most common complication. As our first preference, we use midline closure with tension-free skin margins. Skin on each side of the lesion is undermined far enough away from the lesion to allow the skin to be approximated in the midline without compromising blood supply secondary to tension. If the skin blanches or becomes dusky, then it is necessary to provide more adequate blood supply by freeing up single[683] or double bipedicle grafts. Osteotomy of protruding alae[785] has also been used. Because of the varied nature of open meningomyelocele lesions, we have used multiple closure methods.

Eighty-eight lesions in our Seattle group were covered by skin freed up at the margins, without need for relaxing incisions or creation of bipedicle grafts (65 vertical midline closures and 23 either horizontal or *T*- or *Y*-shaped closures) (Table 6-1). The other 25 required single, horizontal bipedicle grafts and *T* closures (single) or double, vertical bipedicle grafts (21 times) to provide tension-free midline closure.

Complications

Complications have been noted in Tables 6-2 and 6-3. Seven patients (6 percent) developed skin breakdowns and required eight split-thickness grafts; six were necrotic, and the seventh was a wound dehiscence. Sixteen (14 percent) developed minor skin sloughs varying in size from less than a square centimeter to 1 × 2.5 cm; all healed without surgical intervention.

None of the patients developed a CSF fistula. Two patients (1.8 percent) with a single-layer arachnoid-dural closure developed deep CSF leaks underneath their myofascial flap grafts. Both resolved after CSF shunt insertion. One had no other complications; the other developed a shunt-related infection as mentioned above in the section, "Closure of Neural Elements." During the initial shunt procedure and first two revisions, cultures of CSF and parts of the shunt tubing were sterile. *Staphylococcus aureus* was grown from CSF obtained 2 days after onset of fever and illness, during a third revision 2 months after back closure and 4 weeks after the skin breakdown healed. Five (4.4 percent) other children developed CSF infections following insertion of their original

Table 6-2
Complications Associated with Back Closures

Total Number of Procedures	Size of Lesion (cm)	Type of Operative Closure of Skin		Postoperative Skin Breakdown[a] (cms)		Postoperative Infection	Other Postoperative Complications
				Major	Minor		
24	4.0	Vertical,	19	—	1, 1 × 1	—	Tethered cord
						1, postshunt 1, post–back repair	2 later died, AC 5 mo[b] 1, AC, age 1 yr
		H, T, V-Y,	5	1, 3 × 4	—	—	
		Bipedicle,	0	—	—	—	
26	4.1–5.0	Vertical,	19	1, 2 × 3 1, 1.5 × 2	—	—	1, deep CSF leak[c]
		H, T, V-Y,	5	—	1, 1	—	—
		Bipedicle,	2	—	—	—	—
34	5.1–7.0	Vertical,	19	1, 5 × 7+ 2 × 4	1, 2.5 × 1 3, 1 × 1	1, pre–back closure	—
		H, T, V-Y,	5	—	1, 1 × 1	1, pre–back closure	—
		Bipedicle,	10	1, 1 × 6	3, 1 × 1 1, 1 × 1	1, postshunt plus deep CSF leak[d]	

13	7.1–9.0	Vertical,	1	—	1, 1 × 1	—	—
		H, T, V-Y,	6	1, 4 × 8	—	—	—
		Bipedicle,	6	—	3, 1 × 1	—	1, tethered cord 1, died, age 6, AC
7	9.1	Vertical,	4	—	—	—	—
		H, T, V-Y,	0	—	—	—	—
		Bipedicle,	3	—	1, 1 × 1	—	—
21	?	Vertical,	15[c]		—	—	—
		H, T, V-Y,	2	1, 8 × 5	—	—	—
		Bipedicle,	4		—	1, postshunt	—

[a] Major, required split-thickness graft; minor, epithelialized.
[b] One patient had *E. coli* and *S. venticulomeningitis* right after back repair and *S. epidermitis* ventriculomeningitis 1 month later. He was cured and a shunt was inserted. He died 3 months later with apnea and bradycardia thought to be due to AC.
[c] CSF beneath myofascial flaps resolved following CSF shunt.
[d] One patient with a small skin breakdown also had a deep CSF leak, but both resolved. *S. aureus* was cultured during the third shunt revision 2 days after onset of fever and illness after the second revision.
Abbreviation: AC, Arnold-Chiari malformation.[851] CSF = cerebrospinal fluid; H, T, V, Y, V-Y under Type of operative closure of skin = type of wound after trimming excess skin.

Table 6-3
Complications

Complication	Percentage of Cases	Number of Cases
Skin breakdown		
Superficial: spontaneous epithelialization[a]	14	16
Major: requires split-thickness skin graft	6	7
Subcutaneous hematoma (fix with leech)	.9	1
Cerebrospinal fluid leak (beneath myofascial flap graft)[a]	1.8	2
Tethered spinal cord[b]	1.8	2
CSF infection[c]		
Prior to back repair	1.8	2
Post–back repair prior to shunt	.9	1
Postshunt	4.4	5
Subtotal	7	8
Apnea and bradycardia and laryngeal stridor (clinical Arnold-Chiari)	2.7	3

[a] One patient had all three: shunt infection after second revision was detected at third revision at 2 months post–back repair and shunt insertion.

[b] One patient had superficial skin breakdown plus tethered cord. The other tethered cord occurred after myofascial duraplasty.

[c] Two were detected with meningitis treated preoperative with no recurrence. One was with two episodes with post–back repair surgery; one occurred immediately postoperative due to *E. coli* and *Streptococcus*. The other occurred 2 months later due to *S. Epidermitis*. Both were cured; there was a subsequent shunt. Patient died 1 month postshunt with apnea and bradycardia secondary to Arnold-Chiari malformation (postmortem exam). Four patients developed fever and signs of infection postshunt insertion; organisms were *S. epidermiditis* (two), *E. coli*, and *Enterococcus*; the fifth patient had *S. aureus* grown from CSF during third revision.

shunts. These shunts were placed between 2 and 18 days after back closure. Two others were detected to have CSF infection on admission, were treated medically, and then their backs were closed. Neither had subsequent complications, but one is moderately to severely mentally retarded. (This patient had been referred from 275 miles away from our center.) It seems more appropriate to consider these infections as not related to our process for closure of meningomyeloceles. Indolent organisms that may have developed into overt CNS infection could have been introduced at the time of back repair only to become symptomatic when a foreign body, the CSF shunt, was inserted. The frequency of shunt infections after back repair compared with experience with non–meningomyelocele-related shunt procedures is discussed in more detail in Chapter 7. As with CSF shunt procedures, we have used prophylactic antibiotics during repair of meningomyelocele lesions. The only child to develop an unequivocal post–back repair infection was given ampicillin as the only antibiotic. The *Enterococcus* that caused the infection was ampicillin-resistant. It is interesting that this same child returned to the hospital 2 months later with a *Staphylococcus epidermititis* ventriculitis and meningitis. He had not yet had a CSF shunt. The primary author has previously noted the relationship among CNS anomalies, hydrocephalus, and increased risk for purulent meningitis[1053] This patient later developed laryngeal stridor and apnea not relieved by a CSF shunt and died.

Other complications may or may not be related to the technique of open neural tube defects closure. We have observed two of our patients (1.8 percent) develop adhesions and late symptoms of "tethered cord syndrome." To date, one of our two cases of tethering occurred after simple replacements with arachnoid-dura closure. The other was in a $4\frac{1}{4}$-year-old boy who had a 9 × 11 cm open meningomyelocele with kyphosis and a shallow spinal canal. The broad plaque could not be covered by arachnoid or dura mater, and a fascial graft was used to complete dural closure. A 7-cm adhesion bound the cord to the thoracolumbar site of closure and caused progressive spasticity and weakness prior to surgical release. The incidence of tethering may be affected by duration of follow-up as much as by technique of closure so that future studies of populations of patients subjected to different closure techniques need to be undertaken.

No accounts, to our knowledge, report death from later complications of the original defect. The three children in our series to develop fatal Arnold-Chiari malformation symptoms of apnea and bradycardia do not include a fourth who is still in the hospital on monitors. None of these patients manifested symptoms at the time of back repair, and only one did at the time of shunt insertion.

Unfortunately, few reports have sufficient numbers and details about follow-up to allow assessment of the differences in closure methods. McLone[739] reported the following results: 17 of 78 (23 percent) of his cases developed CSF fistulae; five (6.4 percent) required reclosure, and two (2.6 percent) developed CNS infection. Guthkelch and associates[438] presented different results: two of 25 (8 percent) invaginated plaques and two of 25 (8 percent) plaque replacements with arachnoid-dural and myofascial closure developed CSF leaks; and one in each group (4 percent) developed CNS infection. Only one of our patients manifested post–back closure CNS infection (0.9 percent). The majority of infections of the CNS we encountered were detected before back repair or after CSF shunts were inserted. It is not clear from McLone's or Guthkelch and associates' reports[739,438] whether their infection rates included only those infections detected before, or both before and after, shunt insertion. There may be a relationship between shunt infections and the presence of indolent organisms in the CSF of children with recent meningomyelocele repairs that accounts for the higher shunt infection rate reportedly associated with meningomyelocele repair than with shunt procedures performed on children with a closed CNS.[581,716,1052] We recommend, therefore, that as long a time as possible be allowed to elapse between repair of an open meningomyelocele and insertion of a CSF shunt. We now use 1,4:3,6 dianhydro-D-glucitol to prolong this period.[672,1056,1059]

MENINGOCELE CLOSURE

Closure of meningoceles is similar to meningomyelocele closure. Because meningoceles are usually covered with skin and not ruptured, closure is not an urgent matter. Since meningoceles are associated not with paralysis but with the danger of rupture or injury to normal functioning though relatively unprotected nerves, there is usually no difficulty in reaching agreement with all concerned that meningoceles should be repaired. Care must be exercised in trimming the sac to protect neural function by preserving nerves and blood supply. Care must also be exercised in production of a watertight dural closure and eliminating any ectodermal or mesodermal tissue from the nervous system closure. Nonneural elements may later develop into a space-occupying mass within the restructured neural canal.[742,903,1188] Such lesions, along with tethering of the cord, can cause late onset of neural function loss, as is discussed in more detail below.

LIPOMENINGOCELES, LIPOMENINGOMYELOCELES, AND LIPOMYELOCELES

Repair of lipomeningoceles, lipomeningomyeloceles, and lipomyeloceles and lumbosacral lipomas is more controversial than repair of open meningomyeloceles, unless they are causing progressive impairment of function.[43,536,634,742,793,903,1188] The reasons for operating include prevention of future neurologic loss and return of recently lost neural function.[1C12] Hoffman and associates[493] as well as McLone and associates[742] report a higher incidence of permanent neurologic loss after 6 months of age. We, therefore, investigate and repair these lesions when first recognized.

Since these lipomas associated with incomplete closure of the spine arise from those portions of the neural tube developing from canalization and regression (Chapter 3), they are different from meningomyeloceles in several ways. They are extremely rarely associated with family recurrence, they are skin covered, and they are not usually associated with CNS anomalies, including hydrocephalus, the Arnold-Chiari malformation, and mental retardation. They also differ because tethering of the cord by the lipoma or a firm fibrovascular band at the cephalad edge of the open spine defect (usually at the caudal end of the intact spine) will cause progressive loss of neurological function. These fibrovascular bands pass horizontally between the most cephalad open vertebral arches and kink the cord as it passes dorsally between an enlarged subarachnoid space that forms a meningocele and the lipoma.[742,793] A lipoma can be partially intraspinal but mostly extradural, as can be parts of lipomas associated with meningoceles. These lipomas can cause progressive neural function loss in the lower extremities and sphincters by either pressure on neural tissue or producing traction on the cord due to adhesions to myofascia.

Reigel[903] and Shapiro and Fried[1012] also attribute upper extremity and midbrain malfunction as well as lordosis with spasticity and a wide-based gait to tethering. Intraspinal canal extensions of the lipoma can also cause progressive paralysis by pressure on nervous tissue. A third mechanism for production of progressive paralysis is scarring and subsequent retethering after an initial attempt at reconstructive surgery.[742,903,1012,1188] Venes and Stevens[1188] recommend a dural patch and delayed myofascial closure to provide space and prevent retethering. McLone and associates[742] and Reigel[903] stress the need for complete arachnoid-dural closure over a pia-arachnoid closure of the neural plate after removal of lipoma. We have resected as much lipoma as possible and relieved tethering as described by Venes and Stevens[1188] before closing the lesions as for open meningomyeloceles (Table 6-1). None of our twelve lesions has become infected, broken down, or become retethered.

MANAGEMENT OF LUMBOSACRAL MASSES

The initial approach toward management of skin-covered lesions in the lumbosacral area is to define the nature of the spinal dysraphism and lumbosacral mass.[43,634] The second is to accurately identify the extent of nervous system involvement.[793] Surgical reconstitution should consider the possibility of sacrococcygeal cysts that have malignant degenerative potential unless the mass and a tract to the coccyx are completely removed.[634] These benign-appearing lesions are far more sinister than the formidable-appearing sacrococcygeal teratomas.[634] Surgical management of the true lipomas associated with spinal dysraphism should be directed toward (1) release of tethering by the transverse fibrovascular bundle and the lipoma itself as well as by associated defects, such as a shortened and thickened filum terminale or a diastematomyelia[43,742,1012,1188]; (2) reduction of the intraspinal canal lipoma to lessen the chance of pressure on, and destruction of, contiguous nervous tissue, but at the same time, avoidance of excessive removal of the lipoma with resultant damage to functioning nervous tissue; and (3) reconstruction of a pia-arachnoid and dura mater tube around the existing lipoma and nerves to prevent CSF leakage and to lessen the chance of scarring and recurrence of tethering.[742,903,1188] Continued management should carefully monitor sphincter and lower extremity neuromuscular and sensory function to detect retethering of the cord or pressure from lipoma left in situ.

We agree with McLone and associates[742] that children with lipomas associated with dysraphic spinal defects should be followed regularly in a multidisciplinary clinic to monitor lower extremity and sphincteric function and to provide appropriate multidisciplinary management of existing impairments. We conduct detailed range-of-motion and muscle-strength testing on a yearly basis, and, with questionable or definite loss of function, we conduct electromyographic studies to detect deenervation potentials. Routine urinary bladder function studies can reveal urinary bladder and sphincter changes that signal nerve function loss in the presence of normal leg muscle function. In the presence of suspected losses, we carry out computerized axial tomography of the lower spine with matrizamide myelography, as described by Naidich and associates.[793] If suspicious mass or tethering effects are observed, we explore the involved area with the intent to reduce lipoma mass and relieve tethering.

SUMMARY

We recommend early, urgent closure of open neural tube defects of the spine when there is any suspicion that there may be useful function of the large muscles of the thigh or more function in the lower extremity. Such closure is warranted to prevent further damage to the neural plaque from trauma, drying, or infection. Infants with less muscle function can be observed during a reasonable time when long-term plans can be arranged. Closure should include return of the neural plaque to the canal with watertight closure of the arachnoid-dura. If possible, the neural plaque should be entubulated. Preferably, a double-layer myofascial closure should be completed to protect the neural tube and provide extensor erecti spinal muscles. The skin should be closed with a tension-free closure in the midline so that later skeletal surgery can be carried out without concern about blood supply to the overlying skin. Throughout the period of exposure of the nervous system, the infant should be treated as if a bacterial meningitis is present. Pre–back closure cultures and spinal fluid analysis should be undertaken in order to detect and treat infection. Skin-covered lesions of the spine should be investigated thoroughly, and repair should be undertaken before loss of nervous system function.

David Shurtleff
J. Timothy Stuntz
Patricia Hayden

7

Hydrocephalus

Writers throughout the period from 1858 until the present have emphasized the importance of hydrocephalus in the management of meningomyelocele as discussed in Chapter 5. Earlier writers recommended careful selection of cases before back closure because a patient, cured of an open back lesion and protected from the resultant infection with the likelihood of a quick death, could be afflicted with progressive hydrocephalus and horrible disfigurement or slow, painful death.[71,532,594,700,772,1071] However, Dandy's[241b] descriptions of CSF origin, flow, and absorption helped solve this problem in the 1920–1950 era; his concepts led to two new operations for hydrocephalus and shunts to drain CSF. The purpose of this chapter is to present current concepts about management of increased CSF pressure.

Scarff[975] and others perfected the two operations introduced by Dandy. Plexectomy for communicating hydrocephalus and third ventriculostomy for obstructive hydrocephalus were reported to cure hydrocephalus approximately 65–70 percent of the time and were associated with a 5–15 percent operative mortality and considerable morbidity.[975] Nevertheless, they were more successful than the various types of CSF shunts also designed during this same period and based on Dandy's concepts.

Generally, these early CSF shunts failed for eight reasons: (1) lack of understanding of indications for, and limitations of, different shunt

MYELODYSPLASIAS AND EXSTROPHIES: SIGNIFICANCE, PREVENTION, AND TREATMENT
 ISBN 0-8089-1816-8

systems; (2) foreign body reactions to the shunt materials being used; (3) rigid shunt materials that resulted in tissue erosion; (4) metal in contact with CSF that allowed leaking of cations and central nervous system (CNS) damage; (5) inadequate valve and shunt systems that did not allow study of their function once in place, but did allow reflux of blood, urine, or other body fluids back into the CNS; (6) fluid and electrolyte problems due to loss of CSF via external shunts; (7) infection; and (8) shunt obstructions. The latter two problems, discussed in more detail later, are still with us today.

Over the past 30 years, better understanding of the basic hydrocephalic pathophysiology described by Dandy, combined with technical innovations, has improved the results of hydrocephalus management from the 40–50 percent "good" results (better survival and intellectual performance) of the 1950s[975] to the 85–90 percent good results in the 1970s and 1980s.[36,637,730,740,819,901,1058]

In order to explain current management of hydrocephalus associated with meningomyelocele, we will discuss treatment in four parts: (1) clinical pathophysiology, (2) technical management of hydrocephalus, (3) CSF infections and obstructions, and (4) the Seattle experience.

CLINICAL PATHOPHYSIOLOGY

Hydrocephalus is most commonly due to congenital causes such as aqueductal stenosis; it can also be of a congenital communicating nature.[901] There are other considerations, however. Some meningomyelocele lesions have an opening of the central canal draining CSF onto the cephalad surface of the plaque. The hydrocephalus that develops after closure of a meningomyelocele may be secondary to closure of this route through which CSF had been draining. Others have large leptomeningeal surfaces that absorb some CSF. When those surfaces are removed, CSF balance will be disturbed. Trauma from labor and vaginal delivery may produce enough bleeding to add hematogenic inflammation over the arachnoid granulations and later compromise a barely balanced congenital communicating hydrocephalus. These mechanisms, however, are not operative in all cases and do not account for the onset of head growth and accumulation of CSF postnatally in all patients.[901]

Amniotic Fluid Versus Atmospheric Pressure and Head Growth

Two other changes occur simultaneously with back closure: delivery from a confined, fluid-filled space of the uterus into the atmosphere and an abrupt termination of the mother's hormones from across the placenta.

The first alteration removes a constraining force from around the head and allows growth. The bones of meningomyelocele children's skulls are thin and poorly developed, with wider suture separations and larger fontanelles than their normal peers.[1116] The thin, weak skull is more susceptible to intracranial pressure.

Physiological Neonatal Diuresis and Hydrocephalus

Growth of the head frequently will not take place immediately after birth. During the latter portion of pregnancy, ultrasound indicates that previously progressive hydrocephalus can become stable.[402,1221] During the first few days of life, infants often lose weight and dehydrate. In these periods, a negative fluid balance may develop with diuresis due to, first, a decrease in and, then, an abrupt loss of maternal hormones entering the infant's blood from across the placenta. This negative fluid balance seems to affect the formation of CSF so that even the most progessively hydrocephalic infants will show no evidence of increase in their CSF collections until 3–7 days of age at the earliest.

Delayed Onset of Hydrocephalus

Some infants with milder degrees of CSF-absorption deficiencies may not develop symptoms or signs of hydrocephalus for months, and others may not for years. The latest onset of hydrocephalus in our series developed in a 27-year-old woman. Others have reported that only 80–90 percent of infants with meningomyelocele develop overt, symptomatic hydrocephalus in need of CSF shunts.[700,736,901,1113]

Symptoms and Signs of Hydrocephalus

The variability in age of onset and the severity of hydrocephalus requires that the family and practitioner caring for these children, with or without CSF shunts, be aware of the symptoms of increased intracranial pressure. These symptoms and signs can vary from the overt, easily diagnosable symptoms of bulging and tense fontanelle, vomiting, somnolence, and irritability to milder symptoms, including subtle personality changes, lethargy, interference with hand-eye coordination, and decreases in school performance[453,736,901] (Table 7-1).

Maintenance of Normal Head Size

With a better understanding of the subtle symptoms of hydrocephalus, the need for CSF shunts to control head growth *before* the cranial vault develops to adult size was recognized. Even without symptoms

Table 7-1
Shunt Obstruction Symptoms

Mild
- Personality change
- Decreased activity
- Changes in speech
- Decreased school performance: decreased hand–eye and/or visual-motor coordination, decreased Jepson-Taylor, Frostig, etc., test scores
- Decreased social relationships
- Increase in eating and weight gain
- Decrease in eating and weight loss
- Seizures start or increase
- Incontinence increase or onset
- Recurring headache
- Decreased visual acuity
- Papilledema
- Onset of or increased strabismus
- Onset of or increased spasticity in the lower extremities
- Onset of or worsening scoliosis
- Increase in OFC (occipitofrontal circumference)
- Temperature elevation

Moderate
- Above symptoms become worse
- Persistent frontal (behind the eyes) headache
- Infrequent emesis
- Decreased response to lethargy alternating with irritability

Severe
- Somnolence: difficult to arouse
- Pain of headache down neck
- Opisthotonos
- Constant emesis
- Refusal to eat
- Pupils still react, but may be sluggish

Critical (5–30-minute survival)
- In coma or barely responsive
- Pupils dilate, may be asymmetrical, flick or no response
- Vital signs change: blood pressure up, then down; pulse up, then down; respiratory rate irregular
- Probably some irreversible damage

during early childhood and infancy hydrocephalus should be controlled to allow the brain to grow into the CSF cavity. The hydrocephalus should be shunted if the greatest occipitofrontal circumference (OFC) approaches 50 cm before the age of 18 months (Fig. 7-1). Maintaining the maximum occipitofrontal circumference at 50 cm or less during early childhood prevents the following situations: a child with a large cranial vault who will not have potential brain growth to fill the large CSF spaces; a child with a thin brain that is stretched out over large fluid spaces and is, therefore, more susceptible to bleeding; and a child with an excessively large head who will be awkward and more prone to falling and head trauma.

A child's head can be maintained at a normal proportion to his or her body. First, head size can be monitored by measuring head growth and, when indicated, obtaining ultrasonographic or computer-assisted studies of the brain and CSF spaces. Second, if excess fluid accumulation is causing the head to enlarge, then drainage should be instituted to prevent permanent excess fluid. The head size can be allowed to minimally exceed the 98th percentile for an older child or adult since studies indicate that some hydrocephalic brains tend to grow bigger than the mean for unaffected peers of the same age.[303,533,716,1059]

Hydranencephaly and Far-Advanced Hydrocephalus: A Contraindication for Cerebrospinal Fluid Drainage

In more advanced degrees of hydrocephalus, a CSF shunt may be contraindicated. Both ultrasound and computer-assisted tomograms (CT scans) can provide an estimate of brain mass or volume when considered in relationship to head circumference.[533,716,1059] A child who has an excessively enlarged head and no chance of having his or her brain enlarge to any degree after decompression of the hydrocephalus is at higher risk for developing bleeding into the subarachnoid space. An excessively enlarged, soft cranial vault with wide sutures, filled with fluid, will produce a pressure at the opening of the shunt in the head equal to a column of fluid the same height as the distance between that shunt opening and the top of the head.

Intracranial hydrodynamics in a patient with fused sutures differ from those in an infant with open sutures since they involve a closed system with more rigid pressure differentials. The head with an open fontanelle and sutures, along with the accompanying potential for head collapse, is more similar to a column of water with a rubber dam on each end. Normally, brain tissue is subjected to two pressures: the CSF system pressure, which tends to enlarge the ventricles, and the venous drainage system pressure, which tends to reduce the CSF pressure.[447] The pressure

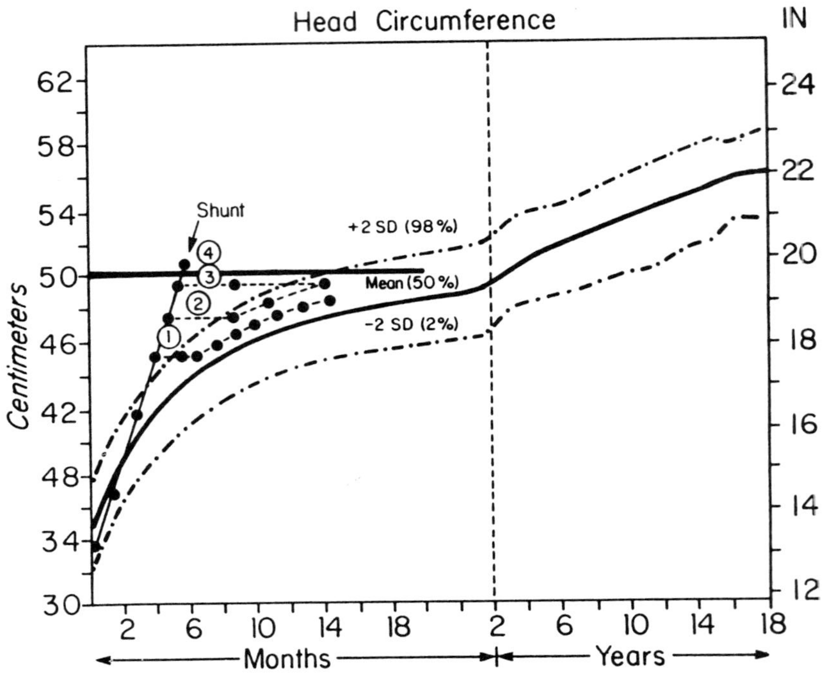

Figure 7-1. Head circumference chart. The child with hydrocephalus and myelodysplasia (usually only meningomyelocele) will be born most frequently with a small head. With time, the head may enlarge more rapidly than normal, stay near to maximum normal (1), or rise above the 98th percentile (2) a spontaneous arrest of hydrocephalus at an earlier age than 3, 3) a spontaneous arrest of hydrocephalus at age 3 or later and cease growing. Line 1 or 2 may be associated with static ventricle: brain ratio. Growth will recommence as soon as the brain grows into any hydrocephalic space. Continued growth of the head (4) that threatens to exceed 50 cm or is associated with symptoms of increased intracranial pressure (Table 7-1) is an indication for a cerebrospinal fluid shunt. (Modified from Nellhaus.[800])

difference between these two systems is responsible to a large extent for controlling the rate of CSF flow across the choroid plexus, ependyma, and arachnoid villi—that is, for CSF production and drainage.[248a] Thus, with the exception of choroid plexomas (CSF-producing tumors), CSF accumulation is dependent on pressure differentials that influence drainage.

In a hydrocephalic child, shunt drainage must compensate for the imbalance between the venous and CSF systems. When it is necessary to reduce the head size, the opening pressure of the shunt value must create a "controlled balance"; however, this balance must prevent fluid drainage to the extent that reduced intracranial pressure will cause intracranial bleeding or such a low pressure that headaches occur with erect posture (low-pressure syndrome). On the other hand, excess pressure will cause continued head growth. The valve transmission pressure must be such that the CSF drains at a rate equal to CSF production, thereby preventing both intracranial low pressure and progressive spinal fluid space and head enlargement.

However, shunt tips with their openings tend to float around in large fluid spaces created with far-advanced hydrocephalus and huge heads. If the shunt opening is at the top of the head and the opening pressure of the valve is moderate or high, then the pressure on the bottom of the child's head will be equal to the opening pressure of the valve plus the weight of the fluid between the opening of the shunt and the bottom of the head. Such a situation may cause continued head growth in the presence of a functioning CSF shunt (Fig. 7-2).

If a valve with a lower opening pressure is inserted to prevent growth, the pressure at the top of the head will become extremely low or negative if the valve remains in the same place and the child's head is rolled over. The weight of the fluid in the child's head will itself exceed the opening pressure of the shunt valve that is at the bottom of the head and cause so much fluid to be drained that a negative pressure will be recorded at the top of the skull (Fig. 7-2). Such a negative pressure may allow protein or blood to ooze or overtly bleed into the subarachnoid space or ventricle.

We have observed these hydrodynamic complications with CSF shunts placed in hydranencephalic or far-advanced hydrocephalic infants for social reasons.

TECHNICAL MANAGEMENT OF HYDROCEPHALUS

Ultrasound, CT scans, and molecular resonance imaging (MRI) allow safer, more frequent evaluation of the hydrocephalic process than was possible a decade ago. Air-contrast roentgenography was more accurate

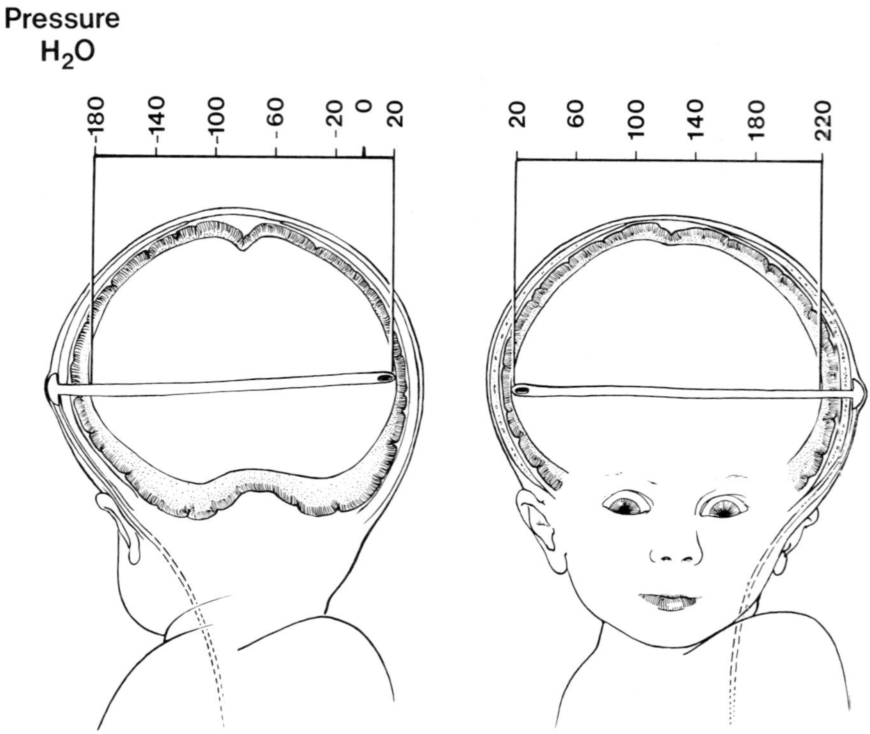

Figure 7-2. Continued head growth in the presence of a CSF shunt. The opening in the cerebral shunt tubing is illustrated as near the cerebral mantle laterally. The opening pressure of the valve is set at 20 mm of water. With the head lying so the shunt opening is at the bottom of the head, the child with a 20-cm head diameter will have a negative pressure of −180 mm at the top of the head (A): 200 mm pressure (column of CSF) minus 20 mm opening pressure of the shunt leaves a column of fluid 180 mm high that must be supported by negative pressure at the top of the skull. This degree of negative pressure may cause exudation of serum or blood into the subarachnoid or ventricle space. With the shunt opening at the top of 220 mm at the bottom of the skull (200 mm column of CSF + 20 mm opening pressure for the valve), such a high pressure may cause head growth (B). Modified from Shurtleff.[1045]

in defining whether or not the patient had communicating versus noncommunicating hydrocephalus, but it was far more likely to involve complications, a subject that will be addressed more extensively later in this chapter.

The safety and ease of both ultrasound for infants with open fontanelles and either MRI or CT for older children allow frequent evaluation and close monitoring of ventricular size as well as repeated evaluations for isolated fluid accumulations such as two-compartment hydrocephalus,[351] hydromyelia, diastematomyelia, intraspinal lipoma formation, and tethering of the cord.[793] Examination of infants pre- and postnatally by cranial ultrasound allows early detection of both enlarging ventricles and the need for a CSF shunt in the presence of questionable and mild symptoms or developmental delay. Repetition of ultrasound and CT studies can also be used to monitor children with and without shunts and thereby assure the physician and family that the ventricles are not enlarging. We have monitored ventricle size in our group of mildly hydrocephalic children being treated with 1,4:3,6 dianhydro-D-glucitol (Ismotic, Alcorn Laboratories, Forth Worth, Texas).[467,672,1056] Cranial ultrasound has also been useful for guiding placement of the tip of the shunt into the frontal horn of the lateral ventricle.[1031]

Following insertion of a shunt, cranial ultrasound and CT scans help to evaluate the degree of ventricle decompression. They permit detection of shunts operating at too high an opening pressure or intermittently so that the ventricles remain too large or at too low a pressure, causing the development of the slit ventricle syndrome, with formation of aqueductal stenosis[353] or adhesions of the ventricle walls and production of isolated compartments that can become symptomatic[351] (Fig. 7-3).

Other complications such as air leaks and bleeding (Fig. 7-4) can be readily demonstrated by CT scans. Despite the efficacy of these procedures, however, the do not provide an explanation of symptoms in all cases.

Gliotic Ventricle Syndrome

After prolonged decompression, a subependymal gliotic layer can develop around the ventricle walls and prevent expansion in the presence of symptomatic increases in intracranial pressure. In such children we have observed headaches down the neck and cardiopulmonary irregularities that suggest pressure on the midbrain. Such a mechanism has caused sudden death in seven of our teenage patients. Three were still alive at the time of entry to the emergency room but did not respond to chemical decompression. They had flat electroencephalographic tracings, and life support was withdrawn. Five of the seven had CSF systems without

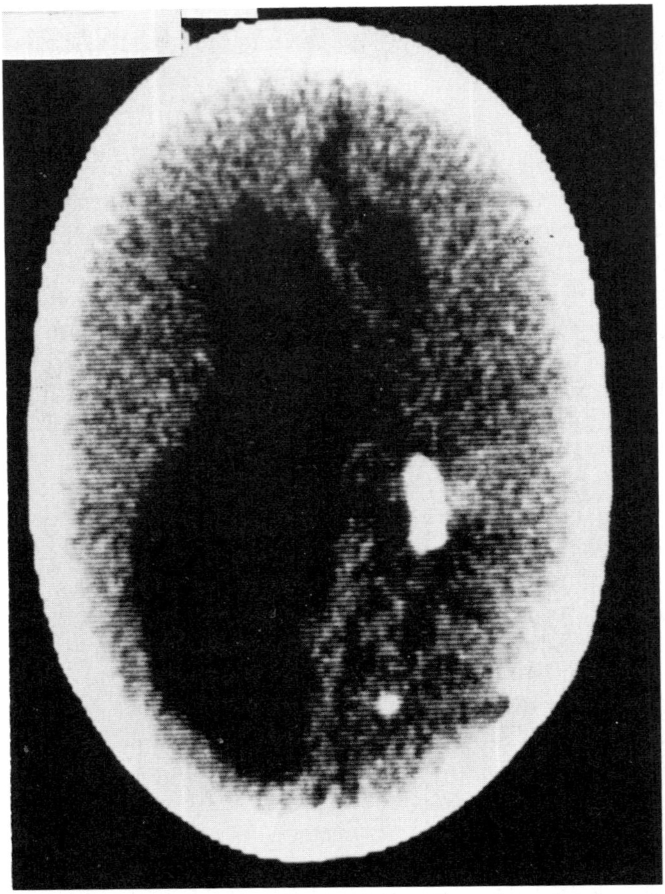

Figure 7-3. Adhesions of ventricle walls and production of symptomatic isolated compartments. This shows a CT scan of a child with a CSF shunt in place for 12 years. She complained of mild intermittent headaches and began to do poorly in school. She also manifested personality changes with irritability and short attention span. Her performance in mathematics dropped more than in other subjects. A shunt study revealed normal pressure, physiologic pulsations, and response to the Valsalva maneuver in addition to a rapid clearance. This CT scan demonstrates the decompressed left ventricle that is shifted to the left and contains the proximal limb of the shunt. The decompressed ventricle via a *Y* connector to the existing left ventricle CSF shunt. She became asymptomatic, and her academic skills improved. Diagnosis was isolated right ventricle hydrocephalus or two-compartment hydrocephalus.

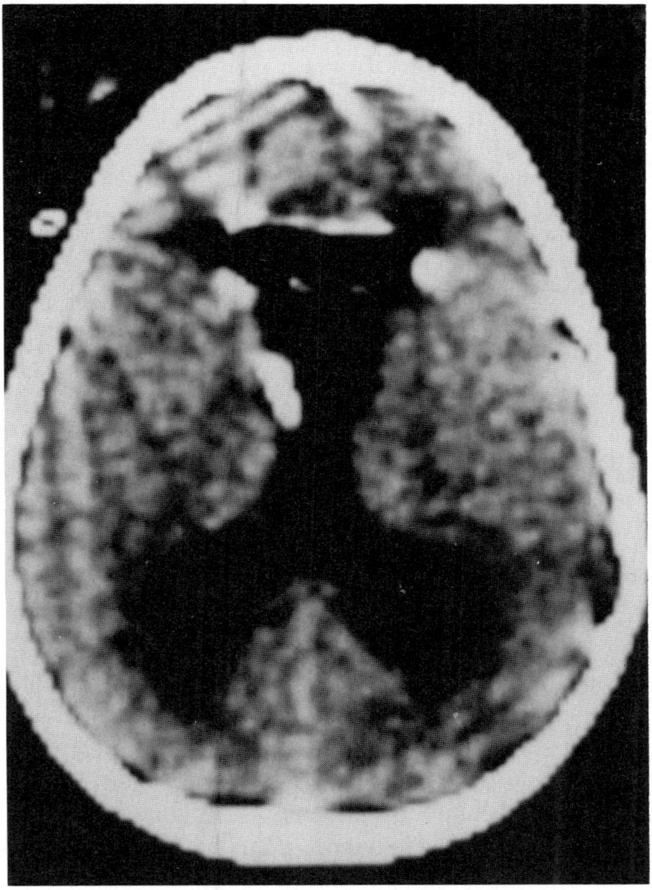

Figure 7-4. Shunt complications: air leaks and bleeding. This CT scan of an 11-year-old patient with a history of 18 months of recurrent shunt infections treated in another facility shows an air-fluid level with blood (white) in the brow-up position. Isotope CSF studies demonstrated the fistula. Antibiotics and a shunt revision after closing the CSF leak cured both the low-pressure headaches in the erect position and the infections. The hydrodynamic principles discussed in Figure 7-2 allowed the negative pressure in the patient's head in the standing position to suck air and bacteria into the head. Normal mechanisms for maintaining intracranial pressure could not compensate for the leak that allowed such negative pressures as to cause bleeding.

reservoirs, and the other two had proximal obstructions. Four had onset of symptoms approximately 1 hour to 20 minutes before arriving in the emergency room. Three were found dead in bed. One died on the operating table during an attempt to locate the tiny ventricles and CSF shunt tubing. Three died during cardiopulmonary resuscitation. An eighth patient with a proximal obstruction responded to 2.5 gm/kg of intravenous mannitol and subsequent shunt revision.

As a precaution against this calamity of sudden death from shunt obstruction in older children, we use a high-enough opening pressure valve to maintain mild hydrocephalus, a shunt system with a reservoir, and, with the earliest onset of headache, a dose of 2.5 gm/kg of 1,4:3,6 dianhydro-D-glucitol. The young man who recovered with mannitol has now avoided severe symptoms on two separate occasions by taking 1,4:3,6 dianhydro-D-glucitol with the onset of shunt obstruction symptoms. On both of these latter occasions, his shunt was obstructed, and he walked into the hospital with only a "pressure" headache partially relieved by the medication, not comatose as on the first occasion.

Shunt Pressure and Clearance Studies

In addition to noninvasive techniques for anatomic studies, we and others have developed pressure and flow determinations to assist in the evaluation of hydrocephalus after a CSF shunt has been inserted.[319,406,416,456,457,471] We have monitored over 360 patients with over 1000 combined pressure-radionuclide clearance studies. Pressure within the shunt system is first determined using a 0.01-cc displacement strain gauge attached to a fluid-filled tubing connected to a 25-gauge needle inserted into the shunt system reservoir. Pressure changes that correspond to heart beat, respirations, crying (Fig. 7-5), and the Valsalva maneuver can be readily seen if the shunt reservoir is in continuity with the cerebral ventricles. In such cases, a direct reading of ventricular pressure can be obtained, or the presence of a proximal obstruction can be identified. Before withdrawing the needle, a sample of CSF is obtained for cell count and culture, and 100 μCi of ^{99m}technetate is injected just before withdrawal of the needle. Then a clearance half time is measured by counting activity over the reservoir for 5 minutes, and the entire shunt system is imaged with a gamma camera.

These studies have demonstrated the following: (1) intermittent, partial shunt obstruction, (2) low pressure as a cause of symptoms, (3) peritoneal loculation, (4) proximal or distal obstruction, (5) breaks or leaks in the tubing that were not palpable, and (6) nonfunction with a patient system but a ventricular pressure less than the opening pressure of the valve. Seventy-two percent of the patients were shunt-dependent,

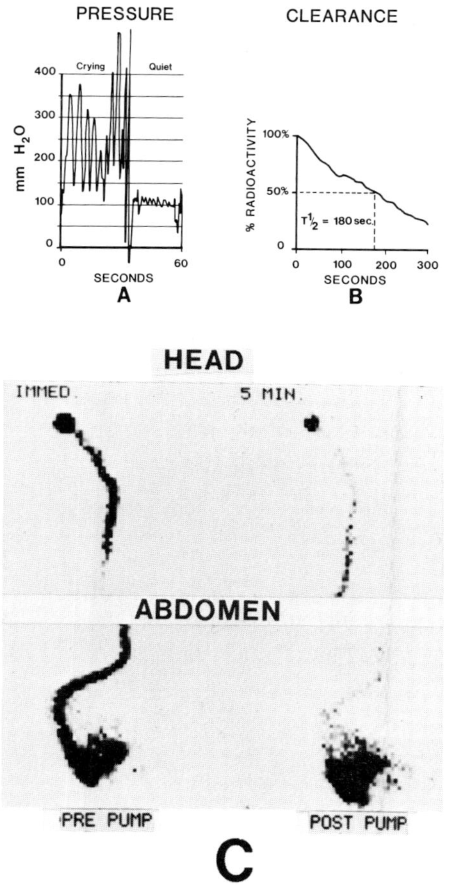

Figure 7-5. Functioning ventriculoperitoneal shunt: crying. Pressure (A) is measured with zero calibrated at the level of the reservoir before the needle is inserted into the reservoir. The pressure wave shows fluctuation corresponding to cardiorespiratory pressure changes (up to 200 mm H_2O). Note the increased pressure fluctuations with crying as a result of the Valsalva effect. Following insertion of the isotope, the half time for disappearance ($T\frac{1}{2}$) (B) was measured at 180 seconds, indicating a rapid flow. Gamma camera pictures of the shunt reservoir and tubing (C) as well as the abdomen both immediately and 5 minutes after isotope injection produced pictures indicating a rapid appearance of fluid in the peritoneal space and diffusion with absorption.

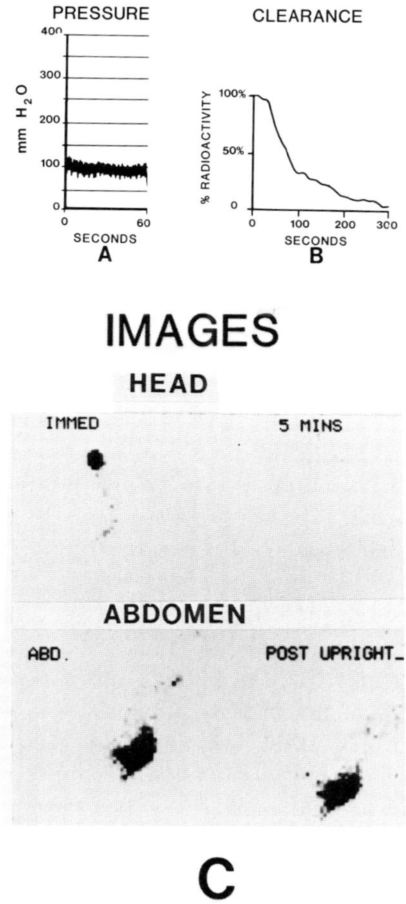

Figure 7-6. Functioning ventriculoperitoneal shunt: rapid radioactivity clearance. Rapid and complete (spontaneous) radioactivity clearance is evident. This illustration is similar to Figure 7-5, but there are wide pressure fluctuations due to heartbeats (A) and a more rapid clearance (B) (C) suggesting a greater need for CSF decompression.

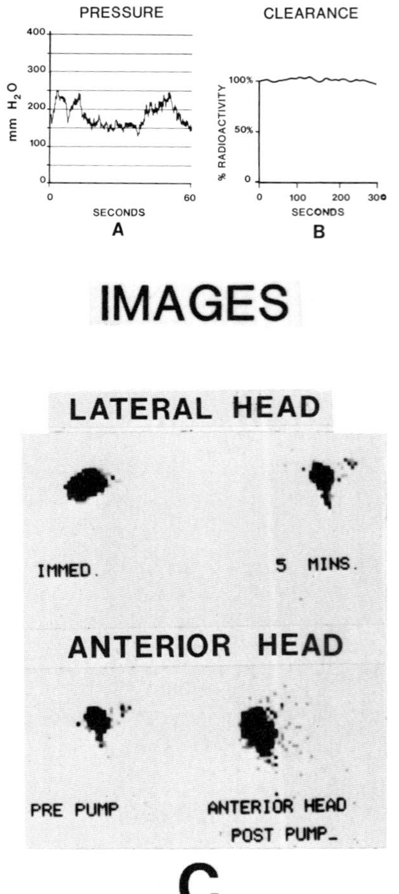

Figure 7-7. Distally obstructed shunt. The pressure is one-and-a-half to two times normal (A), and the half life disappearance is near to infinity after isotope decay is calculated (B). The gamma camera image (C) shows reflux of radioactivity into the enlarged right ventricle. When the shunt was pumped, there was no isotope visible in the distal tubing. Physiologic respiratory, cardiac, and Valsalva pressure changes were recorded along with reflux of isotope into the cerebral ventricle, indicating an open proximal and distally obstructed shunt.

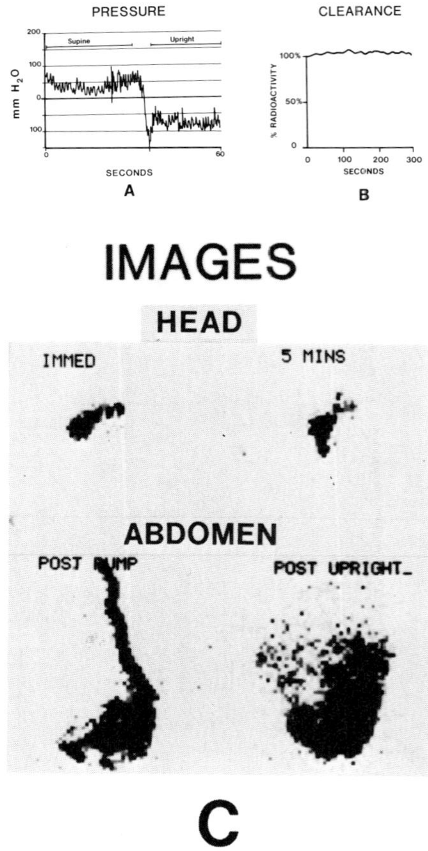

Figure 7-8. Positional low-pressure shunt. Pressure (A) is measured with zero calibrated at the level of the reservoir before the needle is inserted into the reservoir. Radioactivity (B) does not clear when the patient is supine, but does with pumping and upright positioning. Pressure falls markedly from a tolerable normal pressure in the supine position to minus 50 to 100 mm of fluid. As with Figures 7-5 and 7-6, the isotope flows freely through a shunt that is capable of functioning (C). An Antisiphon device (American V. Muller Inc, McGraw Park, IL) (see Fig. 7-11K) or a higher pressure valve needs to be inserted.

demonstrated by normal pressure and rapid isotope clearance (Fig. 7-6) or had obstructed shunts associated with clinical evidence of increased intracranial pressure (Fig. 7-7) or proximal obstruction with a nonphysiologic pressure tracing. Twenty-eight percent had asymptomatic nonfunctional shunts. Six patients have demonstrated low-pressure syndromes associated with headaches in the erect position relieved by lying down (Fig. 7-8). Partial proximal obstruction with normal or low pressure in the shunt reservoir and slow isotope clearance but enlarged ventricles under high pressure is the most difficult to interpret, particularly in the absence of a baseline CT scan or ultrasound obtained during a period of adequate decompression or with a gliotic, stiff ventricle wall (Fig. 7-9). Nonfunction of a ventriculoperitoneal shunt may occur due to increased distal resistance because of loculation of CSF in the abdomen (pseudocyst) (Fig. 7-10).

Of those with normal pressure and no or slow flow, 71 percent remained symptom free for 3–60 months, and 29 percent became symptomatic and required shunt revisions within 1–27 months after having the nonfunctional states of their CSF shunts identified.

We documented periods of alternating normal and high intracranial pressure in hydrocephalic children, an explanation for those patients in whom a temporarily asymptomatic, nonfunctional shunt has been identified.[468] One patient under our care lived for 17 years after shunt removal before developing signs and symptoms of recurrent increased intracranial pressure.

The differential diagnoses among multiple compartment hydrocephalus, low-pressure syndrome, intermittent or partial or complete shunt obstruction, and temporarily or permanently arrested hydrocephalus can be a challenge made much easier to sort out by careful evaluation of symptoms (Table 7-1), psychometric testing, and evaluating anatomy of the ventricles by ultrasound, MRI, or CT scan and pressure/nucleide flow studies.

Shunt Systems

Technical advances in the management and understanding of hydrocephalus have been accompanied by, and to a degree dependent on, improvement in the CSF shunt systems and materials. Scarff[975] criticized the use of CSF shunts when they were in the early stages of development and were complicated by a number of problems, listed at the beginning of this chapter. The large-diameter, tubular shunt, developed by Holter,[816] has been refined by adding a reservoir proximally[929] and by creating smaller sizes and distal tubing that will no longer easily perforate organs or erode skin.[217] The original single tube with a distal slit-core valve

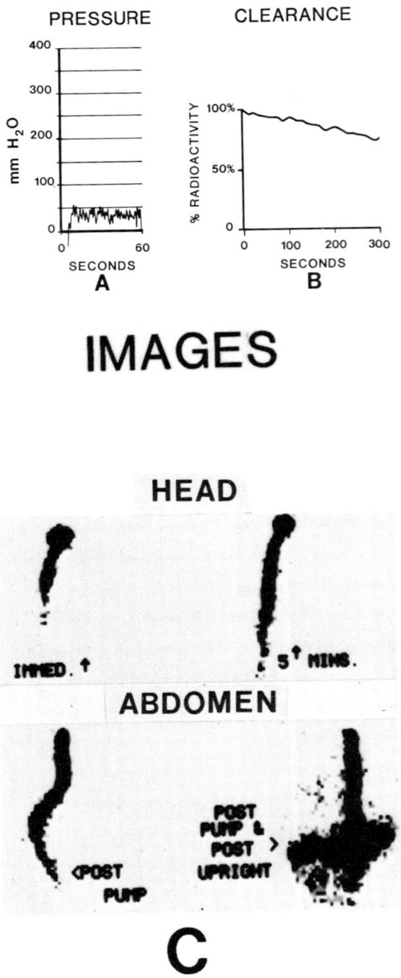

Figure 7-9. Normal or low pressure with slow clearance due to partial proximal obstruction. A previous study indicated this shunt functioned at 130 mm H_2O. T½ is greater than 10 minutes (A) (B). The gamma camera images (C) confirm that the distal portion is patent with rapid diffusion of the isotope throughout the peritoneal cavity. Physiologic respiratory and cardiac pulsations are present with partial obstructions, but oblated with complete proximal obstructions.

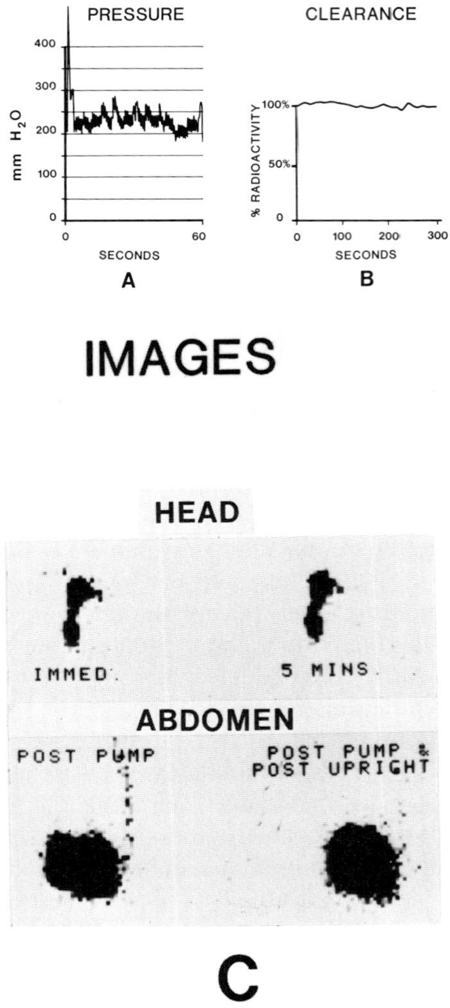

Figure 7-10. Abdominal loculation. The shunt itself is patent, but does drain despite high pressure. The pressure (A) is high with cardiac and respiratory excursions evident; the isotope has a slow flow (prolonged T½); (B) and the gamma camera image demonstrates the isotope is confined to an area immediately around the tip of the shunt (C). Abdominal studies revealed a CSF cyst, as shown in Figures 7-13A and 17-13B.

invented by Heyer[885] has been modified by the adoption of reservoirs, chambers with valves, occluder antisiphon devices, off-on valves, and distal tubing that will not kink or easily perforate organs.[484] The Cordis Company has introduced a valve (Hakim Cordis valve, Cordis Neurological Company, Miami, FL) that we have found handles CSF containing several grams percent of protein and thousands of cells.[222] These valve systems are shown in Figure 7-11. They all are competent, not allowing fluid to reflux back towards the brain, and can be inserted distally into the vascular system, peritoneal space, gallbladder, or pleural cavity.

The choices of shunt system and distal drainage site are as varied as the details of insertion. As a first choice, most centers place a Holter, Hakim, or Heyer system to drain the ventricles into the peritoneal space. We use a Heyer system with a Raimondi peritoneal catheter attached to a Foltz to-and-fro flushing reservoir that, in turn, is attached to a straight ventricular catheter. We use the straight rather than a flanged ventricular catheter because the latter is difficult to remove in the presence of infection and, particularly, if ventricle fluid has caused the material to harden.[999,1039] We use the Foltz reservoir because it allows access to the ventricular fluid spaces for assessment of pressure and treatment of infection as well as for measurement of flow characteristics of the shunt system.[471,657] In addition, with a distal shunt obstruction and high pressure with symptoms of brain herniation, CSF can be aspirated until a neurosurgeon arrives. This latter consideration and the temporary management of the hydrocephalus with mannitol or 1,4:3,6 dianhydro-D-glucital are important since many of our patients live in small, isolated towns and villages spread over a land mass that is 23 percent of the entire United States. Many of our patients may be kept from the nearest neurosurgeon by thousands of miles and, since the only mode of travel may be by airplane or boat, inclement weather. No matter where they live, the parents and patient should be made aware of what kind of shunt is being used. Despite an actual demonstration of a shunt system and provision of a book of written instructions, including a diagram, many of our patients and parents are unable to identify or describe their children's shunt systems. We encourage the use of a medical identification tag or bracelet and provide traveling families with a medical summary including a detailed description of their children's shunt systems.

Without the unique problems presented by our rural population, others recommend a shunt system with a reservoir for access to the shunt for either evaluation[319,787] or treatment of infection.[657,735] Fortunately, some of these systems can be identified by routine roentgenography (Fig. 7-12).

Another advantage of radiopaque shunt materials is that the course and tip of peritoneal catheters can be easily located. Plain abdominal

A

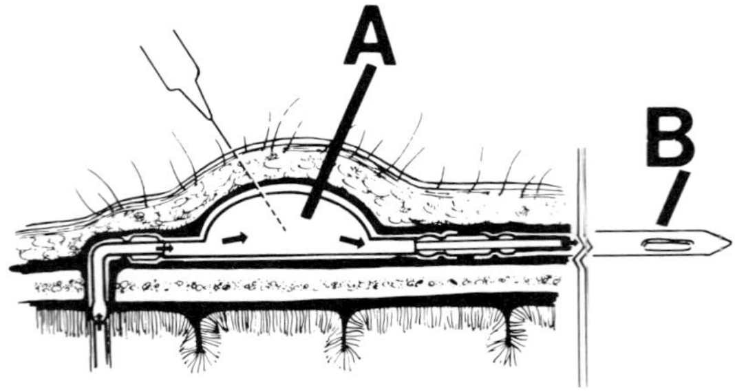

B

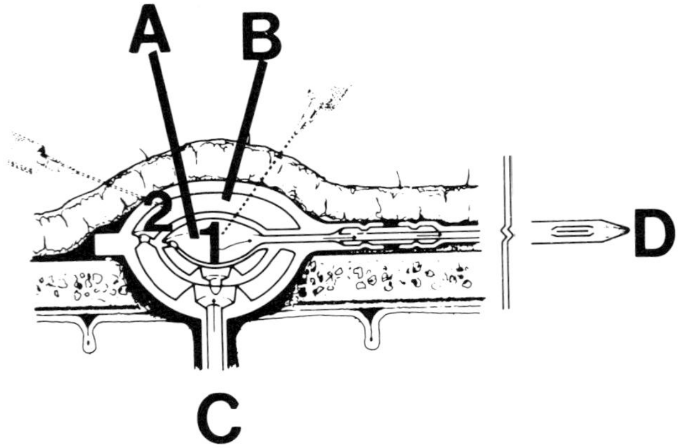

C

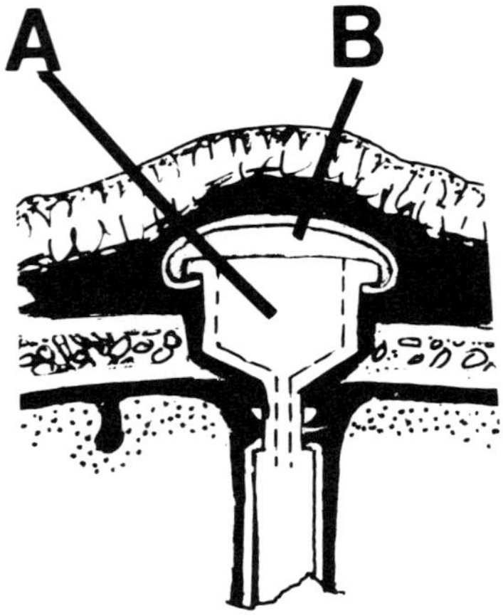

D

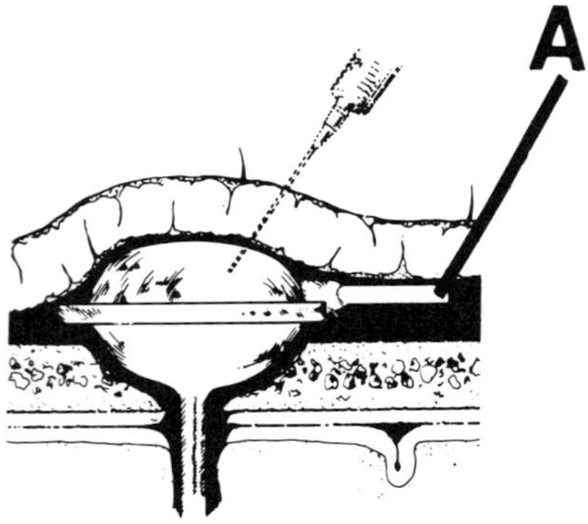

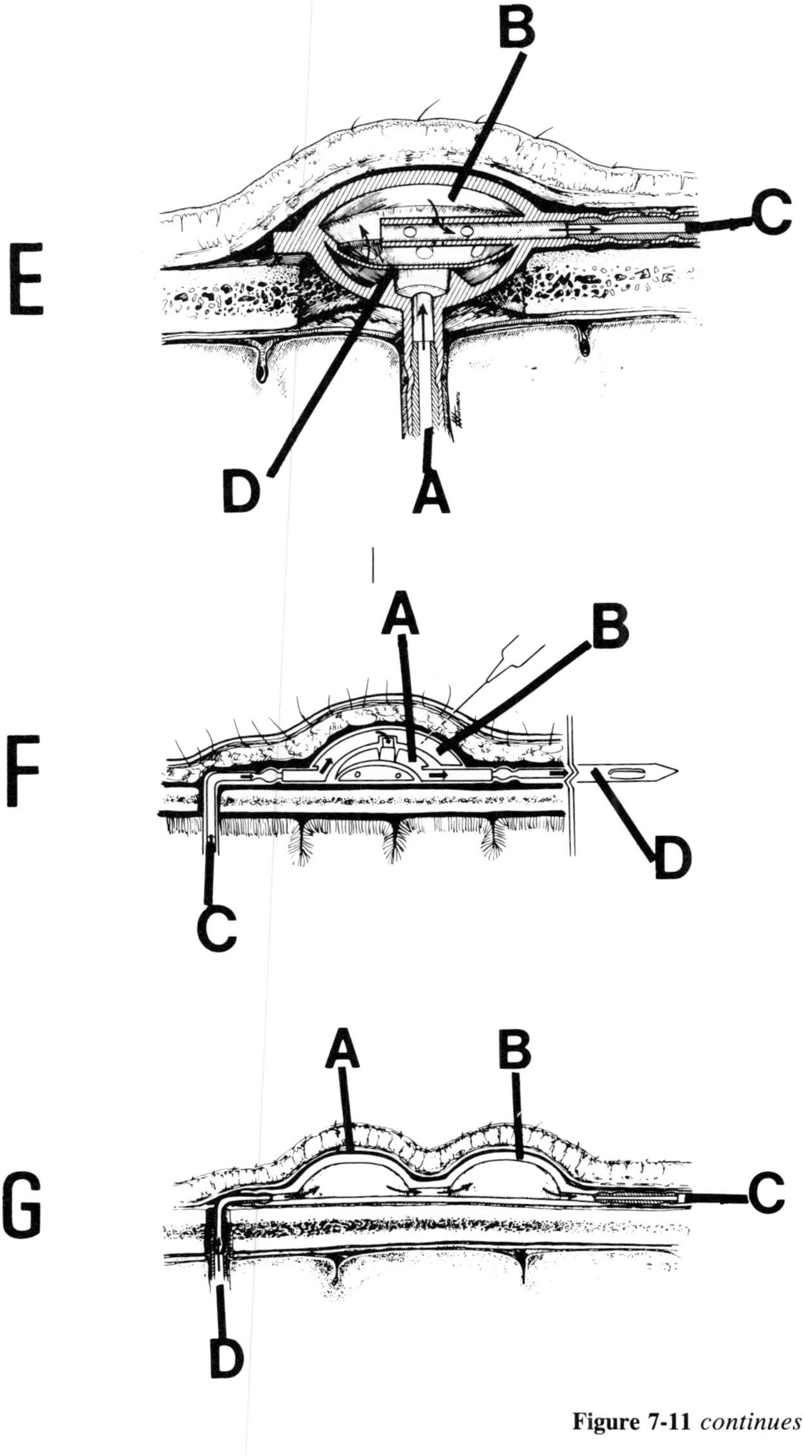

Figure 7-11 *continues*

H

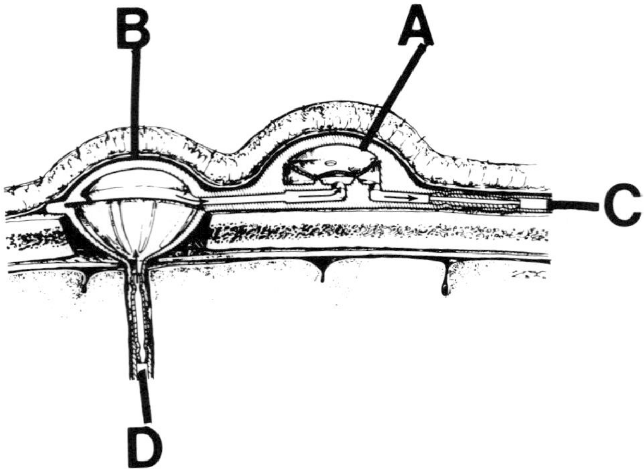

I

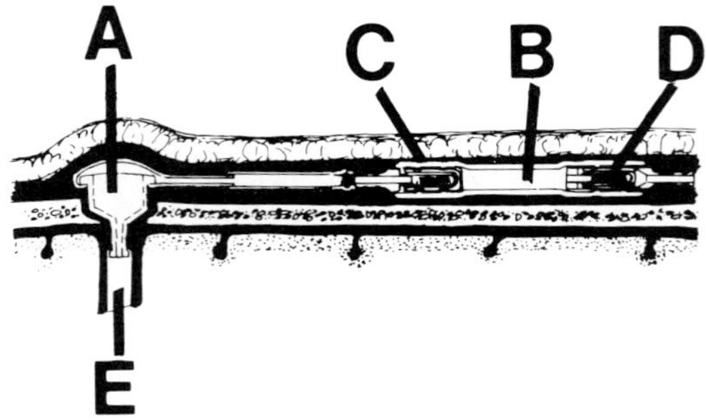

J

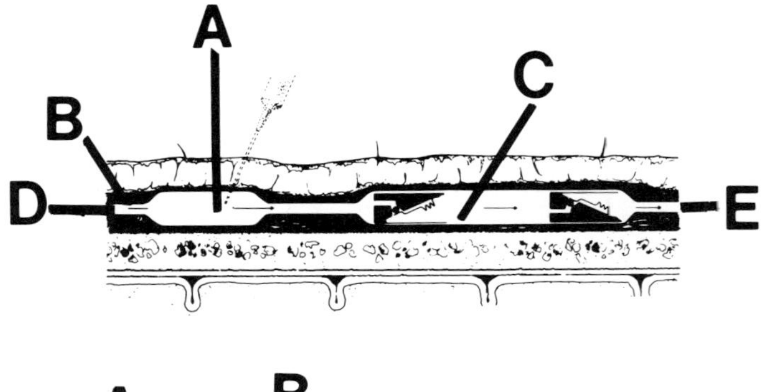

K

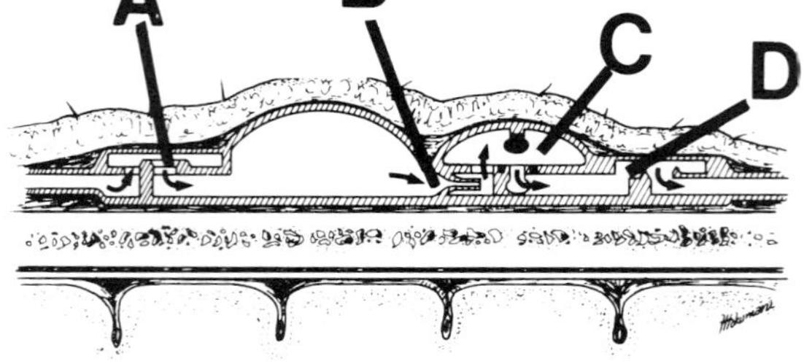

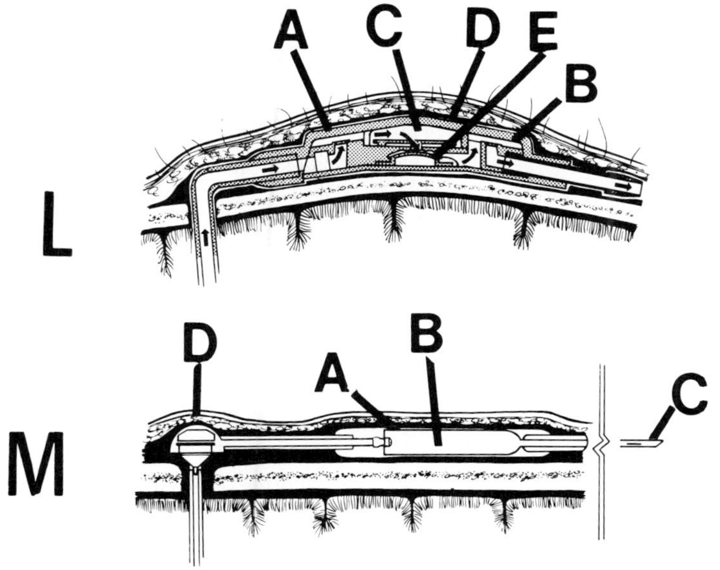

Figure 7-11. CSF shunt valve systems. (A) Foltz to-and-fro flushing reservoir (American V. Muller, Inc., McGraw Park, IL). This device is safely perforable. It contains no valves in the dome (A). The one-way slit valve (B) is at the distal (heart or peritoneal end) of the tubing. With proximal obstruction either internal or by occlusive finger pressure, either injection or dome pressure causes forward CSF flow toward the distal limb. Repetitious finger pressure first on tubing and on dome simultaneously will cause forward "pumping" of CSF. If the dome returns to full position with the proximal tube occluded, then either the tip valve is incompetent; there is a leak in the device or tubing and the defect lies in a pool of fluid; or the proximal "occlusion" is not complete (e.g., there is insufficient pressure to occlude the tube). A firm dome with occlusive pressure on either limb indicates obstruction in the opposite limb. Otherwise, this device functions either with distal limb occlusion or with occlusive finger pressure in a manner described for the converted Omaya Reservoir (Fig. 7-11D) under similar conditions. (B) Mishler-Pudenz double-lumen reservoir (American V. Muller, Inc., McGraw Park, IL). This unit combines an inner distal direction pumping device (A), surrounded by an outer proximal direction pumping device (B). Both reservoirs are safely perforable. Smooth depressing dome pressure may allow the examiner to feel the inner chamber. (1) A needle in the inner chamber aspirates from both chambers. Proximal chamber collapse during aspiration indicates proximal limb obstruction. A firm or resistant inner chamber indicates distal limb obstruction only. Failure of the outer chamber to refill indicates a proximal obstruction of CSF flow. Failure of the inner chamber to refill indicates an obstruction of CSF forward flow in either the outer chamber or the proximal limb. Repetitive pressure on the dome will cause continuous forward CSF flow (pumping). Refilling the chamber can occur with leaks in valves and tubing if they are contiguous with fluid in the presence of proximal obstruction. (2) A needle in the outer chamber aspirates from proximal limb of shunt (C), cerebral ventricle, and one chamber only. Injection or slight dome depression will force CSF simultaneously toward both

Continues

proximal and distal limbs (D) of the shunt limb with proximal limb obstruction. Relatively decreased resistance in either distal or proximal limb will allow CSF to flow preferentially toward that limb also. (C) Rickham reservoir (Codman and Shurtleff, Billerica, MA). This is a metal reservior (A) with a soft cap (B) without side-arm. (D) Convertible Omaya reservoir (American V. Muller, Inc., McGraw Park, IL). This is an all-soft-parts reservoir with optional side-arm (A) for later connection to a shunt system. (E) Standard Pudenz-Heyer one-way flusher (American V. Muller, Inc., McGraw Park, IL). (E) Standard Pudenz-Heyer one-way flusher (American V. Muller, Inc., McGraw Park, IL). Aspirates from proximal limb (A) and cerebral ventricle. Works by injection or with pressure on dome (B). CSF flows distally (C). Needle puncture of the inner or lower chamber may produce valve (D) incompetency by causing permanent diaphragm damage. (F) Double-lumen Mishler-Pudenz reservoir with flat bottom (American V. Muller, Inc., McGraw Park, IL). Both chambers are safely perforable. This has the same characteristics as the reservoir in Figure 7-11B. (G) Braden flushing reservoir (American V. Muller, Inc., McGraw Park, IL). This has two soft compressible domes (A and B) with no internal parts or valves. Constant finger pressure occludes flow through the device, working in a similar manner as the Foltz to-and-fro flusher with occlusive constant finger pressure on domes instead of tubing (Fig. 7-11A). Press first dome A then B for distal (C) flow. Press first dome B then A for proximal flow (D). (H) Coe-Schulte flushing reservoir (Pudenz-Schulte, Company, Goleta, CA). Repetitive finger pressure on distal (more firm) dome (A) causes forward CSF flow (C); constant pressure occludes forward flow more assuredly than pressure on tubing or on Braden dome (Fig. 7-11G) so that simultaneous finger pressure on or injection into the proximal dome (B) forces CSF toward the ventricle (D). Aspiration from either dome draws CSF from the cerebral direction; perforation of the inner distal device chamber may cause damage. (I) Rickham reservoir and Spitz-Holter valve (Codman and Shurtleff, Billerica, MA). In the 1950s and the early 1960s, the Spitz-Holter valve was inserted without a reservoir. Puncture of the soft tube (B) between the metal (C) ends may produce leakage, and repetitive finger pressure there pumps CSF forward toward the distal end (D). With occlusive finger pressure on the tubing, injection or pressure on the cap of the reservoir (A) causes retrograde flow toward the cerebral ventricle (E). Aspiration from the reservoir is also from the cerebral limb. Forced forward injection cannot be accomplished unless there is a central limb obstruction. (J) Hakim-Cordis antechamber (A) and valve (Cordis Neurological Company, Miami, FL). These are rarely seen separately. Only the antechamber is safely perforable. Occlusive finger pressure proximal to the antechamber (B) allows finger pressure on the antechamber or injection to force CSF toward the distal limb. Occlusive finger pressure distal to the chamber (A) allows pressure on or injection into the antechamber to force CSF toward the cerebral limb (D). Aspiration from the antechamber removes CSF from the proximal limb. Repetitive pressure on the soft midsection of the valve (C) "pumps" CSF forward toward the distal end (E). Neither valve, if competent, will allow CSF to flow in a retrograde manner toward the cerebral limb (D). Firm pressure or resistance to injection means obstruction to CSF flow in that component or those components distal to the point of pressure or site of injection. (K) Heyer-schulte all-purpose valve with occluder, on-off control, and antisiphon device (American V. Muller, Inc., McGraw Park, IL). This has three distinct parts

Continues

providing more assurance of occlusion to retrograde flow by finger pressure on the "occluder"(A); a more standard, less variable flow pressure of the Miter valve (B) due to its protection from alteration of materials by body fluids; and a permanent distal flow occluder in the form of on-off control. Valve flow will be effectively stopped by sufficient pressure on the on-off control (C) to engage the radioopaque button (black in illustration) into its seat (the cuff of which is radioopaque and shown as two black dots in the illustration). The on-off control can be opened to flow by first pressing the occluder and then the reservoir. Flow, aspiration, injection, and failure of the reservoir to fill or to fill with imperfections can all be understood by comparing the occluder pressure with proximal limbs and comparing on-off control with distal limbs' finger pressure in the description for the Foltz to-and-fro flusher (Fig. 7-11A). The soft dome of the antisiphon device (D) to the right is pulled down to occlude flow if there is suction from below. Needle perforation of the all-purpose valve should be restricted to the reservoir. (L) Heyer-Schulte low-profile valve (American V. Muller, Inc., McGraw Park, IL). To the left and right are occluders (A and B) similar to the one in Figure 7-11K. A plate (C) in the central reservoir (D) serves as a needle guard and protects the underlying one-way valve (E) from damage. (M) Flat-bottom one-way Denver pump and valve (Denver Biomaterials, Inc., Denver, Co.). The proximal slit valve (A) and one at the peritoneal end (C) of the tubing allow only one-way flow when the chamber (B) is compressed. Proximal to the pump, the Denver system has a metal reservoir with perforable cap (D) similar to the Rickham reservoir (Fig. 11C). Adapted from Shurtleff[1045]

---

films, ultrasound, and computerized axial tomography can demonstrate isolated tubes or the shunt tips in the area of acute symptoms. A 19-year-old woman with a three-generational history of gallbladder disease in seven members of her family, all with onset of symptoms between 18 and 30 years of age, presented with the following symptoms, typical of the remainder of her family: episodic abdominal pain related to eating and pain to the scapula. Her gallbladder study was normal. Abdominal scan of a radionucleide shunt study demonstrated loculation of isotope around the tip of the shunt (Fig. 7-10); an abdominal ultrasound demonstrated a cyst around the end of the shunt tip (Fig. 7-13). Previous lower abdominal symptoms and a 4-cm mass were found to be due to an ovarian cyst, demonstrating no association with the shunt system. Abdominal CSF cyst formation[379] can be a difficult problem and is frequently associated with infection.

CSF INFECTIONS AND OBSTRUCTIONS

Of all the late complications of CSF shunts mentioned by Scarff[975] and listed at the beginning of this chapter, infections and obstructions are still the most troublesome. Moreover, the major cause for morbidity

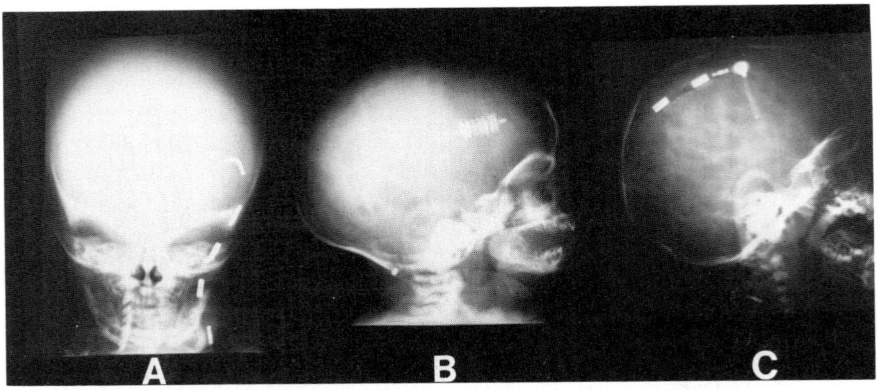

Figure 7-12. Routine roentgenography of a shunt system. (A) Foltz or other Heyer-type domed chamber with Portnoy cerebral catheter; same as Figure 7-11A. (B) Cordis-Hakim valve unit; same as Fig. 7-11J. (C) Rickham reservoir with Spitz-Holter valve, same as Figure 7-11I. Reprinted from Shurtleff[1045].

and mortality with CSF shunts has been identified as infection.[736,981,984,1000,1038,1185]

Most studies describing the follow-up of children born with hydrocephalus or hydrocephalus with meningomyelocele report the intellectual performance of children without taking into consideration whether or not the children had a CNS infection.[36,611,666] Studies of the intellectual performance of children with meningomyelocele[740,1009] or with hydrocephalus of various types[1053] clearly demonstrate that the intellectual performance of those children with significant CNS infections is lower than the performance of those with no infection (see Chapter 16).

Frequency of Infection as Related to Duration of Study

The frequency of infection has been a subject of considerable discussion in the literature. Throughout the 1960s and 1970s, reports of infection varied between 5 and 40 percent.[a] Those reporting a lower infection rate invariably had a short-term follow-up and referred to operative infection rates. Since children require revisions and each revision carries a risk of infection, case infection rates are considerably higher than operative infection rates, particularly for those studies involving long-term analysis[391,492,1051]; therefore, the case infection rate becomes a product of the operative infection rate times the duration of the study.

[a] See references 41, 44, 138, 657, 708, 756, 984, 1000, 1038, 1051–1054, 1056, 1066, and 1156.

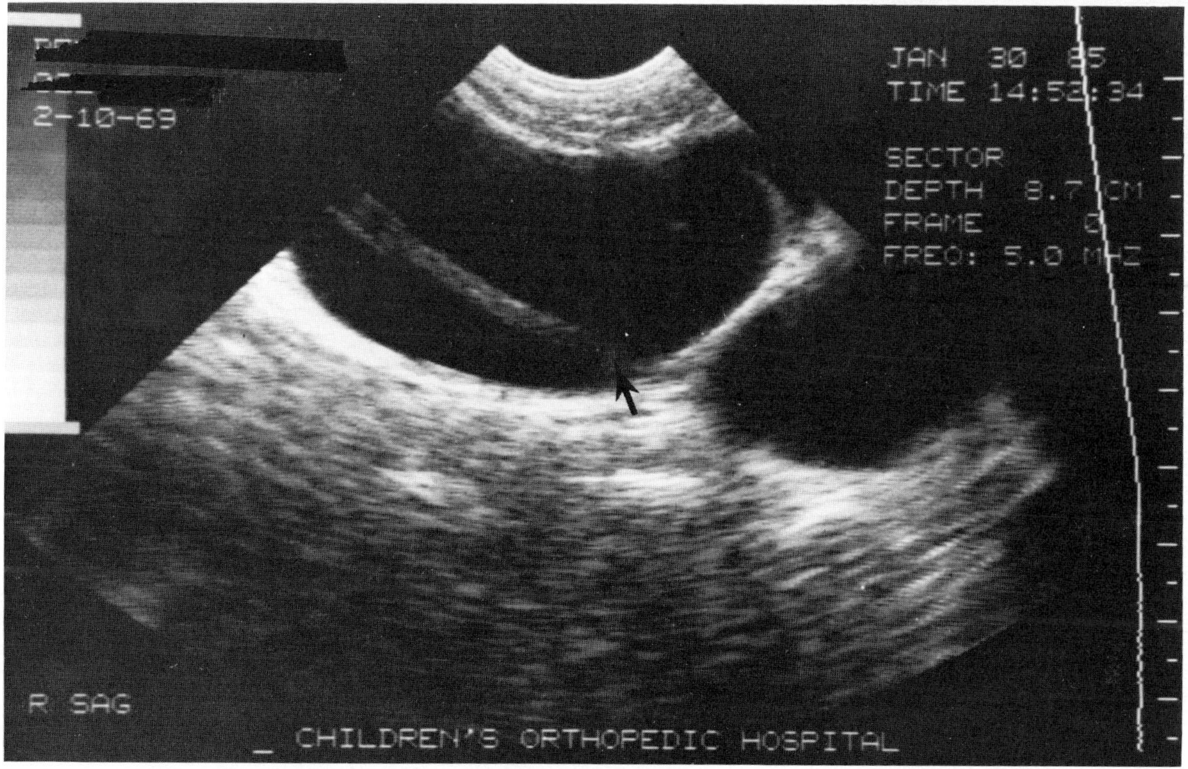

Figure 7-13 *continues*

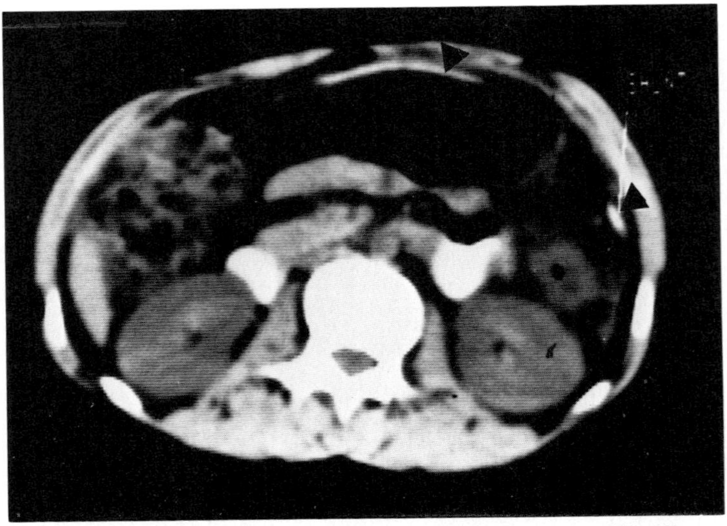

Figure 7-13. Abdominal studies demonstrating a cyst. (A) Ultrasound examination demonstrates a large cavity (black) with a thick wall (white) being transversed by the catheter (white; see arrow). (B) Computer-assisted tomogram of the abdomen demonstrating the cyst (black) with the shunt tube lying along the anterior wall (see arrow). These studies were performed on the same patient in the shunt study in Fig. 7-10.

Types of Infection

Five types of infection have been identified. First, operative infections are the most common. They are arbitrarily defined as symptoms or positive culture within 30 days[391] to 6 months[1185] after the operation. (Our definition is included later under Seattle experience.) Second, delayed shunt infections not related to operations but due to the same types of organisms occur, but with onset of symptoms any time after 6 weeks, up to 7 years. Third, epidemic meningitis due to *Hemophilus influenzae,* beta hemolytic *Streptococcus, Meningococcus,* or *Pneumococcus* occurs more commonly in children with hydrocephalus and CSF shunts.[911,984,1000,1051,1247] Fourth, individuals with ventriculoatrial shunts seem to develop thrombosis and then have blood-borne infections that, in turn, give rise to septic emboli of the lungs and kidneys.[981] Fifth, ventriculoperitoneal shunts would appear to develop complications of infections from organisms that cross the peritoneum or contaminate the CSF shunt as a result of perforation of the intraabdominal organs.[1000]

Severity of Infection

CSF shunt-associated infections have three degrees of severity. First, organisms isolated from the CSF shunt system downstream or outside of the cranial vault do not threaten future CNS function if they are treated adequately and if the infection is not allowed to spread to the CNS or to cause CNS damage from frequent shunt obstruction. Second, low-grade ventriculitis may cause recurrent obstructions and pose a difficult therapeutic challenge,[379,581,1197] but it will not affect the child's mental ability, despite the fact that the child can carry organisms in his or her ventricular shunt system for years. The third type of infection, ventriculomeningitis in association with CSF shunt infection, is far more serious; children with this complication are at a much higher risk for developing cortical damage, as is any other child with meningitis.

Since 1975, both the incidence of CSF infection and the morbidity associated with infection have diminished. The decrease in infection rates is occurring despite an increase in surveillance on behalf of physicians and surgeons who are now carrying out routine cultures on these children much more frequently. Previously undetected low-grade infections that led to shunt obstruction and death are now being detected earlier and more often than in the past because of routine cultures performed at the time of revisions. Early diagnosis and treatment allows for decreased morbidity. In addition, the therapeutic use of intravenous and intraventricular antibiotics associated with either complete shunt revision and replacement or extraventricular drainage (EVD) before replacing the shunt system has decreased morbidity.[541,734,736,1185,1247] Furthermore, detecting those children who arrive for treatment with an infection already existing in the CNS has markedly decreased the morbidity from shunt-related infections. A closed, internalized ventricular shunt system in the presence of ventriculomeningitis has a much worse outcome than if the infection is treated first with antibiotics, and the intracranial pressure is controlled by EVD or chemical agents.[665,1000,1056] The incidence of infection may well be decreased for other reasons, such as improved shunt material, that are associated with decreased frequency of erosion of skin or intestinal organs, improved surgical techniques, decreased use of invasive diagnostic procedures, and improved general attitudes of physicians and surgeons who have developed more caution in the prevention of infection. Whether these practices, in whole or in part, or prophylactic antibiotics have been responsible for the reduction in shunt-related infection has been the subject for considerable discussion.

Prevention of Infections

Haines[446] has reviewed the use of prophylactic antibiotics in neurological surgical procedures. Burke[146] and Alexander and Altemeier[22] demonstrated the effectiveness of systemic antibiotics in the prevention of wound infection if the antibiotics were given just before and during experimental operative procedures on animals. Chodak and Plaut[191] reviewed the application of this concept to general surgery performed on humans and concluded that some effectiveness could be demonstrated for abdominal and vaginal hysterectomies, total hip replacements, biliary surgery, cesarean surgery, and microneurosurgical craniotomy. Geraghty and Feely[392] performed a randomized, controlled trial and found the infection rate was 3.5 percent in the control group and 0.5 percent in the group treated with antibiotic prophylaxis.

Some authors have concluded that systemic antibiotics just prior to, during, and for a day or so after CSF shunting procedures will lower the infection rate.[19,392,518,687,717,965,972,973,1185] Others state that prophylactic antibiotics under such conditions do not, or have not, been proven to lower shunt infection rates.[76,391,446,735,794,984,117,1247] Decreased entry of antibiotics into the CSF has been documented by others.[19,153,361,541,581,717,1193,1239]

SEATTLE EXPERIENCE

Our experience with 1201 CSF shunts included 26 revisions to sites other than the 603 ventriculoatrial or 572 ventriculoperitoneal procedures (Table 7-2). In the 1975–1982 period, 419 procedures were performed, including 118 revisions performed on children initially operated on prior to 1975 or in another hospital (Table 7-3). Only 384 operative procedures performed between 1975 and 1982 were analyzed for the possible effect of prophylactic antibiotics. The 35 revisions not analyzed were performed while the child was being treated for CSF infection acquired elsewhere or associated with one of our own procedures.

Definition of a Shunt-Related Infection

The definition of a shunt-related or spontaneous, delayed infection is arbitrary and varies in the literature. Postoperative infection rates have been reported as occurring by 30 days,[391,1051] by 6 weeks to 6 months,[1185] or by 2 months.[717] Between 1975 and 1982, our case infection rate was 4.7 percent at 30 days, 6.5 percent up to 1 year postoperatively, and 7.5 percent including the three cases detected 1 year or more after the last operation. During this latter period, our operative infection rate was 2

Table 7-2
Total Procedures: 1965–1982

Procedures	Number of Cases
Initial procedures	
VA	212
VP	247
Subtotal	459
Revisions	
VA	391
VP	325
VA to VP	18
VP to VA	4
VP to Vp1	3
Vp1 to VP	1
Subtotal	742
Total procedures	1201

Abbreviations: VA, ventriculoatrial; VP, ventriculoperitoneal; Vp1, ventriculopleural. Reproduced from Shurtleff et al.[1065]

percent at 30 days, 3.6 percent up to 1 year postoperatively, and 4.4 percent including all infections. Because of the marked delay in onset of three infections detected over 1 year after the last operative procedure, we have excluded these three cases from further analysis of operative infections.

Several authors have noted that case infection rates increase with time because of delayed onset of symptoms, delayed infections, delayed diagnosis of indolent infections, and repeated exposure of older patients

Table 7-3
Total Procedures: 1975–1982

Procedures	Number of Cases
Initial VP shunts	170
Revisions performed on these shunts	131
Revisions of shunts placed prior to 1975 or elsewhere	118
Total procedures	419
Revisions performed on known infected cases[a]	35
Total noninfected cases	384

[a] Cases were infected during treatment (such as VP shunt to EVD, EVD to VP shunt, or complete shunt replacement) while on antibiotics to cure the infection. Reproduced from Shurtleff et al.[1065]

to shunt revisions with the attendant risk of infection.[391,492,717,1051] Classifying infections as shunt-related or due to spontaneous late infection is arbitrary.

Infection Rates and Frequency of Shunt Revision

The average number of revisions for the 1975–1982 period was the lowest of any period: 0.77, with a range of 0–6 (Table 7-4). The revision rate for ventriculoatrial shunts in the 1965–1974 period was significantly higher (1.8 per initial shunt) than for ventriculoperitoneal shunts during the same time period (1.3) (Table 7-4), but the infection rate for ventriculoatrial revisions was significantly lower (6.1 percent) (Table 7-5). Ventriculoperitoneal shunts associated with infections needed revisions more frequently (4.07 revisions per initial shunt) than ventriculoperitoneal shunts without infection (0.5 percent) (Table 7-4). Our 4.07 revision rate associated with infected shunt systems is close to the 4.34 revision rate reported by Keucher and Mealey.[581] Shunt malfunction may be more specifically related to infection than commonly recognized.[492,581,1197]

Our higher revision rate for ventriculoatrial shunts compared with ventriculoperitoneal shunts is in agreement with rates reported by most other authors.[492,581,655,1197] The difficulty encountered in isolating low-grade septicemia due to *S. epidermidis*[1051] may explain the 6.1 percent infection rate associated with ventriculoatrial revisions, lower than the rates of infection for initial ventriculoatrial insertions and all ventriculoperitoneal procedures of the same period (15–15.7 percent) (Table 7-5). The ventriculoperitoneal procedures performed during the 1965–1974

Table 7-4
Revision Rates

	Initial	Revisions	Number of Revisions per Initial Shunt	Significance
1965–1974				
VA	212	391	1.8	$\chi^2 = 13.4$; df = 1
VP	77	102	1.3	$p < 0.001$
1975–1982				
VP	156	74	0.5	$\chi^2 = 8.36$; df = 1 $p < 0.01$
VP Infected	14	57	4.07	$\chi^2 = 51$; df = 1 $p < 0.01$

Reproduced from Shurtleff et al.[1065]

Table 7-5
Infections

	Infections	Procedures	Percentage	Significance
1965–1974				
VA initial	32	212	15	$\chi^2 = 0.0009$; df = 1
VP initial	12	77	15.6	p, insignificant
Total initial	44	289	15.2	
VA revision	24	391	6.1	$\chi^2 = 6.9$; df = 1; $p < 0.01$ with Yates[b]
VP revision	16	102	15.7	
Total revision	40	493	8.1	
Total 1965–1974	84	782[a]	10.7	$\chi^2 = 15.5$; df = 1
Total 1975–1982	14	384[a]	3.6	$p < 0.01$ with Yates.[b]
Total 1965–1982	98	1166	8.4	

[a] These were clean procedures without existing infection being treated.
[b] Yates is a statistical computation to correct the Chi Square calculation to avoid any possible bias due to small numbers.
Reproduced from Shurtleff et al.[1065]

interval were generally performed as revisions of obstructed ventriculoatrial systems placed initially. Some may have had undetected low-grade infections that became symptomatic after the ventriculoperitoneal shunts were inserted, thereby possibly explaining why ventriculoperitoneal shunt-related infection rates were so high.

Operative Infection Rate as Related to Year of Study

The overall operative infection rate fell from 10.7 percent in the 1965–1974 period to 3.6 percent in the 1975–1982 period (Table 7-5). Ninety-eight (8.4 percent) infections occurred following a total of 1166 operations performed throughout the entire study and without previously existing infection, as identified by pre- and postoperative cultures (Table 7-5).

The 15.6 percent infection rate following all ventriculoperitoneal procedures for the 1965–1974 period (28 infections and 179 procedures) is significantly higher than the 4 percent rate associated with 99 ventriculoperitoneal shunts performed without intraventricular antibiotic prophylaxis between 1975 and 1982 (groups A and B, Table 7-6). Prophylactic antibiotics were not used prior to 1975. Although the prophylactic regimen combining gentamicin with Staphcillin® (group E) was associated with only a 2.1 percent infection rate, it is not significantly different from the highest infection rate of 5.6 percent associated with no antibiotics (group A) or with any of the other antibiotic regimens (Table 7-6). All the

Table 7-6
Antibiotic Prophylaxis: 1975–1982

Group	Type of Antibiotic Prophylaxis	Total Procedures	Number Infected	Percentage Infected
A	None	36	2	5.6
B	IV only	63	2	3.7
C	IV methicillin plus 10 mg ivent	97	3	3.1
D	IV methicillin plus 100 mg ivent	92	5	5.4
E	IV methicillin plus gentamicin plus 100 mg methicillin and 2 mg gentamicin ivent[a]	96	2	2.1
	Totals	384	14	3.6

Abbreviations: IV, intravenous; ivent, barbotage via shunt into the cerebral ventricle.
[a] The greatest difference is insignificant: $\chi^2 = 0.55$; df = 1; p, insignificant with Yates.
Reproduced from Shurtleff et al.[1065]

Table 7-7
Distribution of *S. epidermidis*

	Type Procedure	Percentage of Isolated *S. epidermidis*
1965–1975		
VA shunt	Initial	71.7
	Revision	66.7
VP shunt	Initial	83.0
	Revision	67.0
1975–1982		
(Prophylaxis groups)		
A		50
B		100
C		50
D		60
E		100
Total		60

Reproduced from Shurtleff et al.[1065]

Staphcillin® prophylactic regimens were associated with infections due to Staphcillin®-sensitive organisms (Table 7-7).

Despite our concerted efforts, we have not been able to reduce our operative infection rate to nil as reported by Malis[687] and Savitz and Katz[972]; to near nil for general neurosurgical procedures, as reported by Geraghty and Feely[392]; or to near nil for artificial hip operations, as reported by Ericson and associates[312] as well as Sandusky.[970] Our overall operative infection rate for the entire series (1965–1982) was 8.4 percent, close to the 7.3 percent for 3951 operations reported by Hoffman and associates.[492] These rates are comparable with other long-term and older studies that range from 5.0 to 15–16 percent.[391,581,717,1185,1197] The overall infection rate of 3.6 percent during 1975–1982 (Table 7-6), as well as the 2.1 percent for the group given both Staphcillin® and gentamicin (group D, Table 7-6), compare with the lowest rates reported for recent studies of ventriculoperitoneal shunt procedures using intravenous prophylactic antibiotics: 2.2 percent,[492] 2.6 percent,[717,972] 3 percent,[76] and 4.54 percent.[19] These rates are close to the 1.8 percent infection rate for 23,649 clean operative cases without insertion of devices reported by Cruse and Foord.[235]

All the studies of shunt-related infections quoted above, with the exception of Bayston,[75] Ericson and associates,[312] and Geraghty and

Feely,[392] are sequential studies comparing more recent operations with prophylactic antibiotics to operations performed previously with older techniques and other, less modern methodologies. These studies all note a significant decrease in postoperative, shunt-related infections over the past 15–20 years.[19,518,717,965,973,1185,1250] Although most authors attribute the decrease in postoperative, shunt-related infections to the use of intravenous prophylactic antibiotics, there are a number of other possible causes. They include the following: (1) more modern shunt materials and operative equipment; (2) more efficient operative techniques; (3) newer operating theaters; (4) more experienced operating teams; (5) shorter operative exposure; (6) more experienced surgeons; and (7) closed preoperative diagnostic techniques such as MRI or CT scan and ultrasound in place of invasive gas contrast roentgenography.[391,717,1185] We believe there are two other significant factors. First, routine preoperative cultures identify existing infections that were previously unrecognized because they were indolent and asymptomatic. In the era prior to obtaining these routine cultures, infections were identified postoperatively and thought to be induced at the time of operation. Second, we believe that pressure and radionucleide flow studies,[471] discussed above as possible causes for reduction in revisions, may also reduce the case infection rate by reducing exposure from open exploration of shunting systems. The many possible factors contributing to decreased CSF shunt-related, postoperative infections obscure the possible contribution of intravenous and/or intraventricular antibiotic treatment. Some of these factors will be discussed below.

Differences Among Surgeons

George and associates[391] reported a 25-fold difference in CSF shunt-related infections between experienced and inexperienced surgeons. Our data suggest there is no difference in postoperative shunt infection rates between senior staff neurological surgeons operating frequently (J. Timothy Stuntz), 3.8 percent, and those operating infrequently (others), 2.5 percent. However, multiple operators, including resident physicians, operated on our patients prior to 1975 and may have contributed to the higher infection rate of that time period compared with the 1975–1982 experience.

Frequency of *Staphylococcus epidermidis* Infections

The organisms cultured from our patients have included *Staphylococcus epidermidis* as the predominant organism, whether or not the patient received any antibiotic prophylaxis, a ventriculoperitoneal or ventriculoarterial procedure, or an initial insertion or revision. These *S. epidermidis* organisms were generally sensitive to methicillin.

Rekate and associates[908] reported an increase in diptheroid organisms cultured on an anaerobic media. They, in addition to Venes,[1185] reported a decrease in *S. epidermidis* infections with intravenous prophylactic antibiotics. Although their numbers and ours are small, we can detect no significant changes between our earlier and later groups.[1065] Indeed, we observed persistent occurrence of *Staphylococcus aureus* and *epidermidis* organisms in postoperative shunt infections. These staphylococcal organisms were generally susceptible to the antibiotics being used for prophylaxis, as reported by others.[391,717]

Presence of Meningomyelocele Versus Uncomplicated Hydrocephalus

Keucher and Mealey[581] and Hoffman and associates[492] report higher postoperative shunt infection rates in children born with meningomyelocele. Our data suggest a higher infection rate of 4.8 percent for CSF shunt procedures following open neural tube defect repair compared with 3.7 percent for children with closed central nervous systems; studies by McCullough and associates[717] and Venes[1185] agree. None of these studies, however, report significance differences. The reduced infection rates in our meningomyelocele patients may be due to our intensive surveillance for infection and treatment following back repair.

Antibiotic Prophylaxis

We could demonstrate no significant differences in CSF shunt infection rates between those receiving no antibiotics and those receiving specifically chosen intravenous antibiotics with or without intraventricular methicillin (Table 7-6). These observations concur with others.[76,392,446,735,794,984,1170,1208] Furthermore, the suggestion that more adequate levels of broader spectrum antibiotics in the CSF may further reduce postoperative CSF shunt infections, as suggested by McCullough and associates,[717] was not borne out by our high-dose intraventricular methicillin or combined methicillin and gentamicin use (Table 7-6).

The past decade has witnessed a significant reduction in mortality, revision rate, and frequency of postoperative CSF shunt infections. Modern revision rates average one to two per patient; infection rates have decreased to an expected 2–3 percent, and mortality can now be expected to result mostly from non–CSF shunt causes, such as complications of the Arnold-Chiari malformation. The effects, if any, of prophylactic antibiotics must be evaluated by large-scale cooperative studies using prospective, randomly selected treatment and control cases.[446,984]

TREATMENT OF INFECTIONS

With the reduction in CSF shunt infections, there have been fewer studies of the treatment of shunt-related infections. Five variables relate to this type of treatment: (1) the organism, (2) the sensitivity of the organism to antibiotics, (3) the penetration of those systemic antibiotics to which the organism is sensitive into the CSF, (4) the type and degree of hydrocephalus, and (5) the type of, and status of, shunt function. These five variables will, in turn, determine whether systemic antibiotics alone or with intraventricular barbotage and shunt revision are necessary.

Our approach to management of CSF shunt infections is outlined in the flow diagram in Figure 7-14. The most important determination is the site of infection. Since there can be total anatomic separation of CSF spaces by complete aqueductal atresia and even multiple-compartment hydrocephalus,[241b,351,353] it is important to distinguish which, if any, compartments are infected. Because of the increased propensity for hydrocephalic children to develop epidemic meningitis[911,984,1000,1051,1247] as well as to have separated CSF compartments, shunt-aspirated CSF can be sterile and free of evidence of inflammation in the presence of purulent meningitis, peritonitis, or septicemia.[1051] Similarly, patients with ventriculitis or shunt infections can have no meningeal component to their infections and, as a result, exhibit few, if any, CNS sequelae, despite severe symptoms of systemic infection.

Recently, we have treated a shunt-dependent child with pneumococcal CSF meningitis and clear, organism-free ventricular CSF and another infant with ventriculitis, manifested by many white blood cells and bacteria, who almost died with severe sepsis. The latter never showed signs of cortical involvement. Neither demonstrated evidence of postinfection or CNS sequalae.

We have also treated several children with blood and shunt CSF cultures positive for *S. epidermidis* for 1–3 $\frac{1}{2}$ years. Repeated psychometric tests demonstrated no change in intellectual performance by these patients. Each was finally cured with systemic and intraventricular antibiotics and removal of the CSF shunt, 7–10 days of EVD, and, while still under antibiotic treatment, reinsertion of other CSF shunt. In one case, *S. epidermidis* organisms were demonstrated to have undergone mutation and developed three strains susceptible to different antibiotic profiles. Another remarkable case was treated for repeated infections with different organisms over an 18-month period in another hospital. Her CT scan is shown in Figure 7-4. Repair of an air-fluid fistula, identification of the organism, and adequate administration of antibiotics cured this child in 11 days. Another patient was identified by isotope studies and cultures to have *Pseudomonas aeruginosa* growing from three isolated

FLOW DIAGRAM OF CSF SHUNT INFECTIONS

Epidemic organisms include meningococcus, B hemolytic streptococcus, pneumococcus, and Hemophilus influenza. The staphylococci and sensitive anaerobic organisms may respond also to system treatment only.

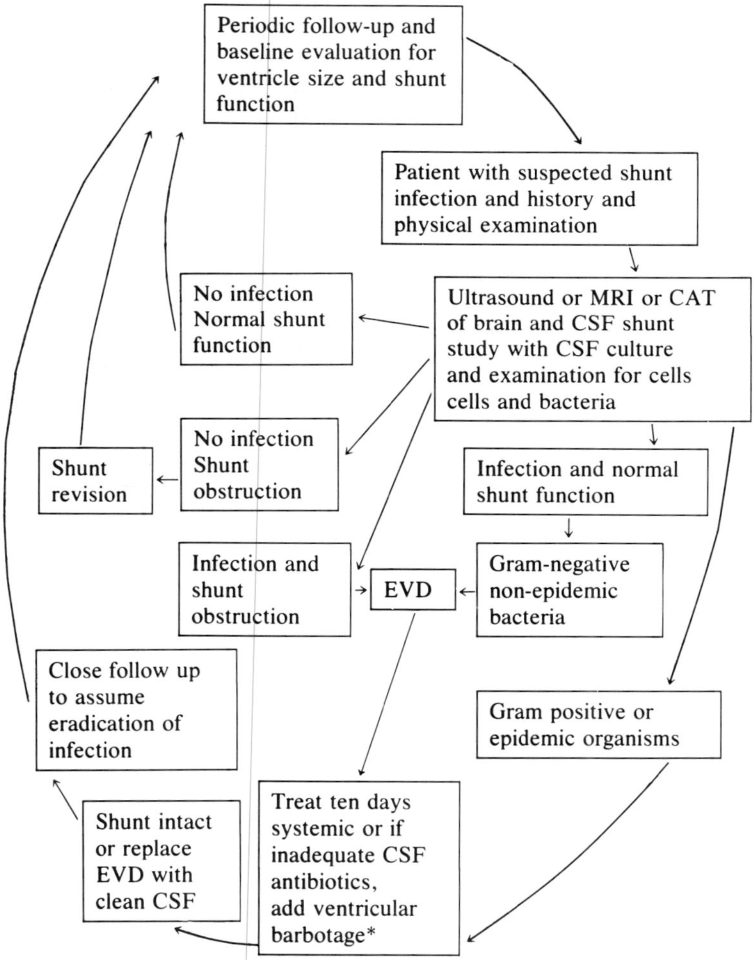

CAT:	Computer assisted tomogram
MRI:	Molecular resonance image
CSF:	Cerebrospinal fluid
EVD:	Extra ventricular drainage
*	See text for selection of antibiotics, also Table 8

Figure 7-14. Flow diagram of shunt infections. Adapted from Loeser et al.[657]

spaces: (1) the ventricular system, (2) the cerebral subarachnoid space, and (3) the spinal subarachnoid space.

These individuals, all unusual cases, emphasize the difficulty in generalizing advice about treatment of shunt-related infections. Nevertheless, it is possible to synthesize these observations with those of others to recommend a useful treatment scheme, summarized in Figure 7-14 as our diagnostic and therapeutic paradigm.

Systemic Antibiotics

Despite poor overall results with systemic antibiotic therapy, this type of therapy is effective in two situations: (1) acute epidemic meningitis due to *Hemophilus influenza*, *M. meningitis*, hemolytic streptococcus, and other common epidemic pathogens would appear to respond to systemic antibiotics in children with CSF shunts as they will in normal children[911,984,1000,1051,1247]; and (2) *S. epidermidis*, in our experience, and as reported by others, has been cured with rifampin given by mouth.[931] In our treatment center, three patients have been cured of positive, CSF shunt–culture, staphylococcal shunt infections with rifampin by mouth and another five with oral rifampin and intravenous Vancocin HCL (Vancomycin, Eli Lilly and Company, Indianapolis, IN). Current recommendations are to combine rifampin with another agent, such as nafcillin or Vancocin® HCL, to prevent the development of resistance to rifampin reported in 25 percent of cases.[320,931]

Systemic and Intraventricular Barbotage

McLaurin[734] reported a high cure rate from combining intraventricular barbotage with systemic antibiotics. We reported a 43 percent cure rate for *S. epidermidis*[1054] and no success for other types of nonepidemic infections.[1000] O'Brien and associates[818] also reported some success with this method of administration. James and associates[539] reported that nine out of ten *S. epidermidis* infections were cured with this method.

Intraventricular administration is indicated only if the organism is susceptible to antibiotics that do not cross the blood–brain barrier in adequate amounts and if the infection is isolated to the shunt system and its immediate environment; the doses we use are listed in Table 7-8. It is inconceivable that a true ventriculomeningitis or even ventriculitis will be affected by intraventricular barbotage if the infection and inflammatory process exist throughout the complicated ventricular system. Diffusion of the antibiotic into such intricate and complicated recesses of the CSF spaces cannot be significant, particularly if it is against the flow of CSF. The pharmocodynamics would be comparable to an attempt at dispersing

Table 7-8
Flow Diagram of CSF Shunt Infections: Antibiotics of Choice in CSF Shunt-Associated Infections

Organism	Antibiotic	Route of Administration	Dosage	Frequency
Staphylococcus	Staphcillin®	Intravenous	100–200 mg/kg/day	q 4–6 hr
	Naficillin	Intravenous or intraventricular	100–300 mg/kg/day	q 24 hr
	Rifampin[a]	Per os	10–20 mg/kg/day	q 24 hr
	Vancocin® HCL	Intravenous	40 mg/kg/day	q 12 hr
Staphylococcus susceptible to aqueous penicillin	Penicillin with aqueous crystalline	Intravenous	25,000–300,000 units/kg/day	q 2–6 hr
B-*Streptococcus* or *Streptococcus viridans*	Penicillin[b] with aqueous crystalline	Intravenous	25,000–300,000 units/kg/day	q 8 hr
E. coli or *Klebsiella* or *Proteus*	Gentamicin	Intramuscular	5–7 mg/kg/day	q 8 hr
		Intraventrocular	2–4 mg/day	qd
Pseudomonas	Gentamicin and/or carbenicillin	Intramuscular	5–7 mg/kg/day	q 8 h
		Intraventricular	2–4 mg/day	qd
		Intravenous	400–500 mg/kg/day	q 4 hr

Modified from Loeser and associates.[657]
[a] Rifampin should be combined with another antibiotic.
[b] Neither aqueous penicillin nor carbenicillin should be administered intraventricularly or intrathecally; both are neurotoxic when injected directly into the central nervous system.

mud into the upper reaches of the Mississippi River by shoveling mud into the river at New Orleans. Dispersion of the antibiotic throughout the ventricular system may be possible with a very slow CSF flow or none at all, as with a reservoir or obstructed shunt without flow.

We have had patients referred to us after poor results with attempted treatment of ventriculitis in the presence of an obstructed CSF shunt and periodic ventricular puncture for CSF drainage with instillation of antibiotics. Ventricular irrigation with gentamicin associated with systemic administration and no shunt revision has been reported successful in four cases by Whang and associates,[1211] an unconfirmed observation. Intraventricular and systemic gentamicin were reported as less successful than systemic gentamicin for ventriculomeningitis and meningitis treated in nonhydrocephalic and nonshunt infants.[714] We have observed suppression of symptoms with intraventricular and/or systemic antibiotics if there is adequate control of CSF pressure. With cessation of antibiotics, infection most frequently recurs.

Systemic and Intraventricular Barbotage with Complete Shunt Removal and Relocation

In 1970, Luthart[679] first reported successful treatment of CSF shunt infections by complete shunt removal and replacement in a different site while administering adequate systemic antibiotics. Perrin and McLaurin[861] recommended immediate shunt removal and replacement in the same site while systemic and intraventricular antibiotics were administered. James and associates[539] reported a 90 percent success rate with the same technique used by Luthart. As noted above in our own experience, resistant staphylococcal and all other types of infections have responded to the combination of systemic antibiotics alone or, if indicated by poor CSF penetration, with intraventricular barbotage of antibiotics with complete removal of the shunt system. We have never cured a CSF shunt infection caused by nonepidemic gram-negative bacteria or *S. aureus* without complete shunt removal.[1000] Review of existing reports /does not enable one to determine whether other forms of treatment (without complete shunt removal) can cure shunt-related infection due to enteric organisms.

Since our last report,[1000] we have treated an additional 19 cases of CSF shunt-related infections. Fourteen have been due to *S. epidermiditis*, the other five to gram-negative infection. These patients have all been cured of their infections. Eighty-one percent are intellectually normal or had no IQ change between pre- and postinfection exams; one is dead from noninfectious complications. Considering the higher mortality rate associated with treatment involved in not removing the shunt, as reported by

James and associates[539] as well as Schoenbaum and associates,[984] we recommend systemic and, when indicated by low antibiotic concentrations in the CSF, intraventricular barbotage associated with complete shunt removal and 7–10 days of EVD before insertion of another shunt in a different site. Rarely, 1,4:3,6 dianhydro-D-glucitol can be used to help control CSF during antibiotic treatment and before reinsertion of a CSF shunt.[672,1059] The theoretical reasons against reoperation[731] would appear to be inconsequential when measured against the real success of adequate antibiotic therapy and complete CSF shunt replacement. Antibiotic administration for *S. epidermiditis* infections can be adequate orally (rifampin) or systemically (nafcillin and vancomycin) or may need to be barbotaged into the ventricular system (methicillin or gentamicin). Variable CSF penetration and, therefore, dosage and frequency can be determined by serial determination of antibiotic concentration at peak and trough levels.[868] The timing of CSF shunt replacement and the use of EVD and 1,4:3,6 dianhydro-D-glucitol can be determined by shunt function, pressure measurements, and clinical response.

SUMMARY

This chapter has reviewed a half century's advances in the understanding and management of hydrocephalus. Original physiologic, nonprosthetic management of abnormal CSF accumulations have given way to the use of many different shunt systems. Noninvasive anatomic diagnostic techniques such as cranial echograms and CT scans have decreased complications associated with older invasive diagnostic techniques. Achievement of adequate CSF levels of antibiotics combined, when necessary, with removal of bacteria-contaminated shunt systems has proven successful in curing shunt-related infections. Combined technological advances and the use of prophylactic antibiotics have reduced shunt-related infections to approximately 2 percent. Currently, we can offer patients and families of patients with hydrocephalus a prognosis of 90 percent or better for prolonged survival with a low morb idity (Fig. 5-1–5-3). Overall mortality and morbidity for hydrocephalus associated with meningomylocele is less dependent on hydrocephalus per se than on other complications associated with simultaneously occurring malformations of the CNS and other organ systems. These other contributors to survival and morbidity will be discussed in later chapters.

David Shurtleff, Julian Ansell
Patricia Hayden, John McLaughlin

8

Exstrophy Lesions

The exstrophic lesions are being considered together in this chapter because initial management depends on different problems and technical solutions than those applicable to the child born with meningomyelocele or an isolated open neural tube defect, as outlined in Chapters 5, 6, and 7. Clear presentation to the parents of all possible courses of action with attendant potential outcomes is, however, necessary with both groups of patients. Parents can then decide whether they should, or wish to, participate in the infant's care.

Unless the extruded intestine of an omphalocele is covered by a membrane and threatens to rupture, the potential for infants with exstrophy to live for weeks, months, and even years without surgery permits a relatively unhurried approach to the assessment of all organ systems. This allows the parents a little more time to make a profound decision for the child with exstrophy. In contrast, parents of a child with an open meningomyelocele must make an immediate decision, within 12–24 hours, because of the risk of infection associated with an open nervous system.[910,1068] Due to danger of infection and attendant tissue damage, however, we recommend a decision about closure of the exstrophy lesion be made within the first few days. At this age, the skeletal structures are more pliable than a few days later, allowing for easier closure as described in more detail below.

MYELODYSPLASIAS AND EXSTROPHIES: SIGNIFICANCE, PREVENTION, AND TREATMENT
© 1986 by Grune & Stratton. ISBN 0-8089-1816-8

EXSTROPHY OF THE CLOACA

Exstrophy of the cloaca presents with the surface of the unfused urinary bladder beneath an omphalocele, between ureteric orifices that are hypertrophied and prolapsed, and above a small remnant of what was to develop into the large colon (Fig. 8-1). One or two appendiceal vestiges may protrude from the right lower quadrant of the colonic remnant, and the prolapsed ileum presents as a central protrusion. Wolferian or Mullerian duct remnants may open onto the surface between the effaced urinary bladder and colonic mucosa. Laterally, there may be halves of unfused external genitalia. Over the sacrum, a soft fluctuant mass may represent a myelocystocele that may or may not be associated with paralysis of the lower extremities.

Because children with exstrophy of the cloaca have multiple-system involvement, these children are evaluated by a pediatrician, a nurse, and multiple consultants (see Chapter 22). Because of the lower motor neuron paralysis, sensory impairment, and pelvic or spine abnormalities combined with genitourinary and gastrointestinal problems, we find these patients and their families are in need of the same spectrum of consultants as those affected with myelodysplasia.

Until Rickham[928] described the first successful surgical closure of a vesicointestinal fissure (also known as exstrophy of the cloaca, exstrophia splanchnica, and triple agenesis of the tail fold[465]), this severe malformation was discussed only in the teratologic and embryologic literature. (Embryogenesis has been discussed in Chapter 2.) The first case report of a surviving, untreated adult was published in 1976.[910] Other reports documented sporadic surgical survivors with death in most cases.[a] We have experience with 12 living of 16 total patients referred for care of their exstrophy of the cloaca. The details of these cases are reported in Table 8-1. Hayden and associates[465] previously reported cases 8 and 12; McLaughlin and associates[727] reported cases 14 and 16.

Most patients with exstrophy of the cloaca die in infancy from electrolyte imbalance following excessive gastrointestinal fluid losses, in part related to short small intestines (cases 8, 10, and 15, Table 8-1).[417,465,550,558,928,1091,1098,1143] Other significant, and at times lethal, congenital malformations include renal anomalies (cases 5, 12, 13, and 16, Table 8-1)[465,727,910,928,1098,1143]; cardiovascular anomalies (cases 1 and 9, Table 8-1)[910]; other gastrointestinal disorders such as duodenal or ileal stenosis[417] or duplication, malrotation, and Meckel's diverticulum (cases 1, 4, 14, and 15, Table 8-1)[910,1091,1098,1256]; and lower extremity paralysis with orthopedic deformities secondary to myelocystocele (cases 1, 2, 7, 9,

[a] See references 112, 355, 417, 465, 476, 550, 727, 1091, 1098, 1143, and 1256.

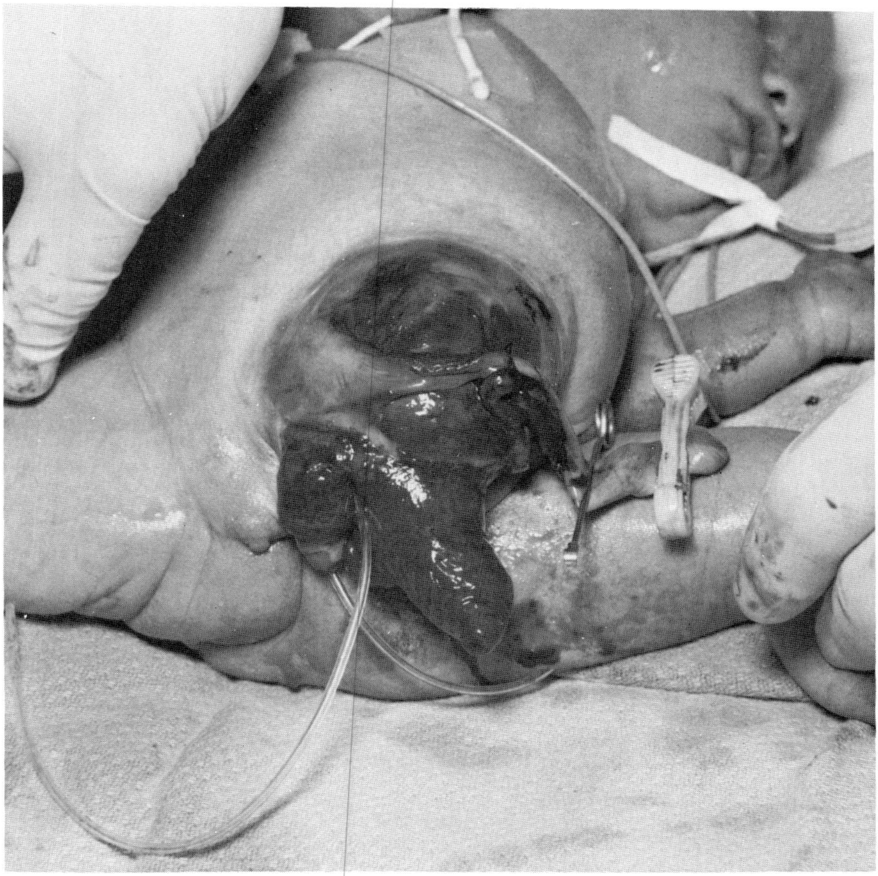

Figure 8-1. Cloacal exstrophy omphalocele. The intestines are visible through the transparent omphalocele at the cephalad region of the lesion. The umbilical cord is closed by both a metal and plastic clamp. It enters the lesion at the interface of the omphalocele and transitional epithelium, which represents effaced urinary bladder that is smooth. The rugated protrusion is ileum that is prolapsed through a small piece of large intestine that is all that remains of what would have developed into the entire large colon and rectum. The protrusion to the right of the ileum is the prolapsed and hypertrophied right ureteral orifice. The plastic tube passes through the penile orifice and out the trigone of the effaced urinary bladder. The partially fused scrotal remnant containing a hypoplastic testis is to the right of the penis. The appendiceal remnants are on the right of the bowel remnant, hidden from view by the prolapsed ileum that also hides from view the left ureteral orifice.

Table 8-1
Sixteen Cases of Exstrophy of the Cloaca

Case Number	Age	Omphalocele	Vesicoenteric Plate	Uterus; Vagina	Penis; Scrotum	Sex	Myelocele
Type 1 variant: Base of urinary bladder and trigone and urethra intact with hypospadius							
1	16 yr	+	+, Base of UB intact, trigone	0	Penis with perineal urethra; bifid scrotum; testes down	M	Lipomeningomyelocele; L5-S1 motor to L1
2	3.5 yr	+	+, Base of UB intact, trigone	0	Hypospadias; absent scrotum; testes up	M	+, Removed when age 1 mo; multiple cysts L5-S1
3	4 mo	+	+	0	Epispadias penis; testes down; fused scrotum	M	0
Type 2 variant: Identifiable external genitalia that can be reconstructed							
4	24 yr	+	+	0	Epispadias penis; bifid scrotum; testes down	M	0
5	9 yr	+	+	0	Diphallus	M	0
6	5.5 yr	Small	+	0	Epispadias penis; diphallus; bifid scrotum; testes down	M	0

Table 8-1 *(continued)*

Other Anomalies: GI Tract	Other Anomalies: Other	Short-Gut Syndrome	Closure of Urinary Bladder	Closure of Colon	Comment/ Outcome
Atretic ileum, resected day 1	Bilateral inguinal hernias; sacral dysgenesis; large ductus and pulmonary artery stenosis	++	Exteriorize, age 1 day; internalized, age 2 mo; ureteroileostomy, age 3.5 yr; cystectomy, 8 yr; developed calcium cysteoxalate stones	Ileostomy, age 1 day; revised twice	Postoperative dehisced treated twice, healed by second intention; IQ, 140 WISC; four orthopedic operations; now WC; osteoknees
Prolapsed ileum with compromised blood supply resected	Talipes equinovarus; left inguinal hernia repair and orchiopexy, age 6 mo	++++	Closed pubis with figure-8 suture; internalized, age 1 day	Ileostomy, age 1 day; revised once; colonic rudiment removed	One orthopedic operation; IQ, 85, SB; cruises
Double-tail gut	0	++, 40 cm	Internalized, age 2 days	Entubulated splayed gut to colostomy on abdominal wall	No wound breakdown
Meckel's diverticulum; atretic duodenum; intestinal infarct, age 15 yr	0	++	Exteriorized, age 1 day; ureteroileostomy, age 5 yr; cystectomy	Ileocolostomy and resection of Meckel's age 1 day	Possible adrenocortical failure; ejaculates; college graduate
0	Incompletely formed vertebrae; two renal masses on left, one in renal fossa, one in bony pelvis, one in renal pelvis	Internalized	Age 3.5 days, phallic halves freed up and joined; Young-Dees vesicourethroplasty and phallic straightening, age 5.5 yr	Ileostomy and herniorrhaphies; intestinal obstruction, age 3.75 yr	Incontinent; normal school class for age; walks with abnormal gait
0	Bilateral inguinal hernias repaired at age 1 yr; orchiopexies; repeat repair of hernias, age 3 yr with phalloplasty with local flaps	+	Internalized age 2 days; halves of penis joined, Young-Dees urethroplasty, and bladder neck suspension iliac osteotomies, age 2 yr; perineal fistula excised, age 3.5 yr; bilateral Cohen ureter reimplants, age 4 yr; left ureteral and bladder stones	Ileostomy, age 2 days, gastrostomy tube; colonic rudiment removed	Walks and runs; normal intelligence

Table 8-1 *(continued)*

Case Number	Age	Omphalocele	Vesicoenteric Plate	Uterus; Vagina	Penis; Scrotum	Sex	Myelocele
7	2.5 yr[b]	+	+	Double uterus and short-right, long-left open vaginal halves; chromosome XX	0	F	+, 17 mo excised because of loss of nerve function
8	1 yr[a]	0	+	0	Rudimentary diphallus; XY chromosome; testes up; age 9 mo	F to M, age 8 mo	+, No neural loss
9	19 mo	Small	+	0	Diphallus; testes up; bifid scrotum not yet reconstructed	M	Lipomyelocele excised, age 3 mo
10	15 days		+	+	Epispadiac penis; bifid scrotum	M	Large; cystic
Type 3: No identifiable external genitalia; complete exstrophy of all three systems							
11	20 yr	Small	+	Widely separated halves of open vagina and uterus	Testes up; XY chromosomes; orchidectomy, age 2 yr	F	+, paraplegia to L5; progressive loss to L1
12	16 yr[a]	0	+	0	XY chromosome at birth	F	L1-2 paresis; 11 × 18 cm
13	7.5 yr	Large		0	0	F	0, No neural loss

Table 8-1 *(continued)*

Other Anomalies					
GI Tract	Other	Short-Gut Syndrome	Closure of Urinary Bladder	Closure of Colon	Comment/ Outcome
0	0	140 cm	Omphalocele excised, age 2 days with internalized bladder and some colon; age 11 mo, colon prolapse via urethra; iliac osteotomies and creation of urethra from colon	Ileostomy and gastrostomy to legs, age 2 days	Nerve function has returned; normal intelligence
0	Vertebral anomalies	++++	Ureteroilestomy, age 9 mo	Ileostomy, age 9 mo; colonic rudiment removed	Maternal noncompliance; died of electrolyte and fluid loss at age 1 yr
0	Talpies equinovarus; T5 distal vertebral anomalies; two-vessel cord; mild pulmonic stenosis	++++, 50 cm	Repaired omphalocele; closed pubis, two "8" sutures; internalized urinary bladder age, 5 days, include piece of colon	Ileostomy, day 5	Now in Native American foster home
0	Two-vessel umbilical cord; bowel transit time, 90–120 seconds	+++++, 10-cm small intestine	0	0	Died of electrolyte and fluid loss at age 15 days
0	Bilateral talipes equinovarus; partial sacral agenesis; hip dysplasias; seven orthopedic operations	+++	Repair omphalocele, age 1 day, urinary bladder excised, age 13 mo; ureteroileostomy revised × four times; right nephrectomy age 10 yr	Ileocecal area closed with perineal pull-through anoplasty, age 2 mo; colostomy to abdomen, age 12 yr	Child abuse in foster home; now in nursing home; IQ, 65, WISC; osteo-knees; seizures; now in WC
0	Bilateral hip dislocations; left pelvic kidney; scoliosis fused, age 14 yr	+++, Improved after ileocolostomy, age 26 mo	Ureterocutaneous colostomy, age 8 mo; ureteroileostomy, age 26 mo; formed uric acid stones	Ileostomy, age 8 mo; ileocutaneous colostomy, age 26 mo	IQ, 96, WISC; psychological problems; WC
0	Bilateral Simian creases; synostosis of 2nd and 3rd toes; left kidney is two separate renal masses; one ureter; splayed pelvis	+	Omphalocele repair; cecum resected, age 2 days; bladder left exterior; bladder internalized with Young-Dees bladder neck closure; bilateral iliac osteotomies, age 9 mo	Ileostomy, age 2 days; colonic rudiment removed	Walks and runs

Table 8-1 (*continued*)

Case Number	Age	Omphalocele	Vesicoenteric Plate	Uterus; Vagina	Penis; Scrotum	Sex	Myelocele
14	2.5 yr	Small	+	Bifid uterus; vagina with proximal plus distal opening	0	F	Lipomatous myelocele excised, age 3 wk
15	2 mo	+	+	Vagina excised, age 1 day	0	F	+, L5-S1 paresis
16[b]	2 wk	+	+	Cervix and vaginal mucosa	0	F	+

Exstrophy was common to all 16 patients; urinary bladder was on each side of primitive ileocecal colon, bifid symphysis pubis, imperforate anus.
Key: +, ++, +++, ++++, mild to severe; BS, Bayley Scales of Infant Development; cruises, walks hanging on; GI, gastrointestinal; L, lumbar, MDI, Motor Development Index; osteoknees, osteomyelitis of the knees; PDI, Performance Development Index; s, sacral; T, thoracic; UB, urinary bladder; WC, uses a wheelchair; WISC, Wechsler Intelligence Scale for Children; SB, Stanford Binet.
[a] Reported by Hayden and associates.[465]
[b] Reported by McLaughlin and associates.[727]

10–12, and 14–16, Table 8-1).[355,417,465,727,910,928,1091,1098,1143] Ambiguous external genitalia in some patients have led to misidentification or purposeful arbitrary assignment of female sex (cases 8, 11, and 12, Table 8-1).[465,910,1143]

The complex array of major malformations associated with exstrophy of the cloaca requires careful evaluation of all organ systems and careful social planning. Otherwise, the affected child will be subjected to major corrective surgery in the presence of fatal anomalies of other systems (cases 8 and 15, Table 8-1), will be assigned inappropriate gender identification, or will be cared for in an inappropriate social setting (cases 8 and 11, Table 8-1).[465,727] Because of the frequent association of numerous major organ malformations and the need for careful preliminary evaluation, we will discuss the major consequences of exstrophy lesion closure according to each potential complication.[343,465,509] As with other major congenital malformations, we discuss etiology, prevalence, and recurrence with families during the initial conference and frequently thereafter.

Table 8-1 *(continued)*

Other Anomalies					
GI Tract	Other	Short-Gut Syndrome	Closure of Urinary Bladder	Closure of Colon	Comment/ Outcome
Small bowel obstruction	Thin undulating ribs; multiple vertebral anomalies T5 and below	++	Internalized and reconstructed vagina, age 1 day	Ileostomy, age 1 day; colonic rudiment removed	PDI 69 and MDI 58 on Bayley; age 13 mo, developed gall stones; cruises
25–30-cm small bowel; distal half dilated; malrotated intestines	Two-vessel cord scoliosis and abnormal vertebrae with 12 ribs; left equinovarus	+++++, 20 minute transit time	Internalized, wound dehiscence; *Candida* urinary tract infection; bladder neck adhered closed	Ileostomy; colonic rudiment removed	Life maintained by feeding intravenously until sepsis and death at age 2 mo
0	Renal hypoplasia on right; renal agenesis Left	++++	0	0	Died with renal failure at age 2 wk

Prevalence

In addition to recent surgical and medical treatments that can potentially keep severely congenitally deformed infants alive, more recent advances in prenatal diagnosis both allow management of the delivery process to improve chances for survival of infants with cloacal exstrophy[476,727] and suggest exstrophy of the cloaca may be more common[413] than the previously reported 1 in 200,000–250,000 births.[31,465,1011] In the decade since our last estimate,[465] we have treated 14 cases born locally among 1.3 million births in our region, suggesting an incidence nearer to 1 in 100,000. Part of this increase in our estimated birth prevalence may be due to more frequent early referral of infants after birth as well as to more cases detected and referred in utero.[727] Hook[503] and Sever[1003] discuss prevalence at birth and among stillbirths and abortuses; they suggest more severe anomalies will cause spontaneous abortion, stillbirth, or perinatal death before referral and, therefore, may be more common than suspected by persons caring for these anomalies in tertiary referral centers.

Recurrence Risk Counseling

As indicated in Chapter 3, the exstrophic lesions are reported most frequently as appearing sporadically, with a recurrence risk of less than 1 percent.[531] Recently, Shapiro and associates[1011] have reported a multicenter study of 2500 index cases of exstrophy of the urinary bladder with a recurrence risk of 1 in 70 for first-degree relatives. Twins concordant for exstrophy of the cloaca have been reported[727,895]; one hypothesis is that exstrophies are caused by the same process that causes twinning (see Chapter 3).[982] Another hypothesis suggests inheritance by non-Mendelian transmission.[1011] The information that exstrophies are infrequent and infrequently recur relieves most families from worry about recurrence and from the guilt frequently associated with congenital disorders, yet also alerts them to the value of prenatal diagnosis for detection of the rare recurrence. Furthermore, early detection with in utero diagnosis allows parents to overcome the shock and grief initially associated with the birth of a congenitally deformed child and enables them to reach a decision as to how their child should be managed during and immediately after delivery; this process is outlined by Haygood and Wahbeh[476] as well as McLaughlin and associates[727] and discussed in Chapter 4 of this text.

Management of the Gastrointestinal Tract

Gastrointestinal anomalies and complications are both the most difficult to manage and the leading cause of death among infants born with exstrophy of the cloaca.[465,910,928,1143] Three of our patients have died as a result of fluid and electrolyte imbalance secondary to the short-gut syndrome. The first patient, case 10 (Table 8-1), was not treated because he had only 10 cm of small intestine. The second patient did so well in a foster home that reconstructive surgery was undertaken at age 9 months. After surgery, she was taken home by her biological parents, became severely dehydrated, and died. The inability of her biological parents to accept her home after closure and a sex reversal may have contributed to her death (case 8, Table 8-1). The third child, who died from ileostomy fluid losses, was sustained by prolonged hyperalimentation after closure of the exstrophy, internalization of the urinary bladder, and creation of an ileostomy (case 15, Table 8-1). Her small intestine measured 25 cm, yet the distal half appeared to be nonfunctional, with dilated loops but neither anatomic obstruction nor capacity to absorb nutrients. The gastrointestinal transit time was less than 20 minutes, and she never tolerated oral feedings. She died with chronic infection associated with wound dehiscence.

The only other case in our series to suffer significant morbidity may have become mentally retarded from fluid and electrolyte loss but also had a history of maternal neglect. She was physically abused and placed in a series of foster homes; she is now in a nursing home (case 11, Table 8-1). An attempt to provide a fluid-absorption surface by using the rudimentary colon in addition to the ileum was not successful in her case, but was in another (case 12, Table 8-1). This segment of colon, however, may be without peristalsis and cause functional obstruction or may have abnormal blood supply and need to be removed (cases 2, 5, 6, 8, 13, and 14, Table 8-1). As illustrated by our only experience with a perineal ileocolostomy (case 11, Table 8-1), such procedures, as reported by others,[910,928,1143] are failures. In case 7, using exstrophied colon, we were able to successfully augment the urinary bladder.

Upper intestinal anomalies, including an intestinal length too short to support life, should be diagnosed by upper gastrointestinal studies before surgery to repair the cloaca. Two types of upper gastrointestinal malformations may require urgent corrective surgery: (1) obstructions caused by stenosis or duplication and (2) upper gastrointestinal bleeding from a Meckel's diverticulum or duplication.

Regardless, careful plans for management of acute illnesses with the potential for increased fluid and electrolyte loss, either due to vomiting or diarrhea, need to be worked out with the family and primary care health provider. Nine of our 15 patients experienced significant small intestine fluid losses. Frequent hospitalizations for fluid and electrolyte replacement must be anticipated. In addition, sodium bicarbonate, sodium, potassium citrate, and calcium solutions for oral use should be prepared at home[114] or prescribed for routine supplemental home use. The exact replacement solution can be prescribed by estimating the electrolyte content and the volume of small intestine drainage. Codeine and anticholinergic agents may also be used to decrease gastrointestinal transit time and decrease fluid and electrolyte loss.

Distal ileum function may be impaired in these patients, leading to poor reabsorption of bile salts and other substances normally absorbed at this level. Consequences may include gallstones (case 14, Table 8-1), calcium oxalate renal stones (case 1, Table 8-1), and potentially, folate and B_{12} deficiency in later years.

Urinary Tract Closure

Information in the literature is insufficient for deriving definitive recommendations for urinary tract management. Perhaps no other malformation better illustrates the need for individualizing management recommendations based on each patient's unique pathology. The varied cases described below exemplify this point.

One young adult has survived to 18 years of age without surgery and with moderate renal impairment,[910] and another, with ureteroileostomy at age 5, has no renal impairment at 24 years of age (case 4, Table 8-1). Despite early ureteroileostomy, two of our patients have needed repeated revisions, have developed nephrolithiasis, and have poor urinary drainage and chronic urinary tract infections (cases 1 and 12, Table 8-1). Another died with renal aplasia (case 16, Table 8-1).

We recommend internalization of the urinary bladder with a piece of the splayed colon, if necessary.[46] Frequent follow-up studies are necessary to detect and treat subsequent obstructive uropathy, ureterovesical incompetence with reflux, and incontinence.[1,821,1233] For these reasons, the family of the newborn with exstrophy of the cloaca should be prepared for careful repeat urinary tract evaluations and several subsequent operative procedures. The only alternative to internalization is urinary diversion. Diversion is always associated with incontinence, and 75 percent of patients develop complications such as nephrolithiasis, infection, and renal failure.[1233] In comparison, Woodhouse and associates[1233] report that ten percent of children with internalized bladders develop continence and only 25 percent develop the complications listed above. With urinary bladder neck-tightening procedures, clean intermittent catheterization, and artificial urinary sphincters, internalization of the urinary bladder should be associated with improved continence and sexuality in the future (see the discussion of exstrophy of the urinary bladder latter in this chapter). Finally, if internalization of the urinary bladder fails, urinary diversion can be done when the child is older and the intestine has grown.

In summary, we recommend complete evaluation of gastrointestinal and renal function and urinary tract anatomy before choosing a method of isolating the urinary tract. Internalization should be attempted, but parents should be informed that it is almost always a multiple-stage procedure; secondary stage procedures may be necessary months to years later. Urinary diversion can always be used if internalization fails. Use of part or all of the colonic remnant to augment the urinary bladder may be considered; the colonic segment may lack peristalsis and, therefore, may not function as an effective urinary conduit. Remnants of the urinary bladder could be used as an urinary conduit to the abdominal wall. Regardless of the type of closure, the short-gut syndrome requires preserving as much ileum as possible. The short-gut syndrome is a particular problem the first few years of life for two reasons: first, the intestine lengthens with growth, and second, young infants have high metabolic water needs that lessen as they grow older.

Genital Reconstruction

Up until the mid 1970s, only Ambrose[30] reported reconstruction of the perineum of a patient with exstrophy of the cloaca. Others have not mentioned experience with reconstruction of the genitals.[343,465,509,910,1143] Our 1973 recommendation to preferentially assign female sex regardless of chromosome sex has now been reversed for three reasons: (1) complete female identification has been difficult to maintain (case 12, Table 8-1); (2) the two males converted to females (cases 11 and 12, Table 8-1) have thin perineal floors with insufficient musculature to prevent intestinal prolapse through the orifice of any perforation made in the perineum in an attempt to form a vagina; and (3) emerging technology may make it possible to reconstruct sterile but functional male external genitalia from silastic inserts and full-thickness, tube pedicle grafts from the thighs.

Instead of converting chromosomal or gonadal males with insignificant penile and scrotal elements to the female role, we suggest identifying the sex by chromosome analysis unless the gender can be easily identified from completely and partially bifid or vestigally remnant reproductive organs (types 1 and 2, Table 8-1). Those with no identifiable reproductive organs (type 3 in Table 8-1) are particularly in need of chromosome analysis, which can be obtained within 24 hours after birth. We do this for two reasons: the chromosomal sex may indicate the fetal hormone present early on during gestation, and, more importantly, we have found that chromosomal sex strongly influences parental expectations. Parental beliefs and views as well as other learning experiences and in utero hormonal effects on brain cells may all influence the child's self-perce-ption. Sex is determined by three additional mechanisms. First, hormones affect genitalia since, structurally, a normal fetus could develop into a male or female; if no male genitalia develop, then the fetus will look like a female. Second, in adolescence, the pituitary releases luteinizing hormone (LH), which is the same in both sexes but will affect the sexes differently according to what type of genitalia exists and whether the individual has eggs or sperm. Third, gamete cells contribute to the sex of the individual. We believe that chromosome sex and parental expectations, reflected in self-perception, are the most important determinants of sex.

The influence of parental expectations is illustrated by case 6 (Table 8-1). The issue of reassignment of the male to a female sex role involved acquiescence of the mother and father. The mother was noted, however, to continue to refer to the infant as "he" and "him" even after the decision to convert had been reached. When the use of the male pronoun was mentioned, the mother admitted to a preference for a male. The operative closure plan was altered to retain the male organs. Currently, he is doing very well with a small, broad penis capable of erection, but he is only a prepubescent boy so that full sexual potential cannot be evaluated. It is now estimated that future phalloplasty will provide him with similar anatomy to sexually functional case 4.

Neurological Complications

Paralysis of leg muscles secondary to a large or small myelocystocele can range from nil to complete. If any function is present, it can be lost progressively (cases 1, 7, and 11, Table 8-1). Progressive paralysis can be stopped by surgical reduction of the cystic mass, with conversion of loculated spaces to free communication with the lumbar subarachnoid space (case 7, Table 8-1). Since early institution of myelocystocele corrective surgery, we have witnessed no significant loss of muscle strength, and three of our young patients with large resected myeloceles are biped ambulators (cases 2, 9, and 14, Table 8-1). These children contrast with two of our older patients who progressively lost so much muscle function they became limited to wheelchairs (cases 1 and 11, Table 8-1). The others have insignificant neuromuscular impairment, no evident myelocystocele, or a high level of paralysis present at birth. Careful neurosurgical dissection and histological study have revealed all of these lesions to be myelocystoceles arising from the ventricles of the conus medullaris. All are distinct from the subarachnoid space and are usually multiloculated. Each contains an ependyma and lipoma or a teratoma. None have contained a neural plaque as seen with meningomyeloceles, but they do contain nerves in the septa and outer walls of the myelocyst.

We have observed no significant central nervous system malformations and found only one case report of associated hydrocephalus.[417] Our one mentally retarded patient experienced prolonged episodes of dehydration and hypernatremia as well as violent child abuse (case 11, Table 8-1).

Musculoskeletal System Management

The unique aspects of musculoskeletal management of children with exstrophy of the cloaca and urinary bladder will be discussed here. The wide separation of the perineal musculature seen with exstrophy of the cloaca is less marked with classical exstrophy of the urinary bladder. The similarity of deformity between the two types of exstrophy is the failure of the public rami and associated soft-tissue structures to fuse in the midline and form the mons pubis (except in rare cases of exstrophy of the bladder without epispadius). As a result, the pelvis is open with the iliac wings flattened. The hip sockets are angulated so that they face posterolaterally rather than laterally. This angulation places the normally true anterior-posterior or truly sagittal plane of hip motion into an anterolateral to posteromedial plane. When walking, the hamstring muscles pull the body forward and to each side, giving the patient with an open pelvis a zig-zag, or waddling, gait. The unfused pubis adds to the waddle. Despite the description of what sounds like a very poor gait, children with only partially connected, unfused pubic rami learn to ambulate effectively.

Most authors recommend bilateral posterior iliac osteotomies in a three- or four-stage closure at the time of initial closure of all of the exstrophies.[1,417,769,821] We use the single-stage closure with bilateral, posterior iliac osteotomies[46,771] and counteract dehiscence of the anterior wall by holding the thighs tightly together with an ace bandage[46] or Buck's traction.[550] Our decision for performing iliac osteotomies is based on "The Pinch Test." This test is performed by squeezing the greater trochanters with the thumb and forefinger of one hand, while placing the forefinger of the other hand between the pubic rami. If the symphyses pinch the forefinger held in between them, the exstrophy can be closed without osteotomies.[46]

Abdominal wall closure is possible by approximation of skin edges, myofascial flaps,[910] or rectus abdominal myocutaneous flaps.[839,1072] Later rebuilding of the male and female escutcheon and external genitalia can be accomplished by thigh, full-thickness pedicle grafts with or without iliac crest.[24,38,638] In case 5 (Table 8-1), we used bilateral fan flaps to the midline, as advocated by Peters and associates.[864] We have not found a need for the more extensive myocutaneous grafts, and we have not been successful with bone transplants in infancy. In general, osseous, myofascial, and cutaneous closures for exstrophy of the cloaca are similar to those procedures used for exstrophy of the urinary bladder.

EXSTROPHY OF THE URINARY BLADDER

Most of this text is about myelodysplasia lesions involving both lower extremity nerve function and control over urine and stool elimination. Although it does not involve neural tube function, exstrophy of the urinary bladder has also been included because (1) it is a major malformation of the embryonic tail bud infrequently discussed in the pediatric literature; (2) it involves major psychogenic growth and development phenomena dependent on learning socially appropriate toileting behavior early in childhood; and (3) special toileting techniques necessary to help these children become continent are common to peers with both types of exstrophy and, to a large measure, those with neurogenic urine and stool incontinence. Self-toileting techniques are discussed in Chapters 9–12. Most of the management considerations discussed in the first portion of this chapter also apply to exstrophy of the cloaca. Below, we will discuss some aspects of exstrophy management, mentioned briefly in the preceding part of this chapter, which are better known from management of urinary bladder exstrophy.

Initial Discussion With Families

Early and frequent discussions about recurrence risk and sexual potential are essential ingredients in the care of children born with neurogenic urinary tract impairment of the sphincters.[285,465] These observations apply to the child with structural malformations of the urinary tract. The embryology, etiology, and low recurrence risk of exstrophy of the cloaca have been covered in Chapter 3 and in the previous portion of this chapter. As with myelodysplasia, it is important to discuss formation, etiology, and recurrence risks (1 in 275) with parents during the first and subsequent contacts. Unfounded fears and concerns of the parents and child can be allayed with accurate information. In addition, the health care professional should introduce the possibility that adults with bladder exstrophy can either father or bear children.[104,454,1233]

The older individuals in our group of patients with exstrophy have manifested a number of psychosexual disturbances similar to those of older patients with meningomyelocele. Most of these older patients have had urinary tract care with little attention to their sexual development. From the earliest contact, all discussions of urinary tract reconstruction should include a discussion of sexual potential. Parents and patients can also benefit from early and repeated descriptions of potential reconstructive procedures for the perineum that will create a more sexually attractive mons veneris and sexually functional penis.[38,454,638,647,864] Parents of females with exstrophy of the urinary bladder must be warned of the frequency of uterine prolapse and difficulty with pregnancies.[104,252]

Urinary Bladder Exstrophy Closure

Primary midline closure of urinary bladder exstrophy with posterior iliac osteotomies, if necessary for tension-free closure,[1,46] can be performed. Aadalen and associates[1] report "nearly" normal continence in 45 percent of their patients and successful closure without significant wound breakdown in 95 percent of 69 cases of urinary bladder exstrophy reviewed between 5 and 16 years postoperation.

Staged repair has been recommended by others and usually includes (1) closure of the bladder and abdominal wall; (2) later bladder neck reconstruction and, if necessary, ureteral reimplantation; and (3) phalloplasty with urethral reconstruction at a later stage.[253,769,821] DeMaria and associates[253] reported 22 patients with continence at an average of 8 years postclosure. Fifteen had normal upper urinary tracts visualized by intravenous pyelography, and all 22 had normal renal function. Only one had required corrective surgery after the initial closure. Oesch and Jeffs[821] reported that they internalized the bladders in 70 (64 percent) of 94 patients presenting with exstrophied urinary bladders and later examined 54 (77 percent) of those patients. Of those examined during follow-up studies, 58 percent (31 patients) experienced complete continence, 18.5 percent (10 patients) partial continence, and 24 percent (13 patients) complete incontinence or diversion. Mollard[769] reported that 11 of 16 patients (69 percent) were continent with neither reflux nor abnormal upper urinary tracts by intravenous pyelography. Lima and associates[650] recommended enlarging the bladder capacity and improving the ease and quality of closure by including human cranial dura mater as an augmentation patch during closure. Light and Scott[647] reported a 90 percent continence rate by applying the AS 752 artificial urinary sphincter to the internalized urinary system and one success by applying it to a bladder constructed entirely of bowel. Others have reported using rectus abdominal myocutaneous flaps for initial closure, but they have not given long-term results on any significant number of cases.[839,1072]

Long-term follow-up results of primary closure and diversion led Woodhouse and associates[1233] to state that most surgeons have given up attempts at primary closure and use diversion as a primary procedure. Follow-up of 29 female and 72 male patients in their 18th year or older revealed 18 percent of primary closure patients to be continent and 75 percent to have normal urinary tracts by intravenous pyelography. None of the patients with ureterocolonic diversions were continent at night. Those with ureteroileal loops required collection devices. Only 70 percent of patients with ureterocolonic and 25 percent of those with ureteroileal diversions had normal upper urinary tracts. In our series of 47 patients closed primarily, 24 (51 percent) are continent; three (6 percent) are too young to evaluate; ten (21 percent) are incontinent; and ten (21 percent) have been diverted. For those who are now incontinent, we anticipate creating continent urinary bladders by either urinary bladder neck-tightening, with or without clean intermittent catheterization, or by using artificial sphincters when these young children come of age (see Chapter 11).

Despite the large number of reports recommending ureterosigmoidostomy for urinary continence with exstrophy of the urinary bladder in patients with an intact anorectal mechanism, we have not encouraged such a method because of secondary electrolyte disturbances,[954] aminogenic coma,[575] and bowel cancer.[181,809,1025,1201]

Rebuilding the External Genitalia and Mons Pubis

Regardless of whether the urinary bladder has been internalized or the ureters diverted, the lower abdominal wall is usually scarred, the mons pubis deficient, the escutcheon separated into widely displaced halves, and the penis short and tethered or the vulva open and facing upward.[38] These abnormalities are distressing to some pubertal and young adult patients. As discussed in the previous section, reconstruction can be accomplished by bilateral local full-thickness skin grafts brought to the midline or by osseous myocutaneous groin grafts.[24,38,638,864] Because of the need for pubertal patients to gain confidence in themselves (see Chapters 19–21), we recommend such procedures on a cosmetic basis to enhance image building.

Female Reproductive Capacity

Five papers report a total of 49 adult women born with classical bladder exstrophy; 16 have given birth to 23 normal children.[104,252,519,872,1233] One gave birth from a single, cornuate uterus.[104] Unfortunately, the postpartum uterine prolapse rate was high.[104,264] We believe the incidence of uterine prolapse will be less in women whose separated pubic rami and perineal structures have been brought to the midline during early closure.

Male Reproductive Capacity

Only two papers describe the reproductive capacity of males born with urinary bladder exstrophy. Woodhouse and associates[1233] report that six of 72 males (8 percent) over the age of 18 years initiated pregnancies. Hanna and Williams[454] studied eight adult males with staged closure of their exstrophied urinary bladders and eight with primary diversions. All were capable of erection, and 10 (62 percent) were married and experiencing satisfactory sexual intercourse. Twelve (75 percent) were able to ejaculate, and three others oozed prostatic secretions after experiencing orgasm. Each of these three had a stenosed urethral fistula, either hypo- or epispadiac in position. Only one of the eight with staged primary closures and four of the eight with diversions had normal sperm counts. All male cases studied had short, normal caliber penises that were adequate for sexual intercourse.[1234] Since all but one of their patients had normal-sized testes, Hanna and Williams[454] suggested that prolonged exposure of the verumontanum and obstruction of the urethra associated with infection may have secondarily destroyed the patency of the vas deferens and, thus, caused sterility. These findings suggest a need to consider protection of the male reproductive system during reconstruction of the bladder neck and urethra as well as to maintain patency of the urethra even with diversion.

Other Complications

Although less common than with exstrophy of the cloaca, similar types of malformations and complications are seen with exstrophy of urinary bladder.[104,158,399,549] Besides those complications previously mentioned in this section, authors have reported Wilms' tumor,[158] double genital tract and uterus,[104,399] and wound dehiscence with urethral fistula formation,[549] in addition to rectal prolapse, imperforate anus, recto-exomphalos, vaginal fistula, vaginal stenosis, absent kidney, double renal pelvis, spina bifida, inguinal hernias, and congenital subluxation of the hip.[104] The frequency of these associated anomalies and the range in expression of severity of the exstrophic lesion itself—from a variant with bladder exstrophy and intact pelvis, mons pubis, and external genitalia to complete exstrophy of the bladder and epispadius[104]—suggest the need for careful evaluation of each patient.

SUMMARY

As with all major defects, complete evaluation is necessary before deriving a set of individualized options and recommendations that can be clearly communicated to the patient and/or family. The initial phase of treatment should consider care of other significant malformations, such as Wilms' tumor, exomphalos, and imperforate anus. Primary management plans should include preservation of the exstrophied bladder, with complete closure of the urinary tract as well as initial reconstruction of the prostatic urethra in the male and all of the urethra in the female. Surgery is also necessary to preserve or create a reproductive system and maintain gastrointestinal function. Counseling should include information and advice about the different self-toileting techniques and the possibility of a satisfactory adult sexual life with the appropriate, sex-related potential for reproduction.

SECTION III

Management of the Neurogenic Bowel and Bladder

Kay Wicks
David Shurtleff

9

An Introduction to Toilet Training

Toilet training is essentially the imposition of social control over automatic bodily functions. Such training is accomplished by using encouragement for the young child to remain clean and free from soiling odor. Fears of social disgrace caused by toileting accidents remain with us throughout our lives. Such fears are indirectly reinforced by jokes about stool and urine. A multitude of commercials implore us to smell clean and convey the message that cleanliness is equivalent to sexiness. Unfortunately, "of all the accidents that trouble a child, fecal soiling is the one that evokes the most intense deprecation from peers and parents, and is the most damaging to self-esteem."[345]345 These socially imposed sanctions place an unique burden on a sphincter-impaired person.

To establish a socially acceptable program that is practical and nonpunitive requires (1) the development of a trusting relationship between a consistent health care provider and the child and/or family for the provision of teaching, intervention, and reinforcement, (2) a developmental approach adjusted appropriately for the individual child in conjunction with patience and willingness to persevere and make adjustments in the program, and (3) a thorough understanding of the specific pathophysiology involved (see Chapters 10 and 11).

THE ROLE OF A PRACTITIONER

A consistent health care provider is critical. A nurse specialist knowledgeable in developmental pediatrics as well as bowel and bladder pathophysiology and management fulfills this role in our clinic. This

MYELODYSPLASIAS AND EXSTROPHIES: SIGNIFICANCE, PREVENTION, AND TREATMENT
 ISBN 0-8089-1816-8

health care provider must work closely not only with the physicians in charge of the case management, but with the child and family. Handling incontinence often affects the family's ability to handle crises. The crisis-prone family that lacks coping resources needs long-standing supervision and support from one trusted individual. Some families, on the other hand, cope quite well and can accomplish a successful daily program readily, but even these families still need guidance from a health care provider willing to encourage progress and make necessary recommendations when interruptions occur in fragile hygiene regimens, as outlined in Chapters 10 and 11.

A DEVELOPMENTAL APPROACH TO TOILET TRAINING

Infancy

When focusing on the developmental progress of a child, the health care provider must be alert to key stages in order to make proper recommendations to a family and child. In the stage of infancy, the baby's deficits become obvious to the parents. Alterations from the normal bowel and bladder patterns, causing loose or constipated stools and dribbling or retention of urine, need early intervention. During this stage, diapers are considered a socially acceptable means for both urine and stool collection, but associated skin irritation from constant soiling necessitates management of diaper rashes.

Parents must understand the causes of perianal skin rashes and sores; soiling without change or eliminating urine with large amounts of bacteria produces skin breakdown. More specifically, the following three main occurrences lead to skin breakdown: (1) production of ammonia caused by the breakdown of urea by bacteria, (2) the lack of normal bladder control mechanisms leading to frequent leakage, and (3) the lack of skin sensation. Insensitivity keeps the infant from fussing or crying and, thus, warning the parent of skin breakdown.

To avoid rashes, parents must keep the skin of the perianal area clean and the urine slightly acid. We recommend maintaining the urine pH below 6, as discussed in Chapter 13. The following hints are helpful: (1) Keep the urine acidic by using an appropriate diet (see Chapters 11 and 13) or ascorbic acid (vitamin C). Parents can obtain test materials that measure the acidity of the urine. These acid-testing materials include a paper tape impregnated with chemicals that will change color when dipped into a liquid (phenothalein papers) and a color chart indicating the pH or degree of acidity relative to the color of the tape. (2) Identify and treat urinary tract infections (UTIs) early. Urine infections can be detected by test tapes; Chem Strip 6 detects leukocyte esterase indicative of pyuria. These tapes are similar to those that measure for acidity. (3) Feed infants a proper, but minimum amount of protein; excess protein is changed into urea, then excreted in the form of ammonia in the urine. (4) Change diapers frequently. Use absorptive disposable diapers with no plastic covers or double- and triple-layer cloth diapers to collect constantly dribbling urine. Emphasis must be placed on changing the diapers frequently, particularly after the infant has been fed. The diapers should be placed in a pail containing one cup of vinegar in a quart of water. Detergents must be removed from the diapers with careful, repeated rinsing. The last rinse may include a solution of vinegar water, which will leave a maximum of acetic acid in the diaper. (5) Use protective ointments (which contain a protective oil or silicone), such as Desitin (Lanolin, Leeming Division Pfizer Inc. Parsippany, NJ), only on healthy baby skin.

Frequently, a rash will begin as redness, pimples, pustules, or patches of red excoriation that bleed easily. If a rash does appear, (1) stop the use of plastic pants or plastic-covered disposable diapers; (2) change absorbant diapers more frequently; (3) expose the rash to air, while using a goose-neck 25-watt lamp at least 12–18 inches distant from the skin, observing *every 15 minutes for redness*; (4) leave diapers off at night, covering the baby with a bath blanket, and use a plastic sheet covered with a terry cloth towel beneath the bottom sheet to absorb urine; (5) clean the baby's perineal area with a mild soap, and wipe with a vinegar-soaked cotton ball after each stool or every 30 minutes if the baby is dribbling urine; and (6) do not use ointments on the rash (ointments can keep water in and macerate skin). Antimonilial and anti-inflammatory agents may be necessary, but they should be in a cream or lotion with an aquaphilic base.

Preschool Years: Pretraining Management

As the child enters the preschool years, it is necessary for the health care provider to maintain frequent contact with the parents to assist them in determining the child's readiness for toilet training. Monitoring individual readiness and educating the parents should be initiated when the child is 12–24 months old, approximately 6–12 months prior to independent toilet training (normally, 18–36 months); the exact number of months of preparation and training are, however, less important than the general readiness of the particular family and child. The first question asked by parents of children born with neurological anatomic abnormalities of urine and stool control mechanisms is similar to that of parents with normal children: "When is my child ready to begin toilet training?" This question requires an individual answer, but in general the following is adequate: "As soon as his or her friends begin, usually between 18 and 36 months."

The difference involved in training the sphincter-impaired child is the addition of a few extra steps, particularly in the area of pretraining management. The focus at this time is on bowel management since this type of program should be intact prior to urinary continence training. To accomplish a successful independent bowel program, particularly if the child shows signs of constipation prior to 18–36 months, establishment of proper stool consistency and of an evacuation time should be emphasized. If these two factors are well managed, it is possible to prevent dilation of the lower colon and rectum, which can cause considerable problems in the bowel training process (see Chapter 10). Prior to an independent urinary continence program, medical management focuses on prevention of complications of the urinary-renal system. Low pressure and adequate drainage of urine must be maintained to insure renal health.

Due to the social attitudes mentioned at the beginning of this chapter, it is preferable that the sphincter-impaired child master self-care prior to normal peer contact in school. Independent urine hygiene for meningomyelocele children, however, can be achieved at the earliest by age 4 for the least paralyzed and by 10 for most paralyzed; on the average it is accomplished by 11–12 years for the least and 15–18 for the most impaired (see Chapter 12).

During the pretraining period, it is essential to provide the parents with education appropriate to their level of understanding and to their child's specific bowel and bladder pathophysiology, including the necessary methods to prevent long-term consequences from the lack of a training program. A family and child's compliance appears to improve if proper education is provided. This teaching must include topics of dietary interventions and toilet training principles as well as mechanics of the bowel and bladder and assisted continence programs. The specifics pertaining to these issues are covered in detail in the following two chapters. Teaching protocols and audio/visual aids are used. A list of teaching aids is provided.[a]

It is important to have several conferences with the parents during this time to continue reinforcement of the premanagement techniques of dietary intervention and timed elimination as well as to review the child's individual problems and, thereby, determine the specific program necessary for continence. Also, play therapy should be initiated with the child if assisted programs using enemas, catheters, or suppositories are required. When the invasive procedures are introduced during play therapy

[a] See references 25, 164, 200, 201, 231, 570, 574, 757, 788,–790, 886, 926, 985, and 1103.

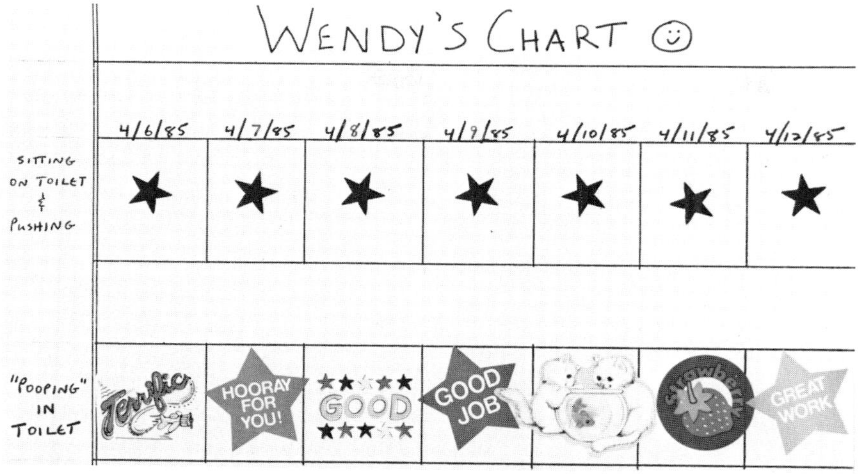

Figure 9-1. Star chart. Wendy's chart illustrates a successful reinforcement chart for a 3-year-old meningomyelocele youngster to reward two expected actions: (1) sitting on the toilet and pushing and (2) "pooping" in the toilet.

using dolls, puppets, and related medical supplies, a child's fear is significantly reduced. As a program is initiated, it is helpful to use simple star charts to reinforce the child's specific behavior (Fig. 9-1). Charts must be individually designed to indicate only the action behavior for the child; for example, "sit on the potty" would be appropriate for the child's star chart. This chart is used to reward the child for an expected behavior. It is equally important for the parent to keep a diary of food and fluid intake in relation to the child's elimination pattern. This record can be designed for bowel or bladder training (Figs. 9-2 and 9-3).

The following questions help parents assess whether or not their sphincter-impaired child is ready for toilet training: (1) Is your child aware of other family members using the toilet? (2) Is your child familiar with words such as *potty* and *diaper*? (3) Can your child sit on a chair with or without a brace or support? (4) Does your child use a sign to indicate that he or she is about ready to have a bowel movement? (5) Is your child able to sit on a potty-chair for 5–10 minutes? (6) Does your child indicate, or have you observed, a regular time during the day when his or her bowel movements seem to occur? (7) Is your child able to remove and replace pants and underclothing despite braces? If the majority of answers to the above questions are affirmative, the child is a candidate for training. In addition, it is important not to start when the child has active medical

A

TIME	Mealtime or Fluid Intake (brief description of meal)	Bowel Program (include suppository, enema, timed toileting, etc)	Results (quantity & character)	Incontinence-Bowel/Bladder (quantity & character)	Physical Activity (brief description)	Comments
6:00am						
7:00					Wake up	
8:00	½ wheat toast and 1 oz. warm Tang				Ready sister to school, Eat, Mr. Rogers	
9:00		Timed toileting on potty Digital stimulation	None		Sesame Street	
10:00	Can of chocolate			10:30—one formed stool accident	Hand crutch practice; then play doll-house; go get sister	
11:00					Play with sister	
12:00	Two bites chili				Lunch and TV	

1:00					Colored; hand crutch practice	
2:00	Four bites chili, 2 oz. Tang				Story with sister, dollhouse and pick up	
3:00					Hand crutch practice; played with new shopping cart	
4:00					Sesame Street	
5:00	Creamed tuna on toast (didn't eat peas)				Dinner and play	
6:00		Timed toileting	None		Played	
7:00	3 oz water				Story and bath	Bran in pudding No go
8:00					Bed	

Figure 9-2 *continues*

B

TIME	Mealtime or Fluid Intake (brief description of meal)	Bowel Program (include suppository, enema, timed toileting, etc)	Results (quantity & character)	Incontinence-Bowel/Bladder (quantity & character)	Physical Activity (brief description)	Comments
6:00am						
7:00						
8:00	Waffle and berry syrup				Woke up. Took sister to school.	
9:00		Timed toileting on potty with digital stimulation times two	2 small, hard formed; 7–8 large, soft formed		Sesame Street. Bath	
10:00					Dress Go get sister	
11:00					Play dollhouse	
12:00	Chili; 4 oz. Hawaiian Punch; wheat toast				Lunch	

1:00		Timed potty same as above	4 large, soft formed or more		Play outside	
2:00	Taco chips				Play inside, practice walking with crutches	
3:00					Play dollhouse Help clean up	
4:00					Sesame Street	
5:00	1/2 hamburger patty; mashed potatoes 1/2 c.; green beans, 1/4 c.				Dinner	
6:00			3 small, soft formed		Potty	
7:00					Bedtime	
8:00						

Figure 9-2. Food and fluid intake in relation to the child's elimination of stool. (A) Illustrates a typical dietary intake of a 30-month-old meningomyelocele youngster with an incomplete program of timed toileting and digital stimulation resulting in an accident. (B) Illustrates a successful program using timed toileting and digital stimulation following each meal for the same youngster.

A

CLEAN INTERMITTENT CATHETERIZATION I & O RECORD

DATE	TIME	FLUID INTAKE	DIAPERS OR PANTS SATURATED	WET	DAMP	DRY	OUTPUT AMOUNT	CATHETERIZATION APPEARANCE
7-4	7:30				X		40 cc	
	12:15	180 cc water			X		30 cc	
	4:30	50 cc milk			X		20 cc	
	8:30						10 cc	
7-5	8:45	180 cc milk		X			50 cc	
	12:30	30 cc pop			X		30 cc	
	4:30	50 cc water		X			15 cc	
	8:00	50 cc pop		X			10 cc	
7-6	10:45	120 cc milk	X				10 cc	
	12:30				X		20 cc	
	5:00 PM				X		20 cc	
	12:30 AM				X		30 cc	
7-7	8:15				X		30 cc	

	12:30	150 cc juice			X		10 cc	
	4:30	50 cc juice			X		20 cc	
	8:30	140 cc water			Went swimming		20 cc	

Figure 9-3 *continues*

B

CLEAN INTERMITTENT CATHETERIZATION I & O RECORD

DATE	TIME	FLUID INTAKE	DIAPERS OR PANTS SATURATED	WET	DAMP	DRY	OUTPUT AMOUNT	CATHETERIZATION APPEARANCE
9-5	8:00	60 cc			X		90 cc	Clear, yellow
	12:30	120 cc				X	60 cc	
	4:00	60 cc + 80 cc				X	70 cc	
	8:00					X	80 cc	
9-6	7:30	120 cc			X		100 cc	
	12:00	60 cc				X	80 cc	
	4:00	60 cc				X	40 cc	
	8:30	80 cc				X	50 cc	
9-7	8:15	150 cc				X	120 cc	Clear
	12:30	100 cc				X	100 cc	
	4:30	50 cc				X	70 cc	
	8:00	90 cc				X	40 cc	
9-8	9:30	180 cc				X	90 cc	

	12:00	60 cc				X	110 cc	
	4:00	90 cc				X	60 cc	
	8:30	60 cc				X	50 cc	
9-9	8:30	120 cc				X	80 cc	Clear
	12:30	80 cc				X	80 cc	
	4:00	90 cc				X	50 cc	
	8:30	40 cc				X	60 cc	

Figure 9-3. Fluid intake in relation to the child's elimination of urine. (A) Illustrates an unsuccessful CIC program. Note the quality of wetness in diaper prior to catheterization (incontinence in this case). (B) Illustrates a successful, socially continent CIC program with Ditropan (Oxybutynin Chloride, Marion Larboratories, Kansas City, MO) and Ephedrine in the same youngster.

issues or is about to have a major orthopedic operation or when the family is having difficulties.

Later Preschool Years: Initiating the Training Process

Once parents, in consultation with the medical team, decide on the right time, a positive, casual, patient manner is most successful for initiating the training process. Furthermore, the following, simple suggestions may help parents: (1) Choose a word for bowel movement that you will be using for the training, and use it consistently when diapering. (2) Choose a potty-chair with arms, and be sure the child's feet touch the floor; or use a box to hold his or her legs and feet in position. In either case, squatting should be approximated. (3) Take the child to the bathroom; close the door; and teach the child how to pull down his or her outer pants first and underpants second, both to around the ankles if possible. (4) Place the child on the potty approximately 15 minutes after each meal or when appropriate for bladder training; this should be for 3–5 minutes initially and then gradually for longer periods of time. (5) Remain with the child while he or she is learning. (6) Assist the child in becoming aware of when he or she is eliminating. (7) Help the child use toilet tissue. (8) Teach the child to flush the toilet. (9) Assist the child with handwashing following toileting. (10) Use verbal praise any time the child is successful.

School-Age Children

As the child develops into the independent school-aged stage, the health care provider must spend time with the child alone, explaining in detail his or her particular disability. Children like to succeed independently during this period and will be apprehensive about accidents that may occur at school, so self-care should be promoted. Individual appointments must be scheduled with the child to provide teaching necessary for achieving independence in bowel and bladder continence. The extent of these sessions depends on the parents' current involvement. Parents should be advised to request that a supportive staff member assist the child at school with any requirements to maintain continence. The United States Supreme Court states that Public Law 94-142 requires schools to provide clean intermittent catheterization (CIC) (see Chapters 2 and 17). It is also necessary for the health care provider to review the child's needs with the school; most parents appreciate this assistance.

The child's needs at school may include architectural changes, supervision of toileting program, and encouragement of positive social attitudes. The architectural set-up in the bathroom must facilitate the child's independence. For example, the child will require a large enough bathroom to allow access if he or she is in a wheelchair. All materials, faucets, and drainage basins must be at a proper level, within the child's reach. In public facilities, a closed toilet area is essential, instead of stalls accessible to curious peers. Supervision and help should be consistent with needs and should be given with firm insistence; this may involve a code or secret signal by the schoolroom teacher indicating an odor or may require actual assistance with the program. Silent computer signals may now be used (see Chapter 17). "Hands-on" help is most often assigned to an educational aid.

In addition to physical requirements, the sphincter-impaired child will have social needs. Schoolmates must be educated to accept appropriate social attitudes. The ridicule and teasing of a sphincter-impaired child with toileting accidents can be as detrimental as physically kicking the crutches out from under a child with paralyzed legs. Moral injunctions and outdated prejudices may give way to more positive attitudes with appropriate education. "The Kids on the Block"[583] puppet presentation is beneficial in creating positive attitudes among peers, as is K-6 "People You Would Like to Meet"[859] curriculum. (Attitudes toward individuals with congenital malformations have been discussed in more detail in Chapter 2.)

Preadolescence and Adolescence

The stress of puberty can precipitate a regression in the preadolescent's or adolescent's ability to perform established continence programs. This may be a manifestation of two similar defense mechanisms: denial of, or withdrawal from, the specific impairment. It is important for the practitioner to help the family understand these defenses and, thereby, avoid anxiety about the preadolescent becoming dependent again. Adolescents will often rebel against the values of all authority figures, including issues and medical staff related to their disability. It is worth checking the adolescent's understanding of particular congenital malformations and specific programs. Adolescents may refuse to carry out a previous regimen, but they may be willing to design a new program to avoid impaction or accidents. This rebellion stage is common with chronically ill or impaired adolescents and is one reason we defer inserting an artificial urinary sphincter or carrying out undiversion until after psychological maturation (see Chapter 18). At this age, techniques for urinary collection need to be changed to become more sexually attractive. (For a more in-depth discussion of adolescence and adolescence and sexuality, see Chapters 19 and 21, respectively).

Effects of Late Referral and/or Inadequate Programs

If the child with sphincter impairment does not adhere to a socially and medically acceptable program for toilet training, one or many complications may evolve. The saddest consequence is the child who presents with socially unacceptable and self-destructive behavioral manifestations resulting from social disgrace. Such patients require referrals to psychological or psychiatric services to improve their damaged self-concepts. School placement may need to be changed in order to provide a fresh start free from harassment (see Chapters 2 and 17). This social disgrace evolves from the child's lack of appropriate hygiene and inappropriate management of incontinence. The incontinence usually stems from inadequate medical recommendations at the various developmental stages. Repeat failures cause depression, rebellion, and lack of compliance by the family and/or child. If a successful bowel program has not been established, obstipation can occur from repeated bowel impaction. This complication, while unresolved, prevents achieving bowel continence (see Chapter 10). Inadequate emptying of the bladder eventually leads to pathologies of the renal system, which obviously are detrimental to the child's health. These complications are just a few, but they point to

Table 9-1
Communication Guideline for Community Follow-up of Bowel and Bladder Impairments

Monitor by Public Health Nurse	Alert Health Care Provider
Level of family's understanding of deficits	Provide summary regarding understanding
Adjustment to disability	Inability to cope
Readiness cues for toilet training	Readiness for training
Family's misunderstanding of toileting techniques	Need for intervention
Bowel and bladder patterns	Constipation or diarrhea or incontinence
Dietary status	Inappropriate diet patterns
Toilet training process	Progress report
Compliance with bowel and bladder program	Need for program changes
Skin care	Unmanageable breakdown
School difficulties secondary to bladder and/or bowel issues	Report on problems
Architectural barriers	Report on problems
Adolescent adjustment	Need for intervention

the importance of working with families and patients to establish a successful toilet training program. A community health nurse referral is helpful if the family needs additional support and monitoring within the home setting. A communication system can be developed for the community health nurse to alert the health care provider to problems (Table 9-1).

SUMMARY

Everyone in our society is expected to be free of soiling odor. Specifics of bowel and bladder pathophysiology and corresponding management are discussed in Chapters 10 and 11; toilet training outcome is reviewed in Chapter 12. Avoiding the social disgrace of incontinence is both essential and possible for the neurogenically impaired. Establishing an acceptable toilet training program requires intervention, teaching, and reinforcement by a consistent health care provider. This program must be initiated in infancy and adjusted appropriately as the child develops.

Kay Wicks
David Shurtleff

10

Stool Management

Although stool control is not as important to health as good urine control, the embarrassment of stool odor is equal to, if not worse than, urine odor. Effective stool management requires clear working concepts of the anatomy and physiology of the gastrointestinal (GI) tract, particularly the large intestine, rectum, anal canal, and the internal and external anal sphincters. Before recommending an appropriate program, the health care provider must understand exactly what is being assessed, that is, not only how the GI tract works, but also what different types of pathology are present. This knowledge will increase the chances of recommending the most suitable program, thereby (1) eliminating excessive trial and error, (2) decreasing complications and patient frustration, and (3) increasing patient compliance. Dietary control, evacuation of the bowel at the same time each day, and behavior techniques are primary considerations in stool management. Seven methods to achieve bowel continence are available for use with the above basic three techniques and are described later in this chapter. Regardless of the techniques employed, the parent or care provider, and eventually the patient, must recognize that accidents will occur, and, therefore, that cleanliness and freedom from odor require vigilance.

MYELODYSPLASIAS AND EXSTROPHIES: SIGNIFICANCE, PREVENTION, AND TREATMENT
 ISBN 0-8089-1816-8

NORMAL ANATOMY AND PHYSIOLOGY OF THE GASTROINTESTINAL TRACT

The GI tract consists of a tube of variable diameter running through the body from the mouth to the anus and is surrounded by three layers of smooth muscle. Contraction of these smooth muscle layers, a process known as peristalsis, exerts pressure on food contents, causing them to flow through the tube. When managing stool continence, it is important to remember that a person's emotional state can affect motility, the movement of food material through the GI tract. Peristalsis and the resultant motility can increase with anxiety, resulting in diarrhea, and decrease with depression, causing constipation. In addition, physical activity can affect intestinal peristalsis and motility, which can be decreased by bed rest and increased by exercise. Digestion and absorption are the two main functions that occur in the tract. Almost all digestion and absorption of food (approximately 95 percent) and water (80 percent) occur in the three sections of the small intestine: the duodenum, the jejunum, and the ileum.[98] After a meal, contractions of the ileum increase, causing the ileocecal valve to open and empty food material into the large intestine; this mechanism is the gastro-ileac reflex. The marked increase in motility occurring after meals, known as the gastrocolic reflex, coincides with this gastro-ileac reflex.

The large intestine, or colon, consists of three relatively straight segments: the ascending, the transverse, and the descending segments (Fig. 10-1). The S-shaped, terminal section of the descending portion, the sigmoid colon, empties into a short section, the rectum, which lies entirely within the pelvis and discharges into the anal canal. The primary function of the colon is to store fecal material. It secretes no digestive enzymes and is responsible for absorbing water remaining in the fecal material presented to the cecum from the ileum. Although the quantity of water absorbed is small compared with that absorbed in the small intestine, the relative amount is crucial to bowel management since it determines stool consistency. If almost all the remaining water is absorbed, then dry fecal pellets and constipation result. If, on the other hand, excess water is not absorbed, diarrhea results. During normal digestion, the large intestine absorbs 90 percent of the water remaining in the contents passing the ileocecal valve—that is, 90 percent of 20 percent not absorbed by the small intestine.[98] The longer stool remains in the colon, the greater the percentage of water absorbed. Rapid transit through the colon will lead to loose, watery stools. Diarrhea is, however, usually due to excess water coming into the large intestine and overwhelming the bowel's absorptive capacity.

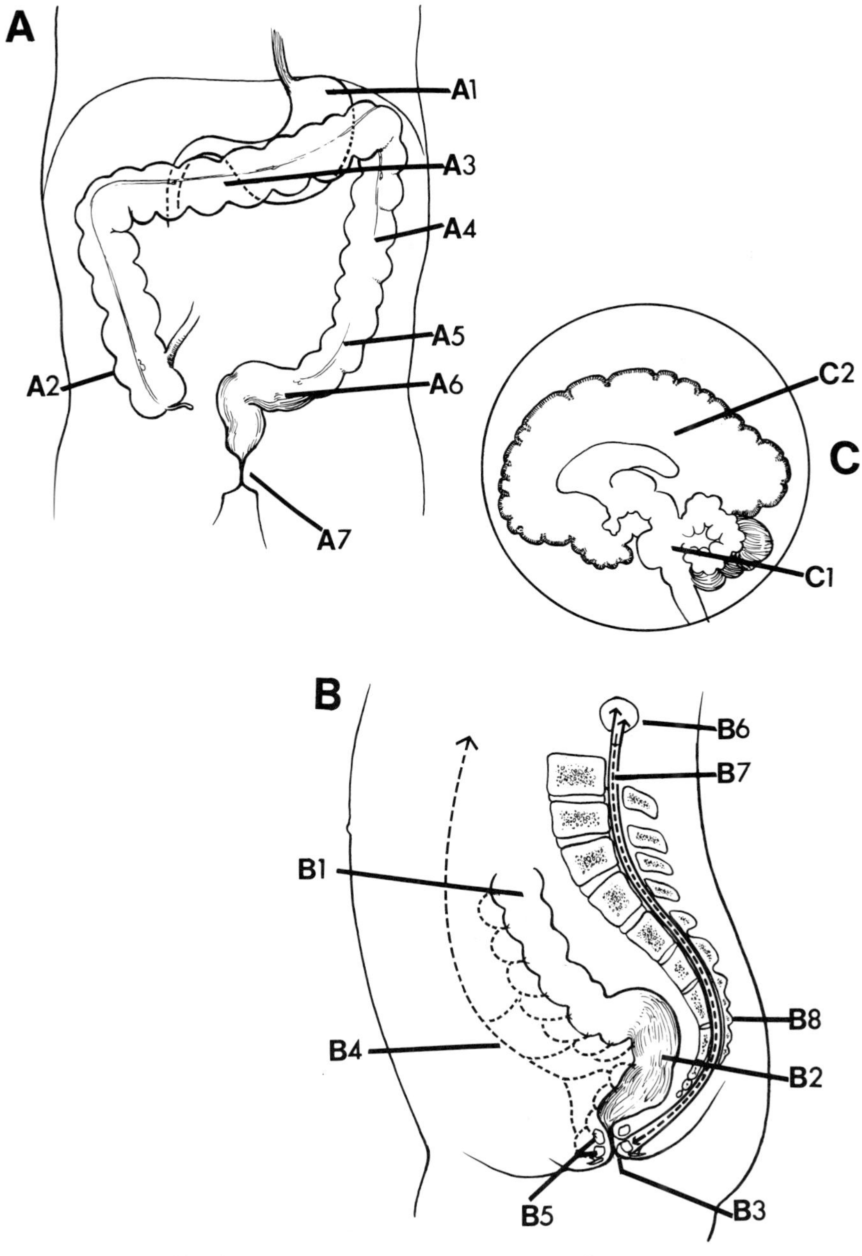

Figure 10-1. This shows the stomach (A1); the ascending (A2), transverse (A3), and descending (A4) sigmoid colon (A5); the rectum (A6); and the anus (A7). Side view of colon (B1) shows rectum (B2), anus (B3), autonomic nerves (B4), circular muscles of sphincter (B5). Also shown is somatic sensory (B6) and motor nerves (B7) and their relationship to the sacrum (B8). The arrows at the top of nerves in part B imply connection of autonomic nerves with reflex arcs at C1 (detrusor arc) and with sensory areas of the cortex (C2) and the connection of somatic, sensory, and motor nerves with the cortex (C2).

NORMAL DEFECATION

The neuroanatomy involved in the process of defecation is illustrated in Figures 10-1 and 10-2. The autonomic, or involuntary, nerve plexus coordinates the autonomic functions of the intestines by innervating the colon, rectum, and internal anal sphincter. The somatic (voluntary), motor, and sensory nerves pass to and from the brain directly via the spinal column. One set of these nerves, the anal sensory, arises in the delicate sensory organs in the wall of the anal canal. When touched, these nerves send different messages to the brain, which normal individuals perceive as gas, liquid, or solid. These differences are learned during prememory toilet training. Even though we read and immediately understand the concepts of anal sensations, we cannot recall how we learned them. Since parents also learned toilet training in infancy before true recall, these aspects of toilet training have not been reduced to physiologic understanding.

The other touch sensory nerves are outside the anus and, like the anal canal nerves, differentiate between touch and pain or hot and cold; the normal person also interprets these as diarrheal (hot) or stool (rough) accidents. The somatic anal motor nerves pass only to the external anal sphincter, which allows direct control over defecation. However, additional sphincter mechanism motor nerves go to the pelvic floor, levator ani, and gluteal muscles and assist in the continence process by pulling the perineum upwards and, with maximum effort, squeezing the buttocks together (as is more fully explained below, under the "pucker" discussion).

The neurophysiological process of defecation (Fig. 10-2) begins as the autonomic sensory nerve arcs coordinate the smooth muscle contraction of the colon, causing peristalsis. This motion, heard and felt as gurgles, cannot be controlled directly, nor can its location be identified as small or large colon. Since colon peristalsis coincides with the gastro-ileac reflex, indirect control over defecation can sometimes be regulated by when one eats. Also, as mentioned earlier, emotional states and physical activity will often affect peristalsis. When peristalsis pushes intestinal contents into the rectum, there is a distinctly different feeling that is associated with the rectum filling to the point of stretching the rectal wall. This combination of colon peristalsis and full rectum is recognized through toilet training as the predefecation urge. During this time, the internal and external sphincters are initially closed, and the resting tonus of the levator ani holds the sides of the anal canal in apposition, keeping it closed (Fig. 10-1). The rectum fills until an autonomic sensory stretch reflex initiates a rectal muscle squeeze, pushing the stool down into the anal canal. The internal anal sphincter is coordinated by the autonomic

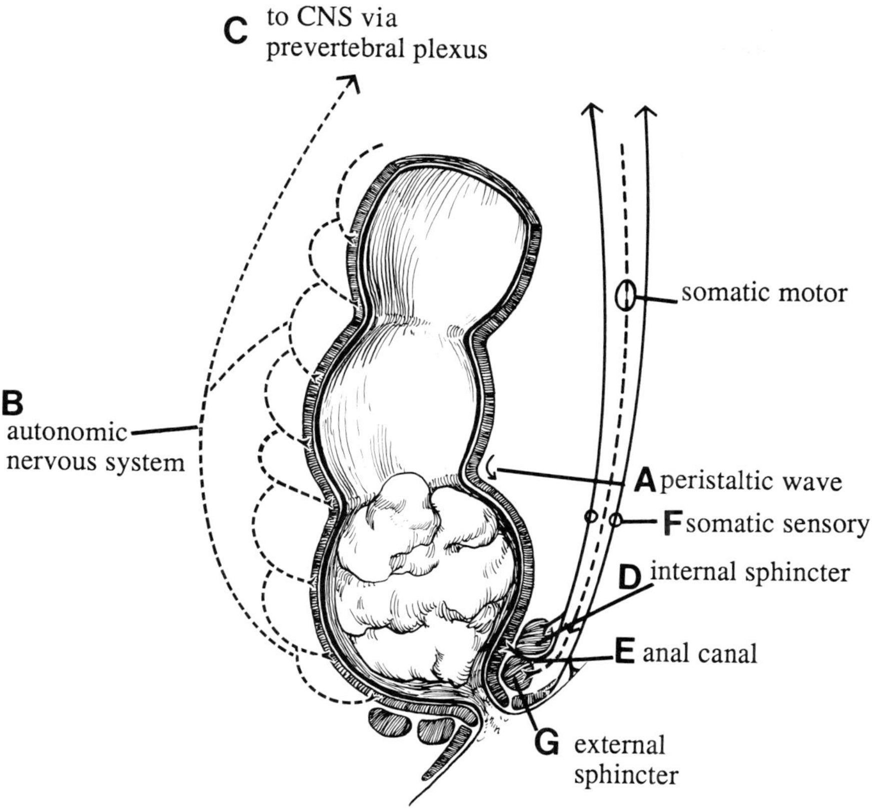

Figure 10-2. The process of normal defecation. As the rectum is stretched by a bolus of stool from the sigmoid colon, a wave of circular constriction (A) moves from the colon toward the rectum, pushing rectal contents into the anus. Automatic nerves (B) control this action and send messages to the brain (C), as the predefecation urge, via presacral nerves that enter the spinal cord in the thoracic and high-lumbar areas. The autonomic nerves also relax the internal sphincter (D), allowing the rectal contents to touch the anal canal and sensory nerves (F), sending a message to the brain via the low-sacral nerves and spinal cord. This message has been learned to distinguish gas from liquid. Stool sphincter (G), levator ani, and other muscles of the anal sphincter mechanism contract or relax to allow passage of contents.

nerves to relax. The eternal anal sphincter remains contracted (Fig. 10-2). This coordination is called the anorectal reflex. The contents of the rectum pass into the anal canal and touch the somatic sensory nerves of the anal canal, causing conscious awareness of the imminent passage of liquid, gas, or stool; this is commonly known as the defecation urge or the actual initiation of the passage of rectal contents.

We react to this urge with the ‘‘pucker,’’ a conscious effort to close the anal sphincter. The pucker occurs in three magnitudes or stages: (1) lightly, by using just the external sphincter, (2) moderately, by contracting both the external sphincter and the levator ani, thereby lifting the perineum up, and (3) strongly, by adding leg and gluteal muscle contraction. (You can feel each set of muscles sqeeze as you pucker with more strength.) Maximum contraction causes a waddling gait, often called the ‘‘outhouse trot.’’ The pucker mechanism will fatigue and finally stop the autonomic defecation process; if this occurs, the stool will be pushed back into the rectum. With continued rectal peristalsis and relaxation of the pucker mechanism, defecation occurs. The defecation act also involves relaxation of the levator ani and the resultant opening of the anal canal. The accompanying Valsalva maneuver increases intra-abdominal and intrarectal pressure, which assists in propelling the stool through the short anal canal. Understanding these details of the defecation process is helpful for stool toilet training, particularly with the types of pathology described below.

DEFECATION PATHOLOGY

Variable intestinal function must be anticipated in everyone, whether colon and anorectal function is normal or abnormal; each person responds differently to environmental influences. The temporary pathological conditions of constipation, obstipation, and impaction as well as diarrhea can be superimposed on the following three types of chronic or static pathophysiologic abnormalities: (1) absence of an autonomic nervous system connection, (2) imperforate anus (Fig. 10-3), and (3) intrinsic spinal cord abnormalities, including a tight, spastic anus (Fig. 10-4) and an atonic or loose anus associated either with constipation (Fig. 10-5) or with frequent stools (Fig. 10-6). We will discuss the types of superimposed pathophysiology before discussing the three types of pathology mentioned above. Parents must learn to recognize the signs of these temporary and superimposed conditions in order both to understand their child's basic or underlying pathology and to teach their child appropriate control.

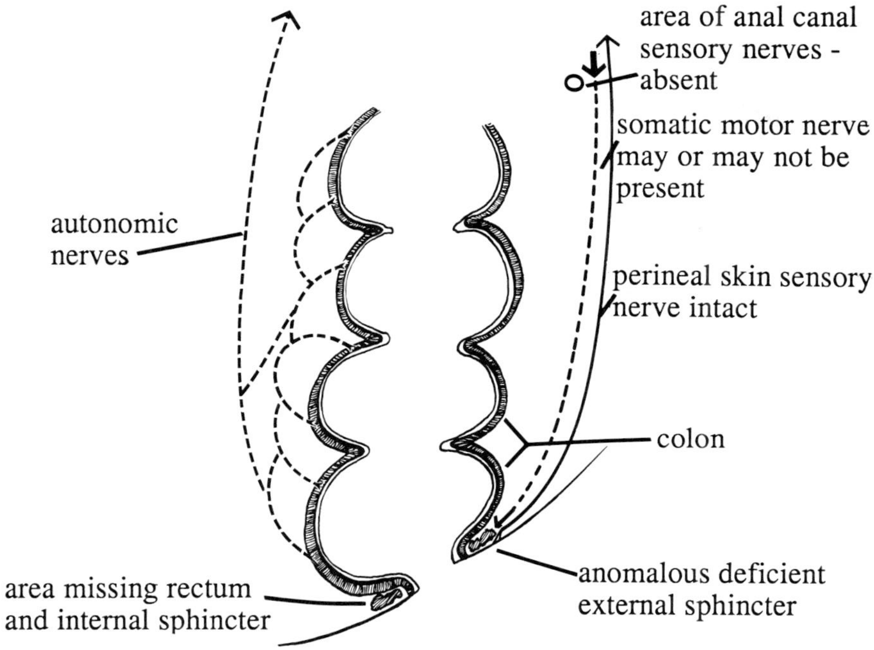

Figure 10-3. This is a postoperative imperforate anus. The autonomic nerve plexus is intact; however, the rectum may have been removed, so the rectal stretch sensation or predefecation urge is absent. The anal sphincter is present in rudimentary form, but rarely is it present in sufficient size to provide a useful function. The anal mucosa and anal sensory organs are always absent, leaving the patient dependent on skin sensation.

Constipation, Obstipation, and Impaction

Most people believe constipation is synonymous with hard stool, but constipation really means the accumulation of stool. Complete and regular elimination of large formed or semiformed stool is healthy, but accumulation of hard formed or semiformed stool is not. Obstipation is severe constipation to the point of colon dilatation. Obstipation leads to a megacolon, that is, an abnormally large colon, as well as "bypass" or "paradoxical" diarrhea interspersed with hard stools. Impaction, an end stage of the above two processes, is a collection of hardened fecal material in the rectum and colon that causes total obstruction. Impaction is associated with vomiting and abdominal pain and may cause intestinal perforation.

It is extremely important to detect constipation since this process, if untreated, can lead to obstipation and impaction. Signs of constipation

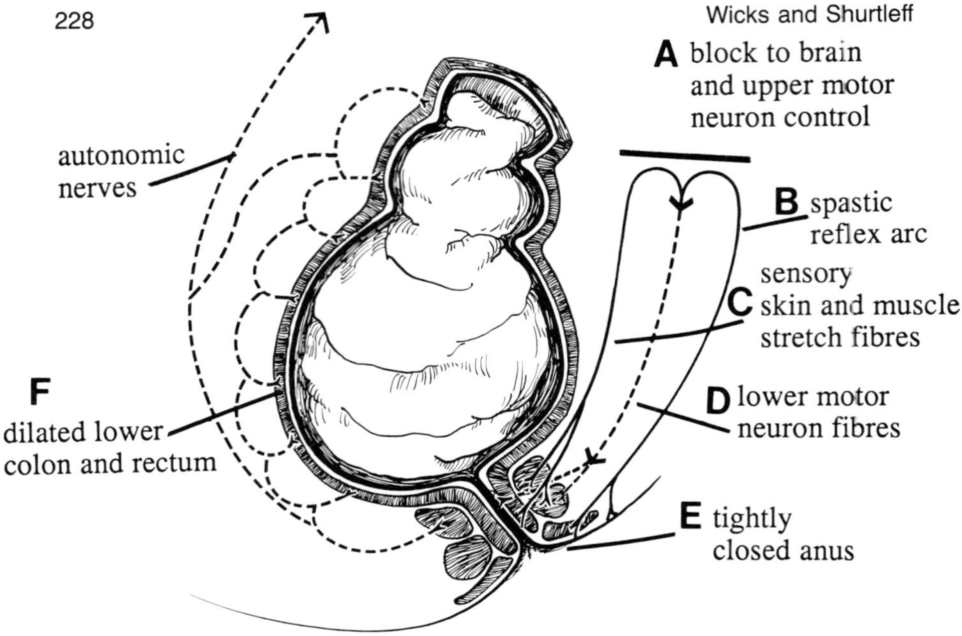

Figure 10-4. Constipation associated with a tight, spastic anus. The spinal cord has been interrupted, so sensory and motor fibers connect to each other in a reflex arc but are blocked from central nervous system reception or upper motor neuron influence (A). Below this block, a spastic arc (B) is established from stretch and sensory input (C) to lower motor neurons (D). Not under control of the brain, this reflex arc accounts for anal wink, frequently misinterpreted during a neonatal examination as evidence for future anal control by the brain. This reflex arc is stimulated to spasm by touch or stretching of anal muscle fibers (e.g., attempt for anal opening with contracture of the rectum and relaxation of the internal-autonomic anal sphincter). This reflex arc produces a tightly closed anal sphincter (E) and impedes emptying of the rectum. As a result of high resistance, the rectum fills, producing dilitation (F). With persistence of this trend, constipation, obstipation, or impaction develop (see text).

include small, hard tools; infrequent and incomplete defecation; and abdominal distention and discomfort. The seven causes of constipation are as follows: (1) anatomic or functional obstruction, (2) low fluid intake, (3) increased loss of fluid from the skin due to a dry, hot climate or fever, (4) low bulk, (5) decreased body activity, including prolonged body rest or incarceration in a body cast, (6) increased consumption of constipating foods, and (7) ingestion of certain drugs that decrease intestinal motility, such as anticholinergic medications. Parents should be warned that anticholinergic medicines prescribed to help dilate the urinary bladder (see Chapter 11) also cause a decrease in intestinal motility and a tendency toward constipation.

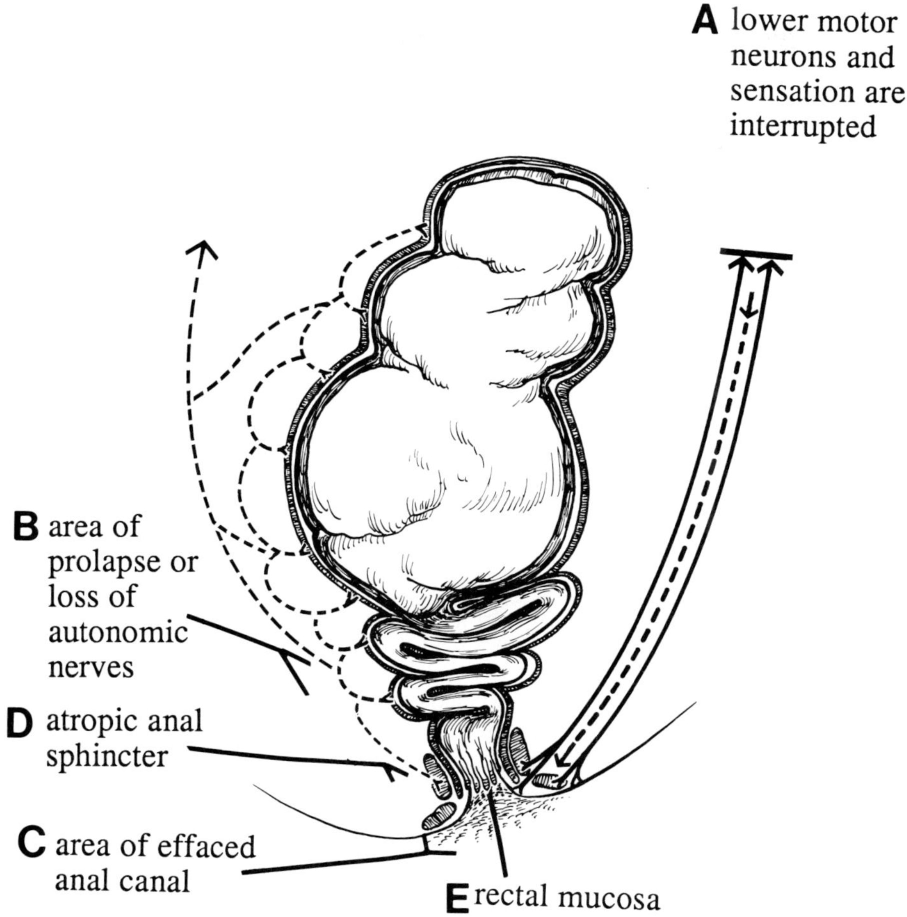

Figure 10-5. Loose anus with obstipation. The lower motor and sensory nerves are interrupted (A) prior to entering the spinal cord. (This is most frequently seen with low-sacral-level lesions.) The rectum does not prolapse out of the anus, but lies folded above the patulous anus (B), producing a flap valve effect. The anal canal is partially or completely effaced (C) with no or little tone because of enervated anal sphincter muscles (D). Deep-red rectal mucosal crypts are easily visible (E) with minimal efforts at spreading the buttocks and opening the anus.

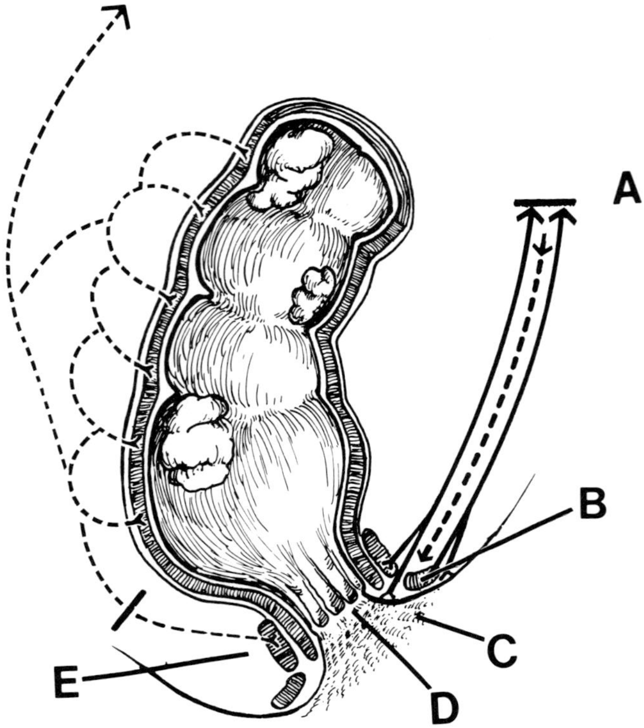

Figure 10-6. Loose, atonic anus with frequent small stools. The anus is identical to Figure 10-5, but the rectum has not become folded, producing a flap valve effect. The lower motor neuron block (A) produces an atrophic open external sphincter (B) with an effaced anal canal (C) with easily visible rectal mucosa or crypts (D). The internal sphincter mechanism (E) is normal or weak.

Diarrhea

Frequent watery stool is the most obvious sign of diarrhea. Causes of diarrhea are as follows: (1) infections of the intestinal tract; (2) dietary influences, such as hot condiments, fresh fruits, chocolate, etc.; (3) lactose or protein intolerance; (4) anxiety; (5) ingestion of certain drugs, such as irritants or antibiotics; (6) impactions causing bypass diarrhea, and (7) the irritable bowel syndrome of adults. Chronic and recurrent diarrhea can be due to infection or an irritable colon subjected to years of chronic constipation. Disabled adults are prone to the latter.

Absence of the Autonomic Nervous System

This type of pathophysiology is more commonly known as congenital agangliosis or Hirschsprung's disorder. Agenesis of the ganglion cells begins in the internal sphincter and involves varying lengths of the bowel. Ultra-short-segment disease pertains only to the distal rectum. However, the majority of cases involve the rectosigmoid portion of the colon in a continuous or skip fashion. The absence of normal peristalsis in the aganglionic segment produces an immobile portion through which stool can be moved only with great force. This segment produces a functional obstruction with dilatation and hypertrophy of the normal proximal bowel. Initial treatment includes resection of the paralyzed portions of the bowel or partial myectomy of the involved, spastic, internal anal sphincter. Management must also include reconditioning of the dilated, hypertrophied, and normally innervated bowel as well as the other toilet training techniques described in this chapter.

Imperforate Anus (Fig. 10-3)

This type of pathophysiology, an abnormal patency of the anus, can be divided into three classifications: high (supralevator), high with either genitourinary or reproductive tract fistulae, and low (intralevator) abnormalities. Associated anomalies exist in many of these children. Patients with imperforate anus present a variety of problems postsurgically, ranging from occasional staining to frequent accidents. Patients with the supralevator type have more incontinence due to the absence of the rectum. Incontinence arises secondary to the following postsurgical anatomical deficits: (1) absent anal canal sensory nerves to differentiate between gas, liquid, and solids; (2) compromised sphincter mechanisms; and, with high lesions, (3) lack of the normal predefecation urge. These patients need individually designed bowel management programs to compensate for these deficits. A program can be designed from any number of the possibilities discussed under the management section of this chapter.

Extrinsic Spinal Cord Abnormalities

The neurogenic bowel, as this type of pathophysiology is more commonly called, is the interruption of the continuity of the sensory and motor nerves to and from the brain. These abnormalities can occur before birth (as with meningomyelocele) or after birth (as with trauma to or tumors of the spinal cord). Regardless of the cause, the degree of nerve injury determines what type of anal sphincter control and what type of voluntary sensation is preserved. Almost all patients with this problem lack delicate anal canal sensation, perianal skin sensation, and conscious motor nerve control over the external anal sphincter and levator ani. More frequently, the intrinsic tone of the internal sphincter remains intact. When this occurs, the anus is effaced, so the mucous membrane of the anal canal is visible. When the sphincter relaxes, the red crypts of the distal rectum are immediately visible (Fig. 10-5 and 10-6).

With impaired nerves of the cord, spastic reflex arcs in the distal sensory and motor nerves maintain anus closure in a majority of patients (Fig. 10-4). The degree of impairment of these cord nerves (upper motor neurons) and the distal nerves (lower motor neurons) determines the degree of spasticity. In general, cord nerve (upper motor neuron) damage with an intact motor and sensory (lower neuron) arc produces the greatest degree of spasticity and the tightest anus. The greater the proportion of distal motor nerve impairment, the less the anal tone. Maximum impairment of the lower motor neuron arc, regardless of the status of the cord nerves, produces the weakest or most flail anus. Generally, the degrees of impairment can be discussed as one of three clinical entities: tight anus with a tendency toward constipation, loose anus with constipation, and loose anus with frequent stools.

Tight Anus (Fig. 10-4)

Patients in this category most frequently have the normal internal sphincter response of relaxation with a spastic external anal sphincter due to the upper motor neuron disruption in the cord. As mentioned above, this pathophysiology usually keeps the anus closed. The rectum fills with stool until the peristalsis of the colon and rectal emptying squeeze become strong enough to force part or all of the contents past the tight sphincter. Some of these patients will be able to feel this rectal peristalsis and filling as the predefecation urge (discussed above). Patients with a tight anus will tend toward constipation, which, unless the rectum and colon are regularly emptied by a bowel management program, will lead to a huge, dilated colon (with obstipation and impaction) and bypass diarrhea. When the colon and rectum have become overdistended, the patient will lose the sensation of the predefecation urge.

Loose Anus With Constipation (Fig. 10-5)

Other patients have weak or nonexistent external anal sphincters as well as abnormal autonomic nerve development in the rectum. The rectal wall collapses upon itself much like an accordian, causing an impedence to the passage of stool and an obstruction above this abnormality. This obstruction is felt on digital stimulation or when attempting to pass an enema tube. The result, as with tight anus, may be a dilated colon proximal to this collapse. Patients with this malformation are missing anorectal stretch-squeeze reflexes, and because the rectum does not fill, the patients will not have predefecation urges.

Loose Anus With Frequent Stools (Fig. 10-6)

Other patients with weak or nonexistent anal sphincters have frequent, small stools. They pass stools from above without impedence. With any physical effort that increases intra-abdominal pressure, they tend to pass any stool present in the rectum, usually in small amounts. The autonomic plexus arc of the anorectal reflex may be intact or interrupted, but there is no or little external sphincter tone. These patients tend not to experience the sense of rectal fullness combined with forceful lower colon peristalsis that other individuals with intact autonomic systems learn to interpret as the predefecation urge.

MANAGEMENT

The goals of management of the sphincter-impaired bowel are two fold: (1) to manage both the specific temporary and static pathophysiology and (2) to prevent potential complications, including social embarrassment. With the above goals established, a plan may be organized to prevent constipation and diarrhea to the maximum extent possible, to manage either when it occurs, and to control incontinence through a bowel training and retraining program.

Management of Temporary Pathophysiology

Preventing constipation and diarrhea is actually a key to avoiding complications and managing incontinence through a training program. Although dietary control over stool consistency can be routinely established, episodes of diarrhea and constipation must be anticipated as responses to ordinary life experiences. Therefore, parents and patients must be taught to expect that retraining the bowel must occur after each episode.

The parent, under the guidance of the health care provider, should initiate maximum prevention of constipation and diarrhea in the infant stage. Even though parents may not understand the implication of total management at this point, they can be taught the signs of possible constipation and diarrhea as well as means for controlling them. (We give the following word of caution: Prior to recommending any suggestions to prevent constipation, the health care provider must examine the child in order to rule out obstipation. If obstipation is a problem, then management must include reconditioning the large colon as well as preventing the underlying cause of constipation. The process of colon reconditioning is reviewed below.)

Constipation Management

Dietary management is the most advantageous initial method of intervention for constipation if the colon has not become dilated. Patients with intact autonomic nervous systems will need large, bulky, semiformed stool to initiate rectal filling and stimulate the predefecation sensation. Dietary recommendations for helping the child produce large, bulky stools are listed in Table 10-1; these foods should be used with the recognition that diet is also important for weight control and urine acidity to prevent urine infection (see Chapter 13). In addition, the constipating foods listed in Table 10-1 should be discouraged. If milk and milk products are determined to cause constipation and thereby must be eliminated, a calcium and vitamin D supplement and stool bulking agents are recommended. Oyster shell calcium tablets are the least expensive source of calcium. Prepared plant fibers and stool softeners are beneficial as bulking agents. Common propriatary names of these hydroscopic agents that hold water in the stool are Metamucil (Psyllium Hydrophilic Mucilloid, Searle and Co., San Juan, Puerto Rico), Effersyllium (Psyllium Hydrocolloid, Stuart Pharmaceuticals, Wilmington, Delaware), Colace (Docusate Sodium, Meade Johnson Co., Evanston, IL), Naturacil (Psyllium, Meade Johnson, Co., Evanston, IL.) and Chronulac (Lactulose, Merrell Dow Pharmaceuticals, Inc., Cincinnati, OH). The deletion of milk and the addition of calcium, vitamin D, and stool bulking agents should be discussed with the care provider.

The above recommendations should be adjusted for the particular child's age and malformation as well as the family's compliance and financial status. It is especially important to remember that children react individually to food. The lists in Table 10-1 include only suggestions on what is helpful in the majority of situations. The diet and individual responses to different foods are so important that parents are often asked to complete a 7–10-day dietary history. The individual diet is then examined, and recommendations are given concerning which foods should be eliminated, decreased, or increased. If constipation is the presenting problem, the specialist should discourage the possible offending foods listed in Table 10-1. Fluids, preferably water, should be increased by at least one glass a day, and other high-fiber foods should be added slowly.

When additional fiber is recommended, families must understand what *fiber* means. It has been defined as cellulose, hemicellulose, pectins, and lignin,[865] all of which are resistant to human digestion. Fiber essentially refers to all foods ingested that reach the large intestine

Table 10-1
Dietary Suggestions for Modifying Stool Consistency[a]

Foods to provide roughage (nonconstipating, bulking foods)[b]	
Breads, cereals and grains	Whole grain breads; unprocessed bran[c]; oatmeal; soy flour; all-bran[c]; puffed/shredded wheat; whole grain or wild rice; popcorn; bran muffins[c]
Nuts[c]	Almonds;[d] coconut;[d] peanuts,[d]
Fruits	Apricots (dried or raw); currants (raw); dates (raw); figs (raw); peaches (raw); prunes (raw or stewed); raspberries (raw)
Vegetables	Kidney beans[c]; lentils[c]; parsley; peas
Soups	Hardy varieties such as minestrone, bean[c], chili[c]
Foods to harden stools	
Breads, cereals, and grains[e]	Refined bread[d], crackers, and breakfast cereals; bagles; cooked, refined hot cereals, e.g., Cream of Rice; white rice[d]; pasta[d]
Dairy and poultry	Skim milk; plain yogurt; ice cream[d]; low-fat cottage cheese; hard-cooked and poached eggs
Vegetables	Tender cooked vegetables; carrots
Fruits	High-pectin fruits; apples (and apple products); bananas
Miscellaneous	Jello; plain candy[d]; jelly[d]
Low-residue diet[f]	
Breads, cereals, and grains	Enriched white bread and rolls[d]; graham crackers; Saltines; refined cereals; waffles[d]; pancakes[d]; biscuits
Potatoes and substitutes	Mashed white potatoes[d]; instant potatoes[d]
Fruit	Strained fruit juices (avoid apple if known to be constipating)
Snacks	Plain crackers; potato and corn chips (observe caloric intake)
Beverages	Milk-free substitutes; tea; water
Soups	Any creamed or broth-based soups without vegetables
Animal protein	Tender meats; fish; poultry
Nonanimal protein	Eggs (not fried)

[a] These recommendations should be applied on an individual basis. Roughage foods with indigestible fiber enlarge the stool. Fatty foods with high oil content soften stools but are not recommended because of their high caloric content. Hard stools are produced by low roughage, low fat, and refined foods. The amount of water and condiments consumed is a key factor, as it can cause consistency changes in stools. In fact, an appropriate amount of water alone can eliminate constipation.
[b] All of these foods have dietary fiber greater than 6 gm/100 gm edible portion.
[c] Caution: may cause flatus, uncontrollable by the sphincter-impaired person.
[d] Use caution with calorie-restricted diet.
[e] Highly refined carbohydrates.
[f] These suggestions include minimal amounts of high-fiber or constipating foods. Use over an extended period of time will require addition of vitamin and mineral supplementation according to the health care provider's recommendations.

unchanged. It includes a wide variety of plants with storage carbohydrates and cell walls resistant to the digestive enzymes in the small intestine. The properties of fiber in producing large, bulky stools include (1) a high hydration capacity, that is, an ability to hold a lot of fluid to prevent the fecal material from becoming hard, and (2) bulky density, which increases stool size. The recommended amount of fiber each day for adults is 30–60 grams. Some nutritionists recommend feeding children 30–40 grams each day, but this has not been documented as being advantageous. The addition of one teaspoon of unprocessed bran twice a day may be the most economical way to add fiber; it may be added to peanut butter, pancakes, muffins, and cookies. The amount of bran may be increased to obtain the desired stool consistency. If the family is eager to add fiber, a number of interesting recipes are helpful.[147] One note of caution is that fiber foods should never be added on top of suspected impaction; the child must be cleaned out first. If parents object to using bran, they may use the other prepared plant fibers mentioned above. Some families use malt and malt products or molasses in various ways to cause regular elimination and soft stools. Their judicious use can be encouraged unless excess weight gain is a problem. The sugars, like pectin, can cause constipation or frequent large stools in certain patients.

When dietary management suggestions have failed to prevent constipation for a variety of reasons, it is important to help parents understand that they themselves have not failed. Frequently, children may be picky eaters or take fluids poorly.

Diarrhea Management

Diarrhea is potentially due to the usual causes noted above. A careful history by the health care provider should eliminate any of these possibilities. Infectious causes can be treated with appropriate antimicrobial or antihelminth agents. Many patients have protracted diarrhea after elimination of the infectious agent. Patients with anorectal disorders may also respond to antibiotics with more diarrhea than normal patients. Dietary intolerances may also cause diarrheal episodes and should not be forgotten in the child with an impaired anorectal mechanism. Wheat may be an offender, and, therefore, its effect should be investigated by careful history, particularly if bran is to be recommended.

After specific causes are eliminated, prolonged or chronic diarrhea can be controlled by increasing the use of constipating foods (Table 10-1) or by one or a combination of the following nonspecific antidiarrheal agents: acidophillus to restore intestinal flora; pectin, kaolin, or other hydroscopic agents, such as Mitrolan tablets (Calcium Polycarbophil, A. H. Robins Company, Richmond, Va.), to absorb water; opiates, codeine, morphine, Paregoric, or anticholinergics to slow intestinal motility; or joperamate hydrochloride and Lomotil (Diphenoxylate hydrochloride, Searle and Co., San Juan, Puerto Rico) to directly relax smooth muscles. These agents should never be used with bypass diarrhea caused by obstipation or to control lactose or protein intolerance. They can be used after elimination of offending infections or chemical agents to assist in reduction of diarrhea due to anxiety or the irritable bowel syndrome. The irritable bowel syndrome of adults must be distinguished from inflammatory bowel disease, diverticulosis, and malignancy before dietary and nonspecific antidiarrheal therapy are prescribed.

Methods for Achieving Bowel Continence

After controlling constipation and diarrhea, it is important to review the basics of toilet training discussed in the previous chapter prior to establishing continence through a bowel training program. It is possible that a child with an impaired sphincter can be taught to pass a firm, high-bulk stool on a regular basis by the age of normal toilet training if the family has complied with pretraining management recommendations including dietary regulations, timed toileting, and behavioral techniques. If the child continues to have accidents or does not have sufficient results on the potty chair, an assisted program should be recommended. These programs require the use of invasive supplies, so it is important to conduct some type of preliminary play therapy with the child (as described in Chapter 9).

There are seven basic methods to assist in achieving bowel continence or emptying on a regular basis. Which of these might be most successful depends on the child's impairments, so a thorough assessment is essential. Certain pathophysiologic states respond more appropriately to specific assisted programs. The helpful checklist in Table 10-2 indicates pathophysiologic factors and programs. A description will follow for the various programs, but it is critical to point out again that the condition of the colon must be determined first. If a megacolon is found, the colon must be reconditioned to reestablish peristalsis, which is essential for any bowel-emptying program. To assess the pathophysiologic states involved and the possibility of a megacolon, the health care provider must palpate the abdomen, perform a thorough rectal exam, and obtain a bowel elimination pattern and dietary history. A supine, flat abdominal plate or barium enema may be necesssary to determine stool distribution and retention. If the rectum as well as the transverse and descending portions of the colon are dilated, the child has a considerable megacolon.

Table 10-2
Diagnosis of Pathophysiologic States That Respond to Specific Management Programs

Examinations	
	Ano-Rectal Examination
____________	Anus has sensation and tone; squeeze normal.
____________	Anus has tone and reflexic closure that is tight, with narrow rim of anal mucosa and rectal crypts not visible; (spastic external or voluntary sphincter); no sensation; no squeeze on command (tight anus).
____________	Intermediate tone to external sphincter; no anal sensation; no squeeze on command.
____________	No external tone or reflex closure; no anal sensation; no squeeze on command. Anal canal effaced; crypts visible; with rectal stimulation, anus gapes open and slowly closes (ano-rectal reflex).
____________	Flail sphincters; open anus with no internal sphincter response; no sensation, no squeeze on command. Prolapse of rectum common.
	Rectal Examination
____________	Empty of stool
____________	Full of stool ____________ stool consistency
____________	Folds of rectum make penetration difficult; use circular motion to find opening
____________	Deep rectal ampula
____________	Deep rectal sensation
	Abdominal Examination
____________	Palpation of hard stool in colon; ____________ location
	Abdominal X-ray
____________	Dilated rectum ____________ portion of colon distended

Special Management Programs[a]

Tight Anus	Loose Anus With Constipation	Loose Anus With Frequent Stools
Rule out megacolon	Rule out megacolon	Dietary management to bulk stools
Dietary management	Dietary management (decrease constipation)	Hydroscopic agents
Timed toileting	Hydroscopic agents	Oral cathartics
Hydroscopic agents	Timed toileting	Timed toileting
Suppository	Oral cathartics	Anal plugs
Digital stimulation	Irritative enema (high)[b]	Expansion enema
Irritative enema	Suppository (high)[b]	
	Expansive enema[b]	

[a] These choices for management programs for specific types of pathophysiology are based on experience. It is important to remember that each child's pathophysiology is individual and needs monitored intervention to determine success.
[b] Use a circular motion to enter high rectum.

Reconditioning a Megacolon

The general recommendations for reconditioning a megacolon are as follows: (1) Stop any bowel program. (2) Begin a low-residue diet, and avoid constipating foods (Table 10-1). (3) Administer a prescribed amount of mineral oil by mouth for 3 or 4 days; it may be necessary to continue the mineral oil for sveral weeks depending on the health care provider's assessment of the consistency and frequency of the stools. (4) Add a water-soluble vitamin to the diet to compensate for alleged problems with absorption secondary to mineral oil; vitamins should be given following the child's meal and 2–3 hours apart from the mineral oil. (5) Administer mineral oil enemas with a straight catheter to the child in a knee-chest position. Two 60–90-cc enemas may be given at an interval of 20–30 minutes twice a day followed by elimination or digital removal of the stool. The hard impacted type stool may take 3–4 days to completely remove. When it has been removed, mineral oil enemas are discontinued. (6) Then administer slowly infused saline enemas at the same time each day, preferably after a meal such as breakfast or supper; retention of the enema for 10–20 minutes is encouraged. The amount of saline given is determined by the age of the child, degree of megacolon, and response. (7) Repeat saline enema cleansing and digital removal of stool until a spontaneous soft stool appears on a daily basis. (8) Continue the use of saline enemas, oral mineral oil, and a low-residue diet until the pattern of spontaneous soft stool is well established. Oral mineral oil may be discontinued before the saline enemas and low-residue diet. This depends on the extent of the megacolon and dietary compliance. The health care provider will indicate the appropriate time to discontinue the reconditioning program and begin appropriate dietary interventions and any necessary assisted bowel programs; usually this will occur in 4–6 weeks depending on the degree of megacolon, compliance, and response of the colon.

Training Programs

After reconditioning the colon, an appropriate training program may be selected from the following seven methods: (1) digital stimulation, (2) suppositories, (3) irritative enema, (4) expansion enema, (5) oral cathartics, (6) anal plugs, and (7) biofeedback.

These methods need to be used in combination with dietary management for maintaining stool consistency and with regular, timed bowel emptying on a daily or more frequent basis. The most convenient time for the individual and family should be selected and must remain constant to within a few minutes. This constant time should be after a meal in order to take advantage of the gastrocolic reflex. If the stool is of a formed, bulky consistency and the child has some anal tone, continence may be achieved.

The first assisted method, digital stimulation, involves initiating the anorectal reflex by inserting a finger, gloved or not, and pressing the wall of the rectum with a gentle, circling movement. This is most beneficial for the child with a tight anus. This process allows the child to release stools from the rectum. The digital (finger) stimulation can be repeated one to three times until results cease. The presence of stool should be checked after each digital stimulation.

Suppositories are also used to stimulate peristalsis and the rectal evacuation. The two types of stimulation are irritation and stretch. Bisacodyl, an autonomic nervous system stimulant, initiates contractions of the rectum and colon. If half of a suppository is prescribed, it should be cut lengthwise, as the medication is in the tip. The suppository should be inserted as far as possible between the stool and the lining of the rectum or colon, not mixed in with stool. If the suppository leaks out, the child should lie quietly for several minutes in a slightly elevated knee-chest position, possibly with the buttocks taped together. Onset of defecation usually occurs within 20–40 minutes, at which time the child should sit on the toilet and be instructed in the Valsalva maneuver. A simple means of teaching this method is to blow bubbles or blow up a balloon; regardless of what toy is used, the child should learn to blow out, gradually increasing the resistance from his or her mouth and throat. Finally, a glycerin suppository is effective in a few children; it aids by stretching the rectum during insertion instead of irritating it.

An irritative enema, such as the Fleet (C. B. Fleet Company, Inc., Lynchburg, VA), hypertonic saline, or bisacodyl, may be used in place of suppository for a stimulant. This type is often preferable to a suppository because of its relatively quick onset of action, 10–15 minutes, and its lack of the mucous produced by most suppositories. The enema should be given 10–20 minutes after meals.

Expansion enemas, given quickly and forcefully in small volumes, can suddenly dilate the rectum and initiate the anorectal defecation reflex. Two Davol bulb syringes (Davol Rubber Company, Providence, RI) can be made into a useful tool for this type of enema; one can be cut to act as a phlange and will prevent back leakage during compression of the syringe (Fig. 10-7). This enema should be given while the child is sitting on the toilet or commode, with the insertion device firmly pressed against the anus and perineum. The solution used in the enema may be water or saline. Several enemas should be administered to ensure complete emptying of the rectum. A rectal examination by a gloved finger should be performed to confirm evacuation.

Oral cathartics can be used to establish regularity. They include

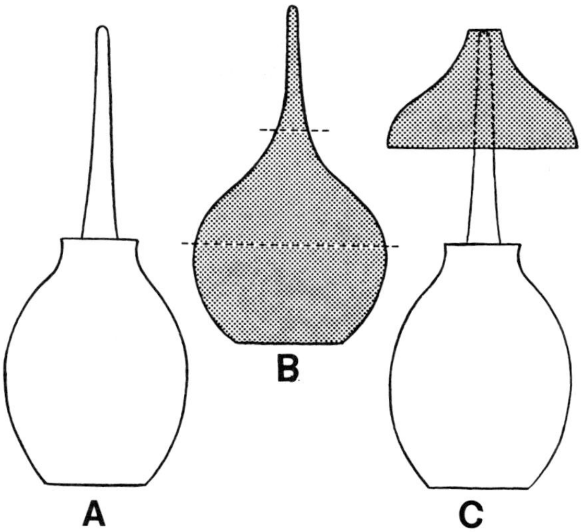

Figure 10-7. Modification of rubber ear syringe for expansion enema. (A) Adult enema syringe, 8-oz capacity. (B) Ear syringe, 3-oz capacity, for infants and small children. (C) B cut on dotted lines and fit over nozzle of A for older children.

Senokot (Standarized senna concentrate, Purdue Fredericks Company, Norwalk, CT), Dulcolax®, bisacodyl tablets, and Perdiem (Senna, William H. Rorer, Inc., Fort Washington, PA). These medications can take effect 6–24 hours after ingestion. Reaction to them is individual, so trial and error must be anticipated before determining the most effective time to administer the dose. Sufficient education must accompany an addition of oral cathartics because compliance can be a problem since the public is well educated by the media that cathartics may be habit forming. Oral cathartics should be used in a time sequence with, and prior to, suppositories, enemas, or timed evacuations so that they work in concert. Unfortunately, gastrointestinal transit time affects oral cathartics and, in some patients, can cause a worse social situation by exacerbating recurrent episodes of diarrhea or loose stools.

Anal plugs can be used to prevent the anus from passing frequent, small stools on exertion. Following early morning elimination, a tampon covered with surgical gel can be inserted into the rectum. The buttocks should be held firmly together and wide surgical tape applied to hold the buttocks together and keep the tampon in place. Identification can be removed from the container and relabeled "anal plugs" to prevent confusing attendants and children (particularly boys).

Biofeedback is the most complicated continence program method. It helps an individual learn voluntary control of autonomic body functions. An anorectal balloon is inserted into the rectum. When it is inflated to simulate rectal filling, the child is taught how to make a squeeze response to this filling by using intact muscles (levators, hamstrings, and/or gluteals, depending on the paralysis). The balloon system used is channeled into a computer, so the child views his or her responses on a monitor screen; the procedure is, thereby, made into a game.

Olness and associates[826] as well as Shepherd and associates[1027] have demonstrated success with the biofeedback method. Shepherd emphasized the need for comprehensive bowel management based on timed, complete, regular evacuation, diet modifications, and biofeedback conditioning. Rectal sensation appeared to be the key factor in the success of this total approach. For those patients who have dilated colons and rectums, rectal sensation must be regained by reconditioning before biofeedback will be beneficial.

Side effects from any of the medications or methods described above are minimal. Burning and cramping may be elicited from the use of bisacodyl suppositories. If this occurs, the amount must be reduced or the method changed. Saline enemas, especially with liquid stool, can cause dehydration and irritation of the colon. Some patients react idiosyncratically to anticholinergics by having diarrhea. Regardless of the initial recommendations for bowel toilet training, the health care provider should stress with the parent or care provider that each child, regardless of the pathophysiology, is unique, and an acceptable program must be learned by intelligent trial and error. Only the rare patient is toilet trained easily.

SUMMARY

Stool management methods include dietary interventions, a consistent evacuation time, and seven specific methods for achieving continence, outlined above. The use of behavioral reinforcement techniques (discussed in Chapter 9) can be a benefit to any of the programs to ensure compliance. Effective management requires not only a thorough understanding of the temporary and static pathophysiologies, but also prevention of potential complications, including social embarrassment and lowered self-esteem. Each child must achieve independent toileting and avoid accidents that may hinder normal socialization. Fortunately, stool management is an individual's secret: sphincter-impaired patients don't have to explain their obvious impairments *unless* they allow themselves to develop odor and staining.

D. Kiko Kimura
Michael Mayo
David Shurtleff

11

Urinary Tract Management

In the toilet-trained individual, normal micturition (urination), like stool control, is a natural body function often taken for granted. However, for individuals with chronic urinary tract sphincter dysfunction, urine elimination can be a life-or-death problem as well as a source of stress, embarrassment, and inconvenience. Chronic urinary tract dysfunction can be a major health concern because renal failure is a life-threatening complication. Since renal impairment can occur without signs or symptoms until late stages, routine follow-up of potential problem patients is essential.

In order to overcome life-threatening and social problems, a urinary tract management program should be established at birth for the infant with urinary tract impairment. The main goal of any such program should be to maintain normal urinary tract function within as normal a life-style as possible. In order to accomplish these objectives, it is important for the health care provider to have a good understanding and working knowledge of normal urinary tract function and the different types of pathology that are possible. Basic knowledge should enable each health care provider to (1) adequately assess urinary tract functioning and status, (2) appropriately prescribe a program that best fits the patient's physiological needs as well as his or her family's life-style, and (3) successfully monitor current bladder management programs.

MYELODYSPLASIAS AND EXSTROPHIES: SIGNIFICANCE, PREVENTION, AND TREATMENT
 ISBN 0-8089-1816-8

NORMAL ANATOMY AND PHYSIOLOGY OF THE URINARY TRACT

Formation of Urine

The kidney filters the blood and then modifies this filtrate by both adding and removing various components to form urine. The rest of the urinary system—the renal pelvis, the ureters, the bladder, and the urethra—are involved in transporting and eliminating the urine as a waste product from the body. In doing this, the urine must be kept at a low pressure and must be kept sterile. It is in the maintenance of sterility and low pressure that the patient with urinary tract anomalies or paralysis is most vulnerable.

Anatomy

The basic anatomy of the urinary system is deceptively simple. However, a detailed look at the anatomy in conjunction with its innervation reveals a complex system that both keeps the body in homeostasis and has many potential causes of dysfunction.

The urine flows into the renal pelvis from the tubules of the kidney. There it is collected, and waves of contraction (peristalsis) transport it down the ureter and into the bladder. The ureter enters the muscular bladder wall at an oblique angle to form a valve that prevents reversed flow (reflux) of urine up the ureter (Fig. 11-1). If the bladder becomes

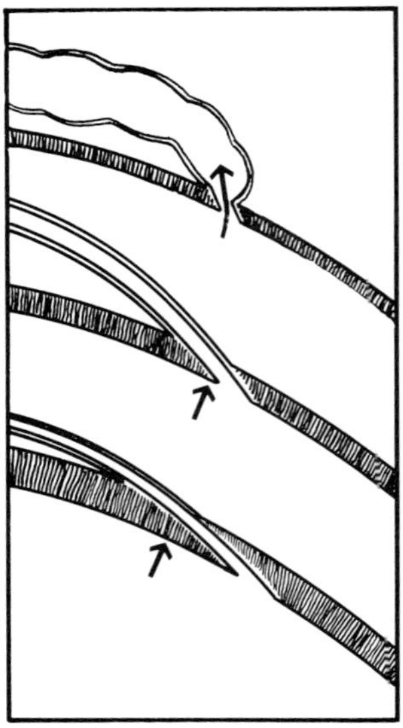

Figure 11-1. Ureterovesicle reflux. The ureter enters the bladder at an oblique angle to form a valve that prevents reflux of urine up the ureter. With distention of the urinary bladder, the bladder wall thins until the flap valve effect is lost, and urine can pass up the ureter directly from the bladder.

overstretched and thin, or if the angle of entry of the ureter is more acute, reflux may occur as urine is forced from the bladder back up the ureters. The bladder stores the urine until voiding, when it is emptied through the urethra.

The bladder detrusor is an elastic, smooth muscle. As the bladder fills with urine, the detrusor relaxes and stretches. This allows a constant tension or force that maintains a low pressure of 15–20 cc water in the bladder as it is filling. During filling, the sympathetic and parasympathetic nervous systems are coordinated. The detrusor is abundantly supplied with parasympathetic fibers that control the emptying process and must relax, while sympathetic systems must hold the urinary sphincter closed.

The sphincters of the bladder outlet (posterior urethra) include the relatively more rigid base, or trigone, of the bladder; the bladder neck (the so-called intrinsic sphincter); and the external striated sphincter. The bladder neck, under sympathetic nervous system control, has the ability to provide constant tension and remain closed as the bladder relaxes and fills. Some of the detrusor fibers are inserted into the urethra from the base of the bladder. When the detrusor contracts, these fibers stretch the relaxed base of the bladder and upper urethra into a funnel shape.

Innervation

The urinary system is innervated by both the autonomic and somatic nervous systems. The nervous system, consisting of the brain and spinal cord, receives, controls, and carries messages to and from the bladder and cerebral cortex via the autonomic and somatic nervous systems. The detrusor reflex arc is mediated via synapses in the midbrain, not in the sacral area of the cord. Although proprioceptive afferents running in the pelvic nerves enter the cord at S2-4, they do not synapse there but instead ascend in the posterior columns to the midbrain before synapsing. The sphincter reflex arc is comprised of somatic nerves mediated via the pudendal nerve entering the sacral cord at S2-4 and has long routed reflexes to the cerebral cortex. The somatic nervous system is the voluntary system that innervates the striated muscle of the external urinary sphincter and is also under control of the cerebral cortex, where somatic nerves also carry afferent sensory messages from the urethra to the cortex. The autonomic nervous system (ANS), not under conscious control, is the involuntary system that innervates the smooth muscle of the bladder detrusor and bladder neck. Within the ANS, two divisions—the parasympathetic and sympathetic nervous systems—play major roles in normal micturition.

The parasympathetic system dominates when normal voiding takes place. These neuromuscular nerve endings secrete acetylcholine, a cholinergic agent that initiates contractions of the detrusor and sustains these contractions during normal micturition. Sensory afferent nerves also travel with the parasympathetic motor or efferent fibers in the pelvis and provide sensation that is interpreted as preurination bladder fullness.

The sympathetic nervous system activates the bladder neck fibers and relaxes the detrusor, preventing emptying of the urinary bladder; this system dominates when urination must be avoided.[1206] These neuromuscular nerve endings produce noradrenalin, which causes muscles of the internal sphincter mechanism that have alpha-adrenergic receptors to contract and retain urine. In addition, the sympathetic afferent nerves carry pain.[1206] These pain sensations and stretching of the peritoneum or abdominal wall are sensations that can be interpreted by the patient with a neurogenic bladder as fullness or the preurination urge. These sensations can enter the cord at the lower thoracic or upper lumbar levels. With higher level lesions, other intra-abdominal sympathetic afferent sensory fibers may be stimulated and are interpreted as bladder fullness by these patients.

Normal Micturition

In the normal infant, micturition is a reflex event. The afferent stretch receptors in the bladder wall sense fullness and send a message that travels via the pelvic nerves up the posterior columns to synapse in the midbrain where efferent fibers arise and travel down in the recticulospinal tracts. At the S2-4 level, these synapse with the cell bodies of the pelvic nerves, sending efferent parasympathetic impulses to the detrusor muscle and thus stimulating it to contract. Combined with detrusor contraction, the sphincters, innervated by the sympathetic nerves (for the bladder neck) and the voluntary nerves (for the pelvic floor), relax in a coordinated manner. In addition to detrusor stretching, other external or environmental stimuli (e.g., changing the diaper) can initiate detrusor contractions and initiate voiding.

In the second year of life, the normal child becomes aware of bladder filling (the preurination urge) and may start to communicate this to the parents. If a detrusor contraction occurs and it is not an appropriate time to void, urinary control may be achieved by willful contraction of the pelvic floor and urinary sphincter. Detrusor contraction itself may be inhibited by local sacral reflexes following sustained voluntary sphincter closure. The bladder pressure will then return to normal, at least for a short time. If this sequence begins at an appropriate time in an appropriate place, the voluntary efferent message to the urinary sphincter mechanisms can be to relax, and the urinary bladder will be emptied by autonomic detrusor contraction. This autonomic aspect of voiding explains why one can sometimes have difficulty initiating the voiding mechanism; only sphincter relaxation is under voluntary control.

Later in childhood, the detrusor reflex is inhibited at the midbrain level by the cortical centers, and the normal adult state is reached. Voiding is then initiated by a voluntary relaxation of the pelvic floor, with the detrusor contraction being the secondary event. Detrusor contractions may still occur at inappropriate moments when the bladder is very full and when other stimuli, such as a cold environment, the sound of running water, the presence of cystitis, etc., are present. When this occurs, the voluntary sphincter contracts to retain urine, suppress the detrusor contractions, and maintain continence.

Most individuals with meningomyelocele do not have normal sensation (preurination urge) although they may feel a vague sensation due to peritoneal stretching (afferents travel via the sympathetics) when the bladder is very full. These sensory deficits cannot be determined until the child can verbalize his or her voiding and filling sensations. Most of these children have no willful control over the voluntary sphincter. In addition, the detrusor reflex may be interrupted so that detrusor contractions occur but are often poorly sustained. Local pelvic floor reflexes are also impaired, and pelvic floor relaxation is not coordinated with the detrusor contraction.

NEUROGENIC BLADDER TYPES

Even when very little interference with the innervation of the muscles of the lower extremities is apparent (since the voiding mechanism is innervated by nerves at the lowest level of the spinal cord), urination may still be impaired. The neurologic level of myelodysplasia lesions is usually even on both sides; however, when it is uneven, the urinary impairment is determined by the better side. The spinal cord lesion can affect the urinary system in several ways, producing a hypoactive, hyperactive, or normally active detrusor and sphincter mechanisms resulting in normal-, high-, or low-pressure systems, continence or incontinence, and ureteral reflex uni- or bilaterally.

Areflexic or Hypoactive Bladder

An areflexic or hypoactive bladder (Fig. 11-2) will dribble at a pressure determined by the resistance of the sphincter mechanism. Usually this resistance is low. The pressure in the bladder will be higher when the sphincter causes increased resistance. The detrusor will not contract, but spikes of pressure can be produced by coughing and body

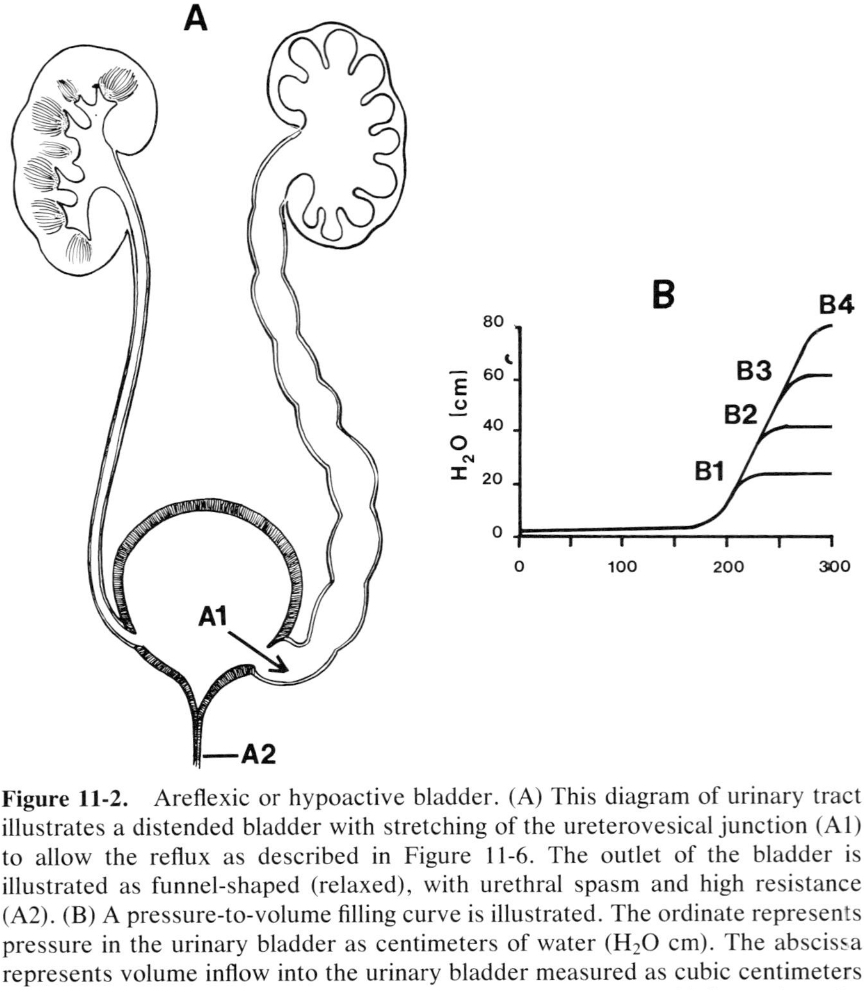

Figure 11-2. Areflexic or hypoactive bladder. (A) This diagram of urinary tract illustrates a distended bladder with stretching of the ureterovesical junction (A1) to allow the reflux as described in Figure 11-6. The outlet of the bladder is illustrated as funnel-shaped (relaxed), with urethral spasm and high resistance (A2). (B) A pressure-to-volume filling curve is illustrated. The ordinate represents pressure in the urinary bladder as centimeters of water (H_2O cm). The abscissa represents volume inflow into the urinary bladder measured as cubic centimeters (volume cc). With the lowest outlet resistance (B1), urine will flow when the ureteral closure pressure is exceeded (20 cm H_2O) (B1). As the outlet resistance increases (B2–B4), a higher volume and pressure is reached before leakage occurs. During leakage, the inflow continues, but the pressure remains constant.

movements that produce increased abdominal pressure. Thus, with low or normal detrusor pressure and increased resistance at the bladder outlet, the urinary bladder will enlarge and may be palpable, but the patient will not be able to empty it. Such systems are susceptible to overdistention, leading to infection and reflux even though the pressure is not high by normal standards. Such patients have overflow dribbling of urine. The capacity of the areflexic bladder varies. Depending on the degree of outlet resistance, extra pressure from straining, coughing, laughing, etc., causes overflow leaking with lesser degrees of increase in intra-abdominal pressure according to the weakness of the outlet sphincter mechanisms.

Fibrotic or Noncompliant Bladder

This type of bladder (Fig. 11-3) is small and noncontractile, but differs from an areflexic or hypoactive bladder in size and filling pressure. A fibrotic bladder is common after prolonged urinary diversion as the "isolated bladder syndrome" associated with recurrent pyocystis. Patients with intact ureters and fibrotic bladders will dribble without spurts of urine. High filling pressures at low volumes can be associated with upper tract dilation due to obstruction at the ureterovesical junction from bladder wall hypertrophy.

Spastic, Hyperactive, or Hyperreflexic Bladder

A spastic or hyperactive bladder develops from an irritable detrusor muscle or uninhibited contractions of the detrusor. If the sphincter mechanisms are weak, absent, or uncoordinated, the bladder will empty with low pressure (Fig. 11-4). If the sphincters have high resistance or are dyssynergic, the system will be high-pressure and will be trabeculated or sacculated (Fig. 11-5). The uninhibited contractions are usually generated at a volume less than capacity and occur with or without coordinated relaxation of the bladder neck and intrinsic urethral sphincter. Since these contractions are acetylcholine-mediated, one method of management includes using cholinergic blocking agents, such as propantheline bromide, oxybutinin chloride, or other medications (see "Chemical Adjunctive Therapy," below).

With hyperreflexia of the detrusor, if the bladder neck and intrinsic sphincter remain moderately spastic or closed most of the time, the patient will have intermittent but frequent passage of small amounts of urine and a moderately high-pressure system (Fig. 11-4). There will be a small amount of residual urine. However, if these detrusor contractions occur with increased sphincter resistance, a high-pressure system will develop (Fig. 11-5). In the latter situation, incomplete voiding will occur frequently, leaving residual urine. The volume is dependent on the relative strength of the detrusor versus outlet resistance. There will be a large amount of residual urine. This is a dangerous situation since absence of adequate emptying can lead to reflux and, with high pressure, a rapidly advancing hydronephrosis (see "Hydronephrosis," below) and hydroureter.

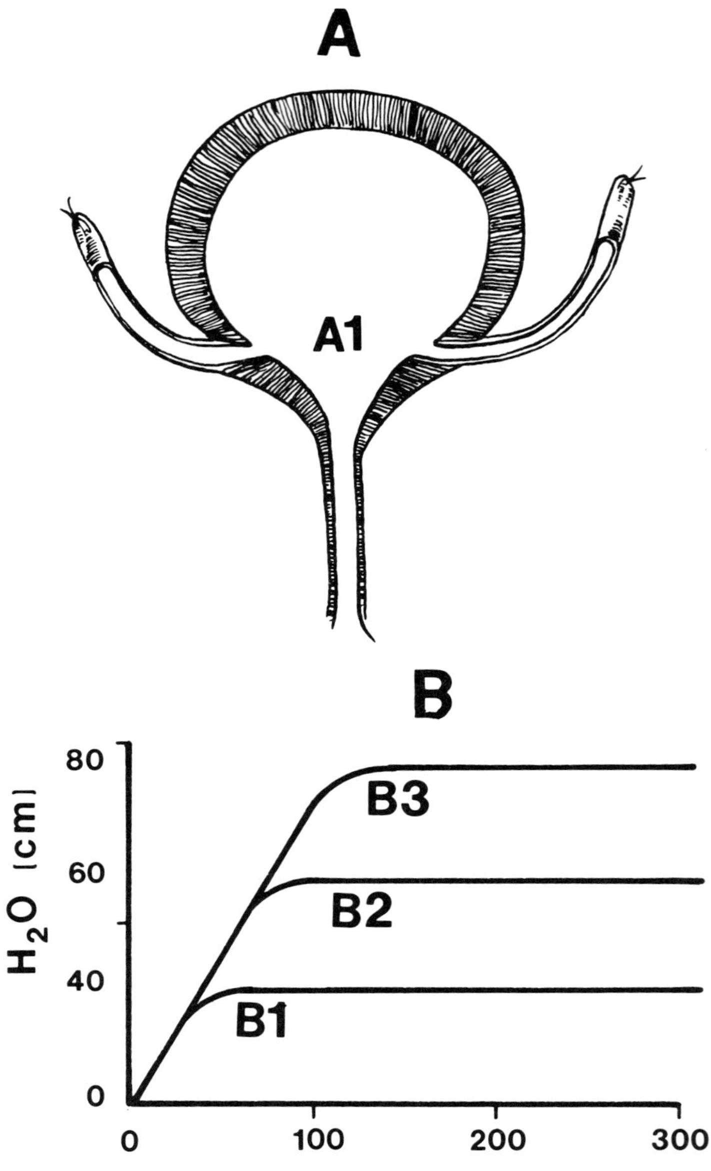

Figure 11-3. Fibrotic bladder. (A) This small, noncompliant, thick-walled urinary bladder may produce ureteral reflux or may have tightly closed, competent ureterovesical orifices (A1). Supravesicle obstruction with hydroureter and hydronephrosis may be produced due to high-urine-flow resistance across the ureterovesical orifices (see Fig. 11-5A2). (B) The abscissa and ordinate are the same as in Figure 11-2. Because of an inability of the urinary bladder wall to accommodate, the pressure rises at a very small total volume infusion (B1–B3). As with Figure 11-2, when the urethral closure pressure is exceeded, urine leaks, and pressure remains a constant (B1, B2, and B3 are curves representing different levels of outlet resistance).

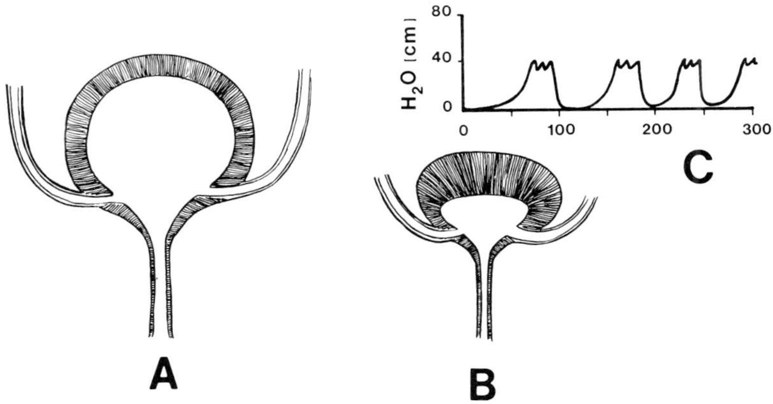

Figure 11-4. Spastic, hyperactive, or hyperreflexic bladder with normal or low outlet resistance. (A) Reflexes mediated by the stretch of the detrusor are present after a small or moderate amount of increase in bladder volume. (B) Reflexes mediated by the stretch reflex of the detrusor are present with a minimal amount of increase in bladder volume. (C) Intermittent detrusor contractions occur at low volumes (C).

Reflexic Bladder

Caused by disruption in the control of the midbrain reflex arc with intact sensory and motor tracts of the cord, the supraspinal bladder is characterized by uncontrolled, involuntary urination. This bladder type (Fig. 11-6) differs from the spastic or hyperactive bladder only in that the bladder will fill nearly full, and then it will completely, or almost completely, empty. The simple reflex arc takes over so that, when the bladder is full, voiding contractions begin, increasing the bladder pressure and resulting in voiding at an inconvenient time. A sudden increase in bladder pressure from an outside pressure, such as a cough, a blow to the abdomen, or a Crede maneuver, may initiate uncontrolled emptying. This type of bladder contracts and empties without dyssynergia. It occurs most often in patients with brain damage or cerebral palsy and is uncommon in those with myelodysplasia.

PROBLEMS ARISING FROM A NEUROGENIC BLADDER

Secondary Changes in the Bladder Wall

Trabeculation (Fig. 11-5A) occurs with repeated contraction of the detrusor against a closed, spastic outlet or an external sphincter that contracts simultaneously (dyssynergia). These circumstances produce

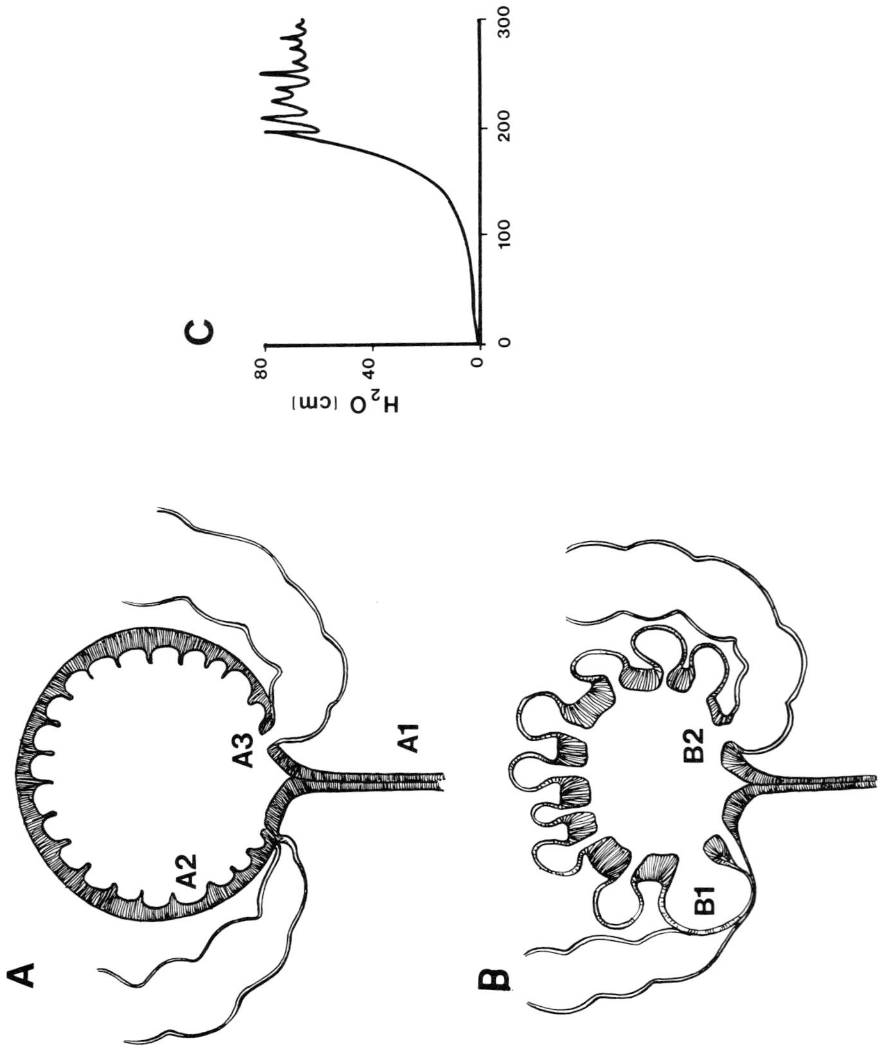

A
A1
A2
A3
B
B1
B2
C
80
40
0
H2O (cm)
0
100
200
300

retention of urine due to incomplete emptying and, eventually, chronic distention. The bladder wall begins to thicken, lose elasticity, and appear irregular on a cystogram. Sacculations (Fig. 11-5B) and diverticula (herniation of the urinary bladder mucosa between the detrusor muscle bundles) occur throughout the bladder, and they may press on a ureter (Hutch diverticulum) and produce an obstruction to ureteral urine flow (supravesicle obstruction) or cause distortion of the ureterovesicle junction and allow reflux with subsequent hydroureter and hydronephrosis (Fig. 11-2A1; Fig. 11-5B1 and B2). With a strong detrusor and a high-pressure system, this type of system can cause rapidly progressive hydronephrosis and hydroureter.

Urinary Tract Infections (UTIs), Urinary Retention, and Reflux

UTIs are almost always ascending; that is, they enter the urethra and ascend up the bladder and ureters to the kidney. The bladder is the only portion of the urinary tract that acts as a reservoir rather than a conduit, and it is the only portion of the urinary system with a retention mechanism. Disturbances in one or more of the nervous systems may cause the bladder to empty incompletely, making it the most vulnerable part of the urinary tract to retention of urine, infection, and increased pressure.

Two of the main urinary tract defenses against infection are (1) unidirectional flow of urine to wash bacteria out and (2) complete

---

Figure 11-5. Dyssynergia with trabeculation and sacculation. (A) Trabeculation of the urinary bladder is caused by intermittent contraction of the detrusor muscle fibers against a tight, spastic, or dyssynergic outlet (A1). Detrusor fibers thicken or hypertrophy with the appearance of an irregular inner bladder wall. The thickened detrusor can cause ureteral obstruction and supravesical dilation of the ureter and renal pelvis (hydronephrosis and hydroureter) (A2) or decompensation of the ureterovesicle valve (Fig. 11-1) and hydronephrosis and hydroureter due to reflux (A3). (B) Sacculation is a more advanced stage of deterioration than trabeculation. The detrusor contractions cause greatly hypertrophied bands of muscle that form a mesh through which the urinary bladder mucosa herniates causing a large number of bulbous outpouchings or saccules. Eventually a diverticulum is produced covered only with peritoneum. If one of these diverticula presses on a ureter, it is identified as a Hutch diverticulum (after the surgeon who first described the entity); it causes obstruction of urine flow down a ureter (B1) or reflux (B2) and hydroureter and hydronephrosis. (C) Urinary bladder pressure in cm of H_2O by volume in cubic cm. A normal filling pressure curve with detrusser contractions that are unable to empty the bladder.

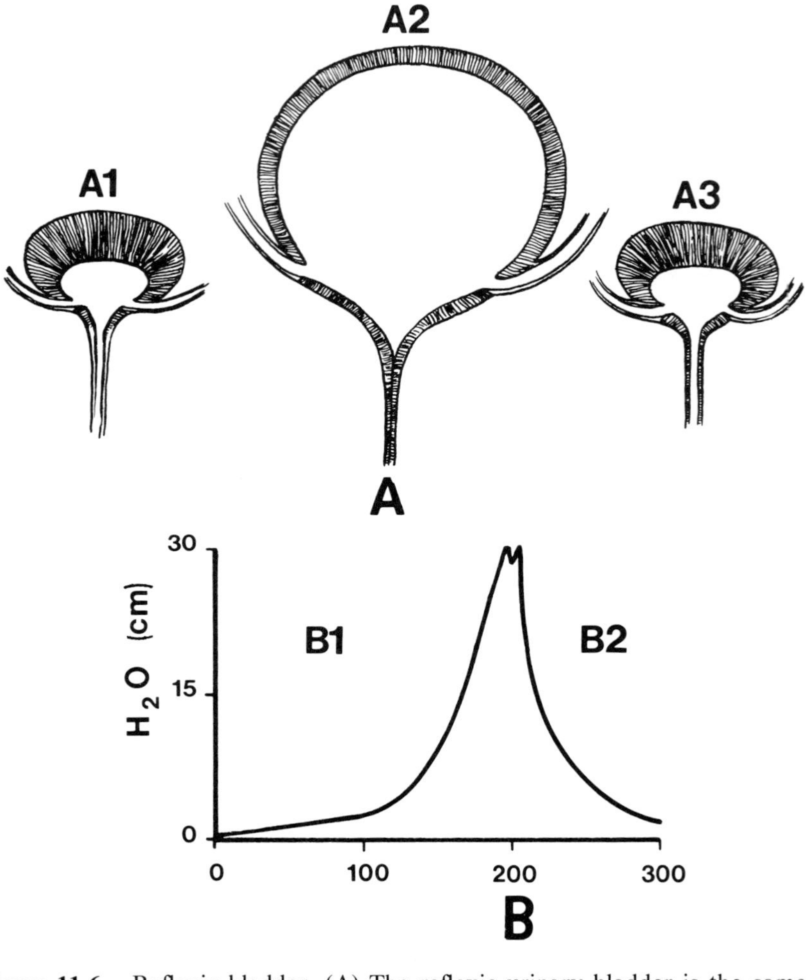

Figure 11-6. Reflexic bladder. (A) The reflexic urinary bladder is the same as normally observed in the normal neonate. The empty (A1) urinary bladder fills to a normal capacity for age (A2) (see Table 11-2) and then responds to a micturition arc by complete emptying with little or no residual (A3). (B) The abscissa, volume of urinary bladder filling, and the ordinate, pressure in the urinary bladder, are the same as for Figures 11-3–11-6. The filling-to-pressure curve is essentially normal for individuals without urinary tract neurogenic or anatomic impairment (B1). The normal micturition reflex then initiates, and the urinary bladder empties adequately (B2) without resistance. No or little (less than 15 cc) residual urine is left.

emptying of the bladder. Thus, one of the first signs of impending problems is a bladder that does not empty completely and carries residual urine (urinary retention). Such a bladder cannot wash out bacteria completely and may also be associated with increased bladder pressure. If ureteral reflux occurs and the pressure remains high in such a system, hydronephrosis and hydroureter will develop.

Symptoms of a possible UTI include any of the following: strong urine odor, cloudy urine, sandy particles, increased urine mucous or wetness, onset of perineal rash, bloody urine, lethargy, fever, and/or chills. When a UTI is suspected, a urine sample should be obtained for urinalysis (UA) and culture and sensitivity tests. Special note should be taken of the collection of this sample. A midstream, clean-catch, voided specimen should be obtained. This can sometimes be obtained by using a Crede maneuver. If the patient is on a clean intermittent catheterization (CIC) program (discussed below) or if the bladder is never full enough to get a good stream, a catheterized sample should be taken. Stick-on collection devices can be used for collection of samples for urine sediment examination, but they should never be used for culture. Suprapubic needle aspiration is most reliable for culture, but it can only be used when an adequate volume of urine will be retained in the bladder during the straining that children exhibit with this painful procedure.

Since bacterial growth is retarded in acidic environments, monitoring urine pH is one preventative method, as mentioned in Chapter 9 and 13. The urine pH should ideally remain between 5 and 6. Should the urine pH be elevated, simple measures to acidify the urine include (1) increasing the intake of cranberry or grape juices, (2) instituting vitamin C, i.e., ascorbic acid, by mouth, (3) reducing the intake of carbonated drinks and citrus products such as oranges, grapefruits, and tomatoes, and (4) limiting the intake of vegetables and peanuts. Because dietary manipulation is required for maintaining stool consistency and a low weight-to-height or weight-to-arm span ratio (see Chapter 13), we prefer to recommend manipulation of urine pH by administering vitamin C.

We also recommend monitoring urinary tract infections at home using the following simple home test method: (1) Test the urine pH. (2) Add enough vinegar to get the pH to between 5 and 6; it is not necessary to add vinegar if the pH is already in this range or lower. (3) Warm the urine solution to body temperature, 98.6°F or 37°C, testing with a thermometer. (4) If the urine clears, probably no infection is present, but if the urine remains cloudy, it may be infected.

Others recommend home use of nitrate test tapes. We use leukocyte esterase as a screening test with microscopic examination of the sediment in the presence of a positive test only. With a positive screening test, culture, colony count, and sensitivity tests need to be obtained. If these tests indicate infection, treatment with an antibiotic is indicated.

Treatment of possible urinary tract infections depends upon several factors. If a positive culture (greater than 10^5 colonies/ml^3) is obtained, the child is asymptomatic, and the UA is within 0–3 white blood cells per cubic centimeter, then such a culture would not be treated with antibiotics. However, if the culture is greater than 10^5/cc and the child is symptomatic or the UA shows significant elevations in white blood cells, then treatment with an antibiotic chosen from sensitivity studies should be instituted. Chronic problems with UTIs may require prophylactic chemotherapeutic treatment and maintenance of an acid urine pH. At times, more complete emptying of the urinary bladder with the Crede method and straining at the end of CIC as well as careful placement of the tip of the catheter at the lowest portion of the urinary bladder may be necessary to eliminate residual urine. A small amount of infected residual urine can provide the nidus for rapid bacterial multiplication and subsequent infection. Prevention of infection includes (1) reducing or eliminating residual urine after voiding or CIC and (2) creating urine not conducive to bacterial growth.

Eliminating the residual urine or facilitating complete emptying can be accomplished by using CIC with Crede and Valsalva maneuvers at the end of urine drainage. Crede and Valsalva without CIC should be used only if minimal pressure will initiate emptying. Considerable pressure during the Crede maneuver can lead to reflux, and excessive Valsalva can cause formation of hemorrhoids.

When using CIC, the catheter may be high up and against the bladder wall, stopping urine flow, thereby giving a false impression of emptiness. Therefore, the catheter should be inserted and then slowly removed, stopping when the urine stops, then reinserting a few millimeters until urine flows again. Alternatively, the catheter can be removed slowly with continued Valsalva or Crede. If the catheter is removed quickly, it will bypass urine low in the bladder or in an open bladder neck, enter the urethra, and give a sense of false emptying. Residual urine can also be considerable when the child is in a supine position and the urine is below the catheter in a lax bladder. Using gravity by sitting combined with Crede or Valsalva after the catheter is properly placed facilitates complete emptying.

In order to inhibit bacterial growth, the urine should be acidified. Creating an acid media entails acidification by diet or adding ascorbic acid (see Chapter 13). A chemotherapeutic agent concentrated in the urine will also inhibit bacterial growth. Furadantin (Nitrofurantoin, Norwich Eaton Pharmaceuticals, Inc., Norwich, NY), Gantrisin (Sulfisoxazole diolamine, Roche Laboratories, Nutley, NJ), or trimethoprim and sulfamethoxazole in one quarter to one third of the therapeutic doses used for tissue infection is adequate.

Hydronephrosis

Increased pressure can cause hydronephrosis, an enlargement of the renal collecting tubules and the renal pelvis. In later stages of hydronephrosis, the kidney substance becomes much thinner, and in the final stage, the kidney becomes a thin-walled sac with very little function remaining. The ureter undergoes the same process at an earlier stage, becoming a large, dilated tube with ineffective peristalsis, causing urine stasis. Infection and obstruction increase the likelihood of urinary stone formation. Stones, in turn, prevent elimination of infection and cause more obstruction.

Loss of Sensation

Another common abnormality with all the myelodysplasias is interference with the bladder sensation so that the patient cannot tell when the bladder is full. Lack of sensation allows the bladder to become too full and decompensate silently without discomfort. A decompensated bladder cannot empty and leads to breakdown of the ureterovesical valve, allowing reflux, infection, and hydronephrosis (Figs. 11-2A1, 11-5A3, and 11-5B1 and B2). With reconstitution of a bladder's filling and emptying rhythm and with increased age, some children with myelodysplasia regain or develop a recognition of the tension within the bladder that able-bodied individuals interpret as urinary bladder fullness. This vague sensation is carried to the consciousness by sympathetic autonomic fibers that enter the lower thorax and upper lumbar region; the sensation may be due to pressure or stretching of the peritoneum or adjacent area. This route should be intact in all children with lower thoracic, lumbar, and sacral-level meningomyeloceles. Lack of appreciation of this vague feeling can be due to chronic distention or to failure to stretch the urinary bladder. Some older patients with various types of meningomyelocele describe this feeling as pain, usually the secondary form of sensation the normally innervated person feels after prolonged retention of urine. The substitution of pain for the sensation of fullness and failure to appreciate any sensation at all despite an adequate filling-emptying cycle occurs with various types of myelodysplasia and has not been adequately explained.

Effect of Medication

Sudden appearance of a tense, palpable bladder may be due to the increase of outlet resistance caused by an increase of bladder neck contraction; this increased contraction may, in turn, be due to systemic administration of an adrenergic nasal decongestant for stuffy nose, head cold, or ear infection. In extreme cases, a decongestant may cause acute retention so that the child is unable to pass any urine, even with increased intra-abdominal pressure or using the Crede method. A child with normal bladder sensation would complain about this distention, but a child lacking sensation may be quite comfortable even though the bladder is becoming overdistended. The obvious treatment in this situation is to discontinue the offending systemic adrenergic agent and use a local drug for nasal decongestion. However, if urethral resistance is decreased, adrenergic agents may assist continence, as is discussed later in this chapter in "Chemical Adjunctive Therapy."

MANAGEMENT OF THE URINARY SYSTEM

We have discussed the potential for urinary infection and obstruction. Early kidney damage involving infection and increased urinary pressure may result in kidney damage from scarring, dilation, stones, loss of renal substance, and, finally, high blood pressure and renal failure. Prevention of these problems is essential for good health. Thus, we began our discussion of urinary tract management by focusing on problems of the urinary system. However, establishing continence may be a necessary first step in avoiding these problems and is essential in the school-aged child. We have divided our discussion of urinary tract management for meningomyelocele children into two phases: precontinence and continence. The first concentrates on the protection of the kidneys; when this is assured, we add the continence program.

URINARY PRECONTINENCE MANAGEMENT (TABLE 11-1)

At birth, a renal ultrasound is obtained to evaluate the urinary tract and to detect any gross abnormalities of that system, including congenital defects; hydronephrosis; an enlarged, poorly emptying bladder; and renal agenesis. In a noninvasive manner, this procedure provides the physician with necessary information for management immediately after birth. A totally destroyed or maldeveloped urinary tract may be a reason for deferring any form of neurosurgical treatment (see Chapter 5). Urinary tract obstruction may develop as a result of birth or operative trauma to the spinal cord and requires immediate drainage to avoid renal damage.

After the repair of the meningomyelocele sac, residual urine is

Table 11-1
Neurogenic Bladder Protocol

	Asymptomatic		Symptomatic
Birth	US to evaluate status of kidney and bladder		
After repair of back	US	If abnormal	Monitor, evaluate PVR
	PVR	If greater than 20 cc	Monitor, use phenoxybenzamine and CIC
	UA	If positive WBC	C&S
At 6 months	US	If increased size	VCUG and UA
	PVR	If increased	Monitor closely
At 12 months	US		
	VCUG (UA, C&S)		
At 18 months	UA (bag)	If positive for leukoesterase or WBC	CIC, C&S
At 2 years	IVP		
	VCUG (UA, C&S)		
	Toilet Training Years		
Yearly	US every 2 years alternating with VCUG every 2 years unless problems		
At 3 years	US		
At 4 years	US		
	Urodynamics (may be done earlier)		
At 5 years	IVP		

Key: US, kidney and bladder ultrasound; PVR, postvoiding residual urine volume; CIC, clean intermittent catheterization; UA, urinalysis; WBC, white blood cells; C&S, urine culture and colony count; VCUG, voiding cystourethrogram; IVP, intravenous pyelogram.

monitored by measuring postvoiding residual urine volume (PVR) by ultrasound; if the residual urine is increased, catheterization should be used since acute urinary retention due to cord shock can occur. If the PVR is greater than 20 cc, then urinary retention is most effectively managed by using Dibenzyline (Phenoxybenzamine, Smith, Kline and French, Philadelphia, PA) (an alpha-adrenergic blocking agent) in a l-mg single daily dose or intermittent catheterization. Rarely, a combination of both is required. Since introducing these methods ten years ago, we have had to perform only two vesicostomies to relieve urine retention.

Baseline Renal Function

Between the ages of birth and 2 years, our patients are routinely followed for urinary tract anatomic changes and function at 6-month intervals. After initial discharge, if the renal ultrasound, blood urea nitrogen (BUN), and creatinine are normal and the urinalysis does not indicate infection, then at 6 months of age, a renal and bladder ultrasound and PVR are obtained. If abnormalities such as increase in size of bladder, kidneys, or ureters are detected, then a voiding cystourethrogram (VCUG), intravenous pyelogram (IVP), isotope renogram, and urine culture and colony count (C&S) are considered, depending on the clinical course. If the PVR is increased at this time, close monitoring is instituted with intermittent PVR checks. Depending on the clinical course, other diagnostic tests are considered.

At 12 months of age, another renal ultrasound and VCUG are performed. A catheterized urine for UA and C&S is also obtained. Appropriate follow-up and diagnostic and treatment measures are taken should there be any indications.

At 18 months, a routine UA is evaluated. If the preliminary report shows an elevation of leukocytesterase or white blood cells, then a sterile urine sample is obtained by catheterization, as discussed above.

At the 2-year check, the routine diagnostic tests are an IVP, a VCUG, an UA, and a C&S.

During the toilet-training years and thereafter, a renal ultrasound to detect upper tract abnormalities is alternated every other year with a VCUG to evaluate the lower urinary tract. This frequency of diagnostic testing is used since changes in bladder function, such as retention of residual urine or reflux, are usually present before hydronephrosis occurs or before changes in kidney function (elevations of BUN or creatinine) can be recognized. When there is a question of functional impairment, we perform nuclear medicine studies such as renal scans and renograms.

An IVP is repeated at 5-year intervals unless there is a question on cystogram or ultrasound examinations.

Urodynamic Study

It is important to know more about the urodynamic balance of the bladder to facilitate incontinence management. At the age selected by the parents for toilet training (see Chapter 9), we perform a urodynamic study with measurement of bladder pressure during filling, taken from a catheter inserted into the bladder (see pressure-tracing, Figs. 11-2–11-6). This pressure is recorded during cineflouroscopy. Unless indicated sooner, urodynamic studies should usually be delayed until the patient is about 3 years of age because the procedure requires cooperation from the patient and is mostly useful for developing a continence management plan. If the upper tracts deteriorate in the first 3 years, urodynamic studies should be performed before intervention (e.g., for reflux) to evaluate bladder wall compliance.

During the first few years, the voiding pattern (that is, whether the child is continuously wet from dribbling, has an intermittent stream, etc.) is not usually of much help when planning since almost all meningomyelocele children will have some leaking, with perhaps a small stream produced by coughing, sneezing, or other stress.

URINARY CONTINENCE MANAGEMENT

The odor-free collection and disposal of urine are the factors determining whether a patient with neurogenic bladder is socially acceptable. Diapers are usually an adequate collection device until the child is close to school age. As mentioned in Chapter 9, continence management of the urinary tract should be started after a satisfactory bowel program is established. It is also important to have a clear understanding of a child's capabilities, both mental and physical, so appropriate and achievable goals can be set for the parents and the child. Some children with significant developmental delay may never achieve independent social continence (see Chapter 12).

Successful attainment of socially acceptable continence requires considerable parent and patient cooperation and understanding as well as a good deal of compulsive attention to the training program. Usually, lack of sensation necessitates voiding by the clock. A patient who cannot get into a wheelchair or cannot easily transfer between a wheelchair and a toilet to void requires special modifications of the continence program. Such a patient may need to try management by CIC, indwelling catheter, or a collection device rather than timed voidings with or without chemicals. Straining associated with wheelchair transfers causes spontaneous urine voiding. Continence programs that can be carried out in the wheelchair without transfer can be more effective.

Clean Intermittent Catheterization (CIC)

Ideal management of incontinence would use the minimum of intervention for therapeutic success. CIC has emerged as an alternative to surgical diversion. Initially, CIC was used to completely drain the bladder and control infection. Today, it is also used for continence since some children remain dry in between catheterizations. Often, the patient who is the most successful with CIC has a bladder of low detrusor tone and high

Table 11-2
Normal Urinary Bladder Capacity by Age

Age (Years)	Volume (ml)	
	Females	Males
0–1	12–21	15–20
1–4	75–90	100–120
4–7	225–305	190–205
7–10	245–310	250–290
10–13	340–485	280–410
13–16	320–405	295–390

This legend was adapted from Gierup[397]: 396 patients were examined 487 times. Micturition volume is only an estimate of bladder volume since residual was not examined after spontaneous voiding.

urethral resistance. Various drugs may enhance and facilitate continence, as is discussed below ("Chemical Adjunctive Therapy"). Infections and other complications are minimized when CIC is instituted early since the bladder can be completely emptied and bladder pressure can be maintained within normal ranges.

For toilet training and continence purposes, CIC can be initiated by the parents or other caretakers as early as age 6–12 months or at the usual age for toilet training, as mentioned in Chapter 9. Each program should be individualized to accommodate the family's life-style and the child's health needs. When CIC is the method of choice for social continence, catheterizations may need to be done only during the waking hours, approximately 2–4 hours apart. Careful attention should be paid to good technique. Renal health may require night time catheterizations to avoid excess stretching of the bladder. Volumes of urine in most children should not exceed the normal bladder capacity for the patient's age (Table 11-2).

CIC is not usually considered successful unless the child is dry for at least 2 hours. However, normal 3-year-old children often urinate more frequently and have occasional accidents.

A few children can be taught to catheterize themselves by age 5. This is an ideal time to begin new habits in preparation for starting school. It also allows the child to take control of his or her own bodily functions, increasing self-image. CIC is the most widely accepted program, and many patients and parents prefer to go directly to this technique rather than try other methods first. Unfortunately, many patients have such lax sphincter mechanisms (or they have reflexic or hyperreflexic bladders) that they are damp or actually wet between catheterizations.

Indwelling Catheters

Indwelling catheters must maintain low pressure and sterility in the upper urinary tract. An indwelling catheter, usually a Foley, can be used. We close all suprapubic cystotomies and use phenoxybenzamine, so we rarely deal with suprapubic catheters. Suprapubic and indwelling foley catheters (urethral) drain urine and keep pressure down, but they usually perpetuate infection, make formation of stones more likely, and cause social problems; they tend to leak and cause both odor and rashes.

Penile Collectors and Clamps

External collectors come in both disposable and reusable styles. Good skin care and appliance care are extremely important when using the external collector. In the male, an external or penile collector can be quite effective on an adequate-sized penis but may need considerable modification to work on a very small child. Penile clamps are only effective for very minimal incontinence, and they have the disadvantage of skin and penile breakdown, especially since most meningomyelocele patients lack penile sensation. A method compatible with sexual function needs to be substituted at adolescence (see Chapter 20).

Timed Voidings

With moderate urethral resistance as well as an adequate urinary bladder capacity that empties almost completely with or without chemical adjuncts, we first recommend timed voidings. The best voiding schedule is usually with the bowel movement in the morning before strenuous activities and at least every 2–3 hours for the rest of the day. However, only a small percentage of patients are socially acceptable on timed voiding. Bladders that will fill and empty adequately are frequently stimulated to empty at inappropriate times by coughing or straining.

The Crede manuever sometimes facilitates emptying. This method is effective in a bladder that appears to have low-pressure retention due to a weak, flaccid detrusor and some urethral resistance. However, this procedure is contraindicated in the presence of reflux or when firm pressure is needed to empty the bladder since pressure exerted on the bladder can cause reflux and, with reflux, be immediately transmitted to the kidney. High-pressure reflux up the ureters will damage the upper urinary tract.

Chemical Adjunctive Therapy

Some situations require drugs to facilitate the desired bladder response. Drug therapy requires an adequate amount of time (4–8 weeks) to ascertain effectiveness both because of the need for dosage adjustments and for a maximum effect on the smooth muscle. Combinations of timed voiding or CIC with drug therapy can provide suitable continence programs.

In the case of *urinary retention* due to excessive urethral resistance, phenoxybenzamine is prescribed to relax the bladder neck and decrease urethral resistance, thereby allowing urine to flow more freely. The dose can be increased until side effects of nasal mucosa swelling or orthostatic hypotension occur. For *urinary incontinence* due to decreased urethral resistence, an alpha-adrenergic–stimulating agent can be prescribed to increase the internal urethral sphincter and the bladder neck contraction. We usually prescribe 25 mg of ephedrine every 4 hours.

Bladder *hyperactivity* is chemically treated with an anticholinergic agent such as propantheline bromide, 7.5–15 mg every 6–8 hours, or Ditropan (Oxybutinin chloride, Marion Laboratories, Kansas City, Mo), 2.5–5 mg every 6–8 hours. A small dose should be used and then increased to achieve the desired effect and avoid the side effects of constipation, blurred vision, dry mouth, flushing, or decrease in perspiration. These agents allow the bladder to relax and increase in capacity, improving urine retention. They also produce a decrease in bladder pressure. Due to the anticholinergic effect of decreased perspiration, the chemicals should be used cautiously in hot climates; also, caution is advised because they decrease gut motility in patients who are prone to obstipation.

Ephedrine and an anticholinergic agent are used in combination therapy, particularly with CIC. However, care must be taken to prevent build up of residual urine on timed regimens.

Anal Plugs and Bladder Stimulators

Anal plugs, presently on the market, produce periodic electrical currents and keep perineal muscles and sphincters contracted. Urinary bladder electrical stimulators cause detrusors to contract. We have not found these to be effective in patients with myelodysplasia.

Artificial Sphincters

To increase urethral resistance, artificial sphincters have been developed by Scott and associates (Scott Artificial Sphincter, American Medical Systems, Inc., Minneapolis, MN).[992] The ideal patient is totally incontinent, voids with no residual urine, has an adequate capacity, and has a compliant bladder wall. If uninhibited bladder contractions are present, they should be controlled with anticholinergic drugs; otherwise, the patient will still experience some leakage and may develop upper tract complications. In this situation, bladder augmentation can be considered. With incomplete emptying, CIC can be combined with an artificial sphincter, but urethral erosion at the cuff site may occur. Infection, need for replacement with growth, and inconsistent or improper use, potentially causing reflux and renal damage, are several reasons for limited use of these sphincters at this time.[398] Our experience with artificial sphincters has been satisfactory only with older teenagers and adults. They should be discussed as potential solutions with families of young patients with incontinence due to minimum urethral resistance not improved by alpha-adrenergic–stimulating medications.

Surgical Diversion of Urine Flow

Surgery use has lessened over the past few years. Surgical diversions (cutaneous ureterostomy, cutaneous vesicostomy, ileal loop, and colonic loop) have been used in the past but are needed now only if the patient's urinary tract has deteriorated despite other treatments. Most recently, bladder augmentation procedures for noncompliant bladders or in combination with reversal of urinary diversions have been successfully combined with CIC or artificial sphincters to produce a continence program. Undiversion is not necessarily for everyone. Careful evaluation by cineflouroscopy and pressure studies of the bladder before and after a series of bladder filling exercises are conducted at home over a period of 6 weeks. These studies should proceed before consideration of undiversion because a small fibrotic urinary bladder, common following bladder isolation, needs to be differentiated from a functional bladder. The small bladder would require ileocystoplasty where the cecum and part of the ascending colon provide adequate capacity. The ureters are attached to the terminal ileum, and the ileocecal valve provides an antireflex mechanism. A bladder with adequate volume and a closed or spastic sphincter may function after undiversion with CIC only. An adequate-volume bladder with a weak or open sphincter would require an artificial sphincter.

Other Surgical Interventions

Other surgical interventions may be necessary to improve continence or renal function. Some children who have incompetent ureterovesicle valves and who have not responded to CIC and anticholinergics to create low-pressure bladders with resolution of reflux will require ureteral reimplantations. CIC and anticholingergics should still be continued after antireflux surgery. In addition, bladder outlet procedures, such as *Y-V* plasty or sphincterotomy, may have to be done prior to insertion of an artificial sphincter to assure adequate drainage when CIC has been socially unacceptable or associated with recurrent prostatitis and epididymitis.

ACHIEVING SUCCESS

Urinary tract anatomy and physiology alone do not necessarily determine the success or failure of any continence program. Each program is unique and must be individualized and fine-tuned accordingly. Consistency and compliance, keys to success, are most readily obtained by asking the parents to keep a record for several weeks of the child's bladder program. Readiness of both parents and child for a continence program must also be assessed through interview. Family and patient desire to achieve continence as well as a thorough understanding of the methods improve the success rate. Good communication and frequent follow-up are essential to help families solve problems. In our program, after an initial evaluation by the consulting urologist, a program is prescribed, and the nurse specialist assigned to the patient works with the family, public health nurses, and school personnel to monitor progress. This specialist modifies any instituted regime, with the advice of a physician, if necessary, to insure maximum success. The need for close contact between the parent and nurse specialist as well as between the school and nurse specialist cannot be overemphasized (see Chapters 2, 9, and 17).

SUMMARY

Our goal is for the child with meningomyelocele to continue in good renal health while achieving a state of social acceptability, cleanliness, and freedom from odor, skin breakdown, and diapers when age-appropriate. We hope that promotion of positive self-esteem and independence, when appropriate, through the effective use of different toileting methods, will positively affect other aspects of each individual's life

David Shurtleff
Michael Mayo

12

Toilet Training: The Seattle Experience and Conclusions

The three previous chapters as well as Chapman and associates' book, *Management of the Neurogenic Bowel and Bladder*,[177] have outlined the pathophysiology and methods for toilet training the patient with anatomic and neurogenic impairment of the anal and urinary tract sphincters. A number of authors describe different toilet training techniques and claim that each works with most impaired children. This chapter discusses the success rates achieved by using all techniques; no single program works for a majority of patients, but each technique works well for a few or some. Our philosophy has been to accept any technique introduced by other centers and, more frequently, by parents or caretakers. Our minimum objectives have been to preserve health, both physical and mental, and provide a program or programs acceptable to both the family and patient.

Preservation of physical health, avoidance of retention (either urinary or stool), and freedom from infection, reflux, and obstipation are readily accepted by parents, by caretakers, and sometimes, by younger patients. However, avoiding the odor of urine and feces, to allow social reception and prevent outright rejection, is very difficult to achieve. We believe the psychological development of the patient is in no way as seriously challenged by any other impairment associated with open spine deformities and hindgut malformations as in the area of toilet training. As

MYELODYSPLASIAS AND EXSTROPHIES: SIGNIFICANCE, PREVENTION, AND TREATMENT
 ISBN 0-8089-1816-8

discussed in Chapters 18–20, adolescent adjustment, the transition from childhood dependence to adult independence, is a goal that must be sought from earliest infancy. Development of a concept of self-worth and sexuality begins in the early years and is dependent, in part, on toileting. A toilet training program, therefore, must be individually designed for patient, family, and social setting.

We cannot analyze each individual method outlined in Chapters 10 and 11 for five reasons: (1) patients with the same motor level of paralysis have different bladder and sphincter malfunction; (2) patients, families, and their local microsocieties differ in attitudes, motivation, acceptance, rejection, understanding, and compliance; (3) different toileting techniques will be successful in the same patient at different times under different environmental circumstances, such as hot, dry weather or intestinal upsets from infectious agents or chemicals; (4) pathophysiology will change with time: frequency of passage and bulk of stool decreases with age; reflux may develop or resolve; and the male prostate provides increased outlet resistance with growth during adolescence; and (5) many of our patients use several methods of toilet training simultaneously. We will, therefore, present our experiences as a general result, with the understanding that multiple methods are used in most patients. The ideal method or methods must be sought for each patient, and an expectation of periodic deterioration with the need for retraining should be included in the overall plan.

In order to explain the success of toileting programs, we will (1) discuss the effect of phenoxybenzamine on urine retention, (2) present a summary of the age at which our patients have first achieved dependent and independent socially acceptable urine and stool hygiene, (3) present data that define how a group of our patients, intensively reported by Okamoto and colleagues,[825] learned various aspects of toilet training and some aspects of urine and stool hygiene separately, and (4) describe what percentage of children in various age groups are independent or dependent and socially acceptable or handicapped by soiling and odor. These data will allow the person organizing a toilet training program for the physically or neurogenically impaired to offer parents, caretakers, and patients (1) an expected earliest age of achievement, (2) the range of ages at which children within subgroups of impairment learn, and (3) the percentage of children in each age group who are independent and socially acceptable at a given point in time.

Criteria for being classified socially acceptable include being free of wetness, soiling, and odor detectable by peers or adult contacts. One accident or less each week is acceptable. The patient must also be free of rash, infection, and retention of urine, which produces reflux, or retention of stool, which causes obstipation. Frequent elimination into the toilet or a commode or using a collection device, such as an external urine collector, diaper, or pant inserts,[177] is acceptable. The choice of the methods, outlined in Chapters 10 and 11, is based on pathophysiology as well as patient and parent preference. We have been strong advocates of any program that allows the patient to remain healthy and socially acceptable.

TOILETING PROGRAMS

Phenoxybenzamine to Relieve Outlet Obstipation

Phenoxybenzamine (Dibenzyline®), an alpha-adrenergic–blocking agent, has been described as useful in treatment of hypertension and relief of urinary tract outlet spasm or dyssenergia (Chapter 11). Between 1977 and 1983, we obtained data on 77 patients admitted to our inpatient services as newborns. Thirty-seven (48 percent) had on arrival, or developed after back repair, either permanent or temporary urinary outlet resistance sufficient to produce increasing residual urine in excess of 30cc. Twenty-one (57 percent) responded to 1–3 mg of phenoxybenzmine (Dibenzyline®) each day by developing residuals less than 15 cc. Ten (27 percent) were treated with clean intermittent catheterization (CIC) alone, and six (16 percent) were treated with phenoxybenzamine and CIC once or twice a day. Parents chose phenoxybenzamine more frequently than CIC because it allowed their infants to be more like their able-bodied peers. (Most later convert to CIC.) Difficulty passing a catheter due to posterior urethral spasm necessitated continued use of phenoxybenzamine in some. Both CIC and phenoxybenzamine have almost eliminated surgical procedures such as suprapubic cystostomy and various outlet-widening procedures. Cystostomy is messy, and outlet procedures destroy the opportunity for effective CIC programs later in childhood.

Earliest Age of Acquisition of Acceptable Toilet Training Skills

During our first study of the acquisition of daily living skills,[1045,1064,1094] we observed that children with meningomyelocele learned toileting skills less well and at a later age than other skills and much less well and later than their peers. We also noted that teenagers, still dependent or with socially inadequate toileting skills, actually lost momentum when learning social skills necessary for interacting with peers.[1041] Adults with meningomyelocele described inadequate toileting skills as their most worrisome handicap.[1057] We therefore redesigned our program in the mid-1970s to emphasize acquisition of daily living activities, particularly toilet training. Since then, we have studied the age at which 525 patients first acquired socially acceptable urine and stool elimination skills (Fig. 12-1). We divided the patients into three groups: those with short leg braces or no ambulatory aids and with sacral-level lesions (S1); those with braces and crutches primarily and with mid- and low-lumbar-level lesions (L3-5); and those primarily in wheelchairs and with high-lumbar and thoracic-level lesions (L2 and up). The patient could be independent in toileting skills or dependent on others either completely or for assistance. By these criteria, 50 percent of all three muscle level groups first achieved socially acceptable toileting by age 6–8 years. Patients in all three groups became socially acceptable for the first time at the same rate until about 10–11 years of age, by which time 75 percent had acquired socially accepted toileting hygiene. The two less severely paralyzed groups then deviated from the more severely paralyzed groups. Thus, by age 13–15 years, all of the former had achieved socially acceptable skills, some with assistance, but not all of the severely paralyzed were socially acceptable by the end of their teen years.

Learning independent toileting skills begins at 4 years for the least paralyzed, at 7 years for those with intermediate degrees of paralysis, and at 10 years for the more severely impaired (Fig. 12-2). As with dependent hygiene, the two least paralyzed groups first achieved independence in toileting skills at about the same rate, with about 50 percent developing independence at 11–12 years of age, 75 percent at 14–15, and 100 percent by 15–18. These rates were insignificantly different for the two groups. Only 40 percent of the most severely impaired learned independence by the end of adolescence, which provided the only significantly different learning curve ($p < .001$).[125]

All three groups first learned stool and urine independent toileting skills at the same rate; the separate stool and urine learning curves are shown for only the mid- and low-lumbar group (Fig. 12-3). When compared with our data from the 1960s and early 1970s,[1094] these data suggest a considerable improvement in the earlier age for first learning both dependent and independent toilet training skills for the two least paralyzed groups, but not for the most severely paralyzed patients.

In order to better understand the reasons for failure to achieve socially acceptable and independent skills for toileting, we examined potential causes for interference (Table 12-1). The most common cause was a physical deformity that prevented or delayed the child from seeing and reaching the perineum or transferring from wheelchair to a toilet. Almost as frequent a cause for failure was family disruption or a combination of family, school, and child failure to comply.

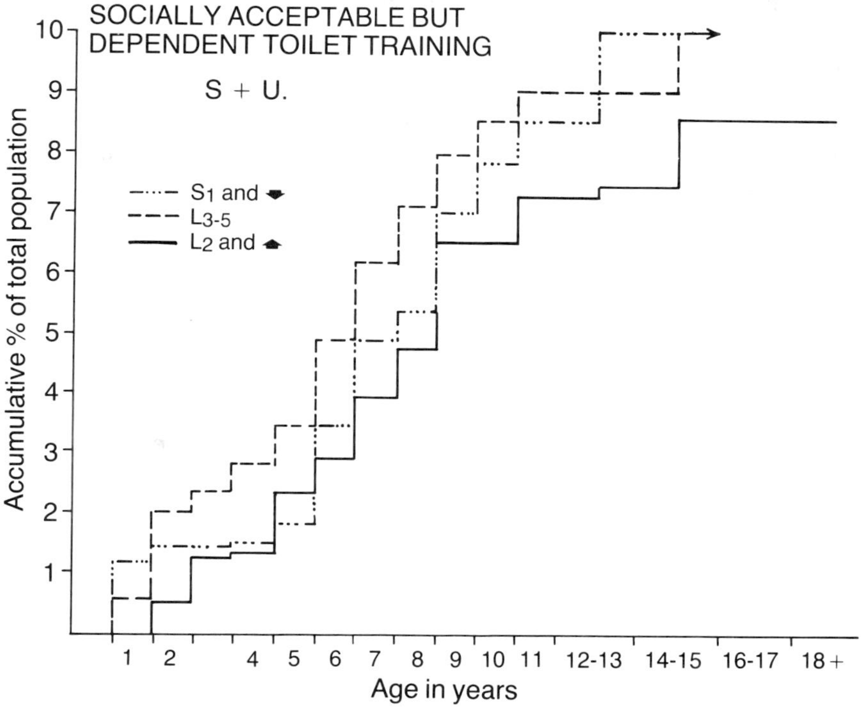

Figure 12-1. Acquisition of socially acceptable urine and stool elimination skills in 525 patients. This computer-generated set of graphs uses the computation of a life table to determine the percentage at risk in each age group who become socially acceptable. The individual either leaves the program or is not old enough to be in the next age bracket is dropped from the analysis without penalty. Once the individual is determined to achieve social acceptance, either by learning toileting skills independently or with varying degrees of assistance from caretakers, he or she is no longer considered in the calculation. Those surviving without learning remain as the denominator in each age group. The numerator is comprised of those learning the task. The percentage calculated from this fraction is multiplied by the remaining proportion of the initial population and added to the percentage of the previous age group having previously achieved socially acceptable skills. Thoracic and L1-2 (L2 and ↑), mid- and low-lumbar (L3-5), and sacral (S1 and ↓) are the three groups. Both stool and urine toileting skills are considered.

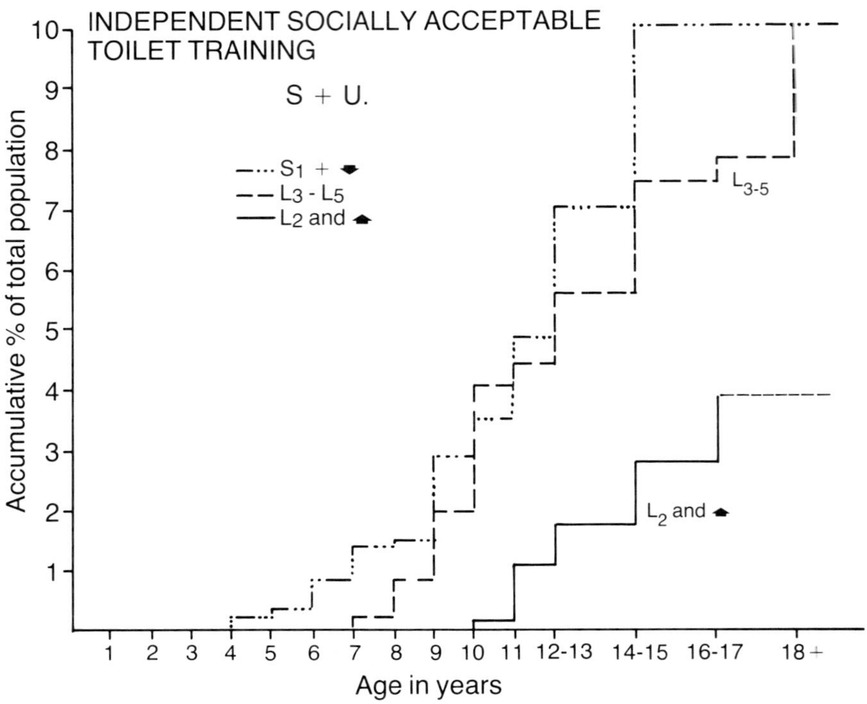

Figure 12-2. Independence in toileting skills. Calculation of these acquisition graphs is by the same method as for Figure 12-1. The only difference is the definition used for determining acquisition; the patients had to achieve socially acceptable toileting skills without assistance. Symbols for the three groups are the same.

These data provide a good estimate of when seriously impaired children can first acquire toileting skills, but provide neither a range of first achievement for similarly impaired children nor a concept of how well they maintain social acceptance.

General Toileting Behavior (Fig. 12-4)

In order to better understand the potential of children with impaired sphincters, we initiated a study of toilet training with a select subgroup of our population.[825] This group had no intellectual impairment (IQ $\geq$ 75), cooperative and compliant families, and either no orthopedic deformities that would interfere with toileting or adequate assistive devices such as extension devices to reach the perineum, access to secure toilets, or commode bars, rails, and side arms, etc. Only patients living within 50

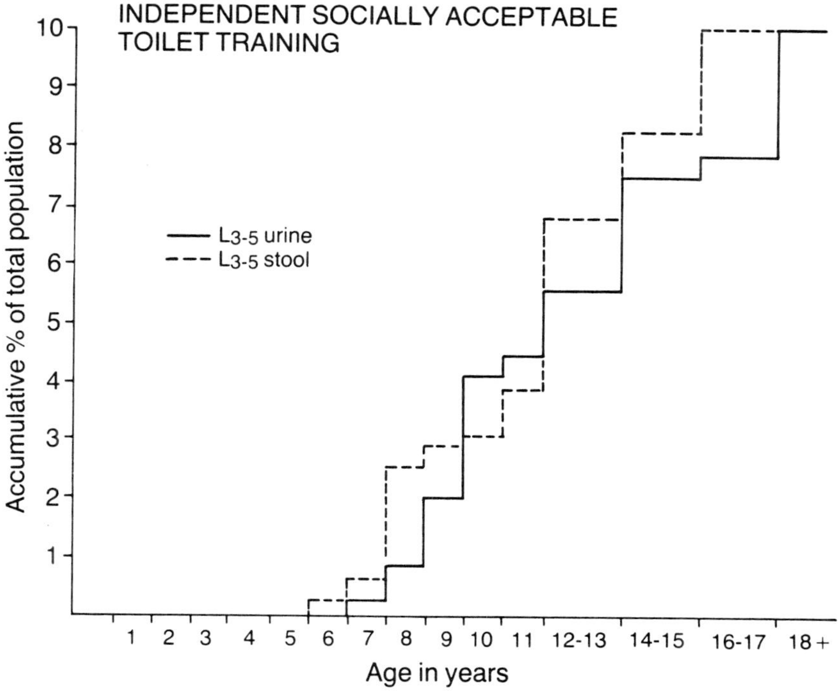

Figure 12-3. Stool and urine independence learning curves for mid- and low-lumbar lesion patients. These two graphs were calculated as for Figure 12-1 but involve only the L3-5 group of patients. Urine and stool toileting skills were analyzed separately, and the definition of acquisition was otherwise the same. Analysis for difference between the slopes of the curves revealed no dissimilarities (see text).

miles of our center whose families agreed were included. One of the authors, Sousa, interviewed in person or by telephone each primary care provider in the home at least every 3 months. Sousa gave parents a standardized question sheet with carefully defined categories and reviewed it with them.[825,1095] We emphasized the necessity to define each achievement as *done routinely*, not as *showing the ability* to do so. Data were collected and entered into a computerized file with demographic and biologic data from our overall meningomyelocele file.[1058] Ages of first routine performance of the first 20 percent, 50 percent, and 80 percent of each task for children in four groups of motor impairment—thoracic, high-lumbar, low-lumbar, and sacral levels of paralysis—were calculated and graphed (Figs. 12-4–12-6).

These data, indicating the potential for children with varying degrees

Table 12-1
Reasons for Failure or Delay in Toilet Training for 1979–80 Review

		Relative Significance		
	Total[a]	Only Factor	Most Significant	One of Several
Entered program late	34	19	1	14[b]
Family or child failure to comply	36	12	5	19[b]
Psychosocial				
Family Stress	44	12	12	20[b]
Divorce	21	(10)	(3)	(8)
Abandonment	17	(2)	(3)	(12)
Mental retardation	31	8	8	15[c]
Physical Disability	47	8	8	31
Kyphoscoliosis	16	(4)	(1)	11
Flail sphincters	10	(3)	(2)	5
High-level lesions with poor sitting balance	9	(1)	(4)	4
Upper extremity spasticity	4	0	0	4
Arthrogrypotic joints	3	0	0	3
Blindness	2	0	(1)	1
Severe Arnold-Chiari malformation	2	0	0	2
Increased Occipito Frontal Circumference	1	0	0	1
Institutional failure to comply	8	2	6	0
Bus	1	(1)	0	0
School	2	(1)	(1)	0
Residential school	3	0	(3)	0
Group home	2	0	(2)	0
Renal complication	9	0	0	9
Recurrent infection	3	0	0	(3)
Renal stones	3	0	0	(3)
Renal failures	1	0	0	(1)
Ammoniacal burns	2	0	0	(2)
Idiosyncratic reaction to medications	6	3	2	1
Totals		64	42	108

[a] More than one cause with relative importance compared to the others not evident.
[b] Mental retardation and multiple physical handicaps were believed to contribute equally to entering the program late and psychosocial family stress in 4 cases and with poor family compliance in another case.
[c] Whether late referral, emotional stress, and failure to comply were the result or were contributing major causes could not be distinguished in 11 paitents.

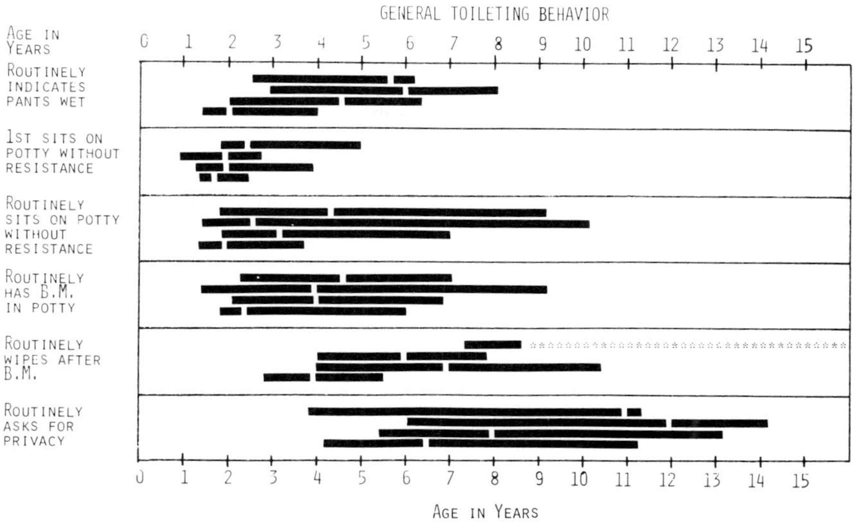

Figure 12-4. General toileting behavior. The age at which 20 percent, 50 percent, and 80 percent of a group of 173 children learned general toilet training skills is indicated by the beginning, white space, and end of the black bars. *** indicate this group never achieved an 80 percent learning proportion. The bars in each category represent, from top to bottom, (1) thoracic and L1-2, (2) L3 and mixed lesions L2-4, (3) L4-5, and (4) sacral-motor-level groups. All patients had neurogenic bladder and bowel dysfunction although some in the sacral group had minimal or no paralysis in the legs. All data were recorded as the child achieved the skill during the 2.5-year period of the study, within 4 months of entering the study, or when the caretaker entered a specific date of achievement in the child's diary. This chart and those in Figures 12-5 and 12-6 were created from data published by Okamoto and associates.[825]

of impairment, are used to teach parents, caretakers, and education and medical therapists the potential of a given patient as defined by his or her age, level of lesion, and type of sphincter impairment.

We constructed graphs for the specifics of general toilet training (Fig. 12-4), for urine (Fig. 12-5), and for stool (Fig. 12-6) and made the following observations. First, all toilet training skills are considerably delayed for all levels of impairment when compared with normal children. Considering the physical and neurologic impairments of these children, such might be expected. However, the second observation, the marked spread over years for first achievement of routine independent performance within impairment groups, is remarkable, particularly since the known causes for failure or delay were eliminated by patient selection. The most marked examples of wide ranges for age of first achievement include (1) first sitting on the potty by high-lumbar-level lesion patients, (2) requesting

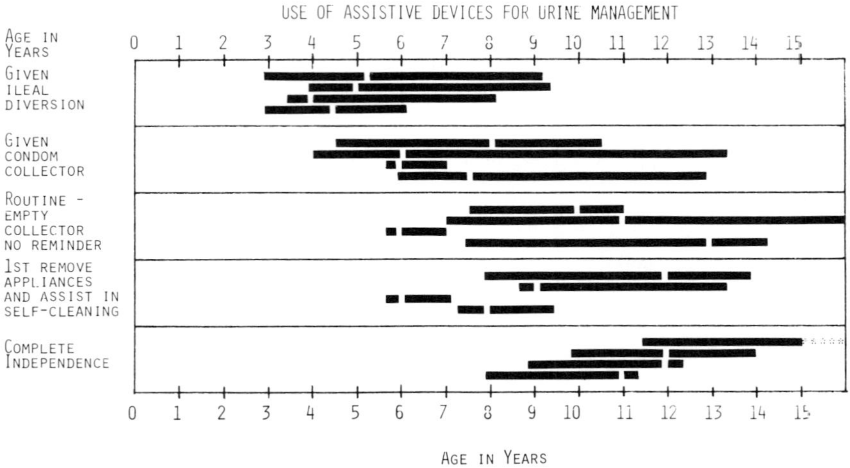

Figure 12-5. Toilet training for urine. See Figure 12-4.

privacy (Fig. 12-4), (3) being completely independent in stool training (Fig. 12-6), and (4) routinely emptying external collection devices by high-lumbar and sacral-level lesion patients (Fig. 12-6). These wide ranges of first routine performance may be due to differences in interpretation by parents or differences in pathophysiology within muscle level groups. Obvious factors causing interference (Table 12-1) were eliminated, however. We suspect a considerable portion of the differences can be

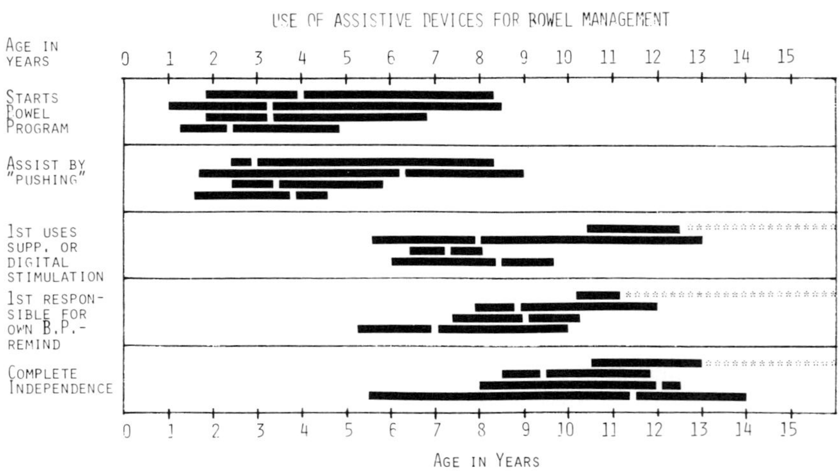

Figure 12-6. Toilet training for stool. See Figure 12-4.

attributed to expectations on behalf of care providers, both parents and professionals.

Since all patients were urged to begin toilet training at the same age as able-bodied peers, but with modifications in technique, acceptance of this recommendation, and therefore compliance, must be questioned. We believe such developmental guidelines as provided by these graphs, despite their imperfections, will assist both parents and professionals in helping sphincter-impaired children achieve socially acceptable toileting skills. We also hope that introducing these guides to parents and professionals will help shift the age of expected achievement of these skills to a younger age. These goals are particularly important if we believe Erikson's concepts about personality development, as discussed in Chapters 9 and 16–19.[314]

Despite our hopes, the age of first achievement of these skills (Figs. 12-1–12-3) and the age of first routine performance (Fig. 12-4–12-6) do not provide the reader with an understanding of what happens as a population of children with sphincter impairment grow older.

Maintenance of Dependent and Independent Stool and Urine Toileting Skills

In order to further refine our understanding of how sphincter-impaired children learn and continue to use complicated and usually only partially successful techniques, we analyzed our success at urine toilet training by prevalence. We determined the percentage of socially acceptable urine toilet-trained children (either dependent or independent) by age groups (Fig. 12-7). We defined socially acceptable as above: free of odor, rash, infection, or evidence of wetness or soiling. We selected children with normal intelligence (IQ $\geq$ 75) and free of either orthopedic deformities or upper extremity neurologic impairment so severe as to interfere with the functions necessary to perform toileting skills. In order to eliminate psychological problems introduced by late onset of toilet training, we selected only those children entering our program under the age of 3 years. We included all forms of myelodysplasia with at least sphincter impairment, but none with exstrophy or imperforate anus. The data in Figure 12-7 indicate that about 50–80 percent of patients are socially acceptable at each age and that independence once attained is not necessarily maintained. Comparison of these bar diagrams with Figs. 12-1 and 12-2 further suggests that initial learning does not mean permanent acquisition of socially acceptable toileting skills. In addition, at ages 3–8, it appears that parents and caretakers are less able to provide adequate toileting for the dependent children since the percentage of socially unacceptable children increases. A similar increase in percentage of

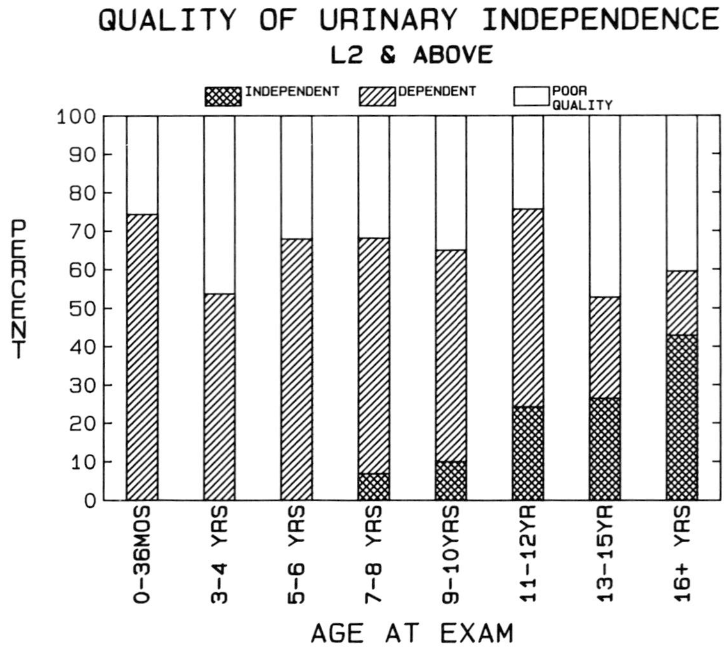

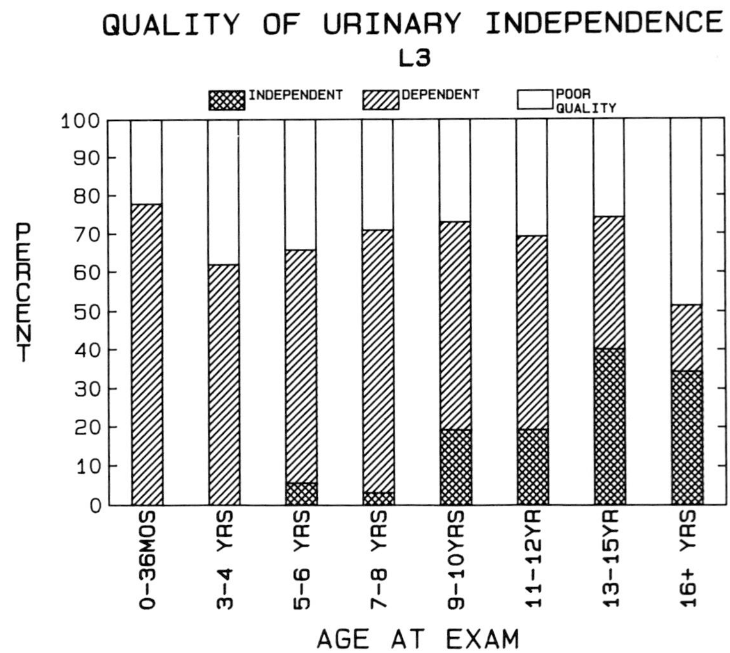

Figure 12-7. Socially acceptable toilet-trained children (dependent or independent) by lesion level: 2094 examinations of 617 patients who entered our program before the age of 3 years were divided into four groups by motor level: (A) thoracic and L1-2, (B) L3, (C) L4-5, and (D) sacral. All had bladder and anal sphincter dysfunction. Each lesion-level group was divided into eight age groups from 0–36 months to 16 years and older. Each age group was divided into three

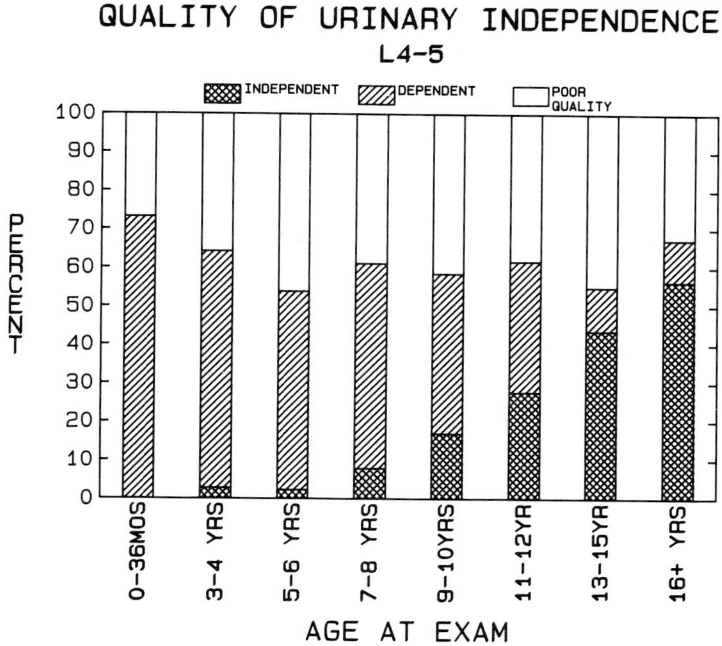

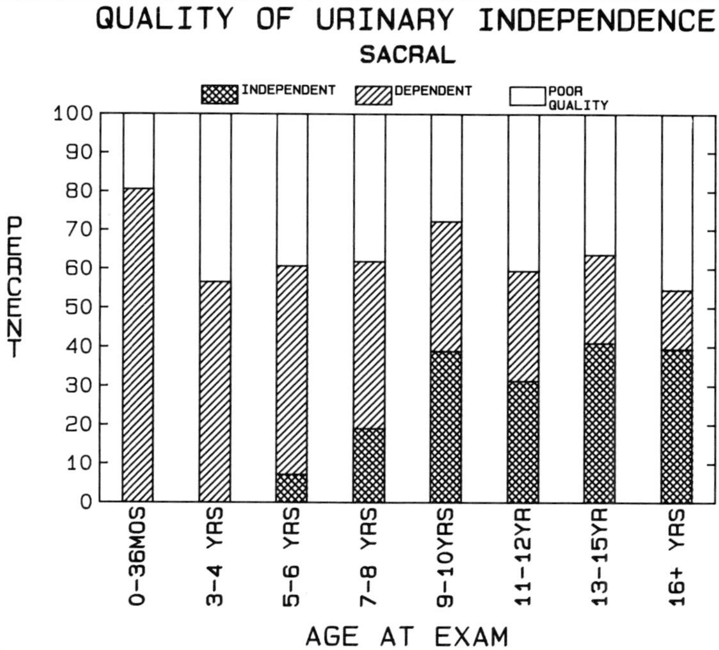

Figure 12-7. *(Continued)* groups according to the quality of toileting hygiene: (1) cross-hatched for completely independent and socially acceptable, (2) unidirectional slant lines for dependent to some degree but socially acceptable, and (3) clear for either dependent or independent but socially unacceptable with poor-quality hygiene. Definitions for independence and social acceptability are the same as in the text and Figures 12-1 and 12-2.

socially unacceptable children occurs in late childhood and early teenage, perhaps reflecting either decreased parental and caretaker assistance or the patients' rebellion against rigid and complicated toileting procedures.

The decreased percentage of more severely involved patients achieving socially acceptable and independent toileting skills is reflected in Figs. 12-2, 12-3, and 12-7. The failure to learn and the loss of ability to maintain toileting skills can be due to one or more complications that develop after achieving socially acceptable and independent skills (Table 12-1).

SUMMARY

These studies outline the current state of our multiple-modality approach to toilet training and a program in transition from emphasis on biped ambulation with its associated benefits (see Chapter 15) to a stronger emphasis on self-care skills. We employ every form of toilet training described in the literature or by patients and parents. We believe adequate toilet training techniques have only been available since the introduction of CIC, urinary bladder augmentation, artificial sphincter, neurohormonal chemicals, and biofeedback. We are not able to report the success attributed to any single type of toilet training program claimed by some adherents. Hence, early in the child's life we initiate a program or programs chosen by the parent or caretaker and based on the patient's pathophysiology. We assign a single nurse specialist to each family and provide both a pediatrician and urologist.

When children arrive at school age, we begin working with school staff and the children directly, particularly when there has been a lack of compliance within the home. We discourage parental participation in toileting activities carried on in the school, often a recommendation that is opposed by both parents and school officials. We believe there can be no more degrading experience than to have parents involved in toileting experiences after the normal age for peers, though assistance during periods of illness or interruptions of routine care are obviously appropriate. A firm goal should be for children to learn how to keep themselves clean at the earliest age possible. Families and schools should provide access to necessary equipment and privacy. At most, sphincter-impaired children should receive a subtle cue when they have malodor. People with unacceptable odor are the last to smell themselves.

We continuously encourage sphincter-impaired children using the techniques outlined in Chapters 10 and 11 to understand the need for self-care independence. We explain the need to provide definitive surgical intervention, such as urinary bladder augmentation or artificial urinary sphincter, only after a child has demonstrated independent self-care and stable maturity. We have witnessed too many children enter a rebellious and self-destructive stage in late childhood or teenage to risk disruption of an artificial sphincter. We prefer to deter insertion of an artificial sphincter for other reasons, including size, development of increased urinary tract outlet resistance with growth of the prostate, and a limited life expectancy requiring revision for any artificial part.

Since we defer definitive procedures until after puberty, and because most people perceive the genitourinary tract as one system, we counsel parents and patients that normal sexual activities can be achieved. Such information about sexual function is rarely requested by parents or patients, but it is of great concern to them. By initiating open discussion of the child's potential and future need for sex-compatible toileting techniques, the clinician can assist the parent and older patient to develop definite social indications for definitive surgery.

As emphasized in other parts of this text, at every opportunity self-concept is *the* most important goal. The area of self-cleanliness in the United States culture is *most* important. An evening watching television commercials will convince the nonbeliever that a young person cannot grow up in our society without smelling CLEAN. We believe that at some time in each child's maturation, he or she will develop the desire to maintain self-cleanliness. At that time, it is the professional's responsibility to provide physiologically sound recommendations and carry out definitive procedures. An individualized program offered to a patient who has been raised with an understanding of the need to anticipate accidents, retraining, and retaining a good self-image will be successful.

SECTION IV

Establishing Lifelong Health Patterns

David Shurtleff

13

Dietary Management

Elsewhere in this text, we have mentioned the importance of diet to (1) avoid an excess weight gain that inhibits mobility (see Chapter 15), (2) control urinary tract infections (UTIs) by producing an acid urine (see Chapter 11), and (3) establish and maintain bowel management by producing a bulky or small hard stool (see Chapter 10). This chapter synthesizes these sometimes conflicting goals and offers recommendations in regard to dietary management.

OBESITY

Obesity and overweight have been identified as significant health problems for children with meningomyelocele.[475,691,925] In addition to causing stress on a compromised musculoskeletal system, excess weight in late childhood is associated with obesity in adulthood and associated diabetes, hypertension, and early death.[272] As with normal children, obesity adds to a lower self-image and is another reason for rejection by peers as young as 6 years of age.[272,924] Because of the negative impact of obesity, the primary dietary goal should be careful regulation of calorie intake according to regular anthropometric measurements in order to maintain appropriate total body fat stores. Other complications such as UTIs and incontinence can be managed with chemical adjuncts or

MYELODYSPLASIAS AND EXSTROPHIES: SIGNIFICANCE, PREVENTION, AND TREATMENT
 ISBN 0-8089-1816-8

Table 13-1
Acid Ash Diet

Potentially acid or acid ash foods recommended to increase acidity of the urine	
Meat	Bread
Meat, fish, fowl, shellfish	Breads, all types; crackers
Eggs	Macaroni, spaghetti, noodles
Cheese, all types	
Peanut butter	Vegetables
	Corn and lentils
Fat	
Bacon	Fruit
Nuts—brazil, filberts, peanuts, walnuts	Cranberries, plums, prunes
	Dessert
	Cakes and plain cookies
Potentially basic or alkaline-ash foods: Avoid or limit these foods to keep urine acid	
Milk products	Vegetables
Milk, cream, and buttermilk	All types except corn and lentils
Nuts	Fruit
Almonds, chesnuts, coconut	All types except cranberries, prunes, and plums
Neutral foods	
Fats	Starch
Butter or margarine	Arrowroot, corn, tapioca
Cooking fats and oils	
Sweets	
Plain candy	
Sugar and syrup	

surgery. An acid ash diet (Table 13-1) is high in carbohydrates and is, therefore, only acceptable for the treatment of UTIs in lean patients. High-bulk diets (Table 10-1) are also high in carbohydrates, as well as fats, and are, therefore, fattening and produce alkaline urine. Stool bulk can be created by low-calorie, bulk-containing foods such as celery, cucumbers, chards, spinach, pickles, and lettuce, or with proprietary agents. In our experience, these low-calorie, bulk foods are not acceptable to children, so we recommend maintenance of stool bulk with proprietary agents such as Metamucil®, other hydroscopic agents, or processed bran (see Chapter 10).

Obesity is not only common, but it is also more apparent in meningomyelocele children because of hypertrophy of shoulder and neck muscles secondary to musculoskeletal deformity and short stature.[179,424,425,475,691,925,1062] Studies of adults with spinal cord injury reveal a 10–30 percent decrease in basal metabolic rate and basal energy expenditure secondary to diminished lean body mass from loss of paralyzed muscle.[67,102,220,226,820,1119] Unfortunately, similar studies of congenital paraplegia in childhood have not been conducted. One can assume, however, that atrophy of congenitally paralyzed muscle and the resultant decrease in activity cause similar decreases in basal energy needs.

Manenica[691] obtained dietary histories consistent with calorie intakes less than two thirds of Recommended Daily Allowance (RDA) recommendations and reported that less than 5 percent of her series of meningomyelocele patients ate more than 75 percent of Beal's standards[77] for adequate nutritional intake. Despite this low calorie intake, many patients were obese.

Manenica[691] reported that it was necessary to lower calorie intake to 7.0 calories per centimeter of linear length to cause weight loss in some meningomyelocele patients, compared with weight loss with 8.0–12.0 calories per centimeter observed with able-bodied obese children[273] and with the normal child's intake of 15 calories per centimeter of height. Manenica's low-calorie intakes[691] are even more remarkable because of shortened linear length associated with myelodysplasia. Rickard and associates[925] also noted the very low calorie intake necessary to reduce weight with meningomyelocele patients. These studies suggest that the decreased basal metabolic rate due to a decreased lean body mass plus decreased activity put the more severely paralyzed child with meningomyelocele at higher risk for becoming overweight.

In contrast, the obese child with normal musculature develops an increased basal metabolic rate and larger lean body mass with resultant increased basal energy requirements just to move about with the larger weight due to increase of total body fat.[272] Unlike their able-bodied peers, children with meningomyelocele and paralysis are unable to significantly increase their basal metabolic rates because they cannot move about like normally muscled obese children. Overweight meningomyelocele children are, therefore, more at risk for continued weight gain and developing obesity. As a result, between 27 and 90 percent of patients with meningomyelocele are reported as being obese.[179,475,691,925,1062]

Definition of Obesity

The definition of obesity and overweight in the meningomyelocele population in terms of total body fat to lean body mass has not been established. Dietz[272] describes 80 percent of visually detectable overweight normal children as having skin-fold thicknesses greater than or equal to the 95th percentile. He states that measurements greater than 120 percent of the average weight:height ratio and clinical examination should be used by health care providers unfamiliar with the use of skin-fold-thickness calipers as criteria for being overweight. Others have recommended against the sole use of skin-fold thickness as a measure of obesity either because of variable inter- and intrarater results[449,699] or because height:weight ratios are a better index of lean body mass and total body fat in obese patients.[356] Upper arm girth has been rejected as a measure of percentage of body fat by some because of the increase in upper extremity muscle mass secondary to use for body transfers and mobility.[691,699,925,1062] Although weight:height ratios are recommended to screen for obesity in a normal population, they are not of use in meningomyelocele children because of their short stature or decreased linear length due to deformity of the spine and lower extremity joints and decreased bone growth of paralyzed extremities.[179,475,691,925,1062] For these reasons, we[691,1062] and others[179,765] recommend substituting arm span for height, stature, or linear body measurements.

Using Englebach's data,[307] we published graphs and tables that demonstrate linear growth of the arms to be more nearly parallel to normal expected linear body growth (stature) for patient with myelodysplasia; the armspan can therefore be substituted on National Center for Health Statistics (NCHS) percentile charts[452] for height.[179,1062] Use of arm span as a substitute for height can be criticized because of the discrepancy in boys, reported in a recent anthropometric study.[311] Engstrom and associates[311] reported 1568 examinations of 160 patients between the ages of 8 and 15 years measured for stature and arm span. Arm span exceeded stature by 1 ± 1.1 cm for 8-year-old boys and increased in a linear mode to 4.5 ± 1 cm by age 15. Arm span was recorded to exceed stature by -0.7 ± 0.7 cm at age 8 years in girls, rose to 0 at 11.5 years, and exceeded height by 6.8 ± 0.7 cm by age 15.

We studied weight divided by arm span squared times 100, an index reported by Roche and associates[942] to have a higher correlation with total body fat than any other anthropometric measurement (Table 13-2). When arm span was substituted for height in this formula for 825 meningomyelocele patients examined 1814 times, we observed inordinately low estimates of fat, particularly for older children. We considered the lower-than-expected weight:arm span$^2 \times 100$ ratios, the lower-than-expected weight:arm span ratios on the NCHS charts, the information about decrease in lean body mass noted above, and the differences in arm-span-to-linear-length ratio reported by Engstrom and associations[311]; these combined considerations led us to substitute .9 arm span for patients without any leg muscle mass (high-lumbar and thoracic levels), .95 arm span for those with partial loss of leg muscle mass (mid- and

Table 13-2
Correlation Between Selected Anthropometric Variables and Total Body Fat

	Age 6–12.9 Years		Age 13–17.9 Years	
	Boys	Girls	Boys	Girls
Weight:Stature^2	0.90	0.84	0.88	0.89
Triceps SFT	0.81	0.79	0.93	0.86
Subscapular SFT	0.84	0.80	0.94	0.87

Key: SFT, skin-fold thickness[292]; total body fat, percentage of body fat times weight in air. Percentage of body fat is calculated from underwater and air body weight minus residual lung volume.
Adapted from Roche and associates.[292]

low-lumbar levels), and 1.0 arm span for those with minimal or no muscle mass loss in our calculations for expected weight-to-linear-growth ratio. We plotted these corrected arm span measurements as a substitute for height on NCHS graphs (Figs. 13-1 and 13-2) and in calculation of weight:height^2 × 100 (Figs. 13-3 and 13-4). These growth parameters appear to more closely reflect the status of body fat stores when compared with skin-fold thickness and clinical impression, as suggested by Roche and associates[942] as well as Dietz.[272]

We recommend, therefore, following each meningomyelocele patient with serial measurements of subscapular skin-fold thickness, linear length measured along the axis of long bones to take into consideration hip and knee joint contractures, arm span measured with a spanner,[691] and weight recorded on a platform scale with patients in their wheelchairs or with their ambulatory aids. The weight of wheelchair and other ambulatory aids is then subtracted.[925] Observations should be plotted on NCHS graphs[452] with arm span corrected by 0.9, 0.95, and 1.0 for severity of each of the three paralysis groups. The relative differences between corrected arm span, weight, and height for the most severely paralyzed group of girls and boys can be appreciated from Figures 13-1 and 13-2.

Subscapular skin thickness is the best choice because extreme use of the upper extremities distorts the triceps skin-fold thickness measurement, and suprapelvic and lower extremity skin and subcutaneous tissues are affected by paralysis, particularly in the higher level lesion patients.[691] Skin-fold-thickness measurements in patients with myelodysplasia alone give too high a suspicion of obesity. Until adequate measures of lean body weight and total body fat of variously paralyzed children are established, we believe weight-to-linear-length ratios using corrected arm span to be a better measure of body fat stores than calculations using uncorrected arm span, linear length, or subscapular skin-fold thickness alone.

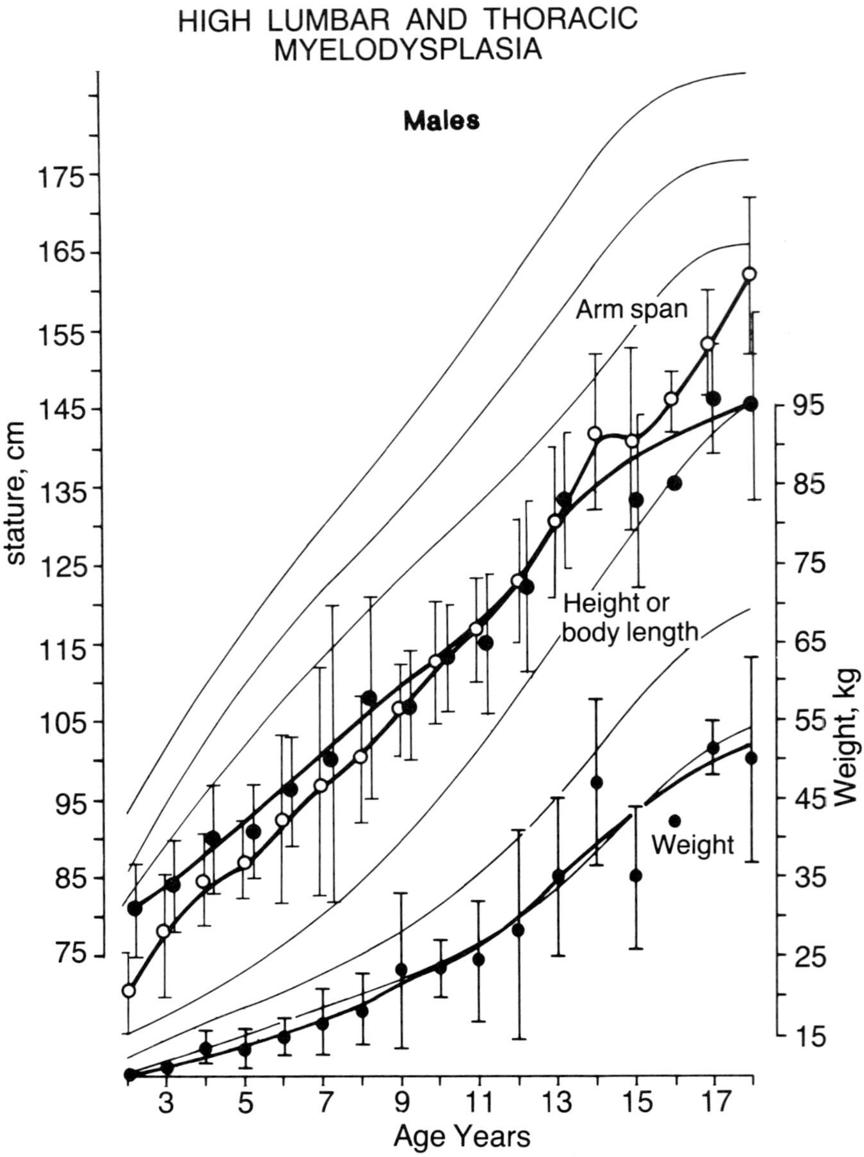

Figure 13-1. Mean height, weight, and arm span graphs for male patients with thoracic- and high-lumbar-level lesions.[452] One hundred and twenty-two weight, 137 arm span, and 121 linear length (height) measurements are plotted on National Center for Health Statistics charts. Arm span measurements have been multiplied by 0.9 to compensate for the decrease in lean body mass and the variation between arm span and linear length, noted in the text. Linear length was measured crown to hip, hip to knee, and knee to heel plantar surface for patients with hip or knee contractures. All data are actual means except for the weight for 3-year-old children, which is an average between 2 and 4 years calculated because one of the 3-year-olds had an outlying, excessive weight that could not be explained but was not thought to be accurate.

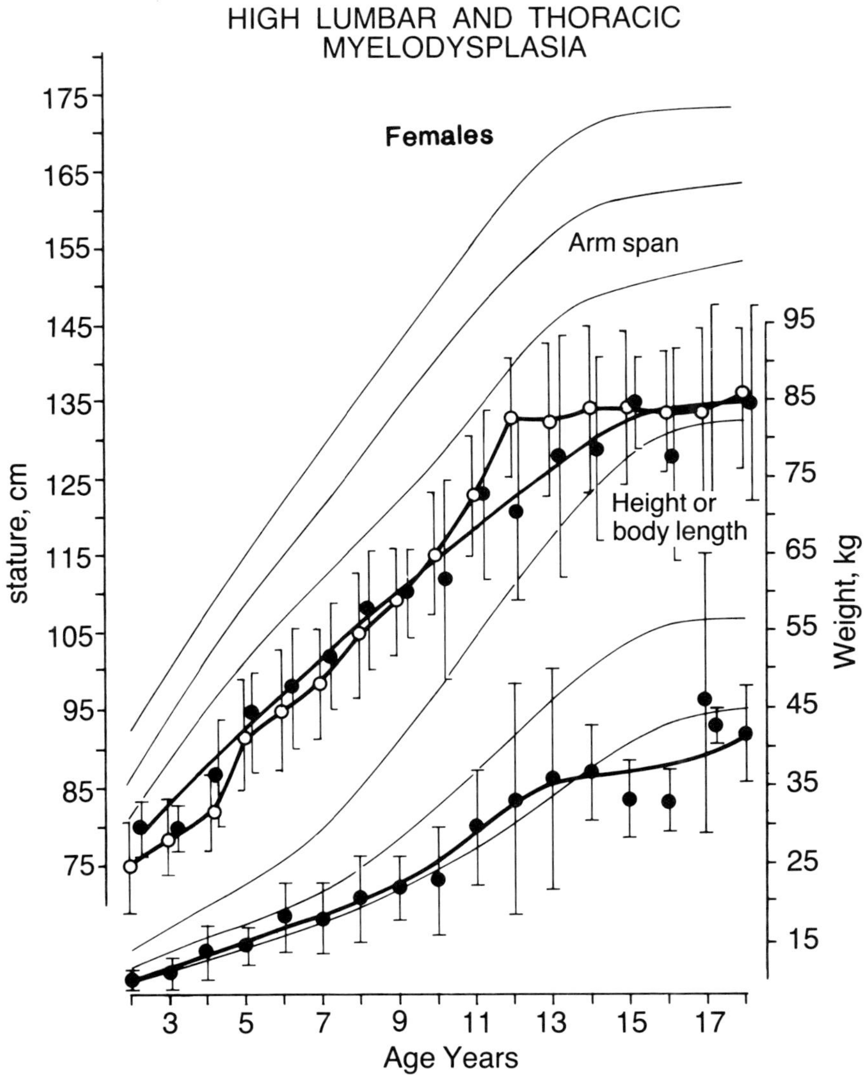

Figure 13-2. Mean height, weight, and arm span graphs for female patients with thoracic- and high-lumbar-level lesions. One hundred and forty-four weight, 159 arm span, and 142 linear length measurements were obtained and plotted, as in Figure 13-1. The weight for 17-year-olds is an average of the 16- and 18-year-olds for the same reason as for 3-year-old males in Figure 13-1.

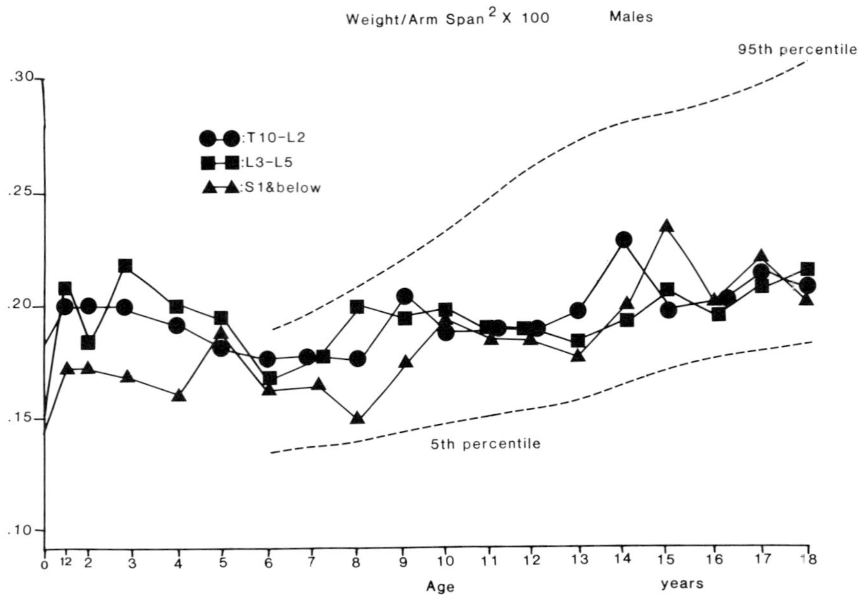

Figure 13-3. Weight: arm span^2 × 100 for males. The mean weight: arm span^2 × 100 index for 1489 measurements was obtained from 432 males born with myelodsplasia. Arm span was multiplied by 0.9 for thoracic and high-lumbar (T10-L2), 0.95 for low-lumbar (L3-5), and 1.0 for sacral-level patients (S1 and below). This index is the best reflection of total body fat.[942] Fifth and 95th percentiles are for normal children, as reported by Roche and associates[942] for ages 6 to 18 years of age. Normative data for below age 6 years do not exist.

Dietary Management: Prevention of Obesity

We begin discussions of decreased energy and, therefore, calorie requirements with parents of infants paralyzed due to any type of myelodysplasia soon after birth (Fig. 13-5). These discussions are continued and eventually include the child. Because of the high rate of obesity among the children of obese parents,[139,272,943] we especially emphasize weight control with such families. Although obesity in normal young children does not result in morbidity,[272] in their paralyzed peers it may contribute to formation of decubiti in insensitive skin, osteoarthritis in neuropathic lower extremity joints, and added stress on upper extremities. We advise a 20 percent reduction in calculated calorie needs for severely paralyzed infants and 10–15 percent for moderately paralyzed infants, based on the calorie need per kilogram of body weight.[699,1119] We warn parents about the tendency for parents to encourage eating[139] and for children[691] to overfeed as compensation for the impairment; we also

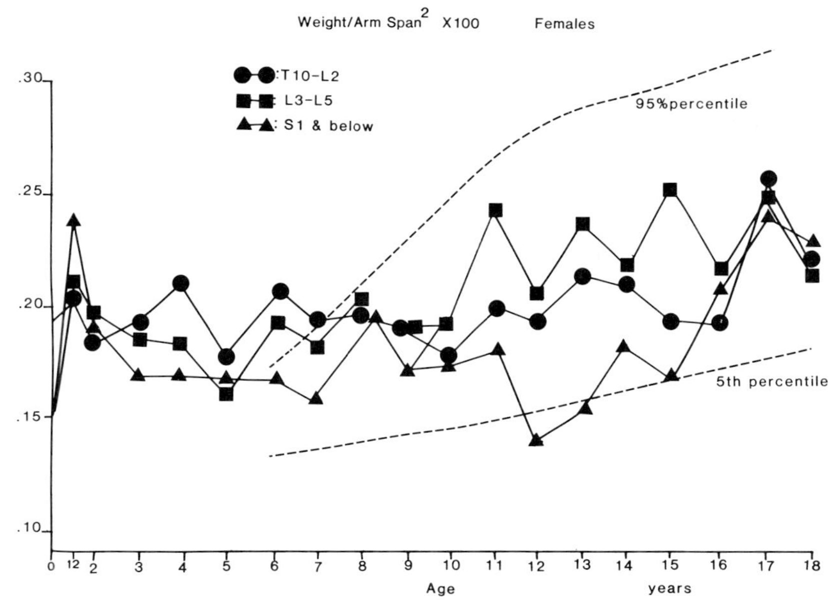

Figure 13-4. Weight : arm span^2 × 100 for females. The weight : arm span^2 × 100 index for 1353 measurements was obtained from 393 females born with myelodysplasia. Calculations and plots are the same as in Figure 13-3.

inform patients and parents that obesity is a defect less tolerated by peers than the impairment itself.[272,924]

Although close monitoring and preventive counsel is the most appropriate objective, we, like others, are not always successful. The main reason for failure is family noncompliance. Another is school lunch programs that offer school children calorie intakes of 1000–1200 calories. One morbidly obese child in our clinic continued to gain despite family compliance. Investigation into the school program revealed the 9-year-old boy was *required* to eat 1200-calorie lunches despite physician orders to the school to restrict his *total* daily intake to 800 calories in cooperation with the family.

Dietary Management: Weight Reduction

Mild to moderate degrees of overweight can be managed by reduction in total calorie intake, as discussed earlier, with elimination of confections and fatty or fried foods.[272] Luncheon meats should be replaced by lean meat and fish (but not halibut, salmon, or shellfish). Milk should be either nonfat or 2 percent butterfat. Gastric fullness and

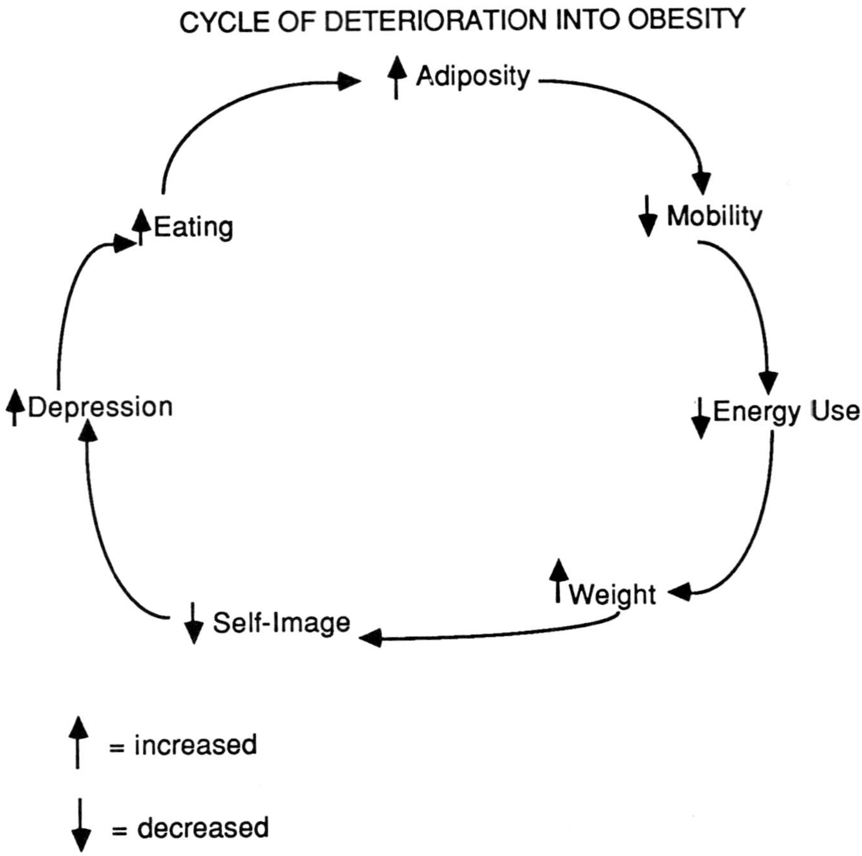

Figure 13-5. Cycle of deterioration into obesity.

resultant satiation can be achieved with satisfying amounts of low-calorie, bulk-containing foods or proprietary agents. More severe degrees of obesity should be managed by a sharp reduction in calorie intake to 500–1000 calories per day (20–25 Kcal/kg/day).[424,425,925]

If corrected arm span measurements are used either in place of linear length or for estimates of ideal body weight to calculate dietary intake, body weight should be further reduced by 20 percent for L2 and higher, by 10 percent for mid- and low-lumbar, and 0 percent for sacral-level lesion patients.[67] Decreased lean body mass with resultant decrease in energy use due to muscle paralysis accounts for the lower estimation.[699,1119] Alternative calculations for weight reduction include 7 calories per centimeter of linear length[425] and should be based on corrected arm span. These calculations will derive 500–1000 calorie per day diets that are, essentially, protein with minimal amounts of carbohydrate and fat. Regardless of the method for selecting a weight-reduction diet, intake should be lowered until urine ketone becomes positive and then maintained for 1 month. Calorie intake should be then increased by 100 calories a day until ketosis is eliminated.

Other nutrients may be absent in such low-calorie diets and, therefore, should be replaced.[272] Dietz[272] recommends daily supplements of 800 g of calcium, 25 mg of potassium chloride, and water-soluble multiple vitamins with minerals along with liberal amounts of sodium chloride in bullion to avoid symptoms of nausea and weakness. The minimum protein intake should be 1.0 g/kg/day. Diets so low in calories are, essentially, the same as liquid-protein weight-reduction diets, which have been associated with arrythmias, sleep apnea, malaise, nausea, and orthostatic hypotension. Rarely, deaths have occurred, but not with medical supervision.[272] To protect against reduction in body protein stores, monthly determinations of lymphocyte count, transferrin, serum albumin, and C3 are recommended by Dietz[272]; determinations of thyroxine-bound prealbumin, retinol-binding protein, and hemoglobin have been recommended by Barton.[67] Electrolyte and mineral disturbances should be monitored by monthly calcium phosphorus and magnesium testing[272] as well as tests for zinc and serum iron.[67] Vitamins K and A should also be monitored monthly if the patient is on a low-fat diet.[67] Water-soluble forms of the usually fat-soluble vitamins may need to be prescribed.

Although no studies have been conducted to measure the effectiveness of exercise in weight reduction programs, we encourage participation in every form of sport and physical activity, including bowling, calisthenics, wheelchair sports, and swimming. Participation in training and competition increases energy use; however, the social diversion of, and motivation in, doing something other than watching and eating are probably more important than the actual energy expenditure.[272] We have observed individual patients become involved in athletic competition with subsequent weight reduction in order to maintain conditioning.

SPECIAL DIETARY PROBLEMS

Dysphagia

Bulbar palsy, a complication of the Arnold-Chiari malformation associated with meningomyelocele, can cause failure to thrive, aspiration, pneumonia, laryngeal stridor, and apnea and cardiac arrest.[342,497,563,646,851] Infants with this problem can have pharyngonasal incompetence with paralysis of the soft palate and laryngopharyngeal dysmobility as well as abductor vocal cord paralysis. Some have gastroesophageal reflux. Any combination of pareses can occur. Recurrent apnea and cardiac arrest or bradycardia can be due to seizure, central nuclei failure, hypoxia, or vagovagal reflex. Aspiration pneumonitis is common. Energy requirements can be increased secondary to respiratory effort and pulmonary infection.

Management includes feeding semisoft solids rather than liquids and, if respiratory distress is too great from abductor vocal cord paralysis, a tracheotomy. Dysphagia may require a gastrotomy and a gastroesophageal plication if reflux presents a problem.[553] With paralysis so severe as to warrant these procedures, we have witnessed only a 40 percent survival rate. Those who have survived have resolved their paralyses and have been deintubated with closure of the gastrostomy and tracheostomy and return to oral feedings. Recently, with severe laryngopharyngeal incompetency in two cases, we have resorted to separation of the larynx from the trachea to prevent aspiration. These two infants are thriving on gastrostomy feedings, and after a few months the paralysis is resolving. We have witnessed the same variability in improvement with other patients with bulbar palsies subjected to posterior fossa decompression (see Chapter 7).

Decubiti

As will be discussed in more detail in Chapter 14, large decubiti are similar to burns as a source of both increased protein loss and increased energy use due to infection.[67,1215] Patients with decubiti may need, therefore, an increase in protein and calories. Vitamins A, C, and K as well as zinc and copper have also been implicated as necessary in increased quantities during wound healing.[67,1215] Parameters of protein body stores as well as direct measurement of the noted vitamins and minerals should be monitored.

Constipation

Dietary management of the neurogenically impaired anus and rectum is covered in Chapter 10 and previously in this chapter. High-fiber diets increase bulk (Table 10-1),[67] but they tend to be alkaline ash, produce an alkaline urine,[1220] and are high in calories. We recommend, therefore, control of stool bulk by chemical adjuncts if the patient has a tendency toward increased body fat stores.

Urinary Tract Infections (UTIs)

Diets to maintain acid urine have been recommended (Table 13-1).[67,656,925] Others doubt their effect.[1126] Baker[60] has suggested an increased need for vitamin C with stress. We recommend maintenance of a urine pH below 6 by chemical means to protect the perineal skin from ammioniacal burns (see Chapter 11).

Fractures

Ascorbic acid has been reported to cause an increase in cation wastage, demineralization, and fractures.[1164] McKibbon and Porter[725] have suggested that an increased rate of fractures occurs due to vitamin C deficiency. Repasky and associates,[912] however, recorded elevated ascorbate levels in meningomyelocele patients and no relationship with frequency of fractures. Low-calorie diets with minimal amounts of fat can inhibit vitamin D absorption; since this vitamin assists in absorption of calcium and decreases osteoporosis and fractures, it should be given as a supplement with water-soluble vitamins and calcium supplements, as suggested above.[272]

Medications

Trimethoprim and Sulfamethoxazole can cause a decrease in folic acid and vitamin K. Metamucil® can cause steatorrhea and social problems due to flatulence associated with neurogenic incompetence. Metamucil® can also lower serum cholesterol. Docusate sodium can cause idiosyncratic diarrhea. Although these drugs and diet interactions are unusual, they should be borne in mind by the prescribing physician.

SUMMARY

Obesity and overweight are acquired handicaps common to the paralyzed child and can be prevented. No good data exist for estimating appropriate lean body or total body mass for children of different ages and with different levels of paralysis. Application of data derived from spinal cord–injured adults and from dietary and anthropometric studies of congenitally paralyzed and normal children and adults suggest that decreased lean body mass is associated with decreased caloric needs and a tendency toward overweight and obesity. Simple substitution of 0.9, 0.95, and 1.0 of arm span for height with high, intermediate, and minimally paralyzed children will allow a fairly accurate estimate of linear-length-to-weight ratios, of the total-body-fat-to-weight divided by corrected arm span squared times 100 formula, and of the height on normal height and weight charts. When combined with subscapular skin-fold-thickness testing, these measurements offer the best estimates of body fat stores. Guided by corrected arm span measures, preventive and severely restricted therapeutic diets can be calculated. The remarkably low energy requirements of paralyzed children require amazingly low calorie intake to achieve weight loss and even to prevent weight gain. For weight loss, we recommend reduction in calorie intake to the extent that urinary ketones are produced. Supplementary vitamins and minerals should be prescribed. Body vitamins, minerals, and protein stores should be monitored, and, in the presence of deficiency, infection, or decubiti, intake may need to be increased. Dietary and medication interactions need to be monitored, and stool consistency and urine infection need to be regulated by chemical adjuncts rather than diet when the patient has a tendency to be overweight or obese.

David Shurtleff

14

Decubitus Formation and Skin Breakdown

Decubitus formation and skin breakdown present only partially solved challenges for prevention and treatment. Decubiti and other types of skin breakdown are common, involving 85–95 percent of patients by the age of young adulthood (Fig. 14-1). Okamoto and associates[823] report skin breakdown observed on 468 occasions during 2116 examinations of 524 patients with myelodysplasia. Pressure decubiti in the perineum and skin breakdown over the gibbus are more common in high-lumbar (62 percent) and thoracic-level (82 percent) than in lower level lesion patients (50–53 percent; $p = 0.03$). Skin breakdown over the lower extremities was equally common in all groups (30–46 percent; $p = 0.16$). It occurred more frequently in patients in the lower level lesion groups who never had perineal decubiti; thus, the total proportion of patients with at least one skin breakdown in these groups was the same as patients with higher level lesions (Fig. 14-1). From age 1 to 20 years, however, only 20–25 percent of patients had skin breakdown at any one time.[823] This prevalence suggests that once most patients develop skin breakdown, they become careful and avoid recurrences. In our clinical experience, few patients developed recurring skin breakdowns.

Breakdown occurred due to excessive pressure (42 percent), a cast or orthotic device (23 percent), urine and stool soiling (23 percent), friction from unguarded activity (10 percent), burns (1 percent), or other, unrecorded factors (1 percent). Other causes of skin breakdown noted in

MYELODYSPLASIAS AND EXSTROPHIES: SIGNIFICANCE, PREVENTION, AND TREATMENT
 ISBN 0-8089-1816-8

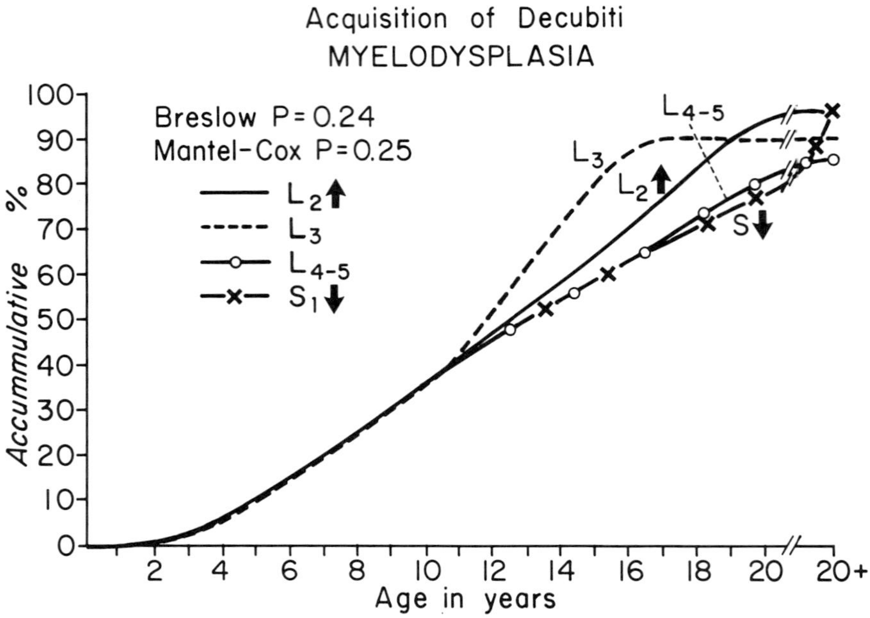

Figure 14-1. Acquisition of decubiti by patients with myelodysplasia. This shows the percentage of accumulation by patients at risk per year of skin breakdown over the back (gibbus), perineum, or lower extremities. Data are from 2116 annual examinations of 524 patients. The curves are adapted from Okamoto and associates.[823]

spinal cord–injured and meningomyelocele patients include obesity, poor sensation, poor vasomotor control with venous stasis, poor blood perfusion, thin tissues over bony prominences postoperatively, and an excessive proportion of weightbearing over pelvic parts with kyphosis (sacrum), scoliosis and pelvic tilt (ischial tuberosities), and lordosis (pubis).[a]

Both decubiti and superficial skin breakdowns are related to age. Young children not yet toilet trained have the largest problem with ammoniacal burns of the perineum, as discussed in Chapter 9. Modern methods of urine collection, including clean intermittent catheterization (CIC), should reduce perineal breakdown. However, an analysis of the rate of acquisition of perineal skin breakdown for 401 of our patients born in 1973 or earlier and 268 born later shows no difference in rates of acquisition of decubiti before and after the introduction of CIC (p = 0.45093; generalized Kruskal-Wallis analysis). The young, active child

[a] See references 242a, 268, 289, 328, 429, 472, 587, 601, 748, 823, 1018, 1076, 1195.

with sufficient motor power is at highest risk for acquiring friction burns of the knees and feet, hot water scalds, and pressure sores under leg casts and braces. Despite our surveillance and prevention methods mentioned below, the same groups of 401 patients born 1973 and earlier and of 268 born later have similar rates of friction burn acquisition ($p = 0.09$).

Older patients, adolescents and young adults, develop lower extremity and perineal skin breakdown from pressure, asymmetric weight distribution, poor blood supply, and abrasion against wheelchair foot rests and orthotic devices. A number of recent improvements mentioned below would appear to have reduced perineal decubiti by 50 percent, but lower extremity skin breakdown rates are unchanged from the rates reported by Okamoto and associates.[823]

The prevalence data reported by Okamoto and associates[823] appear to prevail, perhaps due to the skin insensitivity and poor circulation caused by interference with vasomotor tone.[1196] Lamid and El Ghatit[604] studied spinal-injured patients and noted an increase in decubiti formation among heavy cigarette smokers. Pressure studies in normal pigs suggest that skin and subcutaneous tissues are capable of sustaining 800 mm Hg for 8 hours or 200 mm Hg for 15 hours without breakdown,[242a] considerably more pressure for a much longer time period than expected. Similar studies on humans are not available. Clinical experience, however, suggests that vasomotor and sensory changes associated with interruptions of spinal cord function predispose skin and subcutaneous tissue to breakdown.

Most patients—once they have experienced prolonged hospitalization for serious decubiti or infected skin breakdown that has occurred after minimal trauma—learn to take special precautions and either avoid breakdown or treat skin breakdowns at home without medical supervision[292] (see Chapter 20).

PRESSURE DECUBITI

A true pressure decubitus begins as a breakdown of fat to form a sterile abscess in the subcutaneous tissue, usually over a bony prominence and/or over an area of excess, asymmetric weightbearing. This type of decubitus will present as a small furuncle that ruptures to reveal a remarkably extensive abscess with tracks dissecting for 10–15 cm in all directions (Fig. 14-2). During its initial phase, the decubitus can be felt as a firm nodule that becomes progressively larger. Patients and parents can be taught to roll the skin in susceptible areas between thumb and fingers to feel for the first signs of tissue breakdown. At this early stage, simple relief from pressure will allow resolution.

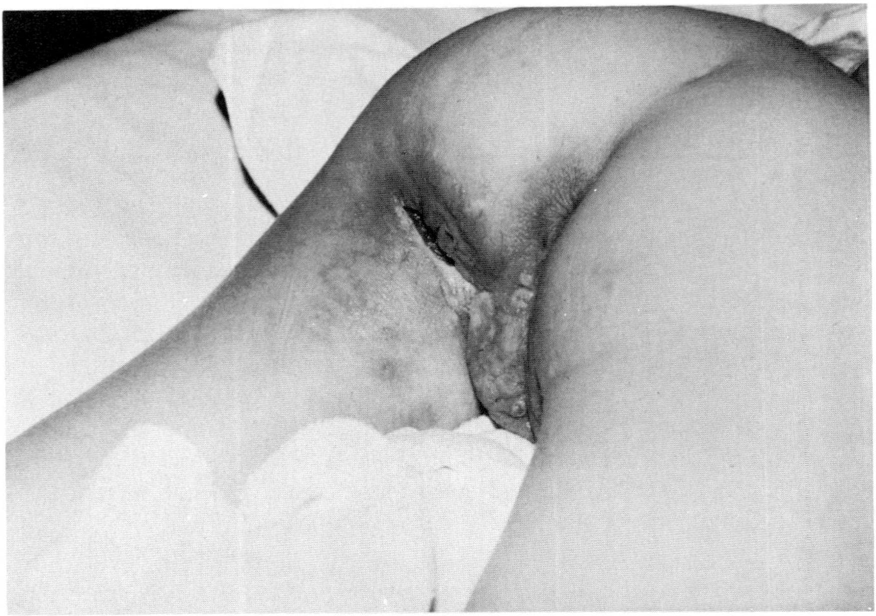

Figure 14-2. Perineal pressure decibitus. This shows the appearance of a pressure decubitus from necrosis of deep tissue subsequent abscess formation, and, ultimately, skin breakdown.

PERINEAL DECUBITI

Skin breakdown in the perineum can be superficial from masceration and ammoniacal burns, or it can be deep tissue breakdown from pressure. Superficial skin breakdowns are shallow ulcers (Fig. 14-3) that are easily distinguished from pressure decubiti. Perineal decubiti are most common during late childhood, adolescence, and adulthood and usually present as subcutaneous tissue breakdown, as described above. They frequently occur after spine stabilization for one of two reasons: (1) The coccyx grows abnormally straight in the presence of severe kyphosis and will act as a spindle protruding through the skin after kyphectomy and correction of the kyphosis. (2) If a scoliotic curve is fused, producing a rigid pelvic obliquity resulting in greater weight on one ischial tuberosity, a decubitus is likely to form. The coccyx should be removed, the protruding ischium reduced, or a Lindseth pelvic osteomy performed to balance the pelvis and distribute weight equally during sitting.[144,242b,651,748,1196]

In order to help prevent such decubiti, we admit patients to our rehabilitation unit after spine fusion. Each individual is measured for a sitting orthosis that will provide an even weight distribution.[289,383] Ideally,

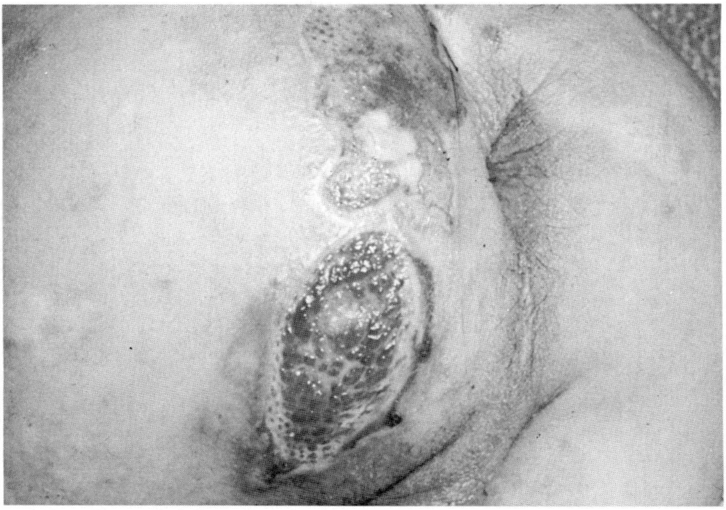

Figure 14-3. Superficial perineal skin breakdown. Superficial skin breakdown over the perineum begins as erythema and edema of the superficial skin and progresses to vesicle or bullous formation. These fluid-filled bullae become quickly infected or are eroded by friction. They then progress to complete destruction of the epithelium, exposing underlying fat. They frequently develop an elevated scarred border.[56]

gel foam or air cell cushions are prescribed in individual designs to prevent perineal decubiti.

TREATMENT OF DECUBITI

Deep dissection of a true decubitus causing destruction of deep soft tissue, hip joints, and osteomyelitis of the pelvis and femur has been described by others,[242b,338,748,1134,1196] and the appearance has been described above (Fig. 14-2). Roentgenograms, sinus tract outlines with water-soluble radiopaque material, and computerized axial tomography helped Firooznia and associates[338] identify four such lesions, as shown in Figure 14-4, among nine patients with perineal true decubiti. Despite aggressive treatment that cured the infection and closed the decubitus successfully, the patient in Figure 14-2 was converted from a brace and crutch community ambulator to wheelchair dependency.

Because of our results with our initial nonsurgical management of decubiti, we have altered our progress. We now recommend surgical closure as soon as the lesion can be prepared. Preparation includes culture

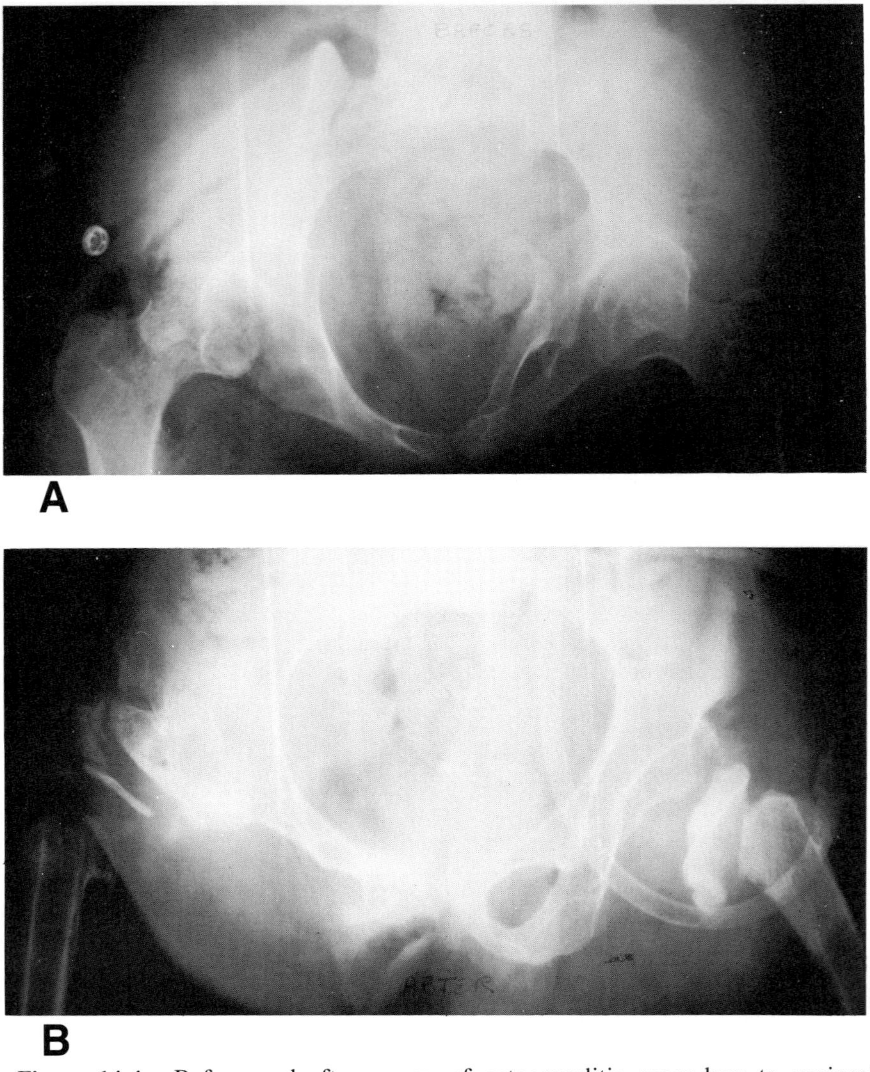

Figure 14-4. Before and after x-rays of osteomyelitis secondary to perineal decubitus. (A) Anterior-posterior film of pelvis of a 19-year-old white male. During final examinations in school, he ignored a perineal decubitus in order to study and maintain a good grade-point average. Shortly after the examinations, he developed severe toxic symptoms and fever. Exploration revealed extensive infection about the hips, osteomyelitis of the pelvis, and extension of the abscess into the pelvis. Following extensive debridement and a prolonged course of antibiotic therapy, the infection was eradicated but he was left unable to ambulate because of the extensive destruction of the pelvis and hip joints. (B) Posttreatment anterior-posterior x-ray of his pelvis.

and initial incision to create drainage. Preoperative detection and treatment of infection; reconstitution of body protein, vitamins C, E, and K, and minerals; extensive dissection to remove all infected tissue; and a bloodless closure are necessary, or breakdown will recur.[242b,338,748,1134,1196] Following prescription of a sitting device, we then prohibit weightbearing on the operative site until 6 weeks of healing. During this 6-week postoperative period, we prescribe a multiple-cell, rotating air-pump mattress with a serial pattern of filling.[242b] Sitting is limited to 30-minute increments, increased by 30 minutes twice a week or when redness disappears in 2–3 minutes after cessation of sitting.

PREVENTIVE SURGERY

A number of different types of neurovascular skin or myocutaneous skin flaps have been reported over bony prominences previously covered by anesthetic skin.[207,268,601,1029] These flaps are recommended to provide sensation and prevent recurrent decubiti. We were unsuccessful in maintaining intact neurovascular bundles over prolonged periods with six patients. They all gradually lost sensation. We have not used muscle-containing flap grafts.[242b] (Types of flaps and grafts for closure of back lesions are discussed in Chapter 6.) Dibbell and associates[268] report successful use of innervated tensor fascia lata grafts to cover excised ischial decubiti with no subsequent breakdown over short periods of time. Daniel and associates,[242a] however, recorded breakdown of muscle at lower pressures and during shorter periods of exposure than for subcutaneous tissue.

FOOT DECUBITI

True decubiti formed on the sole of the feet have been well illustrated and discussed by Menelaus.[748] This type of breakdown first appears as a typical blister that extends. The most common sites are beneath the calcaneus with calcaneal foot deformities, beneath the distal head of the first metatarsal with fixed forefoot pronation, and beneath the distal head of the fifth metatarsal with fixed forefoot supination (Fig. 14-5). The latter two are almost always associated with rigid or semirigid cavus deformity. With a marked rocker bottom foot, hindfoot in equinous, and forefoot in supination, adduction, and dorsiflexion, breakdown can occur over the lateral midfoot.

These plantar foot decubiti are difficult to both prevent and treat. Unfortunately, we are aware of several children and young adults who

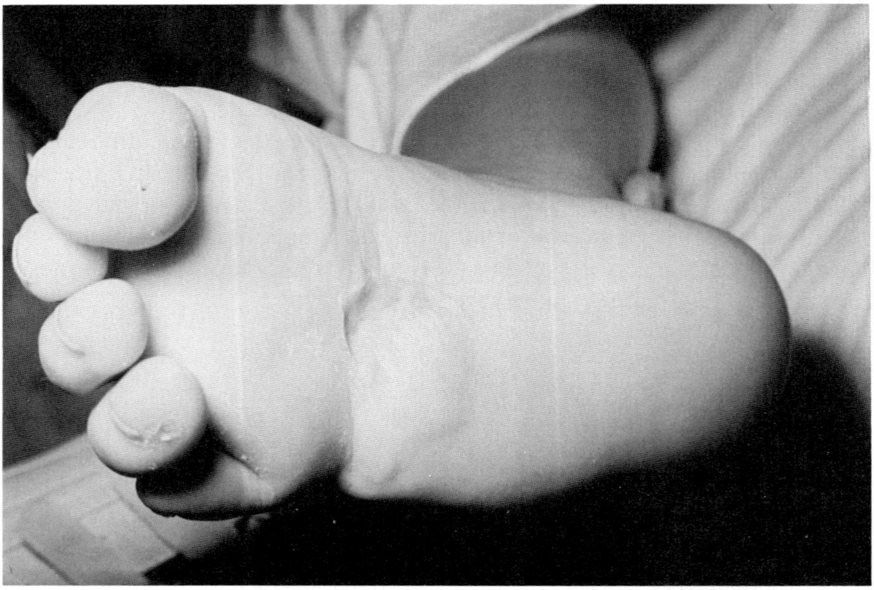

Figure 14-5. Pressure decubitus in the foot. This shows a healed decubitus on the sole of the foot that started as a small ulcer beneath the head of the fifth metatarsal. Orthopedic surgery to realign the foot and construction of a polypropylene shoe insert for more widely distributed weight over the sole of the foot has prevented recurrent breakdown. Although this patient's motor level is S3, the sensory level is L3; a higher sensory than motor loss is a common finding among patients with meningomyelocele.

have been treated by serial surgical procedures, without orthotic management, and have ultimately required amputation. Optimally, the foot should be kept mobile. A shoe insert or an ankle-foot orthosis should be carefully constructed to allow distribution of weight equally along the normal weightbearing surfaces of the foot: the heel, the lateral sole, and each distal metatarsal head.

Healing a decubitus on the sole of the foot has been described as being achieved by release from weightbearing in a walking cast with a window cut around the decubitus, leaving a 1–2-cm margin of healthy tissue.[952] Saucerization of the decubitus with treatment of infection and ongoing wound care is needed. We have had only infrequent success with this method of treatment. Instead, we resect protruding bony parts, dissect the dead tissue, close the wound primarily, and later perform orthopedic procedures to balance the deformed foot, as described by Menelaus.[748]

Postoperative care, as described for perineal decubiti, requires treatment with antibiotics and a 6–8-week healing period followed by cautious and slowly progressive weightbearing in a well-lined silastic or polypropylene orthosis. The most difficult part of treatment is preparation of the orthosis, which should decrease pressure on the breakdown site, redistribute weight evenly on other surfaces of the sole of the foot, and be well padded with a soft resiliant material. We encourage using a thick-soled running shoe with a heel extension to help cushion heel strike and further distribute weight along the entire axis and width of the foot. Another alternative to the form-fitted, silastic, or polypropylene vacuum-prepared foot orthosis is a foam-fitted boot of the type used by skiers.

SKIN BREAKDOWN ON NONWEIGHTBEARING SURFACES

Skin breakdown on a nonweightbearing surface is usually due to a combination of pressure, friction, and abnormal weight alignment. These three factors plus thin, poorly vascularized skin contribute to breakdown of skin over a gibbus. Kyphectomy at birth or later with adequate midline closure of skin prevents such breakdown (see Chapters 6 and 15). We have managed such skin breakdowns with cushions created with a cut-out area to relieve pressure and a polypropylene back shell as part of a back brace or total body garment.

Legs and Knees

Skin breakdown along the legs and knees is frequently due to friction or pressure from a cast or an orthosis. Breakdown is usually superficial and does not need surgery. Offending devices should be removed, and breakdowns should be treated as acute burns. In addition, necrotic material should be removed, culture obtained, and infections treated.[338,1134] We use a sulfur cream and cleansing with 20-minute soaks four times a day. A loose, air-porous bandage should be used when the lesion is not directly exposed to air. With larger lesions, split-thickness or pinch grafts should be applied after a clean granulation base has been established. Braces should be remodeled before being reapplied.

Skin breakdown at the ankle is usually over the malleoli or talus. To prevent both original and recurrent skin breakdown, braces should distribute weight equally along the tibia, fibula, and foot, avoiding pressure on the malleoli. Polypropylene braces have reduced the occurrence of skin problems seen with leather and metal braces. Minor breakdowns are treated as outlined above for similar problems on the leg or knee. Ankle alignment can become so poor, however, that no brace modification can provide a stable weightbearing position and prevent skin breakdown. At that point, realignment of weightbearing by orthopedic procedures is required.[748,976]

Toes

Pressure decubiti of the toes can occur because of hammertoe or claw-toe deformity and because flail toes have been folded under during insertion into a shoe. The former require tendon excisions, ostectomy, or fusion.[748,976] Folded toes can be prevented by extending the tongue of the shoe forward to the level of the toes. The edge of the tongue can be extended by cutting forward from beneath the side flap along the dorsum of the shoe's toe. The laces can be removed, and Velcro straps with *D* rings can be used as replacements (Fig. 14-6). The foot can then be placed flat into the shoe with the tongue completely forward and the side flaps widely open.

Alternatively, rolled moleskin with a flange and five holes cut for the

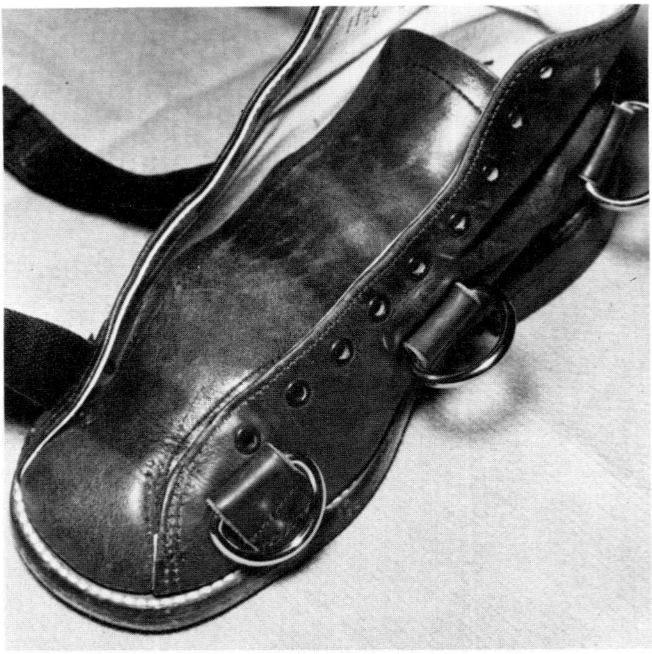

Figure 14-6. Velcro-assisted closure for orthopedic shoe. Removal of difficult-to-loosen laces can lead to incomplete opening of the shoe and folding of the toes. Replacement of the laces with Velcro straps and *D* rings with the smooth side of the grommets on the inner surface will allow easy, complete opening of the shoe. The foot can then be inserted easily with the toes flat.

toes can be prepared and slipped over the toes with a roll underneath the toes to prevent them from curling under. Children wearing ankle-foot orthoses or shoe inserts should have the sole of the foot plate extended to beneath the toes. Compensation for lack of toe extension during gait can be achieved with a curved, thick shoe sole. Toes and feet should be handled as if the patient is an old diabetic. Poor blood supply, dependent edema, and coolness as well as poor air supply render children's feet susceptible to dermatophytosis and other infections. Surgical elastic stockings can improve circulation. Insensitivity and crowding lead to ingrown toenails that should be trimmed frequently. A small piece of cotton tucked under the cover of the nail will prevent bleeding. Parents of and patients with neurogenic feet should be instructed in foot hygiene.

Friction

Both knees and the dorsum of the feet and toes can be burned from friction when patients crawl, creep, or drag their legs across carpets or rough, hard surfaces outdoors. Shoes will frequently slide off flail feet. We encourage using vinyl, artificial leather, or leather patches on the seat, and front surfaces of pants that are long enough to cover the feet. The author learned this simple idea from two adults, one a housewife who used such pants while cleaning her house and the other a sports fisherman at a seaside resort. The former, a woman with meningomyelocele, explained it was too cumbersome to get about the house with her poor balance, braces, and cane in addition to cleaning equipment. She used extra extensions on her vacuum tubing and self-devised extensions on her cleaning utensils to reach up from the floor. The other, a man in need of a full body and leg brace to stand and walk subsequent to recovering from poliomyelitis, explained that, in the fishing village, he felt free from the business-day social requirement to be dressed and upright. With rod and fishing tackle in one hand, he slid along the dock on his leather-reinforced pants, keeping up with his able-bodied peers. In the boat, everyone sat, so he was undetectably different, but comfortably free of his brace.

A combination of contusions and friction burns has produced recurrent deep tissue infection in the patella bursa and knees of two boys with cloacal exstrophy. We have not observed this problem in our other patients with other forms of myelodysplasia. We cannot explain why only these two patients have developed these deep infections. Treatment for friction burns is the same as for the more superficial leg and foot skin breakdowns mentioned above: treatment of secondary infection, removal of necrotic tissues by soaking, air exposure, protection, and, rarely, superficial skin grafting.

Burns

The final skin breakdown problem of patients with anesthetic extremities, burns, is common to able-bodied individuals. Burns occur in insensitive areas at lower temperatures tolerated for longer exposure. These burns can be acquired from floor hot air outlets covered by grids, from automobile hoods, and from covers on motors and heaters in farm machinery cabs. Relatively lower temperatures are tolerated by normal children without producing burns because the discomfort of the heat will cause them to shift their weight. But prolonged sitting without movement by patients with insensitive buttocks can produce second-degree burns.

Tap water scalds are the most common form of burns in these patients and occur on the feet and lower extremities when hot water is added to the bathtub after the patient has transferred into the tub. In addition to proper water temperature checks, the hot water thermostat in all households with children or adults with insensitive skin should be lowered to 120°–140°.[328] A second-degree burn can also be produced over an extensive insensitive area due to an allergic response to fiberglass casts, tape, adhesive solutions, or bandages. Burn treatment is the same as for normal children. Allergic responses should be treated with a corticosteroid added to the antibacterial cream or lotion. The expected healing rate for burns in sensory, vasomotor, and blood supply–impaired extremities will be slow, and there will be a higher incidence of infection. Therefore, partial-thickness skin grafts may be required for smaller lesions, and more careful surveillance and antibiotic treatment may be necessary to prevent secondary infection from extending second-degree to third-degree lesions.

SUMMARY

Modern advances in the care of children with all forms of myelodysplasia have not been associated with a significant reduction in the rate of acquisition of true decubiti and skin breakdown; however, advances in treatment have reduced the frequency of amputation. The patient with insensitive skin and a sitting life-style, orthosis, cast, or asymmetric weightbearing on the sole of the foot should be taught careful surveillance for skin breakdown. Palpation of perineal subcutaneous tissue for the first sign of necrosis is particularly important for the nonambulatory patient. Individualized seats and foot orthoses to improve weight distribution as well as orthopedic procedures to equally distribute weightbearing on pelvic structures and the sole of the foot should be considered for prophylaxis.

Treatment should include presurgical comprehensive evaluation to detect deep tissue and bone involvement. Preoperative and nonoperative treatment of decubiti and other skin breakdown should incorporate all of the following: saucerization, periodic wound debridement, frequent soaking, treatment of infection, and replenishment of protein, vitamin, and mineral stores. Surgical treatment should remove any offending bony prominence, rebalance weight maldistribution, excise all diseased tissue, and provide a covering with good tissue that may include sensation. The covering should be planned with blood supply for future repair in mind. Posthealing management should include surveillance, provision of orthoses to redistribute maldistribution of pressure, protection against friction or burns, and a slow, carefully monitored return to weightbearing and full mobility.

David Shurtleff

15

Mobility

This chapter discusses the relationships among four concerns central to the life of a child with meningomyelocele: (1) functional mobility versus ambulation, (2) the effect of central nervous system (CNS) impairment on mobility, (3) maturation of the impaired musculoskeletal and nervous systems, and (4) development of musculoskeletal complications. We do not emphasize the details of various types of orthopedic operations since a number of texts and articles present evidence for and against specific operative procedures and their indications, goals, and outcomes.[a]

MOBILITY VERSUS AMBULATION

In contrast to the specific skill of biped *ambulation* (or walking), which may require extensive, heavy bracing, effective *mobility* can be viewed as any efficient and effective means of moving about in space that allows the patient to easily go from place to place, explore the environment, grow and develop, and independently pursue an education, vocation, and avocation.[165,238,748,976] Effective mobility includes, therefore, efficient upright ambulation as well as use of wheeled vehicles.

Many authors acknowledge that more severely malformed children with thoracic and high-lumbar meningomyeloceles frequently resort to

[a] See references 143, 144, 165, 238, 595, 748, 749, 786, 976, 1015, and 1141.

MYELODYSPLASIAS AND EXSTROPHIES: SIGNIFICANCE, PREVENTION, AND TREATMENT
 ISBN 0-8089-1816-8

the use of wheelchairs during the second decade of life.[b] Despite this acknowledgement, many of these same authors recommend that most of these children should be taught bipedal ambulation unless they are mentally or severely neurologically impaired. A decision as to the best means for achieving ambulation includes consideration as to the type and timing of surgical procedures as well as the choice of the best orthosis. In addition to various types of short and long leg braces, various authors recommend the following sophisticated ambulatory aids: swivel walker,[748,946] parapodium,[166,780] Verlo I, a platform with a tubular aluminum frame providing body support, (A-frame) or Verlo II (hinged),[1148] stand-up wheelchair,[489] three-point body brace connected to unhinged calipers (another type of solid A-frame),[1127] elastic knee and hip extensors (dynamic orthotic system),[400] A-frame with tubular frame,[166,640,976] reciprocating gait brace,[166,976,1245] and the Rochester variant parapodium.[786]

BODY PHYSIOLOGY

Most of the authors recommending a program that emphasizes upright, bipedal mobility state a number of unvalidated reasons for encouraging their patients to "walk." These reasons include (1) improved body physiology and (2) improved self-image and social interaction. The former can be divided into nine separate issues, the latter into four; all of these issues are discussed below.

Urinary Tract Function

Several authors[166,238,260,748,786,1127] state that the upright stance will improve urinary tract function by providing, through gravity, better drainage. However, no scientific data have been offered to suggest that better urinary tract health occurs in patients who are erect at times rather than totally sedentary. This lack of data may, in part, be due to the formidable problem of separating the effects of standing versus sitting from the effects of neurogenic impairment, degree of obstruction and/or hydronephrosis, type of management, and patient compliance. Asher and Olson[50] found no correlation between ambulatory status and renal function. Furthermore, urinary tract management may even be hindered by ambulation. For example, we have observed that stress incontinence is more frequently a problem for ambulatory patients than for wheelchair patients with similarly affected urinary tracts. In addition, some authors state that braces actually interfere with self-toileting.[143,748,749,1125]

[b] See references 61, 63, 166, 260, 368, 473, 491, 511, 748, 786, 976, and 1125.

Bowel Function

Some authors[166,748,786] have argued that ambulation improves bowel function, also through the effect of increased gravity. However, regular, frequent, and complete emptying of the rectum before a patient with weak anal sphincters exercises and less frequent, but complete, emptying for a patient with a spastic, tight anal sphincter mechanism appears to be more important than whether the patient sits or is erect (see Chapter 10). Whether extensively braced ambulation is an asset or a liability to urine and stool hygiene and health needs to be established, particularly since toileting accidents have been the most socially stigmatizing problem described by our patients (see Chapters 9–12, 20, and 21).[292,1057]

Cardiopulmonary Function

Several authors have described improved cardiopulmonary function for the erect patient when compared with the patient who uses only a wheelchair.[165,595,748,1127] Certainly, thoracic and high-lumbar paralyzed patients expend more energy, but they achieve a much slower maximum pace with braces and crutch-assisted ambulation than equally paralyzed patients in wheelchairs[317,1218]; also, we know of no data to confirm the better cardiopulmonary function of ambulatory patients. Does the active wheelchair athlete involved in racing, field events, basketball, or swimming have better cardiopulmonary status than the passive observer in extensive bracing or a parapodium? The level of everyday activities and energy expenditure is related more to life-style and motivation than to ambulation alone, and this would appear to us to be the significant determinant of cardiopulmonary function.

Osteoporosis and Function

Most authors cite a decrease in lower extremity fractures and osteoporosis as an important physiologic benefit for the weightbearing patient.[166,238,584,595,640,704,786,1127] Others note the increased frequency of postoperative fractures; this factor led us to give up repetitive orthopedic procedures to maintain our patients in a posture suitable for application of the Verlo[1148] or extensive bracing.[327,511,595,749,976] After reviewing the literature and their own experience in 1983, Schafer and Dias[976] reported a higher incidence of leg fractures in thoracic- and high-lumbar-level patients without quadriceps muscle function after spine surgery, removal from a spica cast, and minor trauma. They did not provide data describing the fracture rates for similarly paralyzed ambulatory and nonambulatory peers.

Are fractures less common among those patients in standing or ambulatory programs than among similarly paralyzed sedentary peers? Asher and Olson[50] found no correlation between fractures and the use of wheelchairs. DeSouza and Carroll[260] reported no fractures in seven nonambulators and 38 fractures in 16 ambulators. Our impression is, therefore, that more fractures occur in patients after operative procedures on the lower extremities or during "walking" than in patients who are wheelchair bound and not subjected to operations on the legs.

Lower Limb Deformities

Deformities of the lower extremities, including those following fractures or abnormal bone growth of the femoral neck, lower tibia, or ankle or foot, as well as contractures, are cited as causes for patients to either stop or be unable to achieve useful ambulation.[c] A great proportion of authors writing about orthopedic management of the lower extremities have addressed correcting or preventing these deformities in order to allow patients to ambulate.[165,748] Others[144,260,595,748,976,1141] state that sitting or lying causes flexion contractures of the hip and knee. Dias[265] believes that contractures occur more frequently in the patient who has spasticity and is allowed to sit. He prescribes range-of-motion exercises, a standing orthosis, and night splints to prevent progression of contractures in the child with spasticity.

Our own observations, discussed in detail below, suggest the variability of opinion is due to the development of contractures regardless of level of innervation, age, or type of mobility. A study of patients with meningomyelocele in Seattle and Hawaii revealed no relationship between degree of hip flexion contracture and ambulation.[1241] A more recent study comparing 2583 patient examinations from Melbourne, Australia, and Seattle, Washington, revealed that walking was strongly related to muscle power and program emphasis but not to degree of hip flexion contracture (Fig. 15-1). Even this large number of observations does not answer our question as to the relationship of lower extremity contractures and deformities to ambulation. Nevertheless, growing concern about the effectiveness and complications of orthopedic surgery on the lower extremities has led to a change in emphasis toward operating only for specific indications and minimizing operative procedures in general.[165,166,748,749,976]

The need for limiting operations led Menelaus in 1976 to advocate three principles: (1) select cases carefully to avoid unnecessary surgery; (2) minimize operative procedures by careful timing; and (3) consolidate hip, knee, and foot surgery to one anesthetic and/or one time in a cast.[749]

[c] See references 50, 166, 167, 238, 260, 327, 584, 595, 748, 749, 786, and 976.

Schafer and Dias[976] recommend a minimum time in casts postoperatively and prescribe weightbearing while in leg casts. Several other authors have recommended against surgery to relocate bilaterally dislocated hips because contractures are possible as postoperative complications; also, patients with bilaterally dislocated hips can ambulate almost as well as similarly paralyzed peers with hips in the sockets.[167,260,327,491,511,584,748,953]

Obesity

Obesity or an increase in body weight during the adolescent growth spurt has been given as a cause for ambulatory patients to retreat to wheelchair life-styles.[50,165,260,748] Asher and Olsen[50] pointed out the strong correlation between these two variables. Even they noted, however, that their correlation coefficient was calculated on the weight: linear-length ratio and that this ratio is artificially biased toward obesity by the decreased linear length seen with spine deformity and lower extremity hypoplasia, both known to worsen during adolescence (see below). We recommend that obesity be determined from weight-to-corrected-arm-span ratio and thickness of subscapula fat (see Chapter 13).

Can we attribute the loss of ambulatory ability to obesity? Or is obesity due to an increasingly sedentary life-style? We believe obesity is probably an interactive variable in relationship to wheelchair use; that is, obesity both contributes to, and is worsened by, loss of ambulatory skills. However, a number of our obese patients ambulate, and some of their well-proportioned, similarly paralyzed peers prefer to use wheelchairs. Obesity, addressed in Chapter 13, is primarily a dietary and behavioral issue.

Skin Breakdown

Skin breakdown has not been emphasized as a cause for loss of ambulatory ability. Decubiti have been identified as a direct complication of a sedentary life-style and asymmetric weight distribution.[748,976,1141] Although we agree that perineal decubiti are more common in the patient who is primarily a sitter, Okamoto and associates[823] have documented that lower extremity skin breakdown is common in ambulatory patients due to orthoses and poorly distributed weight on the soles of the feet. We have also witnessed the extension of a skin breakdown over the ischial tuberosity of a patient with long-leg, brace-assisted ambulation lead to a massive abscess formation, destruction of the hips, and loss of the ability to ambulate (Fig. 14-1). Amputation secondary to recurrent breakdown of the sole of the foot has also led to loss of ambulatory ability.[430,1141] The interrelationships between development of perineal decubiti and asym-

A1

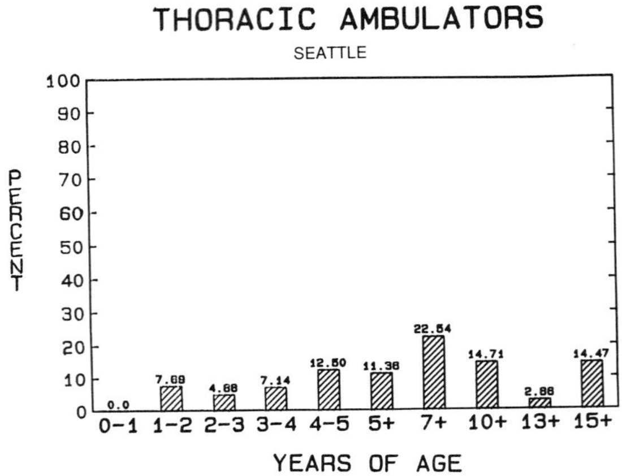
THORACIC AMBULATORS
SEATTLE
PERCENT
100
90
80
70
60
50
40
30
20
10
0
0.0
7.69
4.88
7.14
12.50
11.36
22.54
14.71
2.86
14.47
0-1 1-2 2-3 3-4 4-5 5+ 7+ 10+ 13+ 15+
YEARS OF AGE

B1

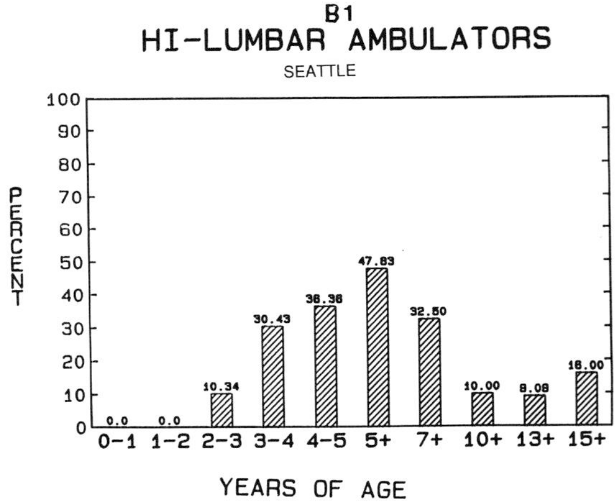
HI-LUMBAR AMBULATORS
SEATTLE
PERCENT
100
90
80
70
60
50
40
30
20
10
0
0.0
0.0
10.34
30.43
36.36
47.83
32.50
10.00
8.08
16.00
0-1 1-2 2-3 3-4 4-5 5+ 7+ 10+ 13+ 15+
YEARS OF AGE

C1

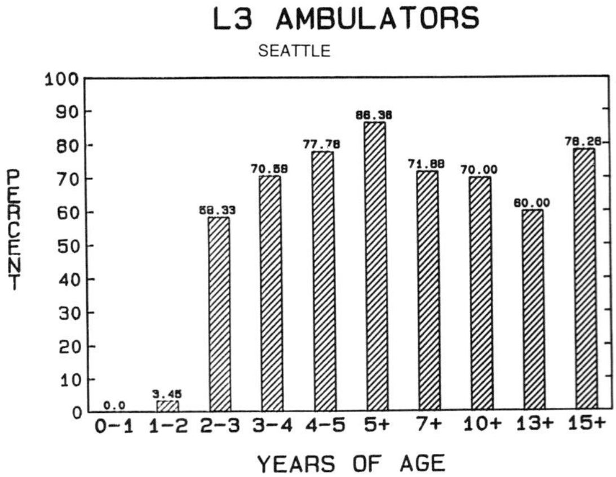
L3 AMBULATORS
SEATTLE
PERCENT
100
90
80
70
60
50
40
30
20
10
0
0.0
3.45
58.33
70.58
77.78
86.36
71.88
70.00
60.00
78.26
0-1 1-2 2-3 3-4 4-5 5+ 7+ 10+ 13+ 15+
YEARS OF AGE

A2
THORACIC AMBULATORS
MELBOURNE

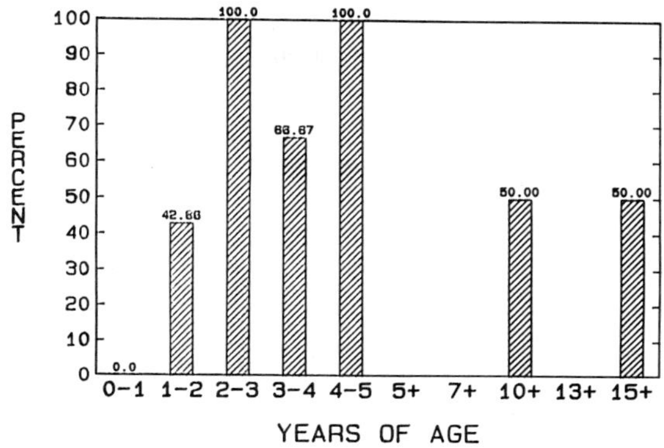

NO DATA RECORDED FOR 13+ PERIOD

B2
HI-LUMBAR AMBULATORS
MELBOURNE

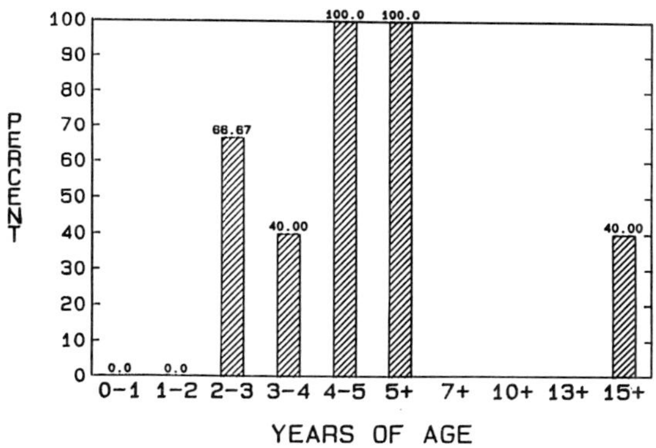

C2
L3 AMBULATORS
MELBOURNE

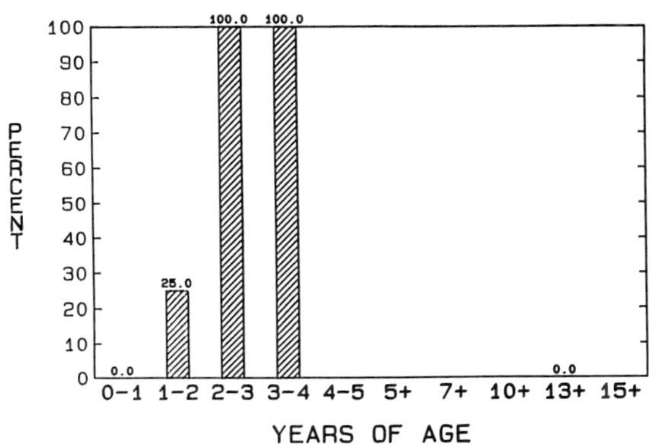

Figure 15-1 *continues*

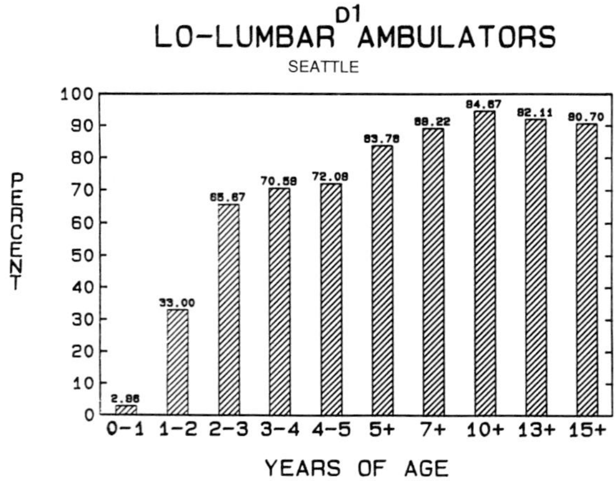

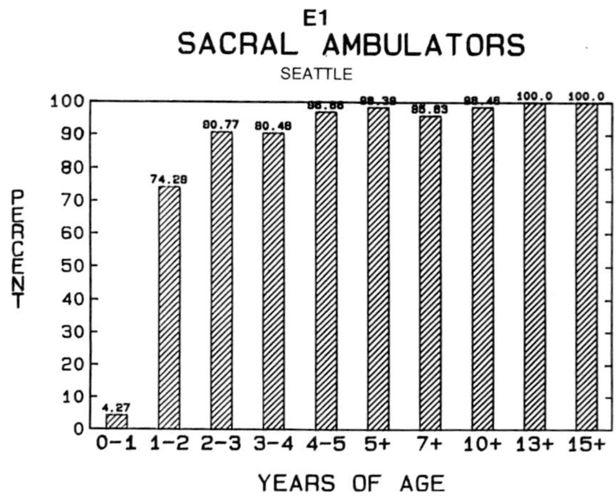

Figure 15-1. Seattle and Melbourne data on walking: muscle power and program emphasis. Five muscle groups from 2,583 Seattle, Washington (1), and 240 Melbourne, Australia (2), examinations of patients were studied. Examinations were recorded not more than once per each patient during any one of the ten time intervals. Ambulators were described as able to get about the home or community using braces and crutches or walkers. Some used wheelchairs for extended mobility or outside the home. Nonwalkers were limited to wheelchair use and standing or demonstration walking at best. (A1 and A2) All patients in these two groups have thoracic level muscle function. (A1) The 491 patient examinations are divided into the following numbers per the ten age groups: 96, 32, 39, 25, 23, 43, 70, 66, 35, 62. (A2) The 41 patient examinations are divided into the following numbers per the ten age groups: 10, 7, 2, 3, 1, 1, 1, 2, 0, 14. (B1 and B2) All patients in these two groups have, in addition, hip adductor and ileopsoas muscle function. (B1) The 287 patient examinations are divided into the following numbers per the ten age groups: 68, 28, 26, 18, 19, 22, 40, 30, 21, 15. (B2) The 29 patient examinations are divided into the following numbers per the ten age groups: 3, 3, 3, 5, 3, 1, 0, 0, 1, 10. The apparent larger percentage of patients over age 5 years in the Melbourne groups with thoracic- and high-lumbar levels (44 percent and 42 percent) compare significantly with the 13 percent and 22 percent

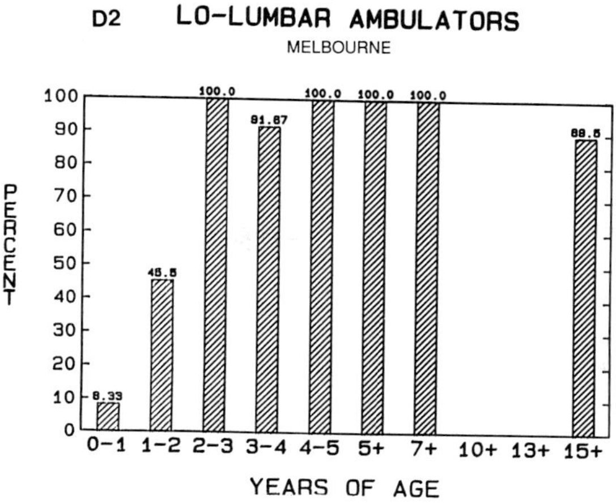

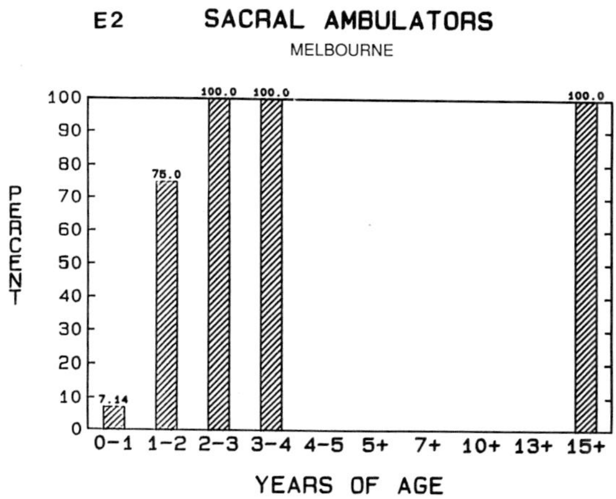

of the Seattle peer groups ($\chi^2 = 24$; df = 2; $p < 0.01$). (C1 and C2) Both groups in this category have hip adductors, ileopsoas, and weak quadriceps muscle function. (C1) The 210 patient examinations are divided into the following numbers per the ten age groups: 41, 25, 9, 10, 9, 22, 32, 20, 19, 23. (C2) The 18 patient examinations are divided into the following numbers per the ten age groups: 3, 4, 3, 7, 0, 0, 0, 0, 1, 0. (D1 and D2) All patients in these two groups have full-strength quadriceps and some have medial hamstring, ileopsoas, anterior tribilias, and gluteus medius muscle function. (D1) The 743 patient examinations are divided into the following numbers per the ten age groups: 145, 89, 57, 56, 42, 73, 101, 75, 38, 67. (D2) The 79 patient examinations are divided into the following numbers per the ten age groups: 24, 11, 10, 12, 1, 1, 1, 0, 0, 19. (E1 and E2) All patients in these groups have more muscle function than the low-lumbar-group D but have some weakness. (E1) The 673 patient examinations are divided into the following numbers per the ten age groups: 136, 54, 52, 37, 32, 62, 96, 65, 27, 51. The apparently larger percentage (80 percent) of Melbourne patients than the (67 percent) Seattle patients who ambulate between 1 and 9 years (7+) of age is not a significant difference ($\chi^2 = 2.8$, df = 1, p, insignificant). (E2) The 73 patient examinations are divided into the following numbers per the ten age numbers per the ten age groups: 28, 16, 13, 5, 0, 0, 0, 0, 0, 11.

metric weightbearing secondary to spinal deformity have not been described, but these factors are common following spinal fusion in our patients. These anecdotal observations, when combined with the frequency of skin breakdown among patients with all levels of paralysis reported by Okamoto and associates,[823] suggest that skin breakdown is another interactive variable that may contribute to, or be due to, a sedentary life-style.

Degenerative Joint Disease

Another physiologic deterioration, degenerative joint disease, has been rarely mentioned[292,748,1064,1141] (see Chapter 21). Lack of proprioception and diminished pain reception combine with a loss of control of the normal heel strike by paralyzed anterior calf muscles to eliminate the cushion effect of the ankle with each step. Rigid ankle braces further eliminate the cushioning effect, producing a jarring impact to the entire leg with each step. This consistent trauma can lead to early degenerative arthritis at the ankles, knees, and hips as well as vertebral disc protrusion. Tachdjian[1141] relates degenerative knee disorders to multiple small fractures, not to neuropathic causes. Regardless of the pathophysiology, these degenerative joint complications can further contribute to the loss of ambulatory ability.

Hand–eye–motor Coordination

The final pathophysiologic condition that may be associated with the ability to ambulate is hand-eye-motor coordination. Some authors[143,165,748,786,1127] state that an upright posture, with hands free for manipulation, improves hand-eye-motor coordination. If so, why doesn't sitting with both hands free lead to the same development? Perhaps only those high-level-lesion children with good hand-eye-motor coordination skills and excellent body control can master upright bipedal ambulation with braces and crutches, reciprocating braces, or parapodiums.[265,704] Wallace[1195] and Menelaus[748] have reported that patients with high-level lesions and upper extremity impairments are less likely to be effective ambulators. To prove that the use of a parapodium or swivel walker improves hand-eye-motor coordination requires documentation of greater improvement than that found in a group with similar impairments documented at the beginning of the study and enrolled in a standard brace-and-crutch or wheelchair program. Poor upper extremity function and body control have been identified as causes for the failure of 35 percent of high-level-lesion patients to ambulate.[266] The relationship of hand-eye-motor coordination to intellectual development is further considered in

Chapters 16 and 17. Because of a lack of information, we can only speculate on the relationships among hand-eye-motor coordination, intellect, and the use of various types of ambulatory aids.

SELF-IMAGE AND SOCIAL ADAPTATION

In addition to the nine pathophysiologic considerations, described above, four social and personality benefits are supposedly derived from upright stance and bipedal ambulation.

Social Interaction

One benefit is the presumably improved social interaction with peers.[143,165,595,748,786,1141] The proponents of this beneficial effect state that a person in a wheelchair is visualized by society as having a crippled mind as well as body. Kopits[595] equates an adult in a wheelchair with a child. As an example, he states a stranger will ask a man standing on a corner for directions, not a person in a wheelchair, implying that the wheelchair-bound person is unknowledgeable as well as confined to a wheelchair. Myers and associates[786] and others[165,595,748] have emphasized the need for children to stand erect in order to interact with their peers at the same eye level. These opinions are not scientifically documented.

Is a sitting position more or less conducive to interaction with peers than braced extremities? As mentioned in Chapter 2, Richardson and associates[924] have demonstrated that abnormal extremities are less acceptable to other children than a child with normal appearing extremities in the sitting position. In addition, as mentioned below and discussed in Chapter 17, individuals in motorized wheelchairs may be better able to keep up with, and thus interact with, their peers (although wheelchair accessibility remains a problem in many schools). Furthermore, most young children interact mainly while sitting during play. Children do not learn to rise from the floor in a parapodium until approximately age 5 years,[786] a definite impairment to multiple-level interaction with their peers during these early years.

While observing a class of children in parapodia in Rochester, the primary author was impressed with the marked agility of two patients and the fearful incompetence of six other children, all with high-level meningomyelocele lesions. The social interactions of the two bright, agile members of the class were in sharp contrast to the other six and probably would have been excellent regardless of their methods of mobility. Their accomplishments and social interactions were similar to those of an outstanding athlete, coach, mother, and business woman who also lives in

Rochester, New York, and uses a wheelchair. A college graduate and businessman and the receptionist for the Governor of the State of Washington are two other agile but similarly paralyzed patients who also function from wheelchairs. The message of these adults to the primary author has been that your self-image, not your method of mobility, is important.

But anecdotes can be found supporting any point of view, and as our society changes to more readily accept the congenitally malformed and provide wheelchair access, we need well-designed, biosocial investigations to answer critical questions about the relationships among social acceptance, personality development, and mobility.

Personality Development

The second most complex interrelationship exists between personality development and mobility. A number of authors quote the need for swift, efficient, and effective mobility to allow children to keep up with their peers and grow and develop normally.[143,165,595,748,786,976] Although some of these authors quote the developmental sequences described by Piaget[866] and Erikson[314] as necessary for personality development, the primary author can find no distinction by any author between effective, alternative methods of mobility and ambulation. A preliminary study by Mazur and associates[704] suggests that patients encouraged to ambulate from infancy may be more independent in skills of daily living than similarly paralyzed peers brought up in wheelchairs. It may be that both parents and children derive beneficial developmental concepts—including improved self-image—even from brief intervals of erect posture each day.[267]

Two studies have documented that children in wheelchairs expend less energy and move quickly to keep up with their nonparalyzed age peers.[317,1218] Other observations from our center demonstrate an outgoing, interactive, and independent attitude developed by very young children provided powered wheelchairs.[150–152] Long-term effects of this experiment are not known, however, and none of these studies have been replicated. Our 10-year study of emphasis on multiple alternative modalities for mobility in place of biped ambulation will be discussed below. Such a concept—multiple modalities for mobility—is not new and is cornerstone of most well-known orthopedic programs for children born with meningomyelocele.[165,748,779,976] Our program has been emphasizing personal worth and acquisition of independent skills for daily living and not encouraging bipedal ambulation except for low-lumbar- and sacral-level patients.

Whether severely paralyzed children should be brought up with upright stance and, if possible, some form of erect mobility remains an unanswered question. What happens to the self-esteem of the older child forced to "retire" to a wheelchair after being brought up in a program that insists he or she must be upright? Does loss of the ability to ambulate cause the adolescent to be depressed? Is the depression associated with the further erosion of teenage self-image the cause for loss of motivation and weight gain? Disabled adults, regardless of the causes for their disabilities, tell us that a good self-image is far more important than the severity of the defect.[292,1057] If we can predict that high-level-lesion patients with meningomyelocele will "retreat" or "resort" to wheelchairs later in childhood,[165,260,491,595,749,976,1125] why should we set them up to fail? Asher and Olsen[50] encourage teaching patients the advantages of wheelchair use as well as the use of braces and crutches. We concur.

Accessibility

A third advantage for the person with ambulatory skills is access to areas inaccessible to people in wheelchairs. Toilet access is an obvious advantage for the disabled person who can ambulate. However, extensive body and leg (hip, knee, ankle, and foot orthosis; HKAFO) braces interfere with undressing, dressing, and therefore, self-toileting.[748] In addition, wheelchair access is less of a problem in some areas of the United States than others because of ranch-style architecture; in crowded cities, on the other hand, apartment buildings and stairs make access more difficult, if not impossible. Access to outdoor recreation on rough ground is also easier in a balloon-tired wheelchair than with braces and crutches or a parapodium.

Do the advantages of brace-and-crutch ambulation exceed those of wheelchair use? With our changing social attitudes toward the disabled and with improvements in orthotics and wheeled vehicles, we need constant reevaluation of the individual patients and their family needs. Access, whether by brace and crutch, parapodium, or wheelchair, is directly dependent on the environment surrounding each individual patient.[61]

Simulation of Normal Development

Our fourth and final concern about adhering to a schedule simulating normal development for bipedal ambulation has been alluded to several times: Are we actually interfering with optimal growth and development by performing surgery and involving a severely paralyzed child in an upright bipedal ambulation program? Are we operating on contractures and deformities that will either spontaneously ameliorate or recur regardless of interventions? For example, some authors recommend hip surgery to correct contractures as early as 10–18 months of age,[143,165,595,976,1014,1016,1141] at a time when our data reveals that contractures are resolving and the accuracy of motor power about the hip is questionable, as further discussed in the third and fourth sections of this chapter. Bunch[143] also alludes to the possibility that orthopedic management may interfere with growth and development and recommends minimizing orthopedic procedures and hospitalization. Menelaus[749] speaks directly to this issue, as described earlier.

In the late 1950s and 1960s, we believed in approximation of the normal sequences for standing and ambulation. The girl depicted as our "star" in various standing devices in our original publication is now a happy, well-adjusted nursing student in a wheelchair full time.[1049] The other "star," depicted in extensive braces, learned to ambulate 100 feet by age 18 years after 23 operative procedures. After achieving a 100-foot "walk," she handed the primary author her crutches and stated she would henceforth use only her wheelchair. Standing in extensive braces has been reported by Dias as a beneficial temporary experience for approximately 65 percent of high-level-lesion young children.[265] Because of many instances of failure and our discouragement with the Verlo standing devices,[1148] we have since altered our program to emphasize factors necessary for achieving independence. These daily living skills are discussed in Chapters 9–12 and 17.

Our studies were expanded to include the ages of first achievement of mobility according to degrees of motor paralysis. The remainder of this chapter will discuss preliminary studies that we hope will lead to a better understanding of effective mobility.

THE EFFECT OF CNS IMPAIRMENT ON THE DEVELOPMENT OF MOBILITY AS REFLECTED IN STUDIES OF GROSS MOTOR SKILLS

Significant delays in gross motor development can be observed prior to sitting and standing among children with meningomyelocele, even those with low-level lesions. Delays in learning gross motor activities were documented in a study conducted primarily by Sousa and associates and partially published.[823,1095] Two hundred patients, aged 3 months to 19 years, with IQs of 70 or more, controlled hydrocephalus, and absence of spasticity and other major abnormalities, were studied. An inventory[1095] was distributed to each family. Forty-five categories of gross motor activity, including the use of braces, ambulation aids, and wheelchairs, were assessed at 3-month intervals by direct examination or discussion with the parents via telephone. From these records, the first age at which the child routinely performed a skill was recorded. In turn, these data were analyzed to determine the age at which 20 percent, 50 percent, and 80 percent of patients performed the task routinely. Criteria were selected from existing assessment tools[26,364,588,1094] (Fig. 15-2). Because of the limited number of patient observations for the large number of variables, patients were grouped according to Sharrard's neuromotor functional classification: group 1 included L2 and above; group 2, L3 and mixed lesions with partial innervation at L2-4; group 3, L4-5; and group 4, S1 and below.[1017]

The delay in acquiring early gross motor skills is more marked among the more severely paralyzed children in groups 1 and 2, but it is also significant for children in group 4 with minimal or no paralysis. This delay has been observed in 35 percent of patients with high-level lesions, and Dias believes that poor control over upper extremity and body tone accounts for why these children cannot learn age-appropriate motor skills.[265] The delay in acquiring independence in motor skills by some patients in each motor group may also be associated with parent and teacher expectations, differences in maturation, and/or other impairments such as stiff joints or lower extremity spasticity.[704] We believe these delays in motor skills may be related to anatomic brain malformations associated with meningomyelocele as well as residua from meningitis or abnormal cerebrospinal fluid (CSF) pressure.

In order to better understand these congenital impairments, Wolf and McLaughlin[1229] studied the manner in which minimally paralyzed children with meningomyelocele have met early motor milestones. Seven children with sacral-level meningomyeloceles were examined at 2-month intervals from age 2 to 12 months of age and again at 15 and 18 months of age. They had difficulty learning head control and sat with rounded spines and shoulders as well as hyperextended necks long after their normal peers. In the prone position, they demonstrate marked neck hyperextension and delayed normal extension along the lumbar and thoracic spine (Fig. 15-3). When reduced to quantitative measures on the Movement Assessment of Infants test (MAI),[176] the ten items for muscle tone were markedly abnormal, indicating hypotonicity. Several patients demonstrated passive resistance to flexion of the shoulder as part of a postural fixation pattern in conjunction with low truncal tone.

Six of the seven children integrated their primitive reflexes by 10 months of age, which is delayed, particularly for palmar grasp. The mean score for acquisition of automatic reactions for meningomyelocele children was markedly below the mean for normal peers. All aspects of head control, trunk equilibrium, and protective responses were acquired late and, when finally developed, were often slow or inconsistent during spontaneous movement.

Low scores on the Motor Scale of the Bayley Scales of Infant Development appeared to reflect poor muscle tone and delay in acquiring automatic reactions. Other areas tested by the Bayley Mental Scale were typically within one standard deviation of the mean.

We believe CNS impairments contribute to the delay in acquiring gross motor skills demonstrated in Figure 15-2. These delays may be related to the impairments that later are measured by hand-eye-motor coordination tests and that interfere with learning (see Chapters 16 and 17). These subtle impairments are in addition to upper extremity, upper motor neuron deficits discussed by Stark[1105] and others.[748,1195] They should be kept in mind—along with obvious deformities of the spine, pelvis, and lower extremities—when designing mobility programs.

MUSCULOSKELETAL DEFORMITIES: FORCES INTERFERING WITH MOBILITY

Little has been documented about the natural history of musculoskeletal deformities that occur secondary to abnormal nervous system function in children with meningomyelocele. Most studies discussing the treatment of or prevention of spine and lower extremity deformities consider the beliefs expressed in the first section of this chapter but do not discuss the CNS impairments that lead to poor motor

---

Figure 15-2. Development of (A) early motor skills and (B) upright motor skills. A study of 200 patients contacted at 2–3-month intervals was done by Sousa and associates.[1095] All lived within the greater Seattle area and were 3 months to 19 years old. The horizontal bars representing the four muscle level groups for each skill are (1) highest have thoracic innervated muscles and high lumbar, ileopsoas, and hip adductors; (2) the second highest have, in addition, weak quadriceps or other scattered but weak muscles about the hip; (3) the next highest bar shows mid- and low-lumbar (L3–5), with quadriceps, medial hamstring, and anterior tibialis functions; and (4) the lowest have more function than the third group but some weakness. The beginning of the solid horizontal bars repreents the age at which the first 20 percent of patients can achieve the given skill; the break in the middle of the bar represents the age at which 50 percent have achieved the skill, and the end of the bar represents 80 percent. Solid bars followed by an asterisk begin with 20 percent and end with 50 percent indicating that 80 percent did not achieve the skill before the last age recorded on the chart. The asterisk lines indicate failure for the group to complete the skill by the age at the end of the chart (e.g., walks holding onto the furniture). Up and down steps includes crawling or sliding. For details of this study, see Sousa and associates.[1095]

A

EARLY MOTOR SKILLS

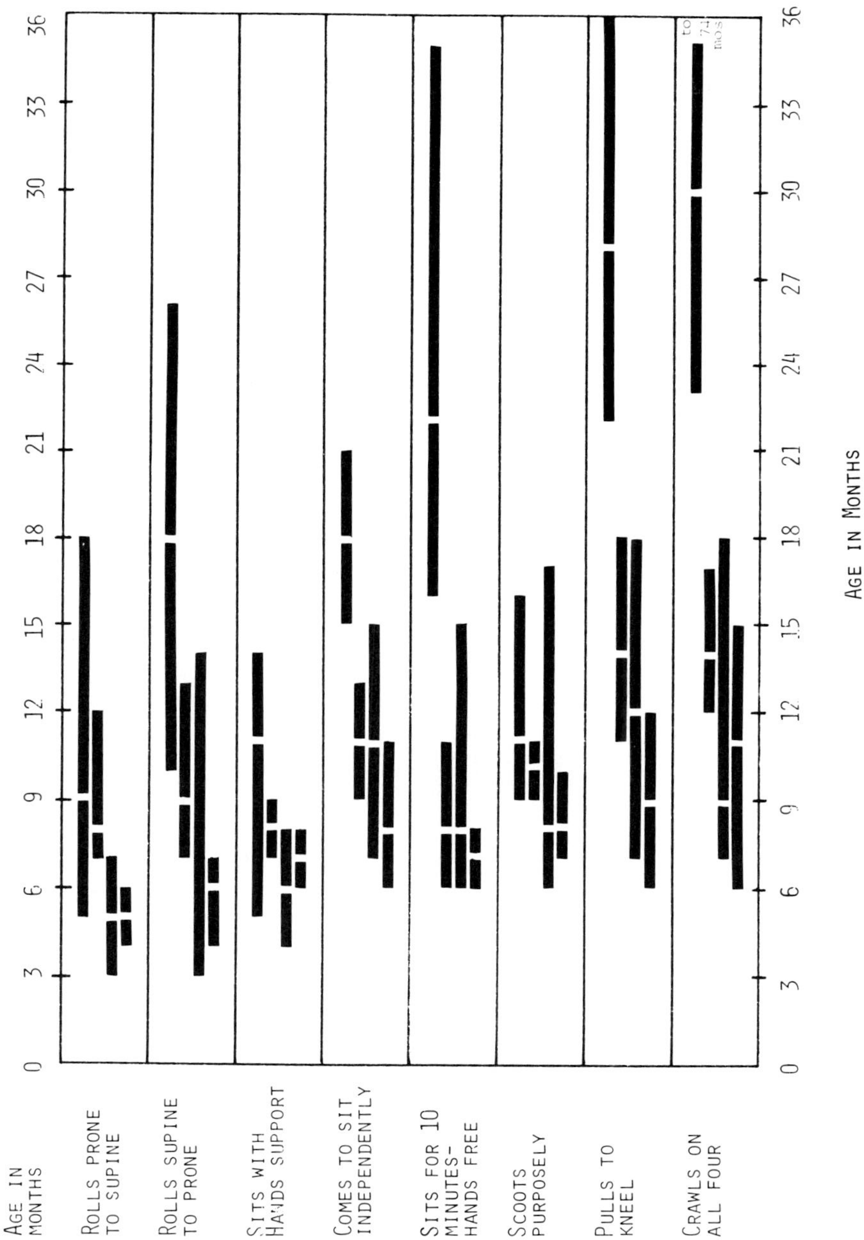

B

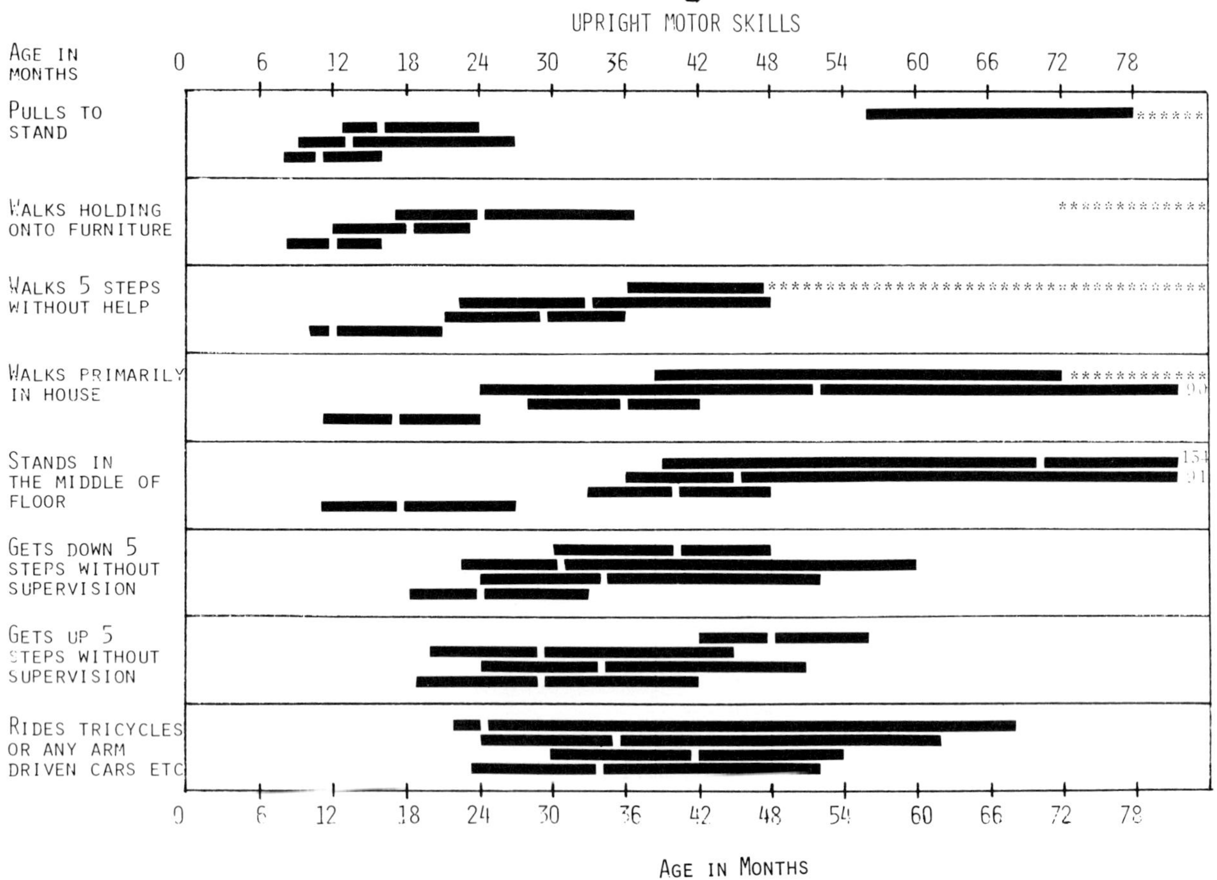
UPRIGHT MOTOR SKILLS
AGE IN MONTHS
0
6
12
18
24
30
36
42
48
54
60
66
72
78
PULLS TO STAND
WALKS HOLDING ONTO FURNITURE
WALKS 5 STEPS WITHOUT HELP
WALKS PRIMARILY IN HOUSE
STANDS IN THE MIDDLE OF FLOOR
GETS DOWN 5 STEPS WITHOUT SUPERVISION
GETS UP 5 STEPS WITHOUT SUPERVISION
RIDES TRICYCLES OR ANY ARM DRIVEN CARS ETC
AGE IN MONTHS

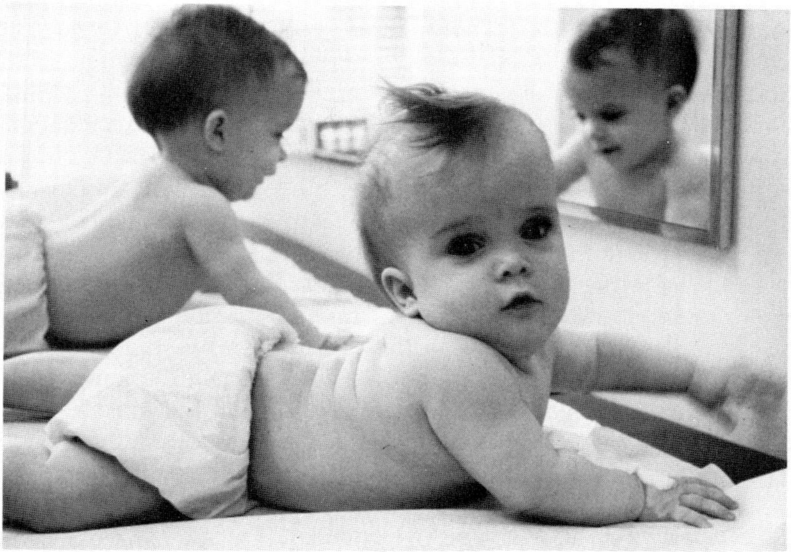

Figure 15-3. Marked neck hyperextension and delayed normal extension along the lumbar and thoracic spine. This photograph shows an 8-month-old infant with lack of proper prone extension. Chest should be clear of mat with back straight. The neck is markedly hyperextended, and the thoracolumbar spine is in marked lordosis. The patient has a sacral-level lesion with weak triceps and good gluteal muscle function. The anatomic site of the lesion is sacral. Hydrocephalus has been well controlled by a cerebrospinal fluid shunt.

control of normally innervated muscles, discussed in the second part of this chapter (see also Chapters 16 and 17). This section will present our observations of musculoskeletal deformities in relation to age according to segmental motor levels.

Functional Motor Levels

Several authors have emphasized that various muscle strengths, which form the basis for the generally accepted motor levels described by Sharrard,[1017] are important to functional outcome.[61,260,511] For example, Huff and Ramsey[511] described the presence of hip abductors as important for the development of an adequate hip socket and gait. DeSousa and Carroll[260] described varying quadriceps and hamstring muscle strengths as important to the development of effective bipedal ambulation. Motor levels have been proposed as criteria for life-and-death decisions by many authors (see Chapter 5). In addition, many use muscle levels to classify their cases into groups for comparison of complications and functional outcome.[50,61,63,165,327,473,491] These authors frequently refer to Sharrard's study[1017] of motor levels in children with meningomyelocele.

The subjective nature of manual muscle testing and the ability of infants and young children to cooperate in certain test movements have led investigators to question the accuracy and predictive value of muscle grading in young age groups. Murdock's study[783] of 95 neonates suggested that the correlation between early muscle strength determined by manual muscle testing and future mobility was poor.

To evaluate the reproducibility of muscle strength evaluations over time, we studied 3084 muscle examinations performed on 825 children with meningomyelocele.[720] 177 of these children with six or more serial exams were studied by calculating the percentages of patients who had examinations at a given age equal to, and within one muscle strength grade of, individual best estimates of ultimate muscle strength. McDonald and associates[720] demonstrated that muscle examinations in infancy, after back closure, precisely predict the median of later examinations after 5 years of age with an accuracy of 54–87 percent (Fig. 15-4A). When plus or minus one grade is used as the criterion rather than a precise prediction of ultimate strength (plus or minus zero grades), accuracy rises to 70–87 percent for various muscles on initial examination in infancy and 87–97 percent after 5 years of age (Fig. 15-4B).

The actual neuromuscular involvement of patients with myelodysplasia may vary from the classic patterns of innervation described by Sharrard[1017]; according to those patterns, an infant has normal function down to a particular level below which there is flaccid paralysis and loss of sensation and reflexes. Stark and Drummond,[1107] as well as Stark alone[1104] and others,[704,1195] have described skip lesions with intact spinal cord segments distal to noninnervated gaps, incomplete lesions with a mixture of spasticity and voluntary level of cord involvement, and lesions resembling complete cord transection. Additional as yet unpublished analyses by McDonald and associates[720] reveal that muscle grade strengths for gluteus medius and medial hamstrings are more highly correlated with hip adductors, ilipsoas, and quadriceps strength than are other muscles previously described as innervated by L4, L5, and sacral roots. Thus, gluteus medius and medial hamstrings may be of functional strength in the presence of weak or absent muscles of the anterior compartment of the lower extremity such as anterior tibialis, which has a lower correlation with hip flexors and adductors. As suggested by DeSousa and Carroll[260] and Huff and Ramsey,[511] further study of exact muscle patterns about the hip is necessary to clarify prediction of ambulation. The differences in the current literature describing ambulation and the effect of treatment, as discussed in the first portion of this chapter, can be explained, at least in part, by the fact that authors have included

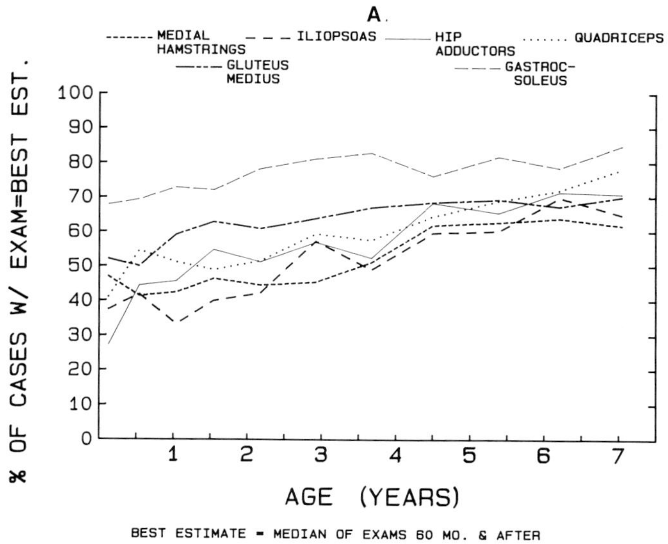

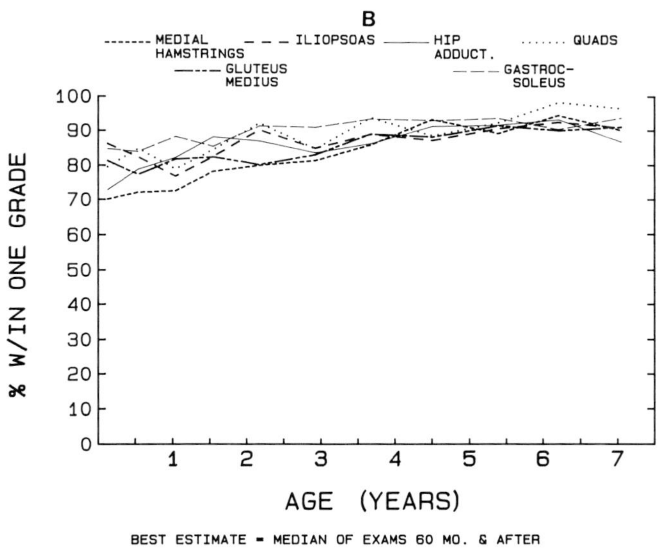

Figure 15-4. Predictive accuracy of initial muscle strength for mean of examinations after 60 months of age. (A) One-hundred-seven patients were examined six or more times. The percentage of patients examined at each age with a muscle test evaluation was based on the rating scale of 0–5, which equalled the median of at least three subsequent examinations performed for each patient after the age of 60 months. All examinations were performed by trained therapists between 1972 and 1984. (B) Plots for agreement of muscle strength examinations similar to part A were used, but accuracy is plus or minus one grade of muscle strength.

Table 15-1
Prediction of Ambulation for Patients With Lumbar Meningomyelocele Lesions

IL 4–5 QD 4–5 MH 4–5 N, 4 3 Comm 1 HH 0 Non		
Il 4–5 QD 4–5 MH less than 3 N, 10 3 Comm 4 HH 3 Non	Il 4–5 QD less than 4 MH less than 3 N, 3 0 Comm 1 HH 2 Non	All less than three quadriceps N, 21 0 Comm 6 HH 15 Non
Il less than 3 QD 4–5 MH less than 3 N, 11 0 Comm 5 HH 6 Non	Il less than 3 QD less than 3 MH 2 or 3 N, 4 0 Comm 2 HH 2 Non	All less than three iliopsoas N, 15 0 Comm 7 HH 8 Non
Il Trans QD 4–5 MH less than 3 N, 19 12 Comm 5 HH 2 Non	Il trans Qd less than 3 MH less than 3 N, 14 0 Comm 3 HH 11 Non	All iliopsoas trans N, 33 12 Comm 8 HH 13 Non
		Separate group: gluteal 2 or 3 Il 4–5 QD 4–5 MH less than 3 N, 20 14 Comm 5 HH 1 Non

patients with gluteus medius function and better ambulatory potential in the same mid-lumbar-level group as patients without abductor power.

Muscle Level and Ambulation

As noted above, most studies emphasize motor power as the single most important determinant of whether patients will be able to ambulate effectively about the house or community. Because of the suggestion that motor power within the segmentally innervated groups described by Sharrard[1017] may affect ambulation,[260,511] Dudgeon and associates[290] have separated our high- and mid-lumbar patients into groups of motor power less than or equal to 3 and greater than or equal to 4 for four major muscles—ileopsoas, quadriceps, medial hamstring, and gluteus medius—and analyzed their relationship to three grades of ambulation: (1) walks about the community, (2) walks only around the household, and (3) is a demonstration ambulator or is nonambulatory. All patients had grade 4 or 5 hip adductor strength. We studied only patients over age 6 with at least two examinations demonstrating consistent muscle strength. The mean data in Table 15-1 suggest that the ileopsoas, quadriceps, and glutei are the most important muscles for achieving biped ambulation. The significance of the medial hamstring may be hidden due to its close association with the quadriceps and gluteus medius. Dudgeon and associates' study[290] of the relationship of muscle strength and ambulation, as well as McDonald and associates' examination[720] of the correlation between the gluteus medius and other hip muscles, indicates that the abductors of the hip are innervated at a higher level and are more important to ambulation than any authors other than Huff and Ramsey[511] have suggested. Dias concurs.[265]

Both of these studies by McDonald and Dudgeon indicate that more data about muscle innervation patterns need to be gathered and analyzed,

---

This includes eight groups of distinct iliopsoas, quadricep, medial hamstring, and gluteus medius powers with no motor power below the knee; all had with full strength hip adductors.

Total number, 85; 738 Seattle area patients; average 3.5 exams each, including all patients seen since 1978.

Key: =, the majority of the patients walk well; ——, the majority of the patients are ineffective walkers; —, patients equally divided between effective and noneffective walkers; Il, iliopsoas; Qd, quadriceps; MH, medial hamstrings; Comm, patients ambulate in the community; HH, patients ambulate in the home; Non, patients are nonambulatory; 1–5, levels of muscle strength (1, weakest; 5, strongest); N, number of patients.

Adapted from Dudgeon and associates.[290]

a task not possible before the age of the computer and large-scale, cooperative studies.

MUSCULOSKELETAL DEFORMITIES

The fourth portion of this chapter deals with the natural history of musculoskeletal deformities acquired as a result of intrinsic bony malformations and abnormal innervation.

Spine

The high incidence of scoliosis, particularly in patients with thoracic and high-lumbar levels of paralysis, is reported by many investigators.[62,684,768,976,1055] Between 80 and 90 percent of patients with thoracic and high-lumbar levels of paralysis will develop scoliosis by the age of 20 years (Figure 15-5). Scoliosis increases throughout childhood in patients with asymmetric innervation and then becomes relatively stable. Scoliosis in lumbar-level patients increases to involve 25–35 percent during adolescence. Kyphosis is present in 20–30 percent of thoracic-level patients by age 1 year and increases to involve 80 percent of patients by age 20. Only 5–15 percent with lumbar-, and 0 percent with sacral-level lesions develop progressive kyphosis.[1055] The underlying causes for the kyphotic and scoliotic curves have been discussed by Bunch and associates.[144] The effect of positioning the paraspinous or lattissimus dorsi muscle posterior to the spine, as described in Chapter 6, remains to be determined. Our clinical impression is that patients who have undergone the procedure during initial back closures have less kyphosis and scoliosis; when present, the curves either stabilize or progress to a lesser degree.

Hips

We have extensively studied the effects of age as well as growth and development on the occurrence of hip flexion contractures. Our study of 6572 hip examinations of 783 patients with various forms of meningomyelocele demonstrates that only some patients in each motor-level group develop hip flexion contractures (Fig. 15-6A). When these data are divided into pre- and postoperative examinations, the significant difference between motor-level groups remains; however, there is an insignificant difference in the proportion of patients with severe or mild forms of hip flexion contracture between the pre- and postoperative groups (Fig. 6B and C).

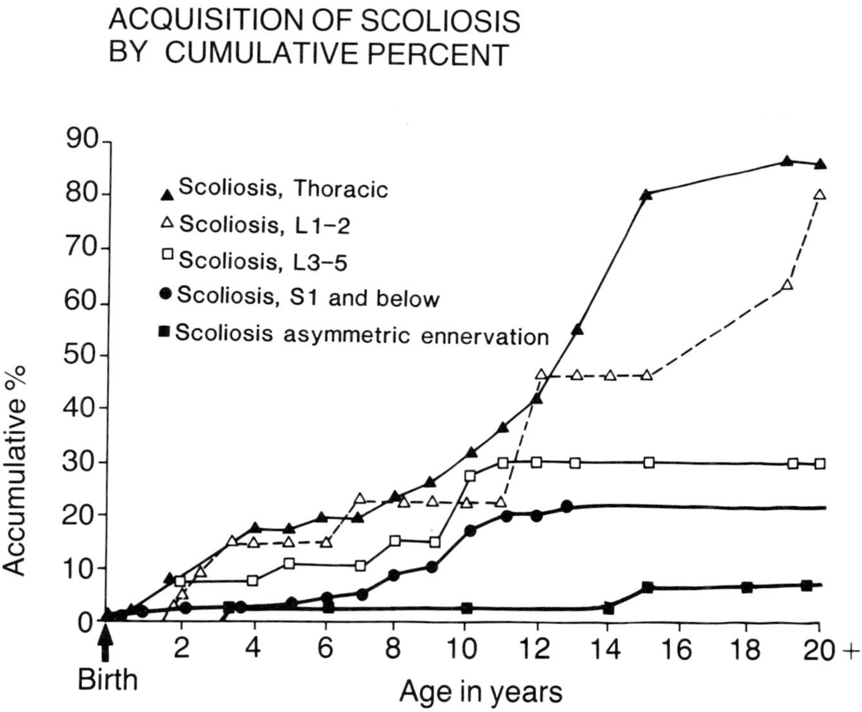

Figure 15-5. Acquisition of scoliosis and kyphosis by cumulative percentage. Kyphoscoliosis was calculated by the actuarial method. The accumulative percentage was derived by computing the percentage of those still at risk (those with newly acquired kyphoscoliosis divided by all at risk) times the percentage of those still remaining at risk. Patients lost to the study because of death or loss to follow-up did not affect the curve. Once the kyphoscoliosis was acquired (scoliosis greater than 30° or kyphosis greater than 30° over six vertebra [gibbus] below T11 or greater than 65° involving more vertebrae), the effect was carried forward regardless if treatment reverted the curve. These curves were plotted from data published by Shurtleff and associates.[(1055)] There are 365 total patients, with 90 in the thoracic; 37 in the high lumbar; 117 in the lumbar 3 (first appearance of quadriceps) to 5 (presence of anterior tibialis but no other muscles below the knee); 90 with sacral level lesions; and 38 with asymmetric innervation.

When we attempted to apply our acquisition analyses by cumulative percentages, as for death in previous studies (see Chapters 5, 12, and 14 Fig. 15-5), we discovered a more rapid acquisition of hip flexion contracture than expected and a nonlinear relationship with age. Therefore, we plotted a prevalence curve of the mean hip flexion contracture by age for all patients with limitation of hip extension of 21° or more in five separate muscle level groups: thoracic, high lumbar (L1-2), mid lumbar

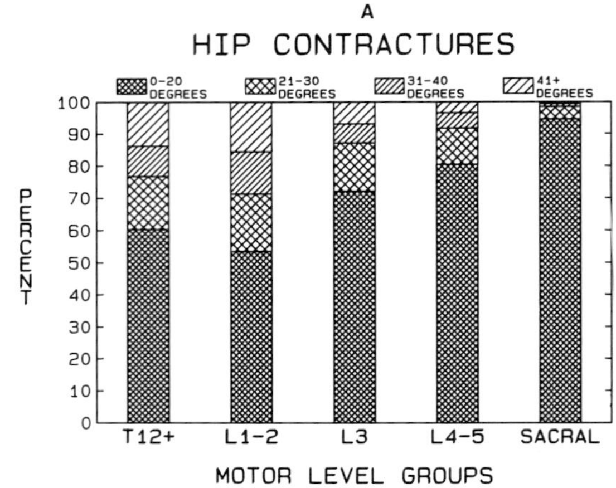
A
HIP CONTRACTURES
0-20 DEGREES
21-30 DEGREES
31-40 DEGREES
41+ DEGREES
PERCENT
100
90
80
70
60
50
40
30
20
10
0
T12+
L1-2
L3
L4-5
SACRAL
MOTOR LEVEL GROUPS

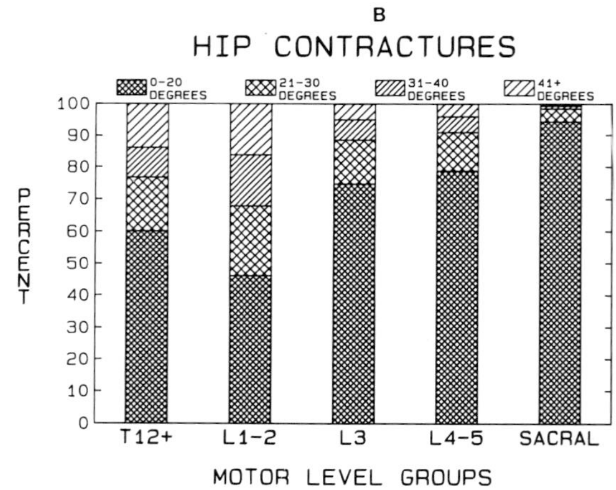
B
HIP CONTRACTURES
0-20 DEGREES
21-30 DEGREES
31-40 DEGREES
41+ DEGREES
PERCENT
100
90
80
70
60
50
40
30
20
10
0
T12+
L1-2
L3
L4-5
SACRAL
MOTOR LEVEL GROUPS

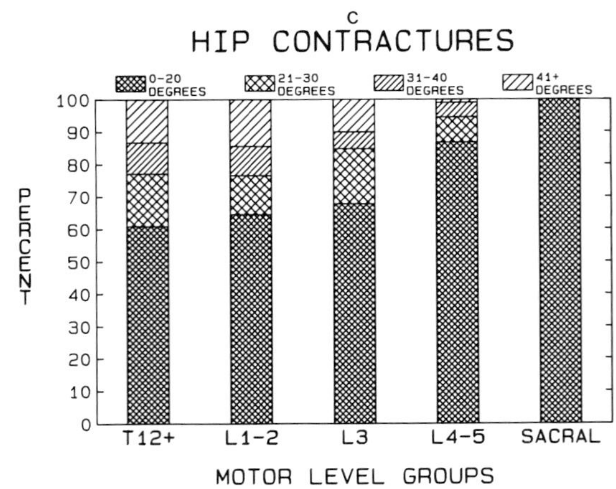
C
HIP CONTRACTURES
0-20 DEGREES
21-30 DEGREES
31-40 DEGREES
41+ DEGREES
PERCENT
100
90
80
70
60
50
40
30
20
10
0
T12+
L1-2
L3
L4-5
SACRAL
MOTOR LEVEL GROUPS

LAMERS 9/9/85

(L3), low lumbar (L4-5), and sacral (Fig. 15-7). Right and left hip measurements from 3167 examinations of 789 patients without prior hip operations were analyzed. Regression curves calculated for the two portions of each curve from 0 to 27 months and older than 27 months were significant for all groups. Further analysis of 2315 hip examinations at all 16 age groups of patients with one hip flexion measurement over the age of 3 years has demonstrated that within all muscle groups some physiologic flexion postures will disappear and not recur as progressive hip flexion contractures; others will reappear by age 3–6 years; and many will entirely or only partially resolve before becoming progressively more severe (Fig. 15-8). These observations probably indicate that the mean of 30°–40° limitation in hip extension seen at birth is really a physiologic postural deformity seen also in normal children[291,441,490] and that it will resolve in most normal children and some patients with meningomyelocele over the next 2–3 years. Positioning and passive range of motion exercises may improve this recovery[1141]; surgery is not indicated until

---

Figure 15-6. (A) Development of hip flexion contractures by motor-level groups (all hips, all examinations). (B) All hip examinations before operation. (C) All hip examinations after operation. (A) All 6,572 examinations of 738 patients seen in Shriner's Unit and the University of Washington Birth Defects Clinics in the Washington, Alaska, Montana, and Idaho (WAMI) Medical School region have been plotted by five muscle-level groups and percentages with four categories of hip flexion contracture. The T12+ group has thoracic-level lesions; L1-2 has hip adductors and ileopsoas muscle function, in addition; L3 level lesion patients have weak quadriceps function added to L1-2 muscle function; L4-5 have, in addition, full-strength quadriceps and medial hamstrings, and some have gluteus medius and anterior tibialis muscle function; and the sacral-level group has more function than the L4-5, but at least some weakness. There are 1511 thoracic, 591 L1-2, 254 L3, 2367 L4-5, and 1249 sacral-level patient examinations. The difference in percentages with the four degrees of hip flexion contractures between the five motor-level groups is significant: $\chi^2 = 485$; df = 12; $p < .001$. (B) The 5,157 hip flexion examinations performed prior to surgery or on patients not subjected to surgery are divided into 1186 thoracic, 361 L1-2, 516 L3, 1805 L4-5, and 1289 sacral patient examinations. These tests demonstrate a similar difference in proportion with hip flexion contractures between levels of lesion ($\chi^2 = 365$; df = 12; $p < .001$). The distribution is, however, not different from the overall group or those obtained postoperatively. (C) The 1415 examinations obtained following operative procedures to relieve hip flexion contractures are divided into 326 thoracic, 198 L1-2, 325 L3, 238 L4-5, and 28 sacral. There is, however, no difference between the percentage of patients with hip flexion contractures of the three degrees of severity in the unoperated and postoperative groups within each motor lesion level.

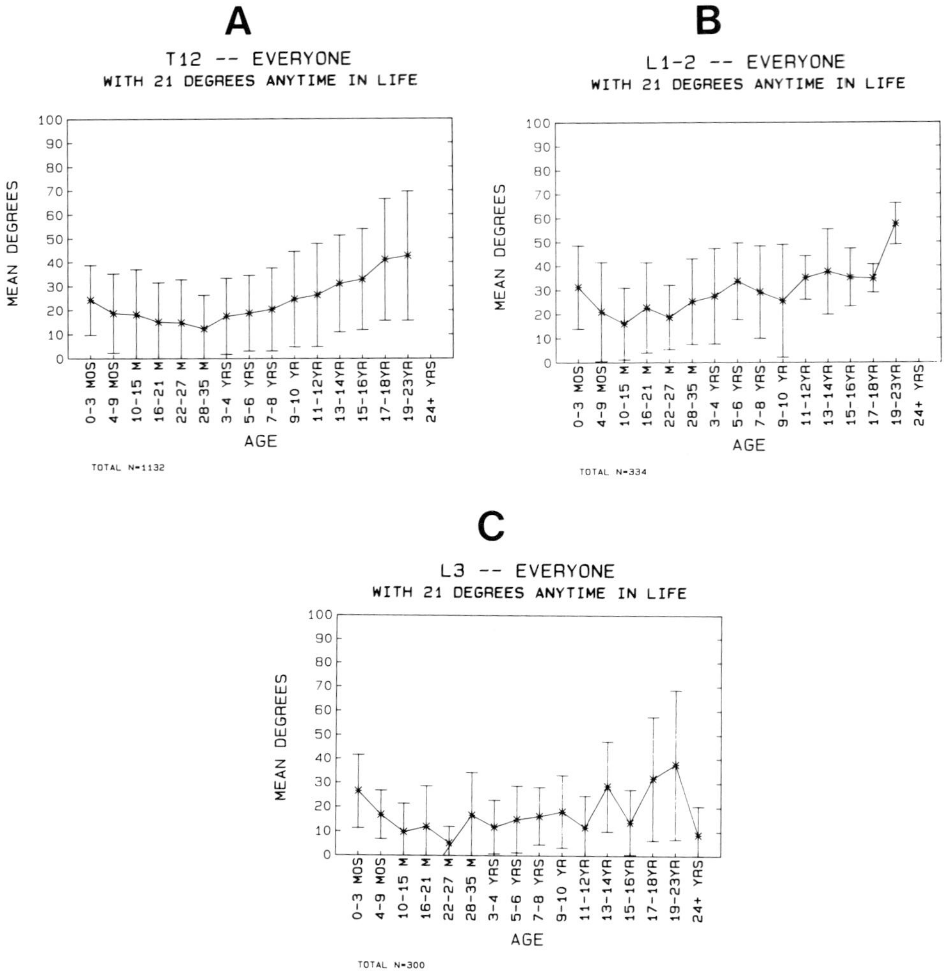

Figure 15-7. Mean hip flexion contracture by age for all patients with (A) thoracic-level lesions; (B) high-lumbar (L1-2)-level lesions; (C) mid-lumbar (L3)-level lesions; (D) low-lumbar (L4-5)-level lesions; and (E) sacral-level lesions. Any patient with one hip flexion contracture (HFC) measurement of 21° or more has been included. The mean degrees of HFC obtained for 16 different age intervals for all patients have been plotted +1 standard deviation for a total of 3167 examinations. None had prior surgery. (A) All patients had thoracic-level motor lesions. The 1132 examinations revealed a significant decrease in HFC contractures from 25° at birth to 12° by age 28–35 months, with a subsequent increase to 43° by age 19–23 years ($F = 11.5$; $df = 20$; $p < .01$). (Where the difference between means (F) exceeds 1.0 and the degrees of freedom are greater than or equal to 20, then p is less than 0.001, when calculated by ANOVAR, Analyses of Variance.) (B) All patients had hip adductor and ileopsoas muscle

D

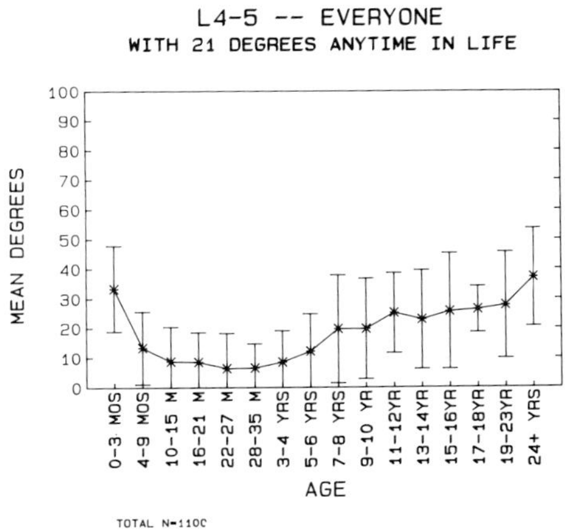

E

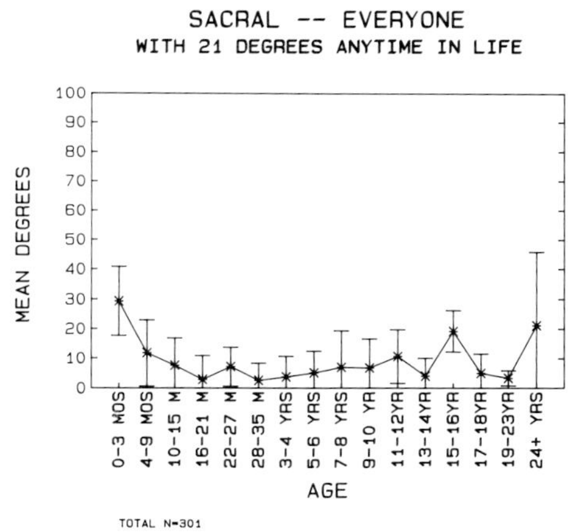

function. The 334 examinations demonstrate a significant decrease in mean HFC from 31° at birth to 27° by age 10–15 months, then an increase to a mean of 58° at age 19–23 years ($F = 3.78$; $df = 20$; $p < 0.001$). (C) All patients had hip adductor, ileopsoas, and weak quadriceps. The 300 examinations demonstrate a significant decrease in mean HFC from 27° at birth to 4° at age 22–27 months, then an increase to a mean HFC at age 19–23 years of 38° ($F = 2.89$; $df = 20$; $p < 0.001$). (D) All patients who had, in addition to the muscle function of group C of this figure, full-strength quadriceps, medial hamstrings, and some gluteus medius and anterior tibialis muscle function are included in these 1100 examinations. The decrease in mean HFC from birth (33°) to age 22–35 months (7°) is significant, as is the increase to 38° by 24+ years ($F = 5.85$; $df = 20$; $p < 0.001$). (E) All patients with more muscle function than group D of this figure, but with some weakness, were included in these 301 examinations. The decrease in mean HFC from 29° to 3° by age 16–21 months is significant, and the increase thereafter is also significant ($F = 38.8$; $df = 20$; $p < 0.001$).

A

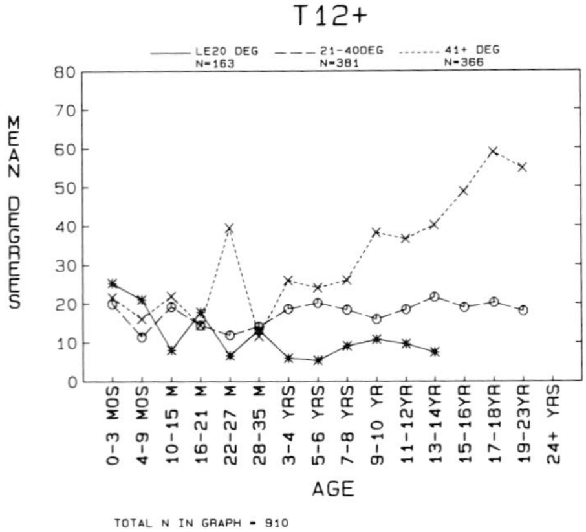
T12+
LE20 DEG N=163
21-40DEG N=381
41+ DEG N=366
MEAN DEGREES
0 10 20 30 40 50 60 70 80
0-3 MOS
4-9 MOS
10-15 M
16-21 M
22-27 M
28-35 M
3-4 YRS
5-6 YRS
7-8 YRS
9-10 YR
11-12YR
13-14YR
15-16YR
17-18YR
19-23YR
24+ YRS
AGE
TOTAL N IN GRAPH = 910

B

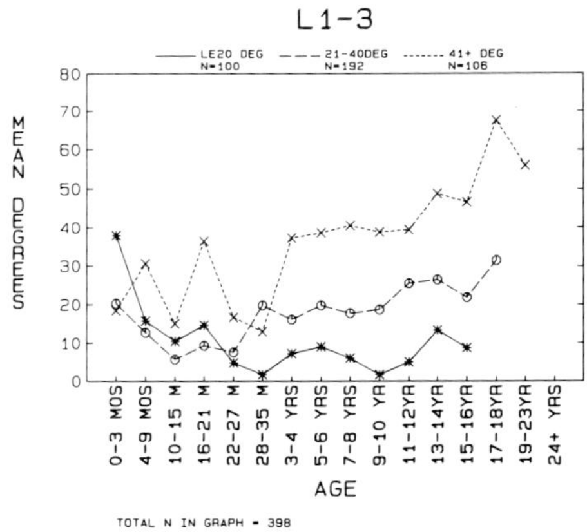
L1-3
LE20 DEG N=100
21-40DEG N=192
41+ DEG N=106
MEAN DEGREES
0 10 20 30 40 50 60 70 80
0-3 MOS
4-9 MOS
10-15 M
16-21 M
22-27 M
28-35 M
3-4 YRS
5-6 YRS
7-8 YRS
9-10 YR
11-12YR
13-14YR
15-16YR
17-18YR
19-23YR
24+ YRS
AGE
TOTAL N IN GRAPH = 398

C

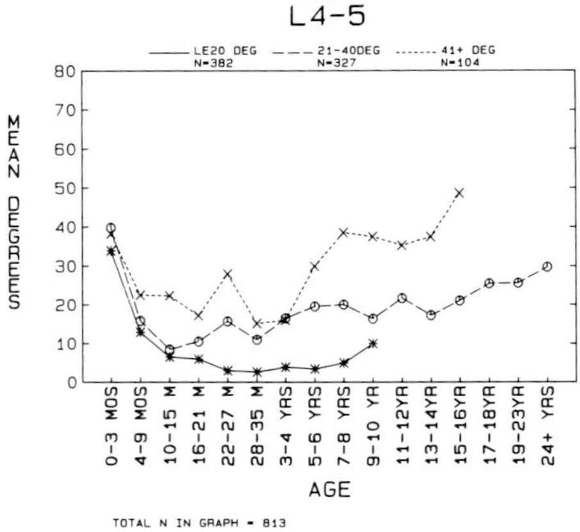
L4-5
LE20 DEG N=382
21-40DEG N=327
41+ DEG N=104
MEAN DEGREES
0 10 20 30 40 50 60 70 80
0-3 MOS
4-9 MOS
10-15 M
16-21 M
22-27 M
28-35 M
3-4 YRS
5-6 YRS
7-8 YRS
9-10 YR
11-12YR
13-14YR
15-16YR
17-18YR
19-23YR
24+ YRS
AGE
TOTAL N IN GRAPH = 813

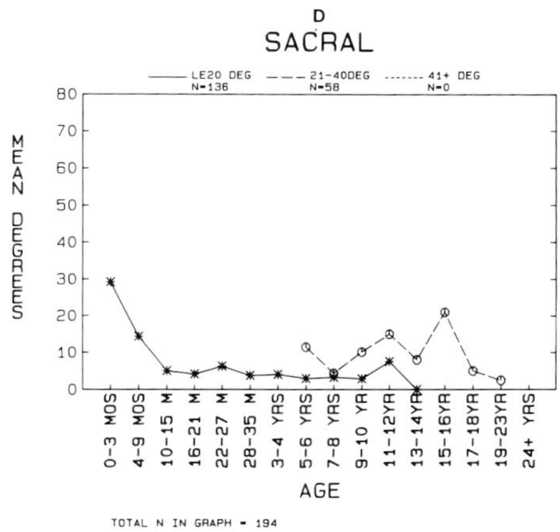

Figure 15-8. Physiologic hip flexion postures or contractures resolve or only partially resolve and then progressively become more severe in patients with (A) thoracic-level lesions; (B) high- to mid-lumbar-level lesions; (C) low-lumbar-level lesions; and (D) sacral-level lesions. All 2315 examinations of patients with a hip flexion measures recorded after the age of 36 months have been plotted. Some graphs are discontinuous because only plots containing a minimum of four observations have been included. All measures were before surgery or on patients who had never been operated on. Of these, 781 were found to have a maximum hip flexion contracture (HFC) less than or equal to 20°; 958 were between 21° and 40°; and 366 were 41° or greater after the age of 36 months of age. Mean degrees per 16 age groups have been plotted. All hip measurements were obtained for patients in these three categories. Statistical analysis was not performed because of small numbers. (A) All patients had thoracic-level motor-level lesions. Of these 910 examinations, 163 were less than or equal to 20° of HFC; 381 were between 21° and 40°; and 366 were 41° or greater after the age of 36 months. (B) All patients had quadriceps (some weak) as well as full-strength thoracic, abdominal, ileopsoas, and adductor muscles. Of these 398 examinations, 100 were on patients with a maximum HFC of 20°, 192 on patients with a maximum HFC between 21° and 40°, and 106 on patients with a maximum HFC 41° or greater after the age of 36 months. (C) All patients had, in addition to the muscle power listed in B, some power in medial hamstrings and anterior tibialis, and some had gluteus medius. Of the 813 examinations in this category, 382 had a maximum HFC of 20° or less, 327 had a maximum HFC between 21° and 40°; and 104 had a 41° or greater HFC after the age of 36 months. (D) All patients in this category had more muscle strength than C immediately above, but some muscle weakness. Of the 194 patient examinations, only 136 were on patients with 20° or less; 58 were on patients with HFC between 21° and 40° as a maximum after 36 months of age. These graphs are reproduced from Shurtleff, et al.[1063]

A

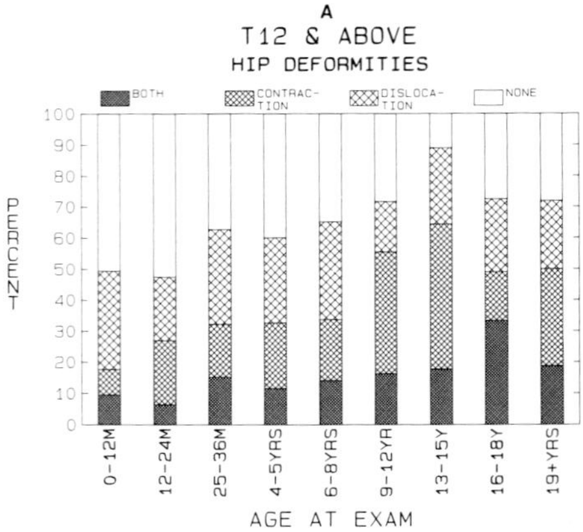

TOTAL NUMBER OF EXAMS = 773

B

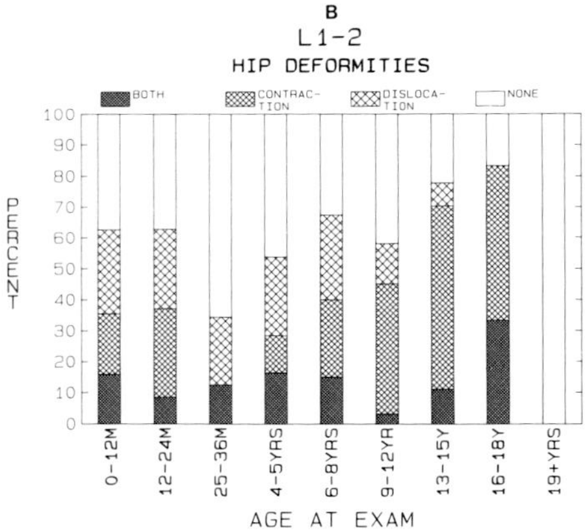

TOTAL NUMBER OF EXAMS = 348

C

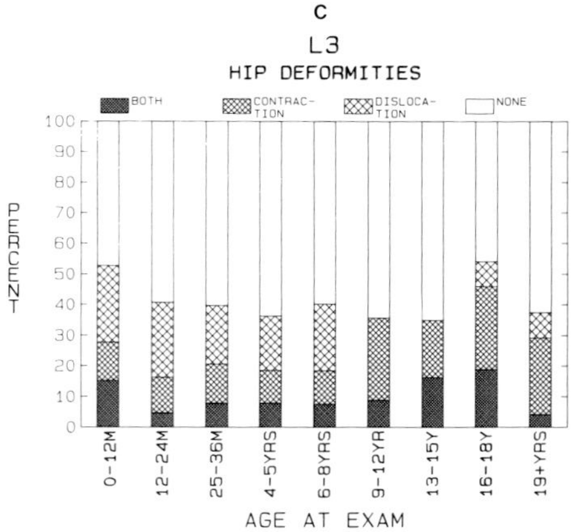

TOTAL NUMBER OF EXAMS = 626

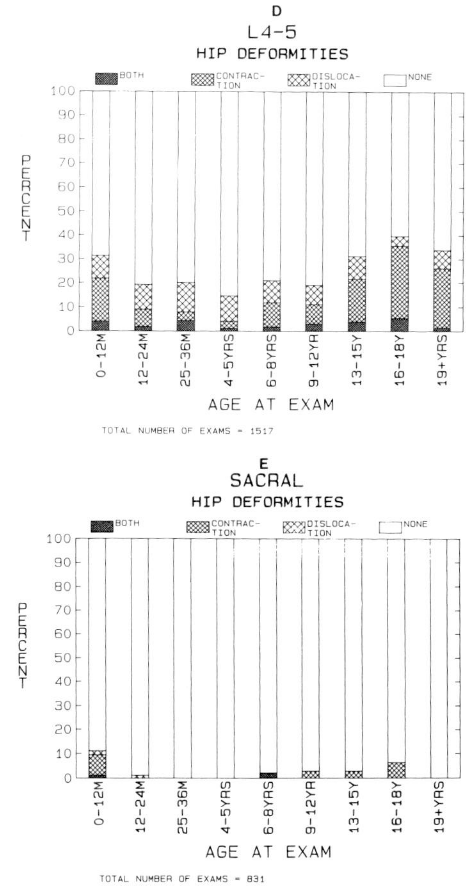

Figure 15-9. Combined hip deformities. (A) All patients have thoracic levels of paralysis. Multiple to single examinations combine for a total of 773. Each of the nine age group bars shows the percentage with some deformity or none. The large cross-hatched areas represent dislocated or displaced hips. The fine cross-hatched areas represent one or more of the following minimum contractures or worse: adduction contractures, (−)10° of abduction; abduction contractures, (−)10° of adduction; flexion contractures, (−)21° or more of extension limitations; extension contractures, (−)80° of flexion or less; internal rotation C, (−)10° of external rotation; external rotation C, (−)10°; displaced hip with one or more of the contractures listed. The bars represent the following number of examinations: 158, 78, 59, 138, 92, 92, 73, 51, 32. The apparent overall increases in both contractures and dislocations or displacement are statistically significant: $\chi^2 = 107$; df = 24; $p \leq .001$. (B) All patients have hip adductor and ileopsoas muscle function. The definition of the cross-hatched areas are the same as for A. The bars represent the following number of examinations: 107, 35, 32, 67, 43, 31, 27, 3, 3, for a total of 348. The apparent decrease, then increase, in deformities of the hip is significant: $\chi^2 = 60$; df = 24; $p \leq .001$. (C) All patients have adductor, ileopsoas, and weak quadriceps muscle strength, but no other muscle function.

(Figure 15-9 continued on next page)

serial examinations demonstrate failure to resolve or worsening of contractures.

In order to assess the frequency of all types of contractures and dislocation of the hips, we combined analysis in five motor-level categories (Fig. 15-9). A total of 4095 single hip examinations for patients without prior hip operations were placed in one of nine age groups from 1 year to 19+ years. Contractures were grouped as follows: flexion contractures of 21° or more, extension contractures of 80° or fewer degrees, adduction or abduction contractures, and external or internal rotation contractures of −10° or more. Dislocations and dislocatable but not dysplastic hips were included. As illustrated in Figure 15-9, 50–60 percent of the three highest, 30 percent of L4-5, and 11 percent of sacral-level-lesion groups had hip contracture, dislocation, or both on their first examinations. With a few age group exceptions that may be explained as due to small numbers, the frequency of hip dislocations appeared to remain the same in age groups within each motor-level group. Contractures, like the previously studied hip flexion contractures, first decreased in frequency, then become more common during later childhood. The lower frequency (35–40 percent) of hip contractures and dislocation among the L4-5 and L3 motor-level groups in later years, compared with the 70–90 percent involvement of the thoracic and high-lumbar groups, may represent the treatment policy in our center. As discussed earlier, we do not operate on hips to correct contractures or relocate hips unless the patient has a mid-lumbar (L3) or lower motor function level and is a candidate for ambulation.

Hip flexion contractures (HFCs) are also noted to recur after hip operations, as demonstrated in Figure 15-10. All patients with hip operations that included HFC as at least one of the indications were

---

Quadriceps power is usually weak. The cross-hatches in the bars are the same as for AW. The bars represent the following number of examinations: 112, 86, 63, 113, 92, 56, 43, 37, 24, for a total of 626. The apparent decrease in deformities from birth to early teenage with a subsequent increase is significant: $\chi^2 = 60$; df = 24; $p \leq .001$. (D)All patients have muscle strength as for C with full-strength quadriceps and medial hamstring, and some have anterior tibialis and gluteus medium function. The cross-hatches in the bars are the same as in A. The bars represent the following number of examinations: 326, 166, 114, 266, 219, 163, 125, 73, 65, for a total of 1,517. The apparent decrease and then increase in deformities is significant: $\chi^2 = 98$, df = 24; $p \leq .001$. (E) All patients have some muscle weakness, but with more function than those in D. The cross-hatches in the bars are the same as in A. The bars represent the following number of examinations: 180, 89, 65, 131, 93, 107, 72, 64, 31, for a total of 831. The disappearance following birth and recurrence in later life is significant: $\chi^2 = 53$; df = 24; $p = .001$.

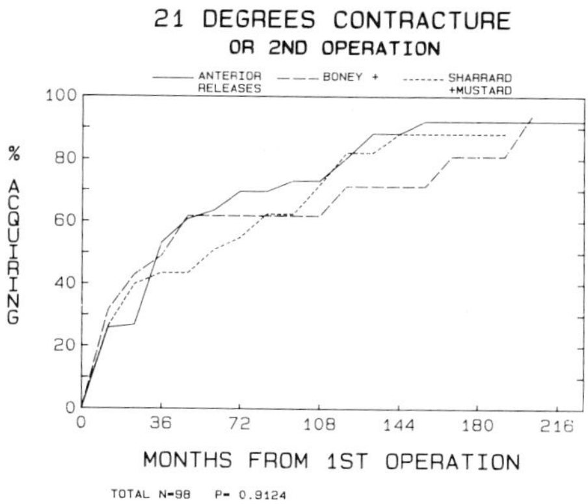

Figure 15-10. Recurrence of hip flexion contractures. HFC was plotted as greater than 20° or as sufficient to require a second hip operation to correct a HFC as the indications for the second hip procedure. Forty-seven patients had soft tissue releases; 20 had bony procedures (9 with and 11 without anterior releases); and 31 had ileopsoas transfers to the greater trochanter (5 Mustard and 26 Sharrard techniques). Time was recorded in months postoperation. The acquisition in percentage of the population at risk is the same as for Figure 15-5[1055]. The approximate chi square (with an inversion of covariance making, 0.4397, df = 2, p = .8026, and, by generalized Kruskall-Wallis analysis, χ^2 = 0.1971, df = 2, p = 0.9124) indicated that the rates of acquiring HFC postoperatively for the three types of procedures were the same for these groups of our patients. Follow-up for the anterior releases ranged from 34 to 218 months, bony procedures from 49 to 193 months, and ileopsoas transfers from 56 to 180 months. The last age group plotted for each graph contains 5 observations.

followed at yearly intervals, and their hip extensions were measured. Patients were divided into three groups: (1) anterior soft tissue releases, (2) femoral osteotomies and soft tissue releases, and (3) transfers of the ileopsoas. By 36 months postoperation, 50 percent of all three groups had 21° or more HFC; by 12 years, 70–85 percent of all three groups had 21° or more of HFC or underwent another hip operation with HFC as an indication.

The only hip procedure not followed by a significant recurrence of HFC has been abdominal external oblique transfer to the greater trochanter in association with several modifications, including adductor recession to the ischial tuberosity and intertrochanteric varus osteotomy.[265,723,1246] Thomas and associates[1162] introduced transfer of the

A

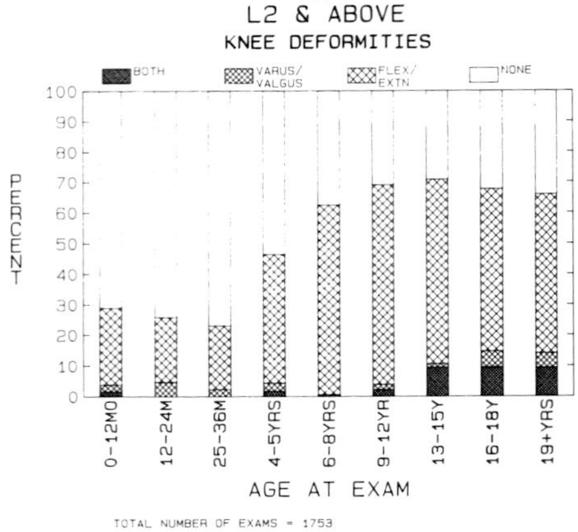
L2 & ABOVE
KNEE DEFORMITIES
BOTH
VARUS/ VALGUS
FLEX/ EXTN
NONE
PERCENT
0-12MO
12-24M
25-36M
4-5YRS
6-8YRS
9-12YR
13-15Y
16-18Y
19+YRS
AGE AT EXAM
TOTAL NUMBER OF EXAMS = 1753

B

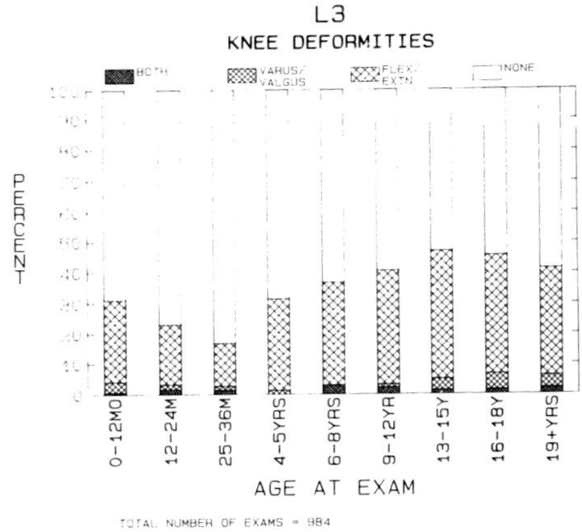
L3
KNEE DEFORMITIES
BOTH
VARUS/ VALGUS
FLEX/ EXTN
NONE
PERCENT
AGE AT EXAM
TOTAL NUMBER OF EXAMS = 984

C

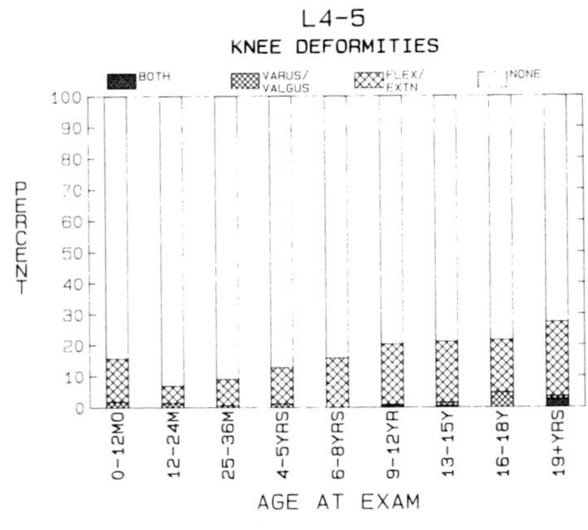
L4-5
KNEE DEFORMITIES
BOTH
VARUS/ VALGUS
FLEX/ EXTN
NONE
PERCENT
AGE AT EXAM
TOTAL NUMBER OF EXAMS = 2399

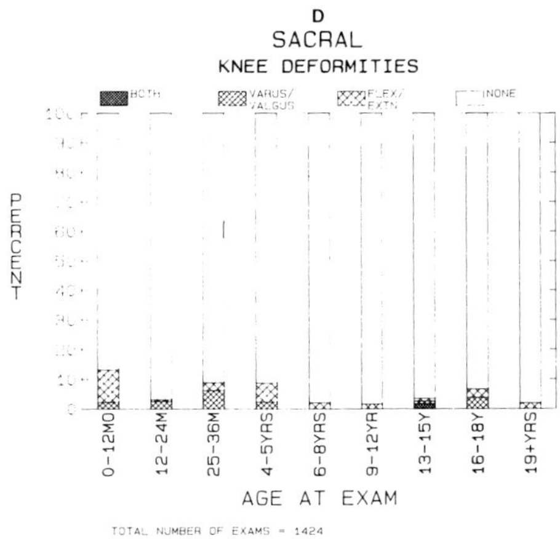

Figure 15-11. Combined deformities of knee extension or flexion contractures and either valgus or varus sufficient to interfere with ambulation. (A) All patients had thoracic-level paralysis or hip adductor and ileopsoas muscle power but no active, voluntary muscle function across the knee joint. Multiple to single examinations per patient combine for a total of 1753. Each of the nine age-group bars shows the percentage with some abnormality or none. The large cross-hatched area represents flexion contractures equal to or greater than (−)20° of extension; extension contractures equal to 80° or less of flexion. The small cross-hatch represents a valgus deformity of (−)20° or more of varus or a varus deformity of (−)20° or more. The black represents any combination of flexion or extension and valgus or varus deformity. The bars represent the following number of examinations: 398, 170, 130, 293, 192, 181, 168, 136, 85. The apparent early decrease, then marked increase, in deformities is significant: $\chi^2 = 321$; df = 24; $p \leq .001$. (B) All patients had hip adductor, ileopsoas, and weak quadriceps. The cross-hatched areas in each of the nine age group bar graphs represent the same deformities as in A. The bars represent the following number of examinations: 174, 130, 77, 162, 136, 96, 81, 77, 51, for a total of 984. The apparent decrease, then increase, in deformities is significant: $\chi^2 = 48$; df = 24; $p \leq 0.001$. (C) All patients have the same muscle functions as in B, with full-strength quadriceps and medial hamstrings; some had gluteus medius and anterior tibialis function. The cross-hatched areas represent the same deformities as in A. The bars represent the following number of examinations: 503, 289, 197, 428, 314, 231, 199, 125, 113, for a total of 2399. The apparent decrease then increase in deformities is significant: $\chi^2 = 105$; df = 24; $p \leq .001$. (D) All patients have more muscle function than for C, but some weakness. The cross-hatched areas represent the same deformities as in A. The bars represent the following number of examinations: 301, 155, 112, 217, 187, 181, 115, 105, 51, for a total of 1424. The apparent decrease from birth with an increase in the late teen-aged years is significant: $\chi^2 = 94$; df = 24; $p \leq .001$.

external abdominal oblique to the greater trochanter in order to add muscle power to the hip with a weak abductor paralyzed by polio. McKay[723] began external oblique transfer, adductor recession, and varus femoral osteotomy to provide hip stabilization in patients with meningomyelocele in 1971. Yngve and Lindseth[1246] confirmed the efficacy of this procedure for producing hip stability when compared with other techniques ($\chi^2 = 6.8$; df = 2; $p < .01$). Later, Staheli[1102] substituted the Pemberton or shelf procedure for varus osteotomy to improve hip stabilization. Other authors[d] have commented on the problem of recurring HFCs and "stiff" hips following operative procedures to relieve contractures and prevent or correct hip dislocation. Hip flexion and adduction contractures are associated with any hip procedure that involves cutting the hip capsule anteriorally and medically.[265] Late onset of stiffness or hip dislocation and recurrent hip dislocation postoperatively may be due to disturbances in sympathetic nervous system control over blood supply, genetic differences in collagen, and, most frequently, overlooked spasticity about the hip.[722] More needs to be learned about why some patients with various forms of meningomyelocele do and others do not develop "stiff," contracted joints of the lower extremities.

Knees

Because we have observed severe knee extension deformities resolve following serial casts and passive range-of-motion exercises, we have analyzed knee deformities as a whole in a similar manner as we have hip contractures and dislocations (Fig. 15-11). The combined deformities of extension or flexion contractures, valgus or varus, and both have been plotted by level of lesion (Fig. 15-11). A total of 6560 examinations of 1187 patients were available prior to operative procedures. Because of the small proportion of patients with deformities and the smaller proportion operated on, we have not studied the effect of surgery. Because of the absence of knee musculature, we combined the two highest level lesion groups (T12 and L1-2) into one group to form four segmental muscle level groups. Since contractures decrease, these data suggest that knee contractures at birth are also physiologic positions and resolve after birth to some extent. Contractures then develop beginning at 4–5 years of age for patients with L3 or higher level lesions and 2–3 years of age for patients with lower level lesions. Contractures are most frequent with thoracic- and high-lumbar-level lesions (65–70 percent) by age 6–8 years, next most frequent among patients with L4-5 lesions (20–25 percent by age 9–12 years), and only sporadic among sacral-level patients.

---

[d] See references 50, 167, 260, 327, 473, 491, 511, 584, 749, 953, and 976.

Valgus and varus deformities occur infrequently in all but the two highest motor-level groups, but they increase slightly in all motor-level groups during adolescence. Varus and valgus deformities may be caused by pathologic fractures or degeneration of knee capsules and joint surfaces from trauma. Some authors have suggested that the knee flexion gait may be due to contractures of the knee secondary to the patient's need to establish a center of gravity over the midfoot[381,976] or secondary to an inability to straighten the hip.[748,749] We believe that the bent-knee gait can be due to foot or hip abnormalities but doubt if they account for the development of contractures. Others state that knee flexion contractures are secondary to weak quadriceps unable to effectively oppose a strong or spastic medial hamstring muscle.[748,862,976] Our data are currently too limited to explain the complex relationships.

Feet

Just as progressive and fixed deformities of the spine are the major interference with function of the patient with a high-level lesion, and just as hips are the problem of the patient with a lumbar-level lesion, so the foot is the site of major functional deformities for the patient with a functioning gluteus medius and a low-lumbar- or sacral-level lesion. In no other group of patients is a careful sensory examination so important. The L4-5 and S1 nerve roots providing sensation to the sole and sides of the foot may be partially or completely nonfunctional, and nerve distribution varies in these patients. If extensive blisters can develop during hikes with poorly fitting shoes on normal people, even partial loss of sensation can contribute greatly to the problem of foot sores aggravated by deformity, abnormal weightbearing, rigidity, and the pressure of orthoses. The primary author has witnessed amputation of feet after multiple attempts at surgical correction of decubitus ulcers; this occurred without the surgeons ever appreciating the complete anesthesia, associated with a low-sacral neurosegmental muscle innervation, of young adults' feet. Plantar decubiti from asymmetric weightbearing on anesthetic surfaces are too frequently covered by skin grafts without surgical or orthotic correction of the weight maldistribution and without postoperative instruction in decubitus prevention. Osteomyelitis eventually develops, necessitating successive partial amputations until weightbearing on skin innervated by an intact L3 level is achieved at the knee.

The deformities of the feet that complicate loss of sensation are of two broad categories: nonweightbearing and weightbearing. The former interfere with wearing shoes in the nonambulatory patient, leaving the patient at risk for abrasion and cold unless expensive shoes are purchased. The latter interfere with alignment of weight or cause abnormal distribution of weight. These two groups can be further divided into flail and rigid deformities, both of which may recur after surgical correction.

Deformed feet are most common in the meningomyelocele patient with innervation at any segmental level proximal to lumbar five (Fig. 15-12). Partially innervated feet develop deformities according to the groups of muscles innervated, and these deformities recur unless the deforming force is removed. Other causes for recurring deformities include the presence of unopposed spasticity due to a tethered cord or other low-spine lesion (see Chapter 6) and skip lesions described by Stark.[1104] In some patients with no apparent muscle function in the feet, rigid fixed deformities occur. These may develop as a result of position, autonomic nervous system abnormalities, or intrinsic collagen characteristics.

The complexity of rotational deformities and the multiple combinations of ankle and foot deformities render discussion of their progress, management, and consequences beyond the scope of this text. We will limit our comments to the frequency of deformities and refer the reader to standard orthopedic texts mentioned earlier[748,976,1015,1141] for detailed discussions of pathophysiology and management.

We studied the occurrence of rotational deformities, talipes equinovarus, valgus, and calcaneus in patients within the four segmental levels of motor function, by the same nine age groups, as for knee deformities (Fig. 15-12). Only 1839 foot examinations of patients were available because we have been recording the details of rotational deformities only since 1979. Deformities were considered rotational if the thigh-foot angle was less than −20° or greater than 50°. ''Clubfeet'' as a category included moderate to severe heel varus, forefoot supination or adductus, cavus, and dorsiflexion of −10° or less. The valgus category included moderate to severe heel valgus, forefoot abductus or pronation, and plantar flexion of −10° or less. Since the clubfoot and calcaneo valgus groups are exclusive of one another, individuals with either of these deformities and a rotational deformity were included in the ''both'' category. The variability in frequency distributions in Figure 15-12 as compared with Figures 15-8 and 15-10 may be due to smaller numbers and more complex deformities.

Deformities sporadically occur among the sacral group of patients. There is an increase in foot deformities during the first 2 years among L3 and L4-5 patients as well as an increase between 4 and 5 years among higher level lesion patients. A decrease in frequency then continues until age 9–12 years among L3 and higher level lesion patients. The decline continues until age 16–18 years of age in the low-lumbar-level group. With the exception of the 16–18-year-old patients with L2 and higher lesions, the frequency of foot deformity is between 20 and 50 percent among all but the sacral-level group. The clubfoot type of deformities are most common among the highest level lesion patients, as are rotational deformities among the older patients with L3 and among the two youngest age groups with L4-5–level lesions. The valgus group of deformities appears to be only slightly more frequent among patients with L4-5 deformities and just as rare as the other deformities among patients with sacral-level lesions. Although clear examples of distinct neurosegmental motor levels and deformities can be recognized when the foot is otherwise flail, it would appear from these data that any type of deformity can be anticipated within any given motor level.

Considerably more observations and more intensive study are needed to better understand ankle and foot deformities. Cases presented in Figure 15-12 have not been studied to determine whether deformities can be attributed only to the natural history or have been altered by physical therapy, serial casts, or surgery.

SUMMARY AND GENERAL RECOMMENDATIONS

This chapter has presented observations that emphasize the variable natural history of deformities secondary to different types of innervation of the lower body and extremities of patients born with meningomyelocele. The primary author believes that a considerable effort should be expended by multiple collaborating groups in order to collect comparable data that will describe the multiple independent, interdependent, and dependent variables that contribute to discussions about mobility. The natural history of individual deformities and their consequences must be studied in more detail before we can judge their significance and develop management plans. Just as teams within centers were developed to assure comprehensive treatment for children with meningomyelocele and other forms of myelodysplasia, so we must now form larger collaborating networks of centers to describe the natural history of individual deformities and the best methods of management.

Because of the large number of variables that affect mobility, a large network is necessary to allow investigators to find comparable cases with similar aspects to compare different types of management and surgery. With computer assistance, large groups of variables, such as those contributing to a specific type of ambulatory program, like upright biped gait, can be matched to those of other programs that advocate different types of programs that may, for example, emphasize seated or vehicle-assisted mobility. Matched groups can then be compared for quality of outcome.

The concept of collaboration, such as produced amazingly complex

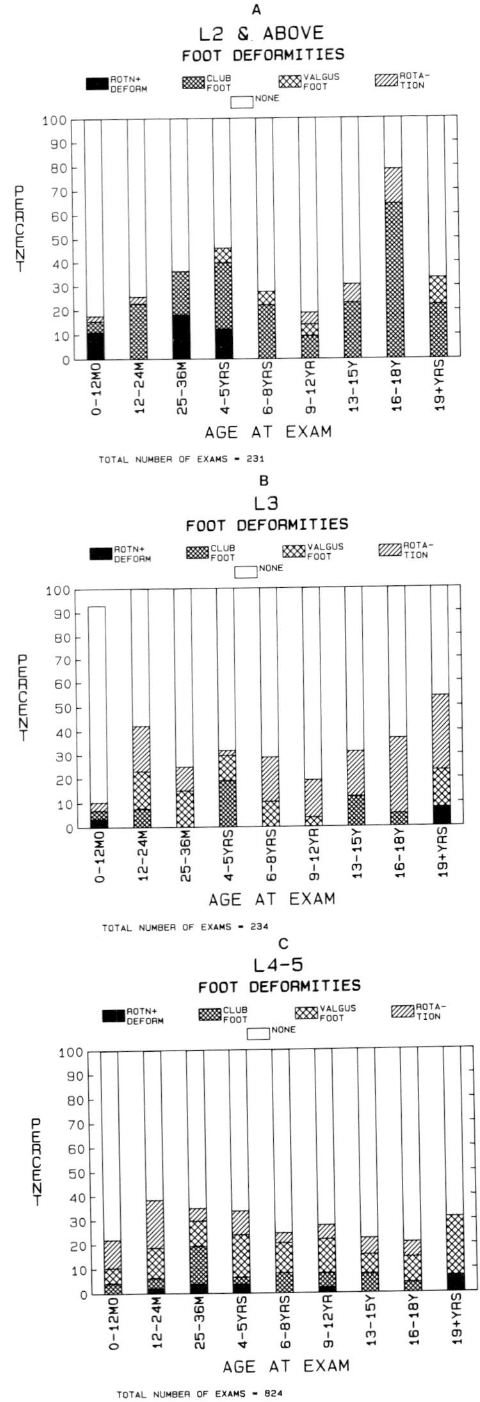
A
L2 & ABOVE
FOOT DEFORMITIES
ROTN+ DEFORM
CLUB FOOT
VALGUS FOOT
ROTA-TION
NONE
PERCENT
100
90
80
70
60
50
40
30
20
10
0
0-12MO
12-24M
25-36M
4-5YRS
6-8YRS
9-12YR
13-15Y
16-18Y
19+YRS
AGE AT EXAM
TOTAL NUMBER OF EXAMS = 231
B
L3
FOOT DEFORMITIES
ROTN+ DEFORM
CLUB FOOT
VALGUS FOOT
ROTA-TION
NONE
PERCENT
0-12MO
12-24M
25-36M
4-5YRS
6-8YRS
9-12YR
13-15Y
16-18Y
19+YRS
AGE AT EXAM
TOTAL NUMBER OF EXAMS = 234
C
L4-5
FOOT DEFORMITIES
ROTN+ DEFORM
CLUB FOOT
VALGUS FOOT
ROTA-TION
NONE
PERCENT
0-12MO
12-24M
25-36M
4-5YRS
6-8YRS
9-12YR
13-15Y
16-18Y
19+YRS
AGE AT EXAM
TOTAL NUMBER OF EXAMS = 824

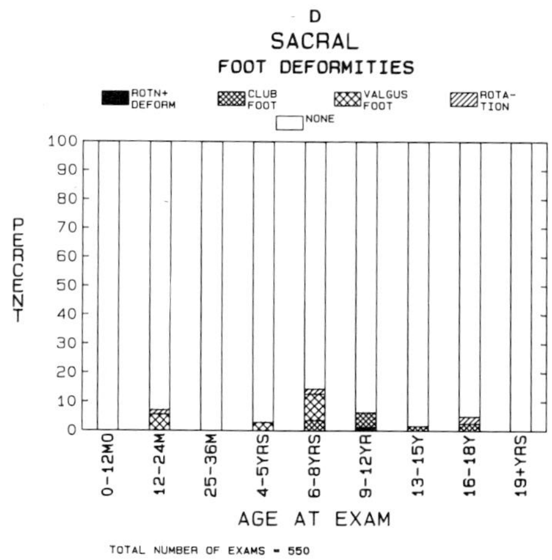

Figure 15-12. Combined deformity of the foot including lower leg and ankle. (A) All patients had thoracic levels of paralysis or functioning hip adductors and ileopsoas muscles. Multiple to single examinations per patient totalled 231. Each of the nine age group bars shows the percentage with some deformity or none. The slant lines represent internal rotation of 20° and more or external rotation of 50° and more. The large cross-hatched areas represent a foot with calcaneous, ankle valgus, or forefoot eversion of moderate to severe degree. The small cross-hatched areas represent heel varus, equinus, forefoot adductus, or cavus of moderate or severe degree. The black areas represent a combination of rotational deformity with either the large or medium cross-hatched areas type of deformity. The bars represent the following number of examinations: 45, 35, 11, 65, 18,21, 13, 14, 9. The variations are significant: $\chi^2 = 63$; df $= 32$; $p \leq .001$. (B) All patients had hip adductor, ileopsoas, and weak quadriceps muscle function. The definitions of the shaded areas in each bar are the same as in A. The bars represent the following number of examinations: 29, 26, 20, 47, 38, 26, 16, 19, 13, for a total of 234. The variations are significant: $\chi^2 = 63$; df $= 32$; $p \leq .002$. (C) All patients had hip adductors, ileopsoas, and strong quadriceps, and some had gluteus medius and anterior tibialis. The definitions of the shaded areas in each bar are the same as in A. The bars represent the following number of examinations: 95, 96, 77, 183, 121, 86, 89, 48, 29, for a total of 824. The variations are significant: $\chi^2 = 74$; df $= 32$; $p \leq .001$. (D) All patients have more muscle function than in C, but all have some weakness. The definitions of the shaded areas in each bar are the same as in A. The bars represent the following number of examinations: 87, 70, 40, 103, 55, 79, 61, 40, 15, for a total of 550. The variations are significant: $\chi^2 = 52$; df $= 32$; and $p = .015$.

journeys to outer space, needs to be adopted for the solution of the biomedical and social problems of our physically impaired youth.[96] The studies in this chapter represent a crude beginning. The computer age has given us the tool to analyze large data sets. The patient with meningomyelocele represents an ideal model with which to develop a collaborative network and study. Others studying childhood cancer and pregnancies have demonstrated the value of collaborative efforts. Until we can establish such a network and develop recommendations based on sound statistical analyses, the primary author is reluctant to offer any advice on the mobility management of children with meningomyelocele other than the various opinions, some conflicting, reviewed in the first part of this chapter. Most of us can agree that the patients with low-lumbar- or sacral-level lesions should be encouraged to ambulate. How and whether to do this with high-level-lesion patients needs to be answered.

SECTION V

Developmental Expectations and Therapeutic/Educational Approaches

Joyce Shaffer, Lynn Wolfe
William Friedrich, Hillary Shurtleff
David Shurtleff, Gayle Fay

16

Developmental Expectations: Intelligence and Fine Motor Skills

The goal of this chapter is not to create a profile typical of the congenitally malformed patient's potential intelligence and fine motor skills but rather to emphasize the need for a comprehensive evaluation of any individual's pattern of strengths and weaknesses. In order to do this, we will identify potential problem areas that may interfere with functional and academic skills. Age-appropriate neurodiagnostic and fine motor skill tests are listed in Table 22-4, and more detailed neurodiagnostic tests are reviewed in Chapter 17 (Tables 17-1 and 17-2). Treatment and educational strategies for dealing with problems are discussed in the Chapter 17 as well.

Parents, educators, and health care providers will be better able to help children with congenital malformations if they distinguish between cognitive and perceptual strengths and weaknesses. As defined by Wechsler,[1204] intelligence is the overall capacity of an individual to understand and cope with the world. It is a multidetermined, multifaceted global entity. Any discussion of intelligence must differentiate among intelligence, intelligence quotients (IQ), and IQ tests. Unfortunately, IQ test scores are often used synonomously with intelligence. In addition, fine motor incoordination and/or impaired visual-perception skills may hamper IQ testing, and testers may assume a cognitive deficit exists when the real problem is an inability to physically respond to visual or spatial tasks.

MYELODYSPLASIAS AND EXSTROPHIES: SIGNIFICANCE, PREVENTION, AND TREATMENT
 ISBN 0-8089-1816-8

INTELLIGENCE

Infant Assessment

Even with normal development, there is poor correlation between preschool test scores and intelligence quotients.[74,122,645] Prediction is probably more accurate for subnormal than for gifted children.[520] The reliability of IQ as a measure of later intellectual function increases with age and does not actually become reliable until 3, 4, or even 5 years of age.[340] The most consistent scores and highest correlation coefficient at all age levels are found in patients with congenital cerebral anomalies.[399] Even if IQ tests did measure potential intelligence fairly well, a total test score does not address the issues of specific learning difficulties, the impact of chronic illness and multiple hospitalizations, and future effects of school, family, and social experiences. However, as we pointed out in Chapter 5, since parents, educators, and health care providers consider intellectual potential when making their decisions about the infant's or child's care and placement, some estimate of this potential is necessary.

Research to Date: Comparison of Studies

Studies of children with meningomyelocele with or without hydrocephalus are difficult to compare for four main reasons, described below.

First, since most studies reporting data on the intellectual functioning of patients with meningomyelocele and hydrocephalus have not controlled for infection and bleeding, considerable confusion still exists as to the functional capacity of these patients without complications of treatment. This distinction is important since the intellectual deficits described as associated with hydrocephalus and meningomyelocele may actually be secondary to central nervous system (CNS) infection or bleeding.[740,1009,1053,1187]

Second, existing literature on hydrocephalus describes heterogeneous samples. Children with hydrocephalus without meningomyelocele have been included indiscriminately with groups of children with hydrocephalus and meningomyelocele.[45,216,526,661,1156] The effects of the underlying disorder that caused the hydrocephalus, the effect of hydrocephalus itself, and the effects of the malformations associated with meningomyelocele cannot be differentiated.

Third, groups of subjects with meningomyelocele have been defined according to functional motor level,[55,1045] sensory level of lesion,[514,1086] and type or anatomic placement of lesion[618,888] and, thus, cannot be compared.

Fourth, multiple assessment instruments used in various studies are not directly comparable. Intrastudy comparisons have assumed equivalence of the Stanford-Binet and the Wechsler Scales,[1057] the Stanford-Binet and the Griffiths Mental Development Scale,[618] and the Cattell Infant Intelligence Scale and the Stanford-Binet.[888] Interstudy comparisons with these tests and the Wechsler Preschool and Primary Scale of Intelligence[1156] or the considerably dated Terman and Merrill Test[666] are equally difficult to interpret. These comparisons also include interobserver differences. While each of these tests is a valid instrument, between-instrument comparisons are not as accurate as intrainstrument studies.

The above problems have made research on verbal-performance differences,[55,450,661,1096,1156] individual subtest differences,[42,1096] and measures of academic skills[42,618,1155,1156] of limited applicability.

Research to Date: Persistent Findings

In spite of the problems cited above, some findings seem to persist. Nonhydrocephalic meningomyelocele children are comparable with their general-population peers in terms of the range of IQ scores; however, in the nonhydrocephalic group, fewer children score in the middle of the curve, and more children score at either end of the curve, particularly at the "dull-normal" end.[274]

Uncomplicated, unshunted meningomyelocele children vary in intelligence scores as a function of the level of lesion.[55,1009] This finding agrees with studies[83,414,423,569,867,1254], cited by Young,[1249] that suggest that active movement during the first 2 years of life may be necessary for perceptual and cognitive growth. However, other studies[119,395,415] reviewed by Young,[1249] including his own research, disagree. In addition, that greater paralysis and associated upper extremity motor impairments depress test scores may be too simple an explanation for three reasons. First, more complications, such as infections, bleeding, and brain malformation, occur with higher level lesions. Second, children with higher level lesions are more likely to have cerebrospinal fluid (CSF) flow abnormalities, which cause cognitive deficits. Gustafson and Hagberg[437] found that their patients with hydrocephalic dementia suffered from general cognitive deficits, including memory dysfunction, as well as decreased perceptual performance and inductive reasoning, but retained verbal ability; after being given shunts, 50 percent of their patients improved, with a significant increase in visual-spatial and perceptual-motor performance. Third, upper extremity abnormalities are not necessarily related to lesion level.

In shunted populations not controlled for infection and bleeding, patients with surgically treated hydrocephalus scored significantly lower (87.7) on IQ tests as compared with their siblings (109.5)[1086] and lower than meningomyelocele patients without symptomatic hydrocephalus (70 versus 90 in Tew and Laurence,[1156]; 87.7 versus 102.3 in Soare and Raimondi[1086]). However, when McLone and associates[740] excluded CNS infection and bleeding, both nonshunted (IQ, 102) and shunted (IQ, 95) children were tested within the average range. In addition, when we excluded these same two variables, our data agreed with McLone and associates' findings.[740]

Seattle Study

Our study of intelligence scores and achievement test data from 60 children born with meningomyelocele was designed with the previously described research problems in mind. We analyzed Wechsler Intelligence Scale for Children (WISC) scores (first test only) and Wide Range Achievement Test (WRAT) scores for children grouped by functional motor activity (L2 and up, L3-5, and S1 and down).[1009]

Seattle Data: The Relationship Between Lesion Level and IQ Scores

We found that in meningomyelocele children, the higher the lesion, the lower the score on the full-scale and performance IQ tests as a whole and particularly on three subtests in those children without shunts. Children with L3-5 and S1-level lesions obtained scores within the normal range. The subtests demonstrating the results of the severity of motor loss were information (range of general factual knowledge), picture arrangement (anticipation of consequences, temporal sequencing, and time concepts), and block design (nonverbal concept formation, spatial visualization, and the analysis of a whole into component parts). Since the latter two subtests are timed tests and require hand-motor function, the lower IQ scores may reflect UE incoordination rather than IQ or intelligence deficits.

In contrast, motor-level function was not related to intelligence scores in our children with shunts. Loss of this predictive relationship with shunting may reflect several factors, including CNS structural differences in those who do develop hydrocephalus severe enough to require shunting, changes subsequent to the brain wall expansion that is characteristic of the hydrocephalic process, or alterations in the corpus callosum with the build-up of CSF.

Seattle Data: The Effect of Shunting on IQ Scores

While previous studies[666,808,1086] report lower cognitive scores in children with shunts than in those without, our intelligence scores did not differ significantly as a function of shunting when functional motor level was not considered. This disagreement may be accounted for by our exclusion of children with infection, bleeding, brain anomalies, and other complications affecting shunted hydrocephalus more frequently than nonshunted hydrocephalus. Earlier studies did not exclude such cases. In our study, shunts were associated with performance IQ scores that were significantly lower than verbal IQ scores.

Seattle Data: Intelligence Profile

The 60 children scored within normal range on five subtests of the Wechsler Intelligence Scale for Children (WISC). Cognitive skills demonstrated by those subtests *not* to be lower than the norms included (1) range of general factual knowledge (information); (2) language development and word knowledge (vocabularly); (3) logical categorical thinking (similarities) (discussed in more detail later in this chapter); (4) social intelligence (comprehension); and (5) visual alertness (picture completion). The high verbal and social skills of these children has led others to describe them as "talkative" or "chatterbox" personalities.[45,445] As elaborated later in this chapter, such "cocktail personality" behavior may mislead health care providers and educators.

On all of the other subtests, the 60 children scored below the norms. Full-scale IQ (92.0) and verbal-scale IQ (95.6) were within the average range. However, performance-scale IQ (89.4) was significantly below the norms. A potentially more useful and empirically more relevant method of analyzing WISC scores is to examine the three WISC factors described by Kaufman.[573] These are verbal comprehension abilities (VCA), perceptual organization abilities (POA), and freedom from distractibility (FFD). Our children were within the average range for VCA. However, the subtests on which they scored significantly lower than the norms were all of those that load on the FFD factor and the majority of the subtests from the POA factor. Other common and underlying traits shown by the lowered subtests are acquired knowledge (arithmetic), integrated (right-left hemisphere) functioning (picture arrangement, block design, and coding), speed of motor response (coding), and memory (digit span, coding, and arithmetic). These results support findings of memory deficits in children with meningomyelocele.[236] Long-term memory deficits would be implied by the low score on arithmetic. Digit span is a measure of short-term auditory memory for numbers. Coding requires short-term visual memory of symbols.

Seattle Data: Verbal Versus Performance IQ

Significant differences between the verbal and performance scores on an IQ test are frequently attributed to the discrepancies between a particular child's learning style and his or her ability to handle varying types of stimuli. The verbal IQ score significantly exceeded the performance IQ score for our total sample (96.6 and 89.4, respectively). Forty percent of the children in our sample, versus 5 percent of the general population, had greater than or equal to a 12-point difference (a significant difference at the .05 level, according to Kaufman[573]) between verbal and performance scores ($p < .001$). In 17 out of these 23 individuals, the verbal IQ exceeded the performance IQ, whereas in six of the cases, performance IQ was significantly higher than verbal IQ.

Since the performance subtests of most IQ tests require complex motor responses, we should consider whether the findings in these studies actually reflect nonverbal reasoning skills that are deficient or whether poor hand function, described below, interferes with adequate measurement of nonverbal skills.

Informal Verbal Assessment and Abstract Reasoning

The clearest concept that emerges from a review of the literature on individuals with meningomyelocele is the need to acknowledge, assess, respect, and work within the framework of individual differences. This need, highlighted by the wide range of scores and large standard deviations reported on most cognitive variables, is especially important when using verbal interaction as an informal method of estimating an individual's scholastic and skill aptitude. This type of common informal evaluation would seem valid since vocabulary correlates highly with intelligence, but it is actually likely to result in expectations of a higher level of overall functioning than could be realized when used to assess individuals with meningomyelocele and/or hydrocephalus. The similarities subtest provides an example of the difficulties. Psychologists tend to interpret an average or better score on this Wechsler subtest as indicative of unimpaired abstraction, but Willner[1222] found that the WAIS similarities score often indicates a facade of, rather than actual, abstraction ability. Rapaport and associates[891] described this subtest as a measure of concept formation requiring definitions based on verbal coherences between objects and their generic terms established in everyday experience (*coat* and *dress* equals *clothing*). These "verbal coherences" become so overlearned that a good score on a similarities subtest may require no abstractive component. Therefore, similarities scores may be no more reflective of abstractive abilities than verbal expression is of global intelligence. As mentioned earlier, the total group was not different from the established norms on only information, comprehension, picture completion, similarities, and vocabulary, with the latter two reflective of verbal expressive skills; all other WISC subtest scores were below established norms. Thus, clinical impressions and informal assessment of these children by the verbal responses would be likely to tap their areas of strength without accounting for their areas of relative weakness.

The practical manifestations of misleading informal impressions can be seen in Sam's case. Repeatedly, this apparently highly verbal patient convinced nurses he understood how to catheterize himself, but he frequently contracted urinary infections. His verbal performance did not reflect his inadequate abilities. Daily sessions with visiting nurses using a highly specialized educational approach corrected the problem. Instructional elements included visual plus auditory instruction, memory devices, repetition of a highly structured technique that remained consistent over time, cueing, fading of instruction, and reinforcement for successive approximation until the young man had mastered the technique. Visual memory devices included posters on the wall detailing an outline of all steps involved. A memory device consisted of charting the time of catheterization, volume obtained, appearance of the urine (to monitor for signs of infection), medications taken, occurrence of diarrhea (a side effect of some of the antibiotics), and steps taken to treat the diarrhea if it occurred. Given the above amount of assistance and daily visits of the nurses, the learning process required a few months in an individual who had been perceived as capable of mastery with three or four demonstrations. It goes without saying that the task at hand was complex (for a more in-depth discussion of bowel and bladder management, see Chapters 9–12), and health care professionals frequently underestimate the complexity of self-care programs they expect patients to incorporate into their daily living activities. However, the example above demonstrates how misleading verbal performance can be and that a detailed educational program for health care may be essential.

Sam's difficulty with learning to catheterize himself may have been due to not only cognitive deficits but also to problems responding physically to the tasks required of him. Functional and academic tasks, like the IQ scores mentioned earlier, can be inhibited by cognitive *and* motoric deficits. For this reason, it is important to distinguish between these problems. Identifying strengths and weakness in these two areas will allow parents and professionals to develop more effective therapeutic and educational approaches to help children with meningomyelocele successfully perform activities of daily living as well as academic tasks (see Chapter 17).

UPPER EXTREMITY FUNCTION, VISUAL PERCEPTION, AND VISUAL-MOTOR COORDINATION

Upper Extremity Coordination

Upper extremity incoordination is an identifiable problem for children with meningomyelocele, and those with hydrocephalus may be at particular risk.[421,1195] This incoordination may be due to (1) cerebellar causes, frequently leading to an ataxic quality of movement and most likely related to the Arnold-Chiari malformation,[1096,1195] (2) a pyramidal cause, possibly secondary to the effects of hydrocephalus on the cortex or to other spinal cord anomalies,[305,1195] and (3) behavioral causes—for instance, these children may have limited opportunities to use their hands for manipulation and exploration since they often use them instead for balance and support.[968,1195]

Fine motor skill involves the use of the hands and fingers in the prehensile approach to grasping and manipulation of objects.[588] Also included in performance may be elements of speed and strength, bilateral hand use, hand dominance, and motor planning ability. Fine motor or upper extremity performance may easily be compromised by neurologically based problems such as tremor, abnormalities in muscle tone, and paralysis or weakness of muscle groups.

For some time, a high frequency of uncoordinated and immature hand function has been identified in children with hydrocephalus and meningomyelocele with hydrocephalus.[445,615,997,1242] More recently, investigators have looked specifically at children with meningomyelocele (with and without hydrocephalus) and have found similar upper extremity incoordination. Sand and associates[968] and Grimm[421] found depressed scores on the Jebsen Taylor Hand Function Test, with Grimm reporting that 82 percent of the meningomyelocele children in that study had scores below the second percentile (−2 standard deviations). All of these authors found Jebsen scores of children with higher lesions and/or more marked hydrocephalus to be significantly lower than scores of those with lower lesions. Sand also showed a negative effect on hand function scores when IQ scores were below 79.[968] This relationship may reflect the more global deficits in children with higher level lesions, as mentioned earlier in this chapter.

Other specific characteristics of hand function also appear to be impaired in the meningomyelocele population. These children show poor timed scores in simple tasks, but they do show some improvement with practice.[41] Their approach to fine motor tasks could be called precise or deliberate, and rarely do they develop continuously flowing movements without considerable practice. Children with meningomyelocele may rely heavily on visual feedback in fine motor control and may lack the kinesthetic awareness that allows many repetitive motor acts to be performed at a more subconscious level.[41] Authors who have suggested that these children have dyspraxia or difficulty planning motor movements may have observed this phenomenon.[140,605]

Delayed development of hand dominance may also contribute to decreased hand skills in this population.[39,997] A large number of children with meningomyelocele show not only mixed hand dominance but also left-handedness suggesting left hemisphere damage.[45,660,997] Delayed development of normal hand dominance may contribute to deficits in bilateral integration, identified by Brunt.[140] The latter deficits may, in turn, interfere with self-care tasks such as shoelace tying and buttoning.

None of the authors who have reported on hand function in this population have suggested a linear relationship between IQ scores and upper extremity performance (other than some indication of predictably poorer performance with IQs below the normal range). These children appear to suffer from specific impairments of motor control and neurologic abnormalities of the upper extremity. Wallace[1195] found that 69 percent of her sample of children with meningomyelocele had neurologically abnormal upper extremities, including pyramidal tract dysfunction, cerebellar ataxia, chorea, and dyspraxia. The type of dysfunction was not related to lesion level. Indeed, clinically, we have frequently come across children with sacral-level lesions and minimal lower extremity paralysis, but with significant upper extremity tremor and incoordination which then interfered with functional skills.

We evaluated fine motor performance, as measured by the Jebsen Taylor Hand Function Test,[547,1150] of 94 of our meningomyelocele patients between 6 and 20 years of age; we performed 244 tests between 1974 and 1984. These children had IQ test scores of 80 and above, as measured on standard tests (WISC, Stanford-Binet), so the effect of impaired cognition on direction following was minimized. Each subject's test scores were evaluated to see if his or her general performance was worse, equal or better than −2 standard deviations below the mean. Serial scores consistently fell in one group or another. In cases where scores showed variation, the most recent scores were considered. If differences between dominant and nondominant hands occurred, the former was considered.

Results (Table 16-1) indicate few differences between the L3-5 group and the sacral group, but marked differences between these two groups and the thoracic-high-lumbar group. A full 67 percent of the high-level lesion children showed impaired hand function, while only 23–29 percent of the lower level lesion groups had impairment. The results also indicate that hydrocephalus, brain anomalies, or complications associated with hydrocephalus may play a significant role in determining upper extremity performance. In all groups, those without shunts showed a much lower incidence of scores below −2 standard deviations than those with hydrocephalus and shunts. While children with shunts and high-level lesions tended to have low Jebsen Taylor Hand Function scores, children with shunts and low-lumbar- or sacral-level lesions frequently demonstrated hand function within 2 standard deviations of the mean. The high percentage of all these children with scores below −2 standard deviations, when compared with the normally expected distribution (2 per-

Table 16-1
Jebsen Taylor Hand Function Test-Seattle Data

	T10-L2 (N = 15)			L3-5 (N = 48)			Sacral (N = 31)			Total Group (N = 94)		
Jebsen Score	With Shunt	Without Shunt	Row Percentage	With Shunt	Without Shunt	Row Percentage	With Shunt	Without Shunt	Row Percentage	With Shunt	Without Shunt	Row Percentage
Above	20%	13%	33%	44%	27%	71%	32%	45%	77%	36%	31%	67%
−2 SD	(3)	(2)		(21)	(13)		(10)	(14)		(34)	(29)	
Below	67%	0%	67%	27%	2%	29%	20%	3%	23%	31%	2%	33%
−2 SD	(10)	(0)		(13)	(1)		(6)	(1)		(29)	(2)	
Column Percentage	87%	13%	100%	71%	29%	100%	52%	48%	100%	67%	33%	100%

cent), continues to indicate, however, that these children (even with lower level lesions) are at risk for hand function incoordination.

Handedness was also evaluated in this group: 22 percent of these children were left-handed, as compared with 7 percent in the general population.[223] Distribution of left handers was fairly even among lesion-level groups. Handedness did not appear to influence performance on the Jebsen Taylor Hand Function Test, with many left handers appearing among the unshunted group and the group performing above −2 standard deviations.

Visual Perception

Visual perception is the visually perceived relationship of the body to its spatial surroundings and to the objects situated within these surroundings[1189] or the cognitive processing or interpretation of information gathered through visual channels. Visual perception enables a child to understand spatial qualities as well as to recognize and interpret forms and symbols.[393] Aspects of visual perception include perception of depth, figures versus the ground, form constancy, visual closure, and position in space.

The question of visual perception function in these children with meningomyelocele is less clear-cut than that of upper extremity impairment, particularly since some studies indicate children with meningomyelocele do have visual-perception deficits, whereas others indicate they do not. First, using the Frostig Developmental Test of Visual Perception (DTVP),[376] Miller and Sethi,[756] Sand and associates,[969] and Tew and Laurence[1156] found that children with meningomyelocele performed significantly below their age level; children with hydrocephalus and higher level lesions demonstrated the most impaired performance.[969] Furthermore, children with meningomyelocele and hydrocephalus have been reported as having deficits in figure-ground concepts as well as being unable to perceive the total spatial configuration of a shape. Investigators felt these deficits could not be attributed to motor deficits.[756,841]

In contrast, when Gressang[420] used the Frostig DTVP, meningomyelocele children with and without hydrocephalus performed within normal limits. Land[605] and Eng[306] found similar performances using subtests of the Southern California Sensory Integration Tests and the Motor Free Visual Perception Test, respectively, with groups of meningomyelocele children. After looking at these studies, we are still left with the question of whether or not these children have specific visual-perception deficits.

Examination of the testing tools used in these studies indicates that Frostig DTVP scores may be biased and are therefore lowered by poor eye-hand coordination. Three of the five subtests require a fairly complex motor response to indicate the child's interpretation of visual material. One of the subtests is even called "Eye-Motor Coordination," indicating the emphasis on the motor response. In the work by Sand and associates,[969] children with meningomyelocele (with and without hydrocephalus) demonstrated the lowest performance in this subtest. In addition, work by Eng[306] demonstrates that children with good eye-hand coordination perform similarly on the Frostig DVPT and the Motor Visual Perception Test, a test with minimal motor response, but children with poor eye-hand coordination show lower scores on the Frostig DTVP than on the Motor Visual Perception Test.

Twenty-five children in our clinic population between the ages of 48 and 108 months and with low-lumbar- or sacral-level lesions were tested with the Motor Free Visual Perception Test. All children had IQ test scores greater than or equal to 80 (based on standard IQ tests). The mean perceptual quotient for this group was 96.3 (test mean, 100; SD, 15). This adds strength to the argument that for children with lower level lesions and adequate general cognitive skills, visual-perceptual performance (with motor components eliminated) tends to fall in the normal range. Larger numbers, including children with thoracic-level lesions, will need to be evaluated to determine if lesion level, hydrocephalus, or CNS complication associated with hydrocephalus influence performance.

There also appears to be a strong correlation between visual-perceptual performance and IQ scores. Tew and Laurence[1156] and Sand and associates[969] found significant correlations between performance on IQ tests and tests of visual perception. This suggests that visual-perceptual skills may be an expression of overall intellectual capacity, that the particular tests we use to measure visual perception require strong perceptual cognitive components, or that the tests we use to measure cognition require visual-motor competence. Children with meningomyelocele should be tested in this area, but test tools must be selected carefully so that they are not invalidated by the requirement to use complex motor responses.

Visual-Motor Coordination

Visual-motor coordination involves elements of both motor skill and visual perception. It implies the pairing of interpretation or processing of visual stimuli with a coordinated motor output or response.[84,458] We will focus on fine motor responses, with skills such as writing, tracing, drawing, and copying representing activities requiring visual-motor coordination. Poor performance in such skills could indicate deficits in the visual perception of stimulus figures and/or difficulty in motor execution. (For a more in-depth discussion of handwriting, see Chapter 17.)

Table 16-2
Beery Test of Visual Motor Integration-Seattle Data[a]

	T10-L2 (N = 11)	L3-5 (N = 42)	Sacral (N = 24)
Mean age of Visual Motor Integration score	141	115	116
Mean delay from chronologic age	60.6	25.2	18.8

[a] All values are in months.

Observations of eye-hand incoordination in this population are common and may be as high as 95 percent.[1045] Sella and associates[997] described problems with handwriting and related them to eye-hand incoordination. Such tools as the Beery Test of Visual Motor Integration reveal significantly lowered scores for children with meningomyelocele[306,740,1086,1096] and depressed scores for these children compared with their siblings.[1086] Soare and Raimondi[1086] and Spain[1096] found that children with meningomyelocele and shunted hydrocephalus had significantly lower eye-hand coordination scores than those without hydrocephalus, but the former's prblems may be due to CNS infections rather than shunts,[740] as mentioned earlier.

The Beery Test of Visual Motor Integration[84] evaluates visual motor response involving processing of visual information and then directing an accurate motor response. We evaluated 124 tests on 81 children between the ages of 4 and 17 years, with standard IQ test scores greater than or equal to 80. In the case of multiple test scores, a mean score for each child was analyzed. Results (Table 16-2) indicate a strong influence of lesion level on this type of task, with more delayed performance seen with higher level lesions. However, even in the sacral-level group, the mean score in visual motor skills was almost 19 months below the chronologic age. Of the total 124 tests evaluated, only 53 (42.7 percent) reflected performance within 1 year of chronologic age. Children without hydrocephalus and shunting were present in the lumbar- and sacral-level groups only. Their scores did reflect better performance than the shunted children.

An apparent relation between age and test scores occurred, with scores for these meningomyelocele children tending to decline with age. For children below 120 months of age, the mean delay from chronologic age was 10.2 months; for those 120 months and above, it was 44.3 months. Of those children with serial test scores, most showed a downward trend, unless all tests were done before 120 months of age, in which case scores tended to be stable. It is not clear whether this finding reflects test construction or represents a specific problem among children with meningomyelocele in interpreting very complex visual-motor information.

SUMMARY

Numerous functional deficits secondary to impairments in upper extremity coordination, visual perception, and/or visual-motor coordination may be seen in the child with meningomyelocele. Young children may be delayed and imprecise in early play skills such as putting blocks in and out of containers, playing with pegs and puzzles, or stringing beads. Children with little success in these skills may shy away from them[39] and be reluctant to play or practice with crayons and scissors as they become older; thus, impairment can accrue. Visual-spatial deficits can impair the ability to easily manipulate a wheelchair or walker and, in conjunction with upper extremity incoordination, can delay attainment of wheelchair transfer skills. Wallace[1195] reports that upper extremity abnormalities are significantly associated with inadequate ambulation (see Chapter 15). These difficulties may, in turn, interfere with education, as is discussed in Chapter 17. In the classroom we see definite impairment, both cognitive and motoric, in writing,[39] in reading comprehension,[247b,300,1085] and in arithmetic. As these children get older and hope to learn to drive automobiles (with or without hand controls), problems with depth perception and inadequate reaction time may keep them from attaining this skill.

Considerable overlap and interplay exists among the concepts of upper extremity function, visual perception, and visual-motor coordination as well as intelligence. This is particularly reflected by school performance (see Chapter 17). When impairments are discovered in a meningomyelocele child's ability to carry out any functional or educational activity, it is imperative that these aspects of performance are broken down as clearly as possible for evaluation in order to plan appropriate treatment or educational approaches. Impairments must be identified as early as possible in order to help children with meningomyelocele avoid functional and educational difficulties later on in life.

Gayle Fay, David Shurtleff
Hillary Shurtleff, Lynn Wolf

17

Approaches to Facilitate Independent Self-Care and Academic Success

In Chapter 16, we identified potential intellectual and physical problem areas that might interfere with functional and academic skills, such as independent self-care and learning at school. This chapter presents practical means of dealing with those deficits. We have combined our discussion of self-care and school since these two important aspects of development overlap. Competence and independence in performing activities of daily living are dependent on motoric skills and essential for normal socialization in school and, thus, for academic success. As discussed in Chapter 2, not only must able-bodied peers be taught to accept children with major malformations, but these children must be made as normal as possible. A child who has not been taught independence may be caught in a negative cycle. For example, a child who is not independently mobile may (1) miss recess and, thus, be prevented from developing normal relationships with able-bodied peers; (2) miss classroom time if classroom activities involve field trips or if the child takes an excessively long time to get to and from the bathroom or to get to different classrooms; (3) miss opportunities for concentrating on schoolwork or for developing a sense of self-worth due to peer teasing; and (4) be prevented from developing a sense of self-confidence to be independent as a result of all of these factors. In order to avoid this negative cycle, children must be encouraged to become independent at self-care skills as early as possible and to become as integrated as possible into local school systems.

MYELODYSPLASIAS AND EXSTROPHIES: SIGNIFICANCE, PREVENTION, AND TREATMENT
 ISBN 0-8089-1816-8

INDEPENDENT SELF-CARE

In the normal population, training in self-care skills automatically takes place in the home, with most children essentially independent with basic personal care skills by the age of 8–10 years. However, research by Sousa and associates[1094,1095] has pointed out that many children with meningomyelocele and intelligence in the normal range show substantial dependence in these self-care areas, particularly in management of bowel and bladder functions (see Chapter 12). This may, in part, occur because teaching independent self-care to children with meningomyelocele may not take place in the home due to (1) low parental expectations for a congenitally malformed child, (2) a protective attitude toward pushing the child, (3) a parental perception that it is faster for the parent to do things for the child, (4) parental difficulty accepting the reality of portions of the congenital malformation, such as urine and stool incontinence; (5) sphincter impairment of a type that renders continence extremely difficult; or (6) other impairments that cause continence programs to fail (see Chapter 12). Despite these obstacles, however, emphasis on self-care training should not wait until a child reaches school. The earliest ages at which independent skills are acquired (see Chapters 12 and 15 and later in this chapter) suggest that a significant percentage of children with sphincter impairment and lower extremity paralysis are delayed in achieving independence in self-care because of attitudes and expectations.

By kindergarten age, normal children are able to fully dress themselves (with slight help with fasteners and possibly a few cues), toilet themselves, eat meals independently, and be mobile. It therefore becomes the responsibility of the health care team working with young children and their families to begin emphasis in this area early and to promote parental expectations of independence in self-care skills. A child's motivation is enhanced by his or her success at tasks, and self-care skills are some of the earliest functional tasks the child acquires. By promoting independent function in these areas, we can hope to not only enhance the child's inner motivation to succeed at an early age, but we can also help parents to see their child as someone who can succeed.

Mobility is an important self-care skill since apathy, particularly lack of curiosity and initiative, may be caused by early restricted mobility.[80,148,150,817,1212] Apathy and restricted mobility are linked with lower school performance and lower IQ scores.[82,150] In addition, curiosity has a positive relationship with IQ scores and performance in school.[150,254,565,593,1212] Although the literature on whether or not purposeful movement during the first 2 years of life affects perceptual and cognitive growth is equivocal, we believe that functional mobility should be stressed in children with congenital malformations so that they can develop optimally.[106,123,150,337,388,548,961,1045,1213]

The solution for these children is to get them as mobile as possible as early as possible (see also Chapter 15); children in walkers and children in wheelchairs may be given motorized chairs. These children might be taught to be mobile as early as most children start to walk—at around 1 year of age. At that time, children get a lot of positive feedback for walking, and they learn not only to be mobile, but also to take initiative, to take responsibility for themselves, and to have self-confidence. We believe that children with meningomyelocele will receive similar positive feedback leading to independence if they also learn to be mobile.

To encourage parents to promote independence in all areas of self-care, we must provide them with appropriate and achieveable expectations for their child. Sousa and associates[1094,1095] have demonstrated that the level of paralysis is crucial in determining the degree of independent function that can be expected, but a wide variability in performance occurs within lesion-level groups. This variability may be due to differences in parental expectation, physical deformity, and/or eye-hand coordination (discussed in Chapter 16).

Okamoto and associates[825] and Sousa and associates[1095] have reported specific expectations for performance of a variety of self-care skills for meningomyelocele children with different lesion levels (see also Chapters 12 and 15). They have documented the ages at which 20 percent, 50 percent, and 80 percent of the children with meningomyelocele at varying lesion levels are able to achieve specific skills. Of importance in their methodology is the identification of not just the age at which the child *can* accomplish the task, but the age at which he or she routinely *does* the task. The latter implies complete responsibility for an activity, which is essential for being independent.

To make this information clinically useful and to allow continual feedback to parents, we converted Sousa's tables into graphic evaluation forms that allow visualization of the child's current performance in the manner of the Denver Developmental Screening Test[364] (Fig. 17-1; Figs. 12-4–12-6; and Fig. 15-2).

Children are evaluated using these forms on a yearly basis, and results are shared with parents. We encourage all children with IQ scores of 70 or above to be in the earliest 50 percent of performance. For skills where performance is delayed, limiting factors are assessed and alternative training strategies are presented. This yearly focus on self-care skills emphasizes their importance to families. Frequently, children can do tasks, but do not do them routinely due to time constraints. In these cases, it is often helpful to teach the parents strategies for improving speed during noncritical times such as weekends and during the summer.

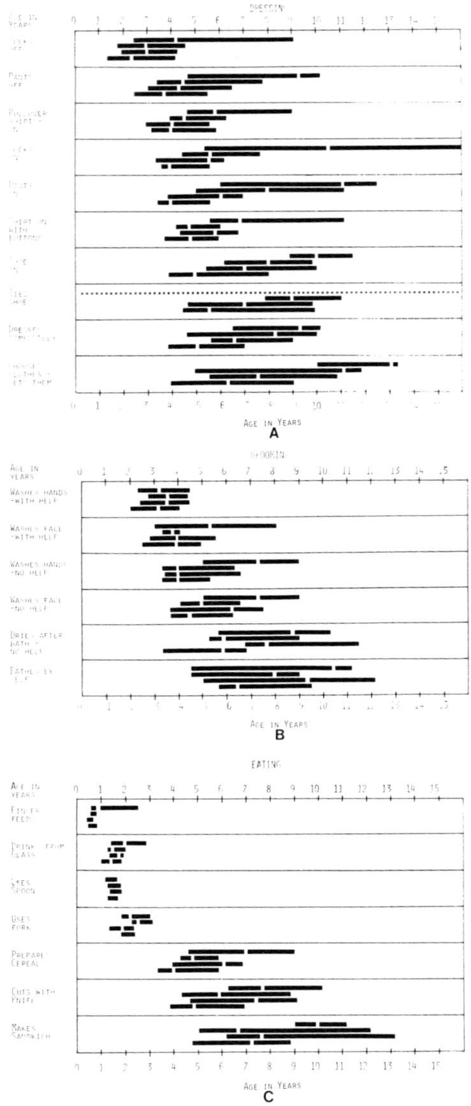

Figure 17-1. Self-care skills. The age at which 20 percent, 50 percent, and 80 percent of a group of 173 children learned (A) dressing, (B) grooming, and (C) eating skills is indicated by the beginning of, space between (white space), and end of the black bars. Triple asterisks indicate that this group never achieved an 80 percent learning proportion. The bars in each category represent, from top to bottom, (1) thoracic and L1-2; (2) L3 and mixed lesions, L2-4; (3) L4-5; and (4) sacral-level groups. All data were recorded as the child achieved the skill during the 2.5-year period of the study, within 4 months of entering the study, or when the caretaker entered a specific date of achievement in the child's diary. These charts and those in Figures 12-4–12-6 were created from data published by Okamoto and associates[825] and Sousa and associates.[1095]

An earlier age of attaining independent care skills not only enhances the child's self-image and independence, but also relieves parents or caretakers of time-consuming, infantilizing care tasks.

As we have seen improvement in personal care skills such as dressing, bathing, eating, and bowel-bladder management, we have become aware that other areas of dependence may keep the young adult with sphincter and lower extremity muscle impairment from active participation in the community; for all of their academic training, many do not adequately know how to use money, tell time and/or understand time concepts, provide their own address and phone number, use public transportation, etc. (see Chapter 19). As these skills are vital to independent community participation, thorough evaluation of performance in these functional community living skills should be a regular portion of periodic assessments. Educators should also be aware of the possibility of gaps in these functional skills.

TREATMENT APPROACHES

When deficits are identified, three specific treatment approaches, described below, may be used at home, in therapeutic situations, or in preschool or school settings. What little literature exists to support the relative value of intervention programs suggests that it is important to consider that programs be implemented early, include parent or caretaker involvement, and continue throughout childhood.[126,135,145,196,259,580,955,980] Unfortunately, these studies of mostly cerebral palsied and mentally retarded children emphasize that social and personal interaction skills are the only sustained benefits observed. Many authors suggest that few, if any, of the studies supporting intervention are scientifically valid.[126,135,333,508,875] Because of the importance of self-care skills and social skills particular to the group of handicapped with sphincter and lower extremity impairments discussed in this text, we believe there is a need for further studies of intervention specifically aimed at studying programs directed at helping them overcome their specific problems. Until then, only generalizations derived from the large numbers of studies of intervention programs for children with other types of impairments can be applied to children with sphincter, lower extremity, and Arnold-Chairi impairments.

DEVELOPMENTAL PROGRAMMING

In the first approach, developmental programming, children are encouraged by parents or other instructors with a "high dose" of normal developmental activity in "at risk" areas, the hope being that additional emphasis and practice in potential problem areas will minimize deficits. Rosenbaum and associates[947] describe such a program for children with meningomyelocele. During the first 12 months of life, parents were given instruction in carrying out a developmental sequence of activities focusing on hand skill and eye-hand coordination. Participation in the program did not improve overall developmental scores, but the authors feel their results suggested some tendency toward higher skills in the eye-hand coordination and performance portions of a developmental test, particularly for children with better potential for mobility. The authors also noted that parents seemed to appreciate having additional information about what to expect from their children as well as structured activities with which to encourage them. Developmental centers and parent-infant classes for congenitally malformed children, in which many of our families become involved, typically use this approach.[508,956] In our area, children with the diagnosis of meningomyelocele generally qualify for these programs and may begin participation even before measurable delays are identified. At this point, no research describes the effectiveness of these programs, although many parents are enthusiastic.

REMEDIATION

The second treatment approach, remediation, is used once a child clearly has problems in a particular area. Age should be considered when using this approach because skills may be more likely to generalize in younger children due to greater central nervous system (CNS) plasticity, a concept believed by some,[1088] denied by others,[333] and questioned by most[126,145,259,508,956,980] as not scientifically documented. Remediation consists of repetition of a set of graded tasks in the domain of concern; for instance, if a child has poor fine motor skills, remediation activities might include putting small objects in containers, stringing beads, pinching clothes pins, etc. Additional practice in such activities theoretically carries over to functional activities such as buttoning and snapping. Studies of children with social deprivation, developmental delay, and cerebral palsy show gains from such activities to be minimal, with little if any carryover.[126,135,145,259,508,955,980] Repetition of fine motor tasks is commonly used with children identified as having visual, perceptual, and/or visual-motor coordination deficits. In such cases, sets of worksheets with tasks of figure-ground discrimination, shape discrimination, or eye-hand coordination are used.[377] Again, improved performance on worksheets theoretically carries over into such activities as reading, arithmetic, and handwriting. Using this approach with meningomyelocele children, Gluckman and Barling[404] used the Frostig worksheet program;

while they found significant improvement in the Frostig test scores, they did not measure changes in related functional academic skills. Therefore, their results may be misleading. Whether or not improved performance on specific worksheets generalizes to general academic function is controversial. Improvement in these test scores may just reflect training the children to take the test, but without carryover into other functional areas.

COMPENSATION

The third approach, compensation, is often used after other approaches have not produced sufficient results or when the child is relatively older or more disabled. Developing methods of compensation is the central element of the philosophy of rehabilitation medicine, and many rehabilitation techniques are drawn upon. Basically, the child's functional performance is evaluated, and areas of functional impairment are identified. Specific strategies are then developed to help the child learn to perform these specific skills as independently as possible or to compensate for the underlying problem.

In the area of dressing, this might include adapting clothing by using Velcro fasteners for someone who cannot button or using Velcro-fastening shoes for someone unable to tie. Special markings might be put on a child's shoes to identify left from right. A child having difficulty orienting clothes for dressing might be shown an orderly sequence for proper placement, possibly with the use of key phrases or mnemonics, and then helped to practice this repetitively. Picture cards or signs may also be created to help a child with sequence.

While no research is available demonstrating the effectiveness of these approaches, case examples are frequent in our clinic. Improved performance is generally seen quickly and easily when appropriate compensations are provided, although general intellectual level seems to be related to the ability to use certain adaptations or devices. Other, more academic approaches, discussed below, may be more appropriate for school settings.

EDUCATION

General instructional formats as well as appropriate classroom placement are crucial in enhancing educational performance and satisfaction in children with both physical and mental impairments. We believe this following information is most useful when it is applied relative to individual situations since children, their families, their schools, and their teachers all differ dramatically.

Preschool Educational Programming

The mandates of Public Law 94-142, discussed in Chapter 2, require consideration of education for preschoolers. Some programs offer services from birth to 5 years of age, others from 3 to 5; some school districts offer home-based programs. From the standpoint of linguistic, cognitive, and preacademic development, center-based programs operating 4 or 5 days a week with parent or caretaker involvement to improve home environment are most effective.[a] Often, the child with physical and mental impairments has little opportunity within his or her home or neighborhood for meaningful play with peers. Contact with a center or special education program can provide such an opportunity. Furthermore, staff professionally trained in the areas of occupational and physical therapy, adaptive education, communication disorders, and early childhood education have the expertise to design programs that achieve developmental learning objectives while at the same time compensating for or going around areas of deficit; for example, computer activities can be used to facilitate perceptual development in a severely physically impaired child. Such program modifications can be taught to parents for continued learning experiences in the home.

These programs are rehabilitative in nature, providing individual or small group therapies and then offering opportunity for supported and educationally programmed transfer and generalization of those skills into preschool classroom activities. This crucial link in constructing a preschool educational program maintains and extends the specific skills being taught in individual therapies as well as ensuring their incorporation into functional strategies. The focus of these programs is more often than not functional insofar as they promote skill in the basic activities of daily living—mobility, orientation, self-care, feeding, communication, and, most important for a child, play. The consensus of most developmental theorists quoted above is that home and community involvement, including play, facilitates the development of symbolic reasoning, communication, and strategy skills. Learning through play with peers (or side by side) offers opportunities for observation of how a slightly more capable peer performs, resulting in teaching and sharing information and skills for instrumental problem solving. These concepts are expressed as the need for total environmental integration for impaired infants and children in order to allow them to attain their maximal capacity.[b]

---

[a] See references 126, 127, 135, 145, 194, 196, 259, 580, 585, 677, 956, 980, and 1109.

[b] See references 126, 127, 135, 145, 194, 196, 259, 580, 585, 677, 955, 980, and 1109.

Classroom Placement and Instructional Format

We provide classroom instructional programs in a variety of formats, each of which can be individually modified to meet the needs of the child with physical or mental handicaps. One format is the mainstream classroom consisting of a teacher trained for either elementary or secondary levels; such classrooms have from 25 to 30 students and can accommodate only children with minimal needs for help with self-care skills. Under the umbrella of special education are a number of other alternatives. A resource room program serves children for periods of time from 30 minutes to 3 hours, offering individualized skill-building programs in all academic areas as well as supplemental instruction augmenting learning activities occurring in the mainstream classroom. Thus, each child with a physical or mental impairment placed in a resource room has dual placement in a mainstream classroom and a resource room. This creates some special problems; logistics of scheduling are extremely important. In order to efficiently instruct, the resource room teacher often groups students according to skill level irrespective of grade. However, without careful consideration of the instructional activities the child is missing in the mainstream classroom, the interface between the two programs is ragged.

To solve these problems, the following are suggestions that one of the authors of this chapter (Fay) has found to be effective. Loss of academic instruction may be exacerbated by children having to miss school in order to attend to special toileting activities, therapy sessions, medical appointments, and surgeries, all of which should be scheduled after classes or during holidays when possible. Otherwise, these children fall further behind in mainstream academics because they are missing the explanatory presentations in certain areas, not because of academic or cognitive deficits. In the worst of cases, there is no consideration toward achieving an effective interface between the two programs, and children are given homework assignments that are (1) incomprehensible because they have not been explained and (2) excessively lengthy because they include all assignments missed as a result of the student being out of the classroom.

Often, through neuropsychological testing, we identify the idiosyncratic learning styles of children with various mental and physical impairments. When interpreting these impairments, we welcome consultations with the mainstream classroom teacher who may have never encountered that type of mentally or physically impaired child. The teacher can be perplexed at the divergence of skills and abilities in such children as well as chagrined at the child's failure to make progress with routine instructional procedures and curriculum materials. The resource room teacher, who as part of the job description allows time for such consultation, can suggest alternative activities as well as assist the mainstream classroom teacher in maintaining appropriate levels of expectation for these children. Specifically, this may include changing assignments, that is, reducing the quantity and complexity of mainstream assignments. At the same time, the subjects may be provided for the impaired student as augmentive materials such as (1) tapes of classroom reading, social studies, or science tests, (2) "written down" or simplified versions of test materials (this is especially important in situations where the child has impaired reading capability, but grade-appropriate math and science skills), (3) computer learning programs that present similar concepts at a slower pace, and (4) project job cards, which enable the impaired learner to independently work with an older student to achieve the learning objective at a simpler level using a parallel activity. Additionally, the teacher can provide direct instruction in those concepts that must be mastered in order to achieve minimal levels of success in the mainstream setting. Finally, it may be necessary to provide an alternative setting and format for evaluating student learning. This latter activity is particularly important for the student who has difficulty with memory retrieval of verbal information or with rate of production. The resource room setting, with its more relaxed, intimate atmosphere, serves to reduce the anxieties associated with evaluation. Furthermore, evaluation measures, administered one-to-one by the teacher or aide, can be oral or via computer or visual aides. The child may receive additional prompts or cueing as is necessary.

At the secondary level in the departmentalized program, resource rooms are used for direct instruction in subject area classes such as English, social studies, science, and math. We recommend that adolescents with mental and physical impairments sufficient to impede their ability to live independently take a combination of special education, distributive education (e.g., focusing on community living, "survival" skills, and vocational education), and mainstream elective classes (see Chapter 19). This enables these children, with their various ability levels and impaired conditions, to each experience unique individualized educational programming suitable for meeting short- and long-range goals.

However, many schools lack careful course planning and monitoring for the impaired because no one school person is assigned as a case manager to organize the student's program as he or she progresses through primary, middle, and high school levels. Unfortunately, the model for provision of services is frequently diffuse, with several specialists attending to different aspects of the student's secondary education. For example, the psychologist monitors ability structure and affective status, the resource room teacher monitors the provision of special education services, and the counselor monitors class selection and scheduling. Team meetings to establish goal congruence and long-term planning often occur only at the insistence of the parents or when the student is in crisis. Under the best of circumstances, the special education teacher functions as counselor and case manager to the adolescent with mental and physical handicaps. In this role, that teacher should organize psychological, academic, and vocational assessments. Since many of these adolescents experience significant psychosocial stress and dysfunction, the case manager should arrange for personality assessment as well as reviews of affective and social status when the student is not making optimal progress. In the best of situations, information from all specialists is integrated at team meetings where short- and long-range goals and goal plans are established. A broad-based program, targeting development in social and affective areas as well as academic, vocational, and community living skills, will use coordinated resources from the community, such as counseling, social skill training, family therapy, and stress management. The crucial variables for successful education of adolescent students with mental and physical impairments are well-managed coordination of activities and continuity in maintenance and fine-tuning of the broad-based educational program; this is the essence of the Individual Education Program (IEP) mandated under Public Law 94-142, the Education-for-All Law (see Chapter 2).

Special note needs to be made of the problems arising from mainstream placement of children and adolescents with mental and physical impairments who are nonambulatory, incontinent of bowel and bladder, or have severe motor dysfunction that interferes with communication or the ability to perform pencil-and-paper activities. Although most school programs offer considerable flexibility in serving these children, many districts experience significant limitations of resources when attempting to serve the more severely motorically impaired child. In some districts these children, contrary to the provisos of Public Law 94-142, are relegated to self-contained classrooms with more severely intellectually impaired students. We believe such a placement is inadequate for the child with normal intellect. The rationales offered by school staff in support of this inappropriate practice are lack of aide time or lack of aides specialized in assisting these children in meeting their basic needs; inability to transport these children from one activity to another or out of the building in case of fire; buildings, classrooms, bathrooms, auditoriums, or lunchrooms that are not wheelchair accessible; and teachers who have neither the experience nor comfort level with these children to assist them in classroom activities or in meeting their personal needs. Such support is a right of the child, regardless of a limitation of resources in the school, as determined by the Supreme Court (see Chapter 2). The failure to accept a physically impaired, normal-intellect child often arises because neither mainstream nor special education teachers have received education or training regarding the sphincter- and motor-paralyzed child. In some unfortunate instances, a teacher's first contact with such children is when they appear in the classroom. This type of circumstance hardly bodes for success for student or teacher.

The reality of successful mainstreaming of highly motorically involved children into mainstream classrooms and resource rooms has been dramatically enhanced by technological advances, combined use of public and private resources to bring those technological resources to the child, and recognition of the long-range individual and societal costs of isolating these children, many of whom can be vibrant and creative.[126]

Electric wheelchairs are an important techological advance, helpful for mainstreaming. Even for kindergartners and preschoolers, they afford an opportunity to easily maneuver throughout the school—providing there are no stairs. Again, under the mandate of Public Law 94-142, fewer schools are inaccessible to wheelchairs. However, this is an area that needs continued advocacy. In the city of Seattle, only four out of 12 high schools are wheelchair accessible. Classroom furniture can be rearranged so children in wheelchairs can easily move about the classroom. Personal needs and supplies should be kept in the teachers' or nurses' bathroom. Children needing direct aide assistance can call through bellboy systems tied to personal "silent" beepers or classroom phones. Computers even make possible vocal responses for nonvocal children through speech-synthesizing systems. The microcomputer has revolutionized the capability of physically impaired children to interact in mainstream classrooms or resource rooms. For students who need additional drill or recursive presentation of new concepts, supplemental computer software is effective. Gaming is a highly motivating format for repetitive practice on skills that need to be mastered, such as reading vocabulary, math facts, or spelling words. Simulation games, via computer, are an excellent method of training reasoning, planning, and learning-to-learn skills. A variety of word processing programs are available for the facilitation of creative and expository writing activities.

If motorically involved children also have significant intellectual deficits, they may need to be put into special resource rooms or self-contained programs that still exist to serve these students. These programs offer not only academic and cognitive remediation, but also an integrated regimen of therapies, including speech, physical, and occupational therapy. Furthermore, in these programs, special curricula and teaching techniques are used. The emphasis is most often on building functional skills that can be used in a variety of real life settings. Even in these more restricted settings, students are mainstreamed out to participate in regular classroom activities as appropriate. Also, other children can be mainstreamed into the self-contained classroom should motor impairments render it difficult for them to move freely about the building.

Thus, the child with physical and mental impairments can be served in various educational settings, ranging from the mainstream to the self-contained. Those children with learning disabilities are thoroughly assessed, and individualized educational programs are designed. These programs use specialized placements, teaching techniques, and curricula. Logistically, the best planned programs interface with mainstream programs to provide the most effective instruction in the least restrictive environment.

Specific Problem Areas (Table 17-1)

Other teaching strategies can be developed for children with physical and mental impairments with the help of neuropsychological testing that identifies an individual's strengths and weaknesses. Because of problems already discussed (see Chapter 16) regarding validity and reliability of traditional intellectual and academic measures for these children, psychologists have begun to rely on the use of the Halstead-Reitan Neuropsychological Test Battery to adequately and systematically measure abilities in a variety of areas. This battery assesses concept learning, logical reasoning, attention, flexibility of thought, language, memory (including short-term auditory and visual memory, semantic memory, memory for learned concepts, and incidental memory), psychomotor problem solving, sensory-perceptual-motor skills, and graphomotor skills. The battery approach is essential to assessing the full range of these children's capabilities while at the same time offering sufficient depth to elucidate a clear idea of competence from the wide variability in performance. Also crucial is an in-depth assessment of academic skills. Because of the heterogeneity of cognitive skill deficits in these children, it is imperative that the skills constructs (or models) for each academic area be carefully behaviorally defined and that testing proceed in a fashion that carefully documents levels of performance in academic areas as well as providing sufficient material for analysis at levels where the skills break down or where the child is unable to integrate a skill into a more complex performance.

Concept Learning

Many children with physical and mental impairments have difficulty learning concepts. Children with meningomyelocele and mental impairment are an example. They are unable to attend to the relevant aspects of a concept-learning activity. They need many, many trials to reach

Table 17-1
Neuropsychological Tests for Children With Meningomyelocele

Potential Problem	Test	Measures
Intellectual	Wechsler Intelligence Scale for Children–Revised	
Adaptive problem solving	Category Test	Strategic behavior; logical reasoning using nonlanguage symbolic reasoning skills; concept learning; memory-proactive and retroactive inhibition
	Factual Performance Test	Psychomotor problem solving
	Trails A/B[a] (color form, progressive figures)	Flexibility of thought, ability to shift between different aspects of a task
	Matching pictures[a]	Ability to integrate visual, spatial, and verbal information in order to solve a task
	Individual performance tests[a]	Perceptual development
Language	Aphasia screening	Review of basic, simple expressive language functions—articulation, naming, labeling, letter recognition, spelling, body part recognition, right/left orientation, arithmetic calculation
	Seashore Rhythm Test	Receptive language
	Speech Sounds Perception Test	
Visual-spatial construction	Aphasia screening	Concentration drawing of simple geometric forms; copying
Sensory-perceptual and motor skills	Sensory perceptual examination	Consistency of response under bilateral simultaneous stimulation; gross motor tapping speed and grip strength; tactile finger and symbol recognition

[a] Battery for 5–8-year-old children.

mastery of a new concept. Even then they are unable to generalize or apply that information to new instances of that concept. Furthermore, because of impairment in the area of memory, they may learn the concepts on one day but be unable to consolidate them into long-term memory and retrieve them the next day. Again, this results in difficulty with transferring and generalizing the information learned to new situations. The implications of this for concept learning are as follows: these children learn best under conditions where distinctive cues are carefully presented, learning activities are broken into simple steps, and frequent opportunities for rehearsal and review are allowed. Once they have achieved mastery, instruction should be directed toward transfer and generalization. Once they have learned a concept and are easily able to apply it across a variety of situations, they should then move on to cumulative review where that concept is incorporated into whatever concepts they have previously learned. Use of this type of instructional format, which is, in effect, the organizational structure of the direct instructional curriculums, should produce reasonably effective concept learning for children having difficulty learning concepts. Also, careful organization and pacing of the increase of complexity in conceptual learning should, with continued experiences of success, reward these children for being more interactive in the learning situation rather than for passively withdrawing in situations that appear overly complex for them.

Writing

Writing includes several skills often taught and measured separately: (1) graphomotor or handwriting skill, (2) spelling, (3) usage, punctuation, and mechanics, (4) creative writing, and (5) expository writing. Often, in assessment, each of these activities is defined as "writing." In the broadest sense of the term, writing is best defined as the ability to express oneself clearly in written prose. However, discussion of the development of these skills in children with motor and mental impairments is clearest when these varied skills are dealt with separately. As an example, children with meningomyelocele frequently have deficits in one or more of the skill areas needed to write adequately.

One of the most common expressions of visual-motor incoordination, handwriting, is an area of significant difficulty for children with meningomyelocele.[39] As a group, they are behind other children.[39,45,514] Anderson[39] and Andrews and Elkins[45] suggest that poor graphomotor skills in this population may be the result of one or more of the following problems: (1) impaired muscle coordination, (2) lack of practice of underlying skills, and/or (3) difficulty processing sensory information and organizing resultant movements. Although many children with meningomyelocele can write cursively, educators note that their letters are not well formed and are larger than their peers' letters and that the children have difficulty with cursive writing and tend to be quite slow.[151] This is unfortunate because it is the subskill on which all other writing skills rest.

Although teachers readily acknowledge the presence of these problems, recognition of their capacity to disrupt the educational process is poorly understood. First, most independent instructional activities entail written drill to provide opportunities to practice and generalize new concepts. The assumption of such educational practice is that printing or writing skills are at an automatic level, thereby freeing the child's attention for concentration on the concepts. However, children with meningomyelocele have such serious graphomotor problems that they must struggle with the letter or number formation aspects of seatwork tasks and, thus, are unable to concentrate on the instructional concepts in the material. Furthermore, their rate of production is so slow that they regularly finish only a third to a half of each assignment. Often, these children are clearly penalized in testing situations where grading is dependent upon speed of production ("timed tests") or upon completion of a certain amount of written work in a specified amount of time, such as in a class period. At the secondary level, many tests are given under those conditions.

When the difficulty in writing seems to be in motor execution, compensation should be considered. This might include the use of an electric typewriter or computer system for word processing since less fine motor control is required. Keyboard guard overlaps that help to eliminate mistakes from excessive or involuntary movement may be helpful in extreme cases of multiple extremity motor impairment such as cerebral palsy. There are a number of systems, such as the Morse Code System (Adaptive Peripheral Inc., Seattle, WA), that interdict the computer keyboard, allowing students a variety of modes of operating the computer if they cannot use a standard keyboard. These include on-off switches that can be operated by head, finger, or toe movements, sip-and-puff devices, and alternate boards that accommodate clumsy or dyspraxic arm, hand, and finger movements. The best of these devices allow the instructor to use off-the-shelf instructional software. This opens the door to a variety of computer-designed instructional remedial materials, particularly in the area of writing skills.

Spelling

Deficits in the area of spelling are pervasive in the population of children with physical and mental impairments. Since processing of sensory information, sequencing, and motor planning skills are frequently impaired in children with meningomyelocele, they are particularly at risk for deficits in this area.[45] Children in the Seattle study, discussed in Chapter 16, performed significantly below the published norms for the Wide Range Achievement Test[546] for spelling (mean, 88.8). These children exhibited a variety of error patterns. Deficits in sequencing affected spelling; for example, *store* was written *stoer*. Some errors related more to a perseverative learning style than to spelling per se; for example, *bloom* becomes *bbloom*, and *summer* may be written as *summmer*. Often, these children can perform relatively well on spelling word lists, but they still are unable to apply their skills to expository or creative writing activities.

Few tests have been developed to assess the full spectrum of writing ability; thus, this area has received little research scrutiny. This is unfortunate because most secondary level educational programs use written tests as the primary media by which students demonstrate their learning of course material. The Test of Written Language[451] is the most comprehensive of existing tests, tapping (1) creative writing, (2) usage, mechanics, and punctuation, (3) spelling, (4) writing vocabulary, and (5) thematic maturity. Since written expression represents a complex and sophisticated integration of cognitive, language, and motor abilities with taught writing skills, it is not surprising that this is the area in which meningomyelocele children exhibit the most striking deficits. However, since the assessment of expressive writing is often omitted from even comprehensive academic assessments, the breadth and depth of these deficits remain unclear. The impact of this impairment is pervasive and far reaching at both elementary and secondary educational levels.

Arithmetic

As a group, children with meningomyelocele are usually unique among the motor impaired because they are relatively farther behind other children in mathematics than one would expect from their IQ scores.[45,1155] Arithmetic skills include not only capability in basic computation, but also in the ability to apply concepts. Deficits in the areas of logical reasoning, adaptive problem solving, visual-spatial reasoning, and perceptual-motor skills often undercut the meningomyelocele child's ability to learn arithmetic skills at an age-appropriate pace. This includes functional arithmetic skills such as the ability to make change, tell time, and use common measurement systems. Heavy reliance on timed tests to measure speeded recall of math facts as well as exclusion of careful and systematic instruction in the area of arithmetic concepts and their applications often exacerbate this situation. We have seen a child with meningomyelocele and hydrocephalus with a normal IQ score take 2 months to learn what another child with an equivalent IQ score will learn in a week.[151]

In general, the meningomyelocele children learn math better if the steps are broken down, slowed down, and repeated. Because of deficits in memory, we suggest providing these children with memory cues. Times tables may be taped to the desks, or number families may be used.[151] Working problems with these cueing devices helps students not only to concentrate on working the problems rather than trying to remember details, but also gives them a sense of accomplishment and self-confidence. After enough practice, students can do the problems without the cueing devices. For children who can't conceptually handle these memory cues, we suggest that calculators be used. Direct instructional curriculum, particularly the SRA Corrective Math Program (Science Research Associates, Chicago, IL), is effective. This program allows a child to move in slow and discrete steps through basic arithmetic concepts of addition and subtraction, multiplication, division, fractions, and decimals. This program has been extremely successful with children who lack a strong visual-spatial base on which to build mathematical concepts.

Reading

Reading is best defined as the ability to decode and to comprehend. Reading uses the subskills of sight vocabulary, word attack (using phonics and structural analysis to unlock new words), context cues (ability to use syntactic and semantic cues to facilitate decoding), and comprehension. A child's inability to achieve a grade- or age-acceptable level of reading can be diagnosed as either an inability to acquire essential subskills in decoding or comprehension or, as is often the case, an inability to integrate subskills into a smoothly integrated reading performance. Such a performance requires attention to visual, auditory, syntactic, and semantic cue systems in the written prose.[396] Therefore, facile reading relies upon highly developed cognitive, perceptual, and language skills. Thus, careful assessment of reading abilities in mentally impaired children will involve a composite battery of reading tests (Table 17-2).

Examination of reading skills of children with meningomyelocele in the Seattle study (see Chapter 16), for example, indicated that they did not perform significantly below the published norms for the WRAT[546] for reading (word recognition, mean 96.8); this test measured only the ability to recognize words, not reading comprehension. The latter should be assessed, particularly since visual-perception problems may lead to deficits in reading comprehension.[247b,300,1085]

Children with meningomyelocele—despite their near-normal WRAT scores, however—are at risk for serious difficulty in the acquisition of

Table 17-2
Reading Tests Useful for Children With Meningomyelocele

Skills Measured	Tests
Sight vocabulary: single words, phrases	Durrell Analysis of Reading Difficulty Gates McKillop Sight Recognition
Word attack skills[a]; phonic subskills	Gates McKillop Sight Recognition Durrell Analysis of Reading Difficulty Woodock Reading Mastery Gallistell-Ellis
Use of context cues	Woodock Johnson
Auditory discrimination; auditory memory	Gates McKillop Auditory Blending and Discrimination Spache
Visual memory	Durrell Analysis of Reading Difficulty
Oral reading and comprehension[b]	Analytic Reading Inventory Durrell Analysis of Reading Difficulty Spache

[a] In order to distinguish whether sight or phonic skills are being used to decode, the test must include nonsense words.
[b] In each test, alternate forms are provided.

reading skills for the following reasons. Perceptual-motor immaturity and deficits contribute to difficulty with letter recognition, particularly those letters that differ only in the basis of their orientation in space: for instance, *b, d, p,* and *q*. The children's ability to scan is also frequently affected. Their ability to move visually across the page with speed is oftentimes limited to taking in only the configuration of one word or a frequently occurring phrase with each movement of the eyes. In the most extreme cases, this impairment is visible as a fixation nystagmus. Understanding and application of phonic and word attack skills not only requires age-appropriate perceptual development, but also loads heavily onto short-term auditory and visual memory, logical and analytic reasoning, and auditory discrimination skills.[396] Integration of decoding with comprehension requires a sophisticated repertoire of strategic behavior and use of varied strategies. Because of impairment in one or more of these basic neurologic functions, comprehension of sophisticated types of reading material is never attained by some children with meningomyelocele.

At the third-grade level and above, reading is a skill necessary for successful and capable performance in subject areas such as social studies, science, and language. Often, children with a good verbal capability but not reading capability cannot keep pace with instructional activities in these areas. Children with deficits in the areas of concept learning experience difficulty with applications and generalization of reading materials. In this situation, access to taped materials may assist these children in independently accessing text information. They also benefit from learning objectives that target the development of well-thought-out plans or strategies for approaching subject area reading activities. For example, in reading a science lesson, the student would first skim headings and bold-faced words, then read carefully through the chapter, and finally underscore unclear areas and sections where teacher assistance was needed. This latter point emphasizes how helpful it can be for the impaired child to have a truly usable version of the classroom text so that it can be annotated for review and organization purposes. This is particularly effective for the student with memory, organizational, or scanning problems.

Reading remediation (Table 17-3) is best undertaken using instructional activities that build subskills such as sight vocabulary, word attack, decoding fluency, and contextual analysis while immediately thereafter requiring that the child apply the skill in oral reading and comprehension. Reading instruction that dwells heavily on subskill acquisition alone without application to general reading comprehension tends to build splinter skills rather than fluent reading capability.[439] In diagnostic reading instruction, the teacher formally and informally monitors percentages of accuracy in decoding, reviews error patterns, and assists students in monitoring their own progress through charts and graphs; this is a successful approach to remediation. Teachers using diagnostic as well as instructional activities soon become able to flexibly individualize their programs by incorporating a wide variety of reading curriculums, including commercial-, teacher-, and student-constructed reading activities. Building motivation and anticipation of success into reading along with independent reading habits is as important as direct instruction in the basic skill. These more important issues are often overlooked. However, it is the hallmark of wise and caring teachers to include objectives in these areas with the hope of instilling a lasting enjoyment of reading.

The Use of Computers

Throughout this discussion of educational instruction, we have referred to the use of computers. Although computers are not a panacea for mental impairment, they are excellent vehicles for interactive learning and for improving concept-learning, attention, and visual-spatial abilities. We believe computers are useful for children at all developmental stages and are particularly effective for children with physical and mental impairments because they combine three factors essential for these

Table 17-3
Reading Remediation

Skills	Program/Activities
Reading development for children unable to use regular textbook series	DISTAR; corrective Reading (Science Research Associates, Chicago, IL)
Sight vocabulary	Games: either teacher-made or commercial using basic Dolch Words (Science Research Associates, Chicago, IL) or simple phonic words; computer-assisted game activities
Phonic skills	
Hearing sounds in words	Lindamood Auditory Discrimination in Depth (Developmental Learning Materials, Allen, Texas)
Blending	Lindamood Auditory Discrimination in Depth (Developmental Learning Materials, Allen, Texas); Orton-Gillingham materials (Educators Publishing Service, Cambridge, MA)
Systematic, slow-paced introduction of basic, phonically regular words	Phonic storybooks (Educators Publishing Service, Cambridge, MA)
Accompanying workbooks	*Cracking the Code* (Educators Publishing Service, Cambridge, MA)
Practice in application of phonic skills	Teacher or commercially available games; computer-assisted games
Comprehension	
Basic development of comprehension skills for language-handicapped children	Comprehension subprograms of *Corrective Reading* (Educators Publishing Service, Cambridge, MA)
General development of a variety of different comprehension skills	Finding the Main Idea, Following Directions, Identifying Basic Facts, Detecting the Sequence (Barnell-Lofts, Baldwin, NY)
Application of comprehension skill to subject area activities	*Be a Better Reader* (Prentice Hall, Englewood Cliffs)
Independent reading—high-interest–low-vocabulary tests	*I Can Read* series (Harper & Row, New York, NY)
Adolescent—high-interest–low-vocabulary materials	Sprint (Scholastic Publications, New York, NY)

children. First, computers are motivating since they are not only visually and auditorily stimulating, but they also employ a game format for repetitive activities. Second, few fine motor skills are necessary for operating computers. Systems have been developed that enable children who cannot access a standard keyboard to use standard software that bypasses the keyboard by employing simple switches; hence, children with upper extremity incoordination are more likely to succeed since they will not be penalized for motor slowness or incoordination and will be able to concentrate on the game rather than on moving appropriately. Third, computer activities offer the opportunity for repeated presentation of instructional activities.

Computer-assisted instruction enhances growth in a number of domains. In motorically impaired preschoolers, programs such as "Facemaker" (Spinnaker Software, Cambridge, MA) and "Delta Drawing" (Spinnaker Software, Cambridge, MA) appear to enhance perceptual skills. "Alphabet Zoo" (Spinnaker Software, Cambridge, MA) and "Kids on Keys" (Spinnaker Software, Cambridge, MA) are examples of many programs that teach readiness skills in a fashion that is novel and entrancing to young children. Abstract reasoning, memory skills, and attention are taught through cognitive skill–building programs such as "The Pond and the Factory."[1136] The LOGO language developed at MIT also teaches skills in these areas, but through the concept of the child as a programmer, who routes a "turtle" across the screen to create magical and exotic figures such as "sprites," all the while exploring spatial and strategic concepts. Academic teaching programs, generally, fall into two areas: drill and practice in a game format as in "Mathblaster" (Davidson and Associates, Rancho Palos Verdes, CA) and simulation games that teach functional applications of skill. Even primary-school-aged children can use word processing programs; easy and accessible is the Milliken word processing program, which uses a picture of a filing cabinet as the graphic presentation of the various aspects of the program's capabilities.

It cannot be stated too strongly: computer-assisted instruction is not a miracle worker but it does offer a window of opportunity for these motorically impaired children to explore and create using systems in which their motor impairments do not impose limitation and constraint.

Behavioral Problems

In our experience, many teachers report that children with motor impairments are extremely dependent, ignore their teachers, talk to their neighbors, can't finish assignments, have cluttered desks, daydream often, and have no sense of time. Children with meningomyelocele as a group are the most notorious. These behaviors may be the result of factors discussed previously in this chapter and in Chapter 16 as well as of a lifetime of success using these maladaptive behaviors with other adults.

Once teachers realize these children have specific behavioral deficits that need to be overcome, teaching strategies can be developed. Teachers who have the most success with these children identify each child's individual problems as well as assets, develop appropriate strategies for each child, and take a firm but considerate approach. We have found that the following strategies are effective: (1) assignments can be broken down into a series of concrete steps and listed for the children to mark off as they progress; (2) if children are particularly distractible, shields may be placed around their desks so that they will not be visually distracted; (3) timers and cues may be used if the children have a poor sense of time; (4) rewards often add needed motivation; and (5) positioning children in front of the class may help them to concentrate on the teacher and class activities.

Although behavioral problems are most often remediated with modifications listed above, they may also be medically treatable. They may be caused by abnormalities in CSF flow in children who are shunt dependent, as is indicated by Gustafson and Hagberg's findings[437] (see also Chapter 7). The authors identified the following specific behaviors resulting from hydrocephalic dementia: disorientation, amnesia, emotional unconcern, lack of insight, psychomotor retardation, and inertia. In addition, adults with occult hydrocephalus suffer from apathy, emotional indifference, lack of insight,[121,437,849] hostility, and aggressiveness.[234,437] Thus, behavioral problems, such as sudden increase in dependence and demanding verbalizations or a decrease in any of the neuropsychological deficits just discussed, may reflect abnormal CSF flow in a child dependent on a CSF shunt. In addition, any child showing changes in personality, greater eye-hand incoordination, sudden decrease in school performance, or lapses in attention may have subclinical seizures. Children with congenital and acquired brain defects are more likely to have seizures.[106,293] Children with a decrease in school performance who are known to have a history of hydrocephalus or seizures should be referred to a physician. Often, relieving a CSF shunt obstruction or adjusting seizure medications can correct behavioral problems, but it may take 3–6 months for a child to overcome his or her behavioral or academic impairments after a shunt revision that reestablishes proper CSF pressure. It may take longer to achieve a proper balance of seizure medications. Therefore, clear communication between families and schools as well as between health care professionals and schools is necessary.

SUMMARY

In this section, we have attempted to define potential intellectual and fine motor skill problem areas pertinent to success at self-care skills and school. Individual strengths and weaknesses must be identified so that appropriate treatment and educational approaches can be developed. Clear communication among various professionals as well as between professionals and families will facilitate not only the development but also the implementation of such approaches. Individual problems must be identified, and approaches should be initiated at an early age since functional and/or intellectual difficulties can compound, affecting self-care as well as academic success and, ultimately, the child's entire life. In addition, ongoing evaluation of each individual's progress is necessary, particularly since children vary so much in their growth and development.

SECTION VI

Psychosocial Adjustment

William Friedrich
Joyce Shaffer

18

Family Adjustments and Contributions

The impact of a congenital malformation is never restricted to the afflicted individual. Members of the immediate family and the larger ecological community[133] of the child are also affected to varying degrees. These relationships and influences are both reciprocal and circular. That is, families are affected by the presence of the congenitally malformed child, and the child is affected by the family's response. Indeed, the satisfactory emotional development of a malformed child is probably more dependent upon the family's responses to him or her than to the extent of the physical defect itself.[88,243a–245b] This chapter discusses pertinent relationships and influences that facilitate good adaptation in one family and maladaptation in another.

Despite the importance of the family's contribution to the development of a congenitally malformed child, relatively little is known about how families of these children actually function.[372] The existing reports of families with congenitally malformed children studied only one family member and/or one specific variable and, thus, had a unidimensional focus. Also, they used only one type of measurement system, such as a questionnaire or interview and thus were unimodal. No prospective longitudinal investigation to date details family adaptation, development, and functioning from the birth of the child to the present.[232]

Most investigators expect pathology in families of congenitally malformed children, as is reflected in their writing. Pathological adapta-

MYELODYSPLASIAS AND EXSTROPHIES: SIGNIFICANCE, PREVENTION, AND TREATMENT
 ISBN 0-8089-1816-8

tions are assumed to be a function of the stress associated with the presence of a child with meningomyelocele.[1152] In fact, a "stress reaction hypothesis" has been developed to explain why the families of congenitally malformed children are frequently seen as maladaptive.[313] However, our clinical experience with families of these children most often suggests that pathological reactions within these families are not uniform. These families and children range widely in terms of their degree of adaptive functioning.[243b] A truly comprehensive model of family adaptation must encompass the range of possible positive and negative adaptations as well as the determinants of positive adaptation.

A much more useful theoretical formulation for research and clinical intervention with families of congenitally malformed children is a competence or coping-based framework. This is a more appropriate alternative to the previously mentioned pathology model in that it emphasizes the tasks and strategies involved in living with congenitally malformed children.[287] Coping, a process not easily described in behavioral terms, varies according to how a family seeks information or takes action (mode), how it solves problems or reduces stress (function), and how adapted it becomes (outcome). With this process, a health care professional can focus on those particular variables or resources that seem to facilitate adequate coping and can answer such questions as the following one: In the separate families of two individuals, each with a similar malformation and an IQ score in the normal range, what aspects of the family account for one child being high on self-help skills and the other child being very low on self-help skills?

In order to identify what facilitates good adaptation in one family and maladaptation in another, we must first describe the stress imposed by the physical malformation. Then we can outline the concept of the family life cycle and how this developmental conceptualization of family growth is useful in understanding adaptation by families with a congenitally malformed child. Finally, we will identify those coping resources that seem to be most useful in helping families with congenitally malformed children.

CHARACTERISTICS OF THE STRESSOR

A congenitally malformed child represents a significant continuing stress within the family and precipitates numerous minor and major crises. These crises compound the normal stress inherent in any family's development and must be considered central to familial functioning. Studies have clearly demonstrated that not only do these families experience increased stress, but frequently the stressors exceed coping resources.[374,502]

A considerable body of stress research has identified characteristics of stressors that make them more or less potent. For example, chronic stress requires a greater coping response than acute stress. This is true of chronic illness, which is a psychological and social phenomenon as well as a physiological one.[698] The predictability or lack of predictability of stressors is also a significant variable in that it is thought that people can more readily cope with predictable stress than unpredictable stress. A considerable body of research[500,971] has shown that life stresses (operationally defined as self-reported life changes) have significant relationships with numerous minor and major health changes, the seriousness of chronic illnesses, and various psychiatric symptoms, including anxiety and depression.

Family investigators identify nine hardships or stressors experienced by families with ill children,[847] including strained family relationships, modifications in family activities or goals, increased burden of task and time commitments, increased financial burden, need for housing adaptation, social isolation, medical concerns, differences in school achievement, and grieving. (Many investigators have found it difficult to determine what is a stressor and what is an outcome.) To some degree, over the family's life span, all of these stressors are operative.

Specifically for families of children with neural tube defects, the initial stress is the actual birth of a child with an obvious physical malformation and possible resultant mental retardation. This stress is unpredictable and chronic in that the family's hoped-for normal child was not born, and the physically malformed child will probably continue to represent chronic and recurrent stress for the duration of the child's life. Initially, confusion, shock, and grief occur.[459,1194] These are often compounded by the issue of selection for life-sustaining treatment.[1058] At our center, we attempt to minimize this initial stress as much as possible through our initial discussion with the parents (see Chapter 5). If the initial decisions at the time of birth are for maximum treatment and retention of custody, the surviving malformed child is a constant reminder to the parents of their sorrow.[1214]

With meningomyelocele, the medically related stress tends to be most intense during the newborn period. The need for constant medical attention and the frequent hospital admissions,[42,370] along with communication deficits between health care providers and families,[244b,459] are additional stressors. Parents are called upon to learn about complex medical procedures, assume home treatment responsibilities, deal with incontinence, lift the growing child, prevent and heal skin breakdown, and handle special equipment needed by the child with paralysis. Limited community resources, the time and effort involved in finding the best care and services, and the financial ramifications of extensive and special interventions are additional stressors on these families.[243a,803,1058] Thus, developmental and medical milestones affect the adaptation response.

The birth of a congenitally malformed child also has repercussions throughout the family's relational networks. The advent of a normal child into a family has a documented negative impact on the marital relationship for the first several years of a child's life.[1132] A physical malformation can presumably exacerbate the initial several-year decline in marital satisfaction; marital satisfaction has been found to be significantly lower in families of physically handicapped, mentally retarded children than in comparison families.[374] Tew and associates[1159] reported less marital satisfaction, a higher rate of divorce, and a lower frequency of remarriage in families of meningomyelocele children than in the control group. The research on divorce rates, however, is equivocal, with approximately half of the studies reporting an increase and approximately half of the studies reporting no difference in overall divorce rates.[959]

Walker and associates[1194] report that some siblings experience marked adverse effects, and many experience anxiety and stress when the meningomyelocele child is hospitalized. The authors also found that, in some cases, older children are called upon to assist in child care to a greater extent than would normally be required. Parents suggest that having a congenitally malformed sibling has resulted in their able-bodied children being more sensitive and understanding of others.

Relationships with relatives, in-laws, and neighbors are affected as a result of the efforts of nuclear family members to cope with the presence of a child with meningomyelocele. Maternal grandparents play a major supporting role, whereas paternal grandparents tend to show far less acceptance. Only 26 percent of families reported receiving help from neighbors while others believed curiosity rather than concern was the dominant attitude of those who lived nearby.[1194] Family social isolation may occur,[284,459] and family routines tend to be disrupted by the need for appointments for medical care and special educational needs.

Toileting programs necessitated by neurogenic bowel and bladder as well as mobility problems provide additional chronic stress as the child develops. The normal child is usually toilet trained and able to walk after the first 2 or 3 years of life, but this is frequently not the case with the child with malformation of the genitourinary tract or lower spine, as noted in Chapters 5–15. Social embarrassment and limits on family opportunity generally persist in what might be termed a prolonged infancy. While no research to date demonstrates a direct relationship between overall severity of the malformation and overall maladaptation in families,[110] one study demonstrates that certain problems, such as toileting and behavior problems, have a particularly deleterious impact on the quality of family functioning and overall marital satisfaction.[375] For these reasons, we have emphasized learning effective mobility (not necessarily biped ambulation) and personal care skills, as outlined in Chapters 9–12, 15, and 17.

The term *chronic sorrow* has been suggested to indicate the ongoing stress and depression families experience in these situations.[1214] At each life cycle transition (see below), such as starting school, becoming an adolescent, etc., the parents reexperience the initial sadness they had at the birth of their congenitally malformed child because they are again reminded of the child's limitations. This phenomenon has important clinical implications. Parents might respond to this reemergence of grief by experiencing their own emotional difficulties or by registering increased concern about their child's progress to the pediatrician or school. The health care professional must be sensitive to the cyclical patterns of grief in parents and must respond appropriately. Genuine educational difficulties (Chapter 17) or learning difficulties due to cerebrospinal fluid (CSF) shunt dysfunction (Chapter 7) must be differentiated from parental grief that is expressed as complaints or concern about an adequate school and a stable state of health.

The cumulative effect of the multiple stressors, most of which are not readily resolved so that their impact persists, is evident in studies finding psychological distress[124] and depression[284] as well as physical illness[803] among family members. The variety of difficulties families confront when raising a congenitally malformed child whose chronic illness requires ongoing care are likely to be evident in the communication difficulties that characterize families under stress.

Family conflict is one of the primary indices of family strains and family breakdown. Nevin and associates[803] use the Conflict Scale from the Moos[774] Family Environment Scale as a measure of family functioning in families with a meningomyelocele child; they report that high-conflict families appear to face a "pile up" of burdens and responsibilities, particularly intrafamily strains, including parent–child, parent–parent, and child–child arguments. Parents in high-conflict families have child management responsibilities and strains that ultimately affect the whole family. There is also an increase in family concern for and about a member who appears to have emotional problems. Nevin and associates[803] further described these high-conflict families as struggling with major family transitions and changes reflective of the ever-changing demands children place upon parents who themselves are undergoing personal and interpersonal changes. High-conflict families score consistently higher on all coping scales than do the low-conflict families and are not to be viewed as dysfunctional or "problematic." The authors described them as family units under stress, struggling to manage hardships. A related bit of research done on families of leukemic children has found that postdiagnosis families of leukemic children report a significant increase in the overall amount of life stress events experienced. These families experience significantly more stress than comparison families, which suggests that one stressful event fosters another.[568]

What is stressful to one family may not be stressful to another family; family A may rate toileting and locomotion problems as much more stressful than family B, which may rate language problems or mental retardation as more stressful. In addition, some evidence suggests that very mild malformations carry with them a certain degree of ambiguity and consequently are very stressful because the family is uncertain as to the appropriate expectations for their child and as to the long-term prognosis for his or her adaptation and coping skills. This concept, known as *marginality*, is so named because marginal differences carry with them a certain amount of stress due to their lack of clear definition.[372]

In summary, a number of variables are related to the relative stress in the family of the individual with a neural tube defect, and a number of particular stresses are germane to these families. The specific stresses and the dimensions along which stressful events can vary in terms of type and severity need to be examined and considered in the clinician's assessment of each family. The investigator needs to include these variables in conceptualizations of how families cope with the chronic stress of a physically malformed child.

THE FAMILY LIFE CYCLE

As any family develops, it moves through a number of transitions and changes. Once a child is born, a family usually makes a number of predictable transitions between the child's birth and the child leaving home somewhere around the end of the second decade of the child's life.[171] These normative transition points comprise the family life cycle. The first transition point requires the two parents to organize around the child and to create a family system consisting of two parents and one child. Once the family has organized around the child and provides a fostering and nurturing environment, 1–2 years will pass; then the family will need to adapt to the next transition, that of the infant becoming a toddler. Following that, the child enters the outside world, usually through the avenue of school. The next transition, around the child's 12th or 13th birthday, is adolescence. Finally, "launching" occurs: the late adolescent is launched into the outside world to begin to develop an autonomous life.

Families with children who have the major malformations discussed in this text are likely to experience difficulty at each of these transition points. We have borrowed from Patterson and McCubbin[847] to present in

Table 18-1
Responsibilities and Challenges in the Care of a Meningomyelocele Child Over Stages of the Family Life Cycle

Infancy (birth to 2 years)
Initial crisis: grieving; intensive medical services including surgery; hospitalizations that interfere with bonding process
Subsequent crisis: delay in locomotion and bowel or bladder training
Preschool (3–5 years)
Ongoing medical monitoring; procurement of therapy services; prolonged dependency of the child requiring additional physical care
Recurrent hospitalizations for cerebrospinal fluid (CSF) shunt revisions and orthopedic procedures
School age (6–12 years)
School programming; ongoing appraisal of the child's development
Establishment of family roles; dealing with sibling discrepancies in abilities; parental tasks
Limited peer involvement
Recurrent hospitalizations for CSF shunt revisions and orthopedic procedures
Adolescence (13–20 years)
Accepting "permanence" of disability
Personal identity
Child's increased size affects care
More need for adaptive equipment
Issues of sexuality and peer relations
Issues concerning loss of biped ambulatory skills
Recurrent hospitalizations for CSF shunt revisions and orthopedic procedures
Launching (21 and beyond)
Discussion of guardianship issues relating to ongoing care of the young adult
Placement plans for the young adult
Parents redefine roles vis-à-vis young adult and themselves

table form the various stressors present at each life cycle phase for families with a child with meningomyelocele (Table 18-1). In addition, these phases and some of the solutions to problems present at each transition point are discussed below.

First, how readily does a parent bond with a child who might be isolated from the parent during medical treatment? What impact might this separation have on getting the parent–child relationship off to a good start? We know little about parents bonding to their congenitally malformed children. Fraiberg[360] has noted that the absence of visual responsivity in blind children requires more effort from the parent and child to bond. This bond will have life-long implications, however.[840] In addition, one of the hallmarks of becoming a toddler is usually the actual act of "toddling," a task difficult or impossible for a child with deficits that impede the normal development of locomotion. Consequently, for many families, transitions through this life cycle would be delayed and would increase the potential of dependency. We have, therefore, emphasized early locomotion with multiple modalities, including the use of braces or a manual or electric wheelchair (see Chapter 15). Six of our children are currently wheelchair mobile at 12–18 months and are, therefore, experiencing brief but increasingly longer periods of time away from their mothers, a normal separation process of toddlerhood.[150]

The school-aged child presents another crisis. Again, parents are compelled to see their child as different from his or her peers. The child is beginning to have to negotiate school and peer relations on his or her own. Can the family enable this transition to occur relatively smoothly, or is this another breakdown in family development?

The advent of adolescence (see also Chapter 19) is a particularly stressful time in any family's life. At this time, the child begins to individuate (become an individual personality separate from the family), and peer relationships begin to exceed family relationships in terms of affective importance. However, physically malformed individuals as a group have less adequate peer relationships than the average person,[3,283,706] and, consequently, the initiation into this life cycle transition point can be considerably delayed (see Chapter 18). Mordock[775] suggests that much of the behavioral disturbance and immaturity displayed by congenitally malformed children is a function of their inability to move successfully through developmental stages as a result of their physical malformation rather than as a result of parental mismanagement. Successful social adjustment includes learning self-toileting skills and establishing sexual relationships. Unmanaged problems associated with the presence of a neurogenic bowel and bladder result in serious social problems starting in the young child and are further complicated by sexual dysfunction in adolescence[177,283,466,1064] (see Chapters 9–12 and 19). Because of insufficient peer relationships, the physically malformed adolescent may turn increasingly toward family for support at this time, but may do so in a way that is simultaneously dependent and ambivalent, thus creating further frustration and stress on the family system. To avoid problems related to stool and urine hygiene, we recommend the toilet training of choice by the family by at least the time of entry into school (see Chapters 9–12).

Finally, the launching transition point is frequently delayed in families with physically malformed children[283,466,1064]; launching is discussed in depth in Chapter 20. Some as yet unpublished research from our center indicates that the families of 17–21 year-olds appear to have the most depressed parents and the most problematic children.[373] This may in part be related to the family's perception that these children are not yet capable of functioning independently; the parents are anticipating a continuation of the chronic strains. With the meningomyelocele patients seen at our center, the much higher dependency rate among teenagers (95 percent) and adults (50 percent) may reflect a later developmental pattern, i.e., a need for longer dependency before the young adult with severe paralysis can achieve independence.[1057] Living arrangements and social and employment opportunities are major problems for many individuals with meningomyelocele. Some are able to achieve true independence with modifications in their living space and the availability of wheelchair-accessible transit systems. Achieving independent employment is complicated by inadequate interpersonal skills,[3] speed and coordination deficits,[1151] and mobility problems.[40] More recently, some improvements in these areas include accessible transportion and the removal of architectural barriers. Employer prejudice is still a problem, however. In general, most jobs for disabled and handicapped workers are available at the labor level in large manufacturing firms[245a] or in sheltered workshops. However, until the larger social system becomes more adept at integrating disabled and handicapped individuals into productive settings, families are going to remain hesitant to "launch" their adolescents. How current changes in our society, as outlined in Chapter 2, and the improved function of our patients, as outlined in Chapters 4–7, will affect adolescence for meningomyelocele children remains to be determined.[426,729]

The concept of a family life cycle is particularly important in the clinician's understanding of the families of physically malformed children. The clinician will more often than not see families presenting with behavioral distress in one or more members at these transition periods. The multiplicity of stressors discussed above would be expected to have a marked impact on the rate of transition in families coping with meningomyelocele individuals. Consequently, the clinican must be sensitive to the impact of these transitions on family development and be aware of how the failure to successfully negotiate a transition can be acutely stressful to the family system.

COPING RESOURCES

As noted above, different families of congenitally malformed children do respond differently to various stressors. However, only recently has attention been given to those variables that appear to moderate or buffer the effects of the stressors germane to individual families of these children. This lack of emphasis is obvious when reviewing the literature, which focuses almost exclusively on the differences between families of physically malformed and able-bodied children rather than relative within-group differences. A more fruitful approach would be to study what it is that discriminates those families of congenitally malformed children that successfully negotiate family life cycle transformations and that respond well to evident stress from those who do not successfully negotiate these transitions or cope.

The impact of a congenitally malformed child on the family system is most likely to be related to the family members' cognitive appraisal of the stress situation and to the family's coping resources.[350] The concept of coping resources presented by Lazarus and Folkman[624] provides a useful basis for understanding the coping process and subsequent familial outcome. These authors delineated six types of coping resources, each of which is assumed to moderate the adverse effects of stress as appraised within the family's cognitive-phenomenological framework. These coping resources include the broad categories of health and energy, problem-solving skills, social skills, social support, material resources, and positive beliefs.

First, health and energy involve an individual's physical and emotional well-being, both prior to and during the course of the stressful event. The study of "chronic sorrow" in parents of retarded children[827,1214] is directly related to such a resource. Second, problem-solving skills involve both global and concrete abilities to research for and analyze information and to generate various sources of action. The ability of a family to solve many of the recurrent problems inherent in raising a congenitally malformed child, such as handling the social embarrassment of incontinence, is related to these problem-solving skills. Third, social skills refer to the ability to communicate and behave with others in ways that are socially appropriate and effective. Social skills facilitate problem-solving in conjunction with other people, increase the likelihood of being able to enlist their cooperation or support, and in general give the individual greater control over social interactions. Fourth, social support means having people from whom one receives emotional, informational, and/or tangible assistance, which may facilitate positive adaptation, as suggested by investigators.[243a,374] Fifth, material resources refers to money and the goods and services that money can buy. Socioeconomic status and family income can have potentially powerful effects on added stress, as can be seen in the studies of Farber,[322] Gath,[389] and Nihira and associates.[810] Essentially, increased income facilitates the family's successful coping in that it allows a family a greater array of medical and educational support systems. The sixth resource area involves positive beliefs. Viewing oneself positively is a very important psychological resource for coping. Included in this category are those general and specific beliefs that serve as a basis for hope and that sustain coping efforts in the face of the most adverse conditions. Hope can be encouraged by the generalized belief that outcomes are controllable, that one has the power to affect such outcomes, that a particular person (e.g., a doctor) or program (e.g., treatment) is beneficial, or by positive beliefs about justice, free will, or cosmic order. Studies of religiosity among families of retarded children[643] as well as parental beliefs in their ability to teach their congenitally malformed child[1131] indicate that this particular coping resource is important.

Mrs. Jones, a 50-year-old single mother and her son, Robert, 17, bring to life some of the concepts we have been discussing in this chapter. Robert is being considered for artificial sphincter surgery. Several stressors exist, including a strained relationship between Robert and his mother, social isolation, and lack of visiting nurse support for Robert once he is back home. From a life cycle viewpoint, Mrs. Jones is moving toward retirement and is less and less open to the responsibilities of a child. She clearly would like to be free of "the burden" as she calls her son. Robert, on the other hand, who should be eagerly looking forward to leaving home and establishing his independence, is poorly equipped socially although he will be graduating from high school with a regular diploma this year. His mother's eagerness to begin her own retirement actually makes it difficult for Robert to be "launched," particularly since he is still ambivalent about his readiness. From a coping resources perspective, the mother's high level of social support from her friends and church are positive signs. But Robert's social support is derived almost exclusively from his mother, and that relationship is strained. Mother and son are intelligent in an academic sense, but both seem to "solve" problems by avoiding or denying their existence. Robert is significantly depressed. In addition, he has only one kidney, so his health and energy are impaired. Mrs. Jones also reports some mild depression and an increase in medical problems pertaining to arthritis. She is stable financially, so their utilitarian resources are adequate. Given this mixture of issues, and the problematic relationship between Robert and his mother, we recommended conjoint therapy for both mother and Robert before surgery is considered an option. Robert needs to be able to perform as a responsible adult to care for his sphincter. Such a reciprocal or circular arrangement among child, family, and medical problem with its solution is evident in this example: Robert needs to be independently capable of caring for his sphincter before he can receive a sphincter that will enable him to be continent and more likely to develop self-confidence and an adequate self-image and, thus, become independent. Appropriate counseling preoperatively may facilitate a greater likelihood of success.

Clearly, the concept of coping resources has considerable utility in the study of familial adaptations to congenitally malformed children, as the family's differential response to stress is not solely related to the potential child marker variables of age, appearance, and severity of malformation. Future study of these families should present a more integrated perspective, assessing the relative impact and potential interaction of each of these six (and, possibly, additional) coping resources within family adaptational response.

SUMMARY

This general overview of family adaptation to a physically malformed child emphasized the importance of a coping model when studying familial adjustment. We have deemphasized research focusing on individual members of a family and emphasized that the clinician and the investigator need to view the entire familial system as a coping entity that is traversing family life cycle transitions with some degree of success or failure. The concepts of family life cycle and coping resources have been introduced to facilitate the reader's understanding of the family's adjustment to this chronic stress. Elective surgical procedures, as illustrated, should be considered within the framework of the family's ability to handle this type of stress at a particular point in its life cycle.

William Friedrich
Joyce Shaffer

19

Adolescent Psychosocial Adaptation

Although adolescents have been traditionally portrayed as subject to a large number of problems and driven by impulses they are unable to control with ordinary psychological means, this perspective is changing to become more positive. For example, Erikson[314] described adolescence as a normative crisis, "a normal phase of increased conflict characterized by seeming fluctuation in ego strength and yet also by a high growth potential." In addition, Offer[822] discussed adolescence as a transitional period presenting the adolescent with a special burden, challenge, and opportunity. According to Offer, adolescents must develop an independent personality, increase their self-confidence, establish comfort and strength in their abilities, make important decisions about their futures, and free themselves from earlier attachments to their parents. This appears to be a substantial list of challenges, but human history leads one to conclude that the majority of teenagers cope with these tasks successfully. In fact, Belsky and associates[86] indicate that among 14–18 year-old adolescents, few, if any, serious disagreements with parents occur. This concept of adolescence as a transitional crisis is directly related to the concept of family life cycle (presented in Chapter 18). According to Offer,[822] families routinely negotiate life cycle transitions with a reasonable degree of success.

Is this current, more positive view of adolescence also true of congenitally impaired adolescents? To what degree is adolescence in an

MYELODYSPLASIAS AND EXSTROPHIES: SIGNIFICANCE, PREVENTION, AND TREATMENT
 ISBN 0-8089-1816-8

individual with an impairment a normative crisis? To what degree is it more difficult to surmount than for an able-bodied adolescent? These questions are difficult to answer with the currently available literature, mainly because the nature of the population has recently altered drastically in two main directions (see Chapter 21). First, in previous eras, repeated infections and far-advanced hydrocephalus led to death or to bedridden, severely mentally retarded individuals with disturbed cerebrospinal fluid absorption. However, due to the advances in surgical intervention described elsewhere in this text (see Chapters 4–8), individuals with these problems currently achieving adolescence and adulthood outside of institutions tend to be *more* physically impaired than independent survivors of previous eras.[292] Second, due to improvements in the same surgical interventions mentioned above and better selection, many complications, such as hydrocephalus, paralysis, etc., can now either be controlled or avoided; thus, *current* surviving infants and young children tend to be *less* severely impaired than patients who are currently adolescents and young adults. Third, the improvements in educational, vocational, and social opportunities discussed in Chapters 2, 16, and 17 should allow the impaired child to become a less disabled teenager. In general, more congenitally malformed individuals now survive infancy and will enter society with better capabilities.[292,729]

The best available data[40] indicate that adolescence for the congenitally impaired is typically a very difficult time and psychologically more problematic than Offer's normative crisis. Anderson and Clarke,[40] in a landmark study, assessed the psychosocial adaptation of over 100 late adolescents and young adults with physical impairments. In this chapter, we will focus on those of their results that are most relevant to teenagers. They interviewed 119 adolescents (15–19 years old), including people with cerebral palsy and meningomyelocele, and their parents. They collected data pertaining to the attainment of independence and responsibility, quality of social life, heterosexual relations, and psychological adjustment and rated their subjects accordingly: just under half (49 percent) were satisfactorily adjusted, and the remainder (51 percent) had "some" or "marked" problems, compared with only 15 percent of the control group. (Additional validation for these prevalence figures comes from teacher ratings and self-report questionnaires.) The main problems were anxiety, fearfulness, and depression coupled with low self-esteem and self-confidence. Antisocial behaviors were significantly less prevalent in the control group. The authors also attempted to determine those individual and familial factors associated with the presence of psychological problems. Cortical damage, seizure disorder, lower IQ, and severity of malformation were related to increased problems, but not uniformly. Depression in mothers, unsupportive families, and enrollment in special schools were similarly related. However, about one half of the subjects had no apparent psychological problems, despite the presence of predisposing factors in a number of them.

Anderson and Clarke's findings[40] are similar to previous reports. Among older meningomyelocele patients, Shurtleff and associates[1057] described the largest problems as low self-image, depression, and poor motivation for achievement. "Delayed adolescence" occurred because physical impairment interfered with mobility, socialization, and acceptance into the process of growing up.[1064] Craig and Van Natta[227] found symptoms of depression, as measured by the Center for Epidemiologic Studies-Depression (CES-D), to be significantly related to the degree of disability. Hayden and associates[466] described the lack of appropriate chores, decreased opportunities to interact and compete with peers (see Chapter 16), and uncertainties about bowel and bladder continence (see Chapters 9–12) as the greatest impediments to emotional growth in a physically handicapped group of teenagers with meningomyelocele. Other problems faced by adolescents with paraplegia include concerns about evolving sexual changes (see Chapter 21), intellectual function (Chapters 16 and 17), stature and mobility (see Chapter 15), details of continuing to cope with the chronic problems generated by the condition itself (see Chapter 21), and the psychosocial impact of all of these factors.[464] Social isolation of adolescents with meningomyelocele has been reported in Australia,[705] England,[673] and America.[466] Finally, Dorner[283] reported that "some degree of misery was very common" in adolescents with meningomyelocele. It is interesting that suicide, a growing problem among able-bodied adolescents, has not been reported nor noted among our population with congenital impairments.

In addition to the practical issues and concerns listed above, adolescents with congenital impairments may have other reasons for emotional difficulties, including problems with body image, cognitive development, establishing a personality independent from the family, and peer social support.

BODY IMAGE

Body image is directly related to egocentricity, a style of thinking in which a person interprets everything that happens in the world as if it were directly meant for the self. Elkind[299] indicated that egocentricity is rampant during adolescence, much as it was earlier during infancy and toddlerhood; thus, adolescents are, in general, acutely aware and vehemently insisting that everybody is looking at, and all behavior is meant for, them.

Due to typical concerns about acne on the face and secondary sexual characteristics becoming noticeable, the able-bodied adolescent's body image is in a state of flux, resulting in considerable anxiety.[578] In addition, the congenitally impaired individual must grapple with a physical defect. Because our society emphasizes physical fitness, athletic prowess, and physical attractiveness, the physically impaired adolescent is left with a body image that is not congruent with what is considered "normal" or desirable (see Chapter 2). Individuals with a very well-developed sense of self and the capacity to separate their personal worth from their physical characteristics may deal with this inconsistency successfully, but most adolescents are not yet this sophisticated. Instead, the physically impaired adolescent may readily believe that disabled body equals disabled person. In fact, in some of the only research done in this area,[578] the chronically ill and disabled adolescents reported significant distress over body image. This particular variable was most significant for groups with visible impairment, such as rheumatology, which caused distress and great dissatisfaction with body image and self-esteem.

The successful resolution of distress over body image is expected when the able-bodied adolescent is less disturbed by developing secondary sexual characteristics, has stabilized in terms of physical growth, and has increasing cognitive maturity, especially an awareness of self-worth as being based not only on physical appearance, but also on a number of less tangible variables. Adolescents with congenital impairments simply have more to overcome since they must learn that a malformed body does not necessarily equal a malformed person. Opportunities for school achievement, career or job advancement, and better peer relationships might facilitate this understanding, but they are usually lacking for most adolescents with congenital impairments.

In an eloquent discussion of the illusory nature of self-esteem in the impaired individual, Anderson and Clarke[40] present three cases: two adolescents were the most physically active and peer-involved and did well in school, but evidenced lower self-esteem than a more impaired adolescent who had slightly more cognitive impairment and a poorer family. These examples underscore the complexity of psychosocial adjustment in impaired adolescents, with body image being only one of the many contributors and, even then, not always a predictable one.

COGNITIVE DEVELOPMENT

According to Piaget,[866] the child becomes progressively more cognitively sophisticated, eventually learning how to think about the world like an adult. Formal operations, a level of cognitive development equivalent to that supposedly used by adults, is characterized by the individual's capacity to formulate hypotheses about his or her own behavior, to act according to a future time perspective, and to think in an abstract fashion. Although latency-age children still use concrete operations and can sometimes delude themselves into thinking that malformations are only temporary, adolescents use formal operations and, thus, realize that their impairments are going to be with them for the rest of their lives.[847] As an example, adolescents with meningomyelocele must realize that they will chronically and consistently have to deal with all of the concomitant issues that comprise their clinical pictures, such as decubiti, obesity, toileting accidents, urinary tract infections, shunting complications, scoliosis, arthritis, limited mobility, subtle impairment of intellectual function, etc. (see Chapter 21).

A common outcome of this stage of cognitive development is a decrease in hope for change. Beck[79] identified one of the most important contributors to depression: hopelessness. In fact, his "hopelessness scale" is a much better predictor of suicide than depression itself. It is not hard to extrapolate from Beck's findings of hopelessness and its relationship to depression; if adolescents feel no hope for change in their condition, at the very least they will experience a depressive episode of uncertain length and may spend much of the rest of their life coming to terms with this hopelessness.

At the stage of formal operations, an awareness of an individual's pattern of cognitive strengths and weaknesses would be particularly helpful along with creative problem solving from people working with the individual. This is evident and essential in the school setting.

In early childhood, efforts at remediation of academic and learning skill deficits seem warranted as described in Chapter 17, but over time, many of our patients experience difficulty overcoming the schools' efforts to remediate fixed deficits when it would be more appropriate to facilitate an increased ability to appropriately compensate for their deficits. Many of our impaired adolescents refuse to be babysat and insist that their parents get them reevaluated. One young man, during the bus ride to his school for the physically handicapped, enjoyed helping a younger student in her effort to learn state capitals, but was also annoyed that he had never been taught the same subject himself.

Instead, his teachers kept focusing on reading and math remediation. He insisted his parents arrange for an evaluation by a neuropsychologist, who provided suggestions for better schooling. Similar suggestions are described in detail in Chapter 17. It is refreshing to learn of a young impaired adolescent capable of being so assertive as to define his school experiences and obtain parental and school support in these efforts. Unfortunately, professionals too frequently experience encounters with overprotective parents and undermotivated students.

If the school is unresponsive to the requests of the student, the advocacy of the parents, and the recommendations of the neuropsychologist, moving to another school may be the preferred resolution; however, this may also present difficulties since another school district is also likely to require the student to take reading and math remediation. This occurred with the young man mentioned above; even after graduation from high school, when he entered community college, his teachers insisted on reading and math remediation in lieu of using creative teaching techniques that would compensate for his deficit skills as well as teach him new information. In some situations, legal recourse may be the only alternative (see Chapter 2).

We believe parents and older impaired individuals need to take an active role in the process of deciding what education is appropriate. Unfortunately, parents are too often intimidated by education professionals and do not use the power inherent in the IEP required under the Education-for-All Law (see Chapters 2 and 17).[245a] We are not suggesting that negotiating an appropriate, career-oriented education will be an easy task. Nor are we implying that school personnel are to blame for the child's failure to thrive in an academic setting. However, there are multiple ways to learn the contents of a worthwhile book, to learn how to live and earn a living, and to communicate the understanding of concepts.

For both the impaired adolescent and the parent, active problem solving as well as learning a vocation, compensation, and an avocation are recommended as a potential antidote for a sense of hopelessness and associated depression resulting from school and social failure. In addition, health-care and education professionals will be better able to help impaired adolescents and their families by using creative, flexible approaches and teaching the adolescent how to obtain appropriate medical care on the open market. Some useful approaches to education have been outlined in Chapter 17.

Individuation

Competence is judged in terms of the success with which the adolescent has been "launched" (see Chapters 18 and 20) into roles outside the family. In fact, texts on adolescent psychology leave readers with the impression that the major function of the family during this developmental phase is to give the adolescent someone to leave. The emphasis is on breaking ties and establishing independence from parents and from unrealistic parental expectations that foster dependency.

Investigators are beginning to become increasingly aware of the importance of the family in adolescent development. The family has always been seen as an instrument for the transmission of values and skills from parents to children. The family systems perspective views each family member's behavior as both contributing to and constrained by an ongoing family pattern.[494] Both individuality and connectedness in family relationships are important in adolescent development.[85] Family systems–oriented therapists stress the importance of the balance between individuality and connectedness in the family as a predictor both of family health and of adolescent individual competence. What are the developmental needs of the adolescent who is beginning to "leave home"? Minuchin,[764] a family systems theorist, suggests that individuated family relationships, characterized by separatedness in the context of connectedness, facilitates this leaving process, giving the adolescent permission to develop his or her own point of view within a secure base that allows the adolescent to explore worlds outside the family.

The important question here is, to what degree do these criteria characterize congenitally impaired adolescents within their own family? The balance between separateness and connectedness is important when examining the relationship of impaired adolescents with their family. Our clinical impression is that families with impaired adolescents emphasize connectedness and deemphasize separateness, resulting in the adolescent becoming more and more fused with the family and less and less separated from it. This situation may, in turn, prevent individuals with impairments from joining the ranks of adolescents who have left home, established identities, and achieved autonomy.[283,466] Reasons for emphasis on connectedness are numerous, but they may be as simple as a normal protective response from the parent who is reacting in a realistic way to the special needs associated with the physical malformation. This initial effort to be supportive could evolve into an overprotective stance.

Mothers of congentially impaired children are routinely accused of being overprotective, but overprotectiveness here is not a simple response of a neurotic mother who needs to keep her child infantile; instead, each member of the family system plays an integral role. First, the impaired adolescent's difficulties will frequently require extra assistance. Second, the parent who responds, usually the mother, is often able to feel that her presence has an impact; thus, a "professional" parent,[324] as defined in Chapter 2, may develop. Third, this feeling of being capable may assume critical importance if the second parent, usually the father, is peripheral to the family and, thus, unsupportive. The impaired child may be the parent's only source of emotional support. In fact, the quality of the marital relationship has as much bearing on the development of overprotective parenting as does any other factor. The cycle of overprotectiveness can be interrupted if the overprotective parent develops a positive, involved relationship with the other parent or with some significant other, so that social support can be derived from another adult rather than the meningomyelocele adolescent.

In addition, for the moderately and severely impaired individual, independence is problematic for very real and practical reasons, and adolescence accentuates the need for parents to search for creative solutions as adulthood approaches. As Darling and Darling[245a] describe, normalization is likely to be threatened. Problems raised by the impaired child's continuing dependence must be faced. Parents must eventually make decisions about their child's future. At this time, "seekership"[245a]—reading books, consulting experts, writing letters, making telephone calls—should be prominent as parents assist the impaired adolescent in grappling with issues of living arrangements, independently obtaining medical care, and finding employment opportunities or other services necessary for independence.

PEER SOCIAL SUPPORT

Peer relationships appear to be most important for allowing an adolescent to connect with the outside world. In fact, the most notable social phenomenon of adolescence is the emergence of the marked importance of peer groups.[86] Usually, if adolescents have an active peer relationship and a well-developed social network, they develop opportunities for separateness apart from the family in addition to the connectedness that still remains with the family. However, studies noted previously have reported social isolation as a significant problem for impaired adolescents. As Anderson and Clarke[40] illustrate in *Disability in Adolescence*, many impaired adolescents have impoverished peer relationships. In their sample, a majority reported at least one friend, but almost four in ten were rated as at least somewhat disliked by peers and almost three of four as at least somewhat solitary; these descriptions, done by teachers, compare with one in ten and two in ten, respectively, in normal children. That teachers tend to have lower expectations for less attractive children may partially explain these findings (see Chapter 2). In addition, as discussed in Chapter 17, bussing and classroom changes may keep children with meningomyelocele from being able to form peer networks.

Due to social isolation, the average adolescent with congenital impairment does not have the necessary opportunities for separateness and has fewer opportunities for identity formation and role taking, two tasks necessary for normal development. Studies of physically impaired, latency-age children indicate that children with significant peer relationship function the best.[372] Consequently, if physically impaired adolescents report that their social networks are impoverished, an apparently valid assumption is that their emotional development is disabled. However, although social isolation and emotional retardation generally do occur, some of the adolescents with congenital impairments seen in our clinic surmount the difficulties presented above, establish peer relationships, and experience normal emotional development. Families and professionals responsible for physically disabled adolescents should assist in the development of social peer groups or entry of the disabled into able-bodied peer social activity. Impaired children brought up with such goals will become peer interactive adolescents, sometimes in activities of which their parents will disapprove.

The absence or diminished presence of peer influences makes the family uncomfortable and also makes the adolescent even more dependent on the family for social support. Individuation from the family cannot proceed in the "normal" fashion for an obvious reason: it is psychologically difficult to leave a situation if there is nothing to take its place.

SUMMARY

We conclude that the outcome for adolescents with congenital disabilities must be programmed in childhood. We highlighted four important variables that contribute to the difficulties many congenitally impaired adolescents do have to negotiate; recommended active problem solving, which often includes compensation for fixed disabilities; and suggested that the delay in traversing adolescent hurdles characterizing individuals with congenital disabilities will tend to require greater parental involvement than would be true of able-bodied adolescents.

Joyce Shaffer
William Friedrich

20

Young Adult Psychosocial Adjustment

Since individuals with congenital disabilities are delayed in resolving issues of adolescence (see Chapter 19), some of this resolution is still in process during early adulthood. Consequently, development of the disabled young adult tends to be delayed and confounded by efforts to work through issues of adolescence. Yet the adolescent task of establishing a separate identity is very different from the young adult task of "launching,"[719] which is described in greater detail later in this chapter. Existing research has some limits in defining the issues of these disabled young adults because of the tendency to combine this age group with adolescents and because of the nature and severity of the problems in individuals with congenital impairments reaching young adulthood today.

The launching of a disabled young adult has been most extensively reported for populations with meningomyelocele and will, therefore, be used as an example throughout this chapter. As explained in Chapters 1, 2, 5, 19, and 21, current populations of meningomyelocele are larger in number and more severely malformed than in previous eras.[292,426,729] These individuals may be so different as to represent a "new disease."[637] Thus, adult psychological adjustment needs to be highlighted to establish necessary areas of research to describe this "new" population and to facilitate a proactive approach in the planning of total care of these impaired individuals. For instance, what are the relative effects if any, of psychological and the medical aspects described in Chapter 21 have on the quality of life of these impaired young adults?

MYELODYSPLASIAS AND EXSTROPHIES: SIGNIFICANCE, PREVENTION, AND TREATMENT
 ISBN 0-8089-1816-8

We believe that these congenitally impaired adults do not differ substantially from the able-bodied in their goals for maximal development, health, happiness, and inclusion within the mainstream of our society, despite potential delays in development, particularly during launching,[719] (Chapters 16, 18, and 19).

According to McCullough,[719] during this family life cycle stage the adult must (1) move toward independence and make decisions about future life goals, including occupational choices; (2) explore and consolidate friendships and choose a possible mate, usually leading to marriage and some state of connectedness with an in-law family plus an eventual new role as parent; (3) address a new state of relatedness with parents and other family members on the basis of mutual adulthood, usually leading to confusion for the young adult as well as for the other family members; and (4) achieve financial independence. In addition, the young adult may (5) produce offspring and, thus, address yet another state of relatedness (parents become grandparents, etc.). Given the "delayed adolescence" characterizing individuals with this congenital malformation,[1064] delayed progress into and through the launching phase seems likely since mastery of one stage is required before moving on to the next.

OCCUPATION AND FUTURE LIFE GOALS

In the previous chapter, we introduced a landmark study conducted by Anderson and Clarke[40] on late adolescents and young adults with physical handicaps. In this chapter, we will focus on the results that are relevant to the latter group. Anderson and Clarke[40] followed young people from England and Wales through what the authors called the "transition year," the period between leaving school and obtaining job placement. This particular study provides an opportunity to examine some dimensions of the qualities of life-style experienced by young physically malformed adults. For example, the authors note that common stressors for these individuals were anxieties caused by long delays prior to their first job placements. Additional stress came from their perception that their abilities were not being fully used as well as concern about whether or not their abilities *could* be fully used.

These concerns might be valid, based on the literature of individuals with meningomyelocele. Our initial survey reviewed individuals born during the preshunt era prior to 1955.[1057] Among these adult meningomyelocele patients, 53 percent were fully integrated with complete self-help skills and were gainfully employed, functioning as housewives, or in higher education; 15 percent had partial self-help skills and were in job training; and 32 percent were in custodial care or living at home with no program. In a more recent review of young adults, we found that 25 percent of our patients were employed.[292] In a group of adults with meningomyelocele without hydrocephalus, Barden and associates[63] reported that one third of the patients with meningomyelocele were in full-time employment. When housewives and part-time employees were included, one half of their patients were considered active in some functional role in society. Similarly, Evans and associates[318] reported that 74 percent of all and 54 percent of the more severely disabled of their disabled men and women with meningomyelocele work regularly. Tew[1151] concluded that deficits in speed and manipulative skills would make one third of his population unlikely to obtain competitive employment and that, therefore, they should be educated to occupy their leisure time fully. (Reduced mobility has also been cited as limiting the employability of these individuals.[40]) In England, 50 percent of the adults were employed or in vocational training courses[663]; over 70 percent were employed in Wales.[613] In Australia, 17 percent were in "open employment."[705] Of the 24 Australian individuals who had left school, nine had attended a rehabilitation center and were disappointed with the time spent there; their expectations of the center's functions and of what they would learn there were not fulfilled, and they experienced problems in communicating with the staff. McAndrew[705] quoted one man as saying: "I feel I didn't gain much there. I would like to have done more office work, but was not given much and never told why they took me off it. Everyone makes smashing suggestions, but nothing is ever done or followed through. It is confusing and disappointing."

All of the authors in the above paragraph were describing a population of individuals from the preshunt era. During the early shunt era, between 1955 and 1975, shunt placement was complicated by shunt dysfunction and central nervous system (CNS) infection. Patients were often institutionalized in homes or schools for the handicapped. Thus, one might expect that adults born during this period would be more severely handicapped than those born during the preshunt era. Our more recent study included individuals who had been shunted during the early years that shunts were available.[292] Of these individuals, only 25 percent were employed.

The employment rates cited for persons with paraplegia vary from 14 to 44 percent in studies reviewed by Trieschmann.[1168] Obstacles to employment cited were financial disincentives to productivity, lack of complete services of the state-federal Vocational Rehabilitation program, and negative attitudes of employers. Unless facilities receive federal funding, no federal law prohibits private employers from denying employment to handicapped individuals.[1205]

Unemployment for young adults with meningomyelocele may be due to a variety of additional factors, including medical problems[663,705] and severe health problems, some involving prolonged hospitalization.[40] Anderson and Clarke[40] cogently suggest that difficulties inherent in moving from pediatric specialists to general medical care providers less familiar with the particular needs of individuals with meningomyelocele exacerbates the medical problems of these young adults.

Evans and associates[318] correlated increasing disability with decreased probability of employment, increased time off work, and increased chance of never working. Our recent survey is consonant with this finding.[292] Mental retardation was reported in up to 36 percent of adult patients outside of institutions and surviving from the preshunt era.[239,318,613,1057] The discrepancy between rates of retardation in these studies is most likely explained by different methods of selecting patients and different definitions of mental retardation. We recently defined 15 percent of our young adults as retarded, with IQ scores below 80.[292] Tew and Laurence[1153] reported that 73 percent of adolescents had an IQ below 90, an IQ score that usually predicts the student will not be able to pass the English General Certificate of Education, implying a mental disability. In comparison, however, Lonton and associates[664] reported that 52 percent of their meningomyelocele young adults were undertaking or had passed these examinations and were undertaking, or had completed, higher education. Smith[1073] reported that 83 percent of 124 meningomyelocele adults age 16–73 years had completed secondary school qualifications in Scotland. Approximately 40 percent had pursued higher education. Our most recent study is in agreement with Smith; 87 percent of our patients either completed high school or obtained an equivalent graduation certificate from a community college, and approximately half had gone on to higher education.[292] Lower than average visual, perceptual, and clerical skills, along with deficits in speed, precision, and manipulation, still hindered the education and regular employment of individuals with meningomyelocele and hydrocephalus.[841] In addition to neurologic impairment and poor educational preparation, other factors accounting for unemployment included lack of mobility[1073] and psychiatric disturbance.[705,1041,1057]

Another important issue described by Lonton and associates[664] is the perception that disabled adults are not consistent workers. Between 16 and 45 percent of working adults with meningomyelocele report frequent unemployment.[318,663,664,1073] However, over 95 percent of those employed had less than 28 sick days per year.[1073] Most patients reported a positive attitude by employers and co-workers and a willingness by employers to modify the work place for those with walking aids or wheelchairs.[663,1073]

According to McAndrew,[705] intellectual ability was more important than physical disability for individuals working in open employment in

Australia; to enter open employment, the young person had to couple intelligence with energy, determination, and a competitive spirit. In some instances, these qualities would need to be supplemented with appropriate advocacy to overcome employers' resistance. For example, one wheelchair-bound young man encountered multiple difficulties, described below, when first getting hired.

When this young man first moved to a new community, he immediately recognized an existing job as one that he could handle with ease. The only requirements were to stuff various papers in a plastic container, which then had to be hung on each resident's doorknob in the apartment complex in which he lived. Since this apartment complex was wheelchair-accessible with slightly over 200 apartments, this part-time job seemed tailored to his needs. However, when he called the employer, a newspaper company, two obstacles existed. First, ten other doors on this route were outside the apartment complex and not wheelchair-accessible. Second, an able-bodied individual was already performing satisfactorily on this route; however the company agreed to put the young man's name on a waiting list with top priority for that specific newspaper route because of its wheelchair accessibility.

However, what sounded like an amicable solution was no resolution at all. Rather than rely on that company's memory, the young man called them every month or so to see if the route had yet become available. Each time they assured him it had not and acknowledged the agreement to give him first consideration for that specific wheelchair-accessible route when the current carrier resigned. And so the pattern continued for approximately 2 years, until the route had been reassigned to a new carrier other than himself.

His attempt at problem solving this unexpected incident was only met with frustration. As he ascended the administrative ladder of the company, information gathered about the chain of events finally revealed that, although this particular route was to be saved for this particular wheelchair-bound individual, the field supervisor had independently decided that "the route would be too hard because of the wheelchair." In spite of admitting that the long-standing promise had been broken, the people in highest authority in that company refused to correct this error at the young man's request; in addition, they were unresponsive to intervention from other responsible community individuals and to the lawyers whose aid he enlisted.

When this depressing situation was mentioned to the young man's physician, the physician called the company, and within a few hours, the company director called the young man with an apology, an offer to begin the route as soon as the young man wished, and a rearrangement of the route to include only wheelchair-accessible doors. In addition to the energy, determination, and competitive spirit described by McAndrew,[705] the proper advocate was also essential in this one instance. Only the physician succeeded in convincing the employer that meningomyelocele, hydrocephalus, and use of a wheelchair do not necessarily preclude adequate job performance.

"Delayed adolescence" might be another factor influencing the low rate of employment among adults with meningomyelocele. The narrowing of educational and vocational alternatives occurs as the able-bodied adolescent explores options and as various choice points approach. However, congenitally malformed youth are often denied the needed exploratory experiences so important to this stage. They also do not achieve the level of vocational development their able-bodied counterparts do. Developing and shaping personal identities through work experiences are often blocked. In some communities, efforts are made to remedy this situation. For example, Seattle-area schools offer work-study experiences in an attempt to facilitate transition into the work place. Ryan[958] described a summer work program at the Institute for Rehabilitation Medicine in New York, providing counseling, career seminars, and job-seeking-skills workshops in conjunction with training on the job site. The disabled youth obtained paid work experiences, opportunities to integrate into the work world, and a realistic evaluation of performance and enhancement of skills, work habits, and knowledge of career possibilities. Data were not cited on the effectiveness of this approach with severely disabled young adults.

In summary, the literature indicates that individuals with meningomyelocele fall short of their able-bodied peers in the key factors of ability and freedom to move toward independence and make decisions on future life goals. The poor employment picture described for individuals of the preshunt era was, as anticipated, worse in the one study of individuals born during the early shunt era.

FRIENDSHIPS AND MATES

Young meningomyelocele adults also experience social isolation: about 50 percent of those surveyed were judged to be severely socially isolated.[284,705] According to McAndrew,[705] 26 percent had not been visited, gone to visit, or otherwise been out with a friend in the year prior to interview. Eight to 25 percent indicated they had no close friends.[284,613,673,705] Dorner[283] described misery to be more common with meningomyelocele individuals than with "normals" (85 percent and 50 percent, respectively). He also stated that 5 percent of the males and 25 percent of the females had had suicidal ideation, with one female making a suicide attempt.

Among our population of older meningomyelocele patients, the largest problems were poor self-image, depression, and poor motivation for achievement[1057]; intelligence and level of paralysis showed a significant positive association with good adjustment in adults.[1041] However, McAndrew[705] reported that the environmental support systems available to the individual since birth, not the severity of the disability, determined the ability to cope with physical and emotional situations. According to his young adults, regular school placement was the preferred preparation for life in the community. The most important lesson they learned in regular classes was about social relationships: 'the basics of getting on with people,'' ''respect for others' feelings,'' ''what is acceptable and what is not.'' The disadvantages they ascribed to the schools for the physically handicapped included poor academic standards, divorce from the normal community, and excessive sheltering.

When Anderson and Clarke[40] followed their sample of young adults past the ''transition year,'' they did not find substantial differences in the overall quality of their social life from year 1 to year 2. In general, the situation was rather poor, with less than one fifth of the subjects thought to have a satisfactory social life. Lack of peer involvement, the most common source of stress among these young adults, affected over 60 percent of the sample to some degree and 40 percent to a severe or very severe degree. The most extreme difficulties with this stress occurred in moderately or severely malformed individuals who had attended special schools so they were both less mobile socially and had fewer opportunities to make friends while in school. The authors conclude that ''it is a cause for great concern that both the psychological well-being of the disabled and the degree of social isolation related so closely to achieving a satisfactory job placement, when the long-term prospects for many are so poor in this respect.''

Social isolation has also affected the long-term physical health of these individuals. Lynch[680] described a biological basis for the human need to form loving human relationships; failure to fulfill this need may result in poor health. Yet, less than a third of those with meningomyelocele marry,[63,318] and of the 11 marriages in Barden and associates's group,[63] 64 percent divorced. Between 25 and 51 percent reported having had a relationship with the opposite sex.[284,613,705,1057] Although all expressed interest in the opposite sex,[284] with so few of these individuals employed, the opportunities for social contact decreased drastically after they left school.

Less than half were members of groups or clubs.[705] McAndrew found that two thirds of his group were in clubs catering primarily to the able-bodied since they viewed clubs and social groups for the disabled as fostering and emphasizing their differences. Half of this study group were opposed to such clubs. Only 22 percent of Evans and associates' group belonged to a group for the disabled.[318] Interaction with the able-bodied would be hampered by lack of equal access to community life. Private owners of hotels, recreation facilities, restaurants, etc., are not prohibited by federal law from denying housing or services to handicapped persons either in the USA or other countries.[1205]

Attitudes further compound social integration. Rating scales designed to measure attitudes of the nonhandicapped toward the handicapped[1251] have found a preponderance of negative attitudes. When positive attitudes were present, they were generally distorted and stereotyped. Stereotypes and prejudices (including the self-defeating attitudes and behaviors of some disabled persons) tend to limit opportunities for handicapped individuals (see Chapter 2).

MUTUAL ADULTHOOD

According to McCullough,[719] the change in relatedness as an able-bodied child moves into young adulthood can be particularly confusing to parent and young adult alike. The degree to which young adults have mastered adolescent tasks in the formation of their own identities will determine how dramatic changes in family relationships will be at this point. The parental response to these changes in their offspring will also influence this adjustment. Each developmental shift precipitates problems relative to unresolved issues of previous stages. In that meningomyelocele individuals are delayed in their progression through these stages, difficulties in transition might be expected. For many, this would be accentuated by finding themselves graduated from high school into the state of being unemployed and lacking job skills. Stress in mothers of these young adults might be related to having a family "off schedule," that is, "having a child who does not become successfully independent when expected."[466] This might be likened to the stress of a "nonevent." Young adults might be expected to respond to the "nonevent" on a personal level as well as with an awareness of parental distress.

Anderson and Clarke[40] noted that some significant sources of stress in these young people resulted from disturbed family relationships, "in some cases resulting in general family strife or continuous tension, and in others in the silent misery of the handicapped young person." In contrast, according to Dorner[284] and McAndrew,[705] young adults with meningomyelocele believe they had reasonably good relationships with their parents in terms of doing things together and finding their parents easy to talk to. More parental encouragement to take part in social activities, do school work, and foster independence, particularly in daily living activities, would have been appreciated by McAndrew's group,[705] though a third of them believed they had been given all of the encouragement and help possible. In addition, the severely malformed often are realistically dependent for advocacy,[754] physical care, and resolution of complex issues made difficult by their subtle intellectual deficits.

FINANCIAL INDEPENDENCE

In our young adults with meningomyelocele, 24 percent lived alone, 33 percent with partners or friends, 36 percent at home with parents, and 8 percent in institutions.[292] In contrast, Lonton and associates[664] reported that 86 percent live with parents in England. Able-bodied individuals in the United States experience longer periods of financial dependence on parents when pursuing a professional education. However, this is generally time-limited, goal-oriented, and socially acceptable. With meningomyelocele individuals, the situation is more ambiguous, characterized by temporal uncertainty, and less socially acceptable because it represents the inability or failure of the young adults to become stable income creators for themselves. Lack of protection against denials of housing to the disabled[1205] exacerbates financial dependence. Unless facilities receive federal funding, no federal law prohibits private realtors or property owners from denying housing to individuals in the USA.

THE NEW GENERATION

While McCullough[719] considers the onset of parenting (and the concomitant redefinition of intergenerational relatedness) to be a task of the young adult, apparently few individuals with meningomyelocele have achieved it. Of 29 surviving patients, three married females had a total of nine children.[63] Thus, only 10 percent of that study group became parents and initiated this transition to the family system. Evans and associates[318] found that the degree of physical impairment affected the onset of parenting: 96 able-bodied patients had between them 75 children (the authors did not indicate the number or percentage of the 96 individuals who had had offspring); in marked contrast, of the 96 with disability, one man had one child, and 15 women had 25 children. Therefore, 17 percent of the disabled group had become parents. Sexuality with meningomyelocele is discussed in more detail in Chapter 21.

SUMMARY

Much is yet to be learned about the adjustment of adult meningomyelocele patients. Few studies have been done on this population specifically. Yet advances in medical and surgical care have increased the numbers of these individuals surviving to adulthood as well as the percentage of those who have done so with significant physical impairments but still able to survive outside of institutions.

Asch[49] stated that since the malformation itself has been found to dominate the awareness of the able-bodied and to obscure the importance of other attributes of people with handicaps, most psychologists have not included handicapped people in their research. However, we need to know whether existing psychological theories and research methods can account for the experience of disabled people. Similarly, investigators have rarely included the experience of people with disabilities in their research on gender and race and have focused more on the impact of the handicapped on the nonhandicapped than vice versa. Asch[49] suggests that we are relatively ignorant of the experience of disabled children and adults in family, school, work, and play as well as of the incidence of psychological and social problems among disabled people.

More research including the handicapped, particularly on the adults with meningomyelocele specifically, is necessary. Research to date on young adults with meningomyelocele describes delayed progress to and through the launching stage of the family life cycle. This social deviance is evident on all five of the tasks required of the young adult, as described by McCullough.[719] Thus, at this point in time, it's essential to anticipate and plan for the needs for goods and services that this increasing population is likely to experience as adults.

In a review of the literature, Varni[1181] stated that little research had been reported on interventions intended to mitigate the apparent negative effects from meningomyelocele on the psychosocial functioning of the meningomyelocele patients and their families. He found that efforts had been exclusively directed at improving the competence of meningomyelocele individuals and/or their parents in some particular illness-related area rather than using traditional psychotherapeutic techniques aimed at improving their psychosocial status.

Darling and Darling's work[245a] is a striking exception. They very cogently point to the need for practical interventions, such as providing information, assisting in advocacy for this relatively powerless minority in American society, and facilitating access to goods and services such as respite care. In addition to these suggestions, we recommend research to assess coping styles, resources, and effectiveness of coping[624] in mengingomyelocele individuals and their families, with interventions as indicated by research findings.

SECTION VII

Long-Term Management

David Shurtleff
Kevin Dunne

21

Adults and Adolescents With Meningomyelocele

Successful surgical treatment of infants born with severe forms of meningomyelocele, reviewed in prior chapters, dates back only one generation; therefore, cumulative experience regarding adolescents and adults with meningomyelocele is limited. As mentioned in Chapter 20, most studies of this population have involved individuals with less severe forms of the congenital malformation or with complications that can now be avoided. Children in treatment programs since the mid-1970s will experience different long-term consequences of their congenital paraplegia. The treatment of children with various types of myelodysplasia can be divided into three eras. First, the preshunt era occurred prior to 1955. Most survivors were severely mentally retarded from uncontrolled hydrocephalus or afflicted with mild, arrested, or no hydrocephalus. The former were institutionalized, so those in the community were mildly affected. Second, during the early shunt era from 1955 to 1974, available treatments were limited, infection common, and orthopedic and urologic therapy evolving. As a result, many treated survivors suffered from central nervous system (CNS), genitourinary, and orthopedic problems that can be avoided in the third, current era. The many advantages to this modern treatment period have been described in prior chapters. Although treatments are evolving rapidly, there remains a large number of children yet to become adolescents with the same spectrum but not the same severity

MYELODYSPLASIAS AND EXSTROPHIES: SIGNIFICANCE, PREVENTION, AND TREATMENT
 ISBN 0-8089-1816-8

Table 21-1
Factors Interfering With the Health Status and Social Adjustment of Adolescents and Adults With Meningomyelocele

Factors	Percentage
Decubiti	85
Obesity	70
Urine leak	62
Scoliosis (symptomatic)	60
UTI	43
Hydrocephalus	40
Arthritis	35
Mental retardation	15
Prolapse of perineum	13
Poor self-image	10

Data are from Dunne and Shurtleff[292] from an interview survey with 37 adults aged 19–41 years of age.

of complications as today's teenagers. Undoubtedly, they will be presenting their problems to physicians in the future. Therefore, this chapter will discuss the problems of these teenage and adult patients who are survivors of outdated treatments.

To have paralyzed legs requiring braces or a wheelchair for mobility, to lack voluntary control over bowel and bladder function, and to lack the sensation necessary to protect half of one's body from injury are barriers to completing the primary tasks of adolescence (see Chapters 9–12, 14, 15, and 19); that is, establishing an identity and becoming independent are hampered.[a] In addition to a number of studies by others, our 20 years of clinical experience provide the basis for the following review.

We have combined our adolescents and young adults into one population in this chapter since medical management pertaining to these two groups is similar, unlike psychosocial adjustment (discussed separately in Chapters 19 and 20). We discuss below a number of separate abnormal aspects of growth, development, and physical health of an individual born with meningomyelocele; these factors directly influence adjustment to adulthood and emphasize how the growth and hormonal changes of adolescence affect the physical well-being of these patients. In addition, we list (Table 21-1) and discuss the most significant health and social adjustment problems for young adults aged 20–30. Others have reported similar problems among adolescents and adults, but have

[a] See references 110, 156, 283, 285, 318, 466, 613, 705, 817, 1045, 1064, and 1125.

emphasized, in addition, subtle impairment of intellectual function,[18,239,318,613,841,1009,1057,1195] seizures,[106,293] painless loss of motor function,[1064] delayed or abnormal development of psychosocial and psychosexual behaviors[110,285,318,466,1057] (Chapters 19 and 20), and perineal prolapse.[292]

PRIMARY NEUROLOGICAL CONCERNS

Hydrocephalus was reported as a cause for sudden death in two adolescent patients cared for in our center in 1977.[1064] Since then we have observed a third. Only three of 20 adolescents were reported as shunt dependent in 1979 by Hayden and associates,[466] and records of our 20–30-year-old population in combination with individual patient records reveal that 30 percent have cerebrospinal fluid (CSF) shunts and 10 percent have enlarged heads and/or headaches suggestive of increased pressure. One patient known to us developed symptoms of increased pressure at 17 years of age, 15 years after removal of a CSF shunt, because of infection. Another with mild cephalomegaly required her first CSF shunt at 27 years of age. Lorber and Pucholt[670] report that 17 percent of 11–20 year-old patients are no longer shunt dependent. Lonton and associates[664] describe hydrocephalus as causing decreased motor abilities and decreased visuoperceptual performance among 11 percent of young adults aged 18–25 years. Some of our female adolescents and adults with marginally adjusted hydrocephalus have complained of headaches premenstrually. We have successfully prescribed diuretics such as chlorthiazide or 1,4:3,6 dianhydro-D-glucitol in usual doses for these headaches (see Chapter 7). Using computer-assisted tomography (CT scans) and radionuclide and pressure studies, hydrocephalus and shunt status should be ascertained as a baseline during optimum shunt function and whenever the adolescent or adult patient has symptoms, no matter how subtle. We are aware of two adult women with headaches not relieved by insertion of a CSF shunt following only a single study showing enlarged ventricles. Two other adults developed pain, paraesthesias, and weakness in their arms. One was studied and found to have hydromyelia, and symptoms abated after CSF shunt decompression. The other adult (Fig. 21-1) developed severe bulbar palsy after a chiropractic adjustment and is now bedridden. He had previously been an ambulator without aids.

Other Neurologic Problems

Epilepsy has been reported in 10–30 percent of patients.[68,106,293,507,666,902] Seizures may be shunt obstruction symptoms, can be associated with brain malformation, or can remain as residues of past

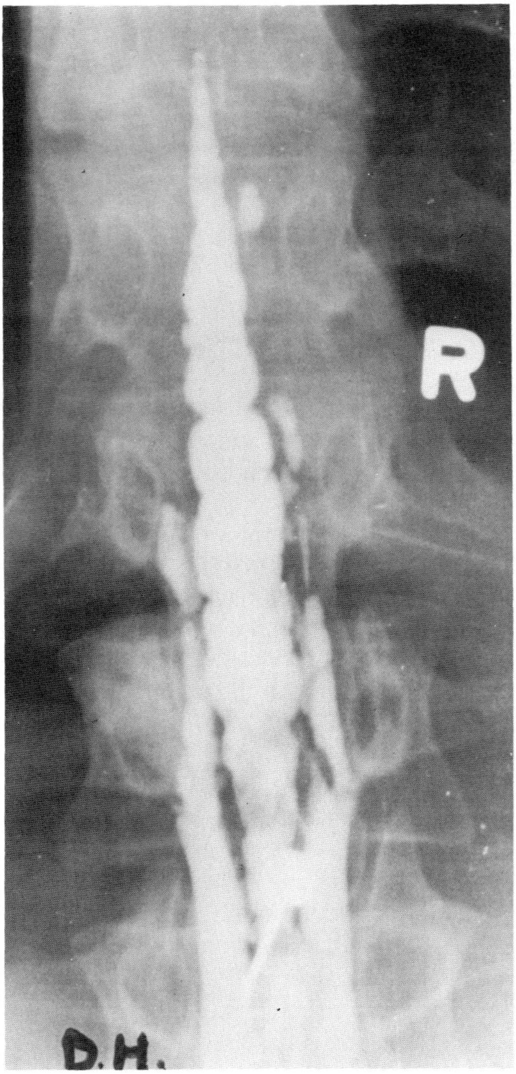

Figure 21-1. An adult with syringobulbia. This shows a thoracocervical myelogram demonstrating a hydromyelia of the central cervical and high thoracic cord (central eliptical white shadow) within a thin-walled cord (between the central and lateral white shadows). Radiopaque dye (white) is also in the subarachnoid space of the cord and is seen as the lateral white shadows. The patient developed weakness and paresthesias of the upper extremities. Following a chiropractic adjustment he developed extensive bulbar palsies and upper and lower extremity paralysis, rendering him bedridden.

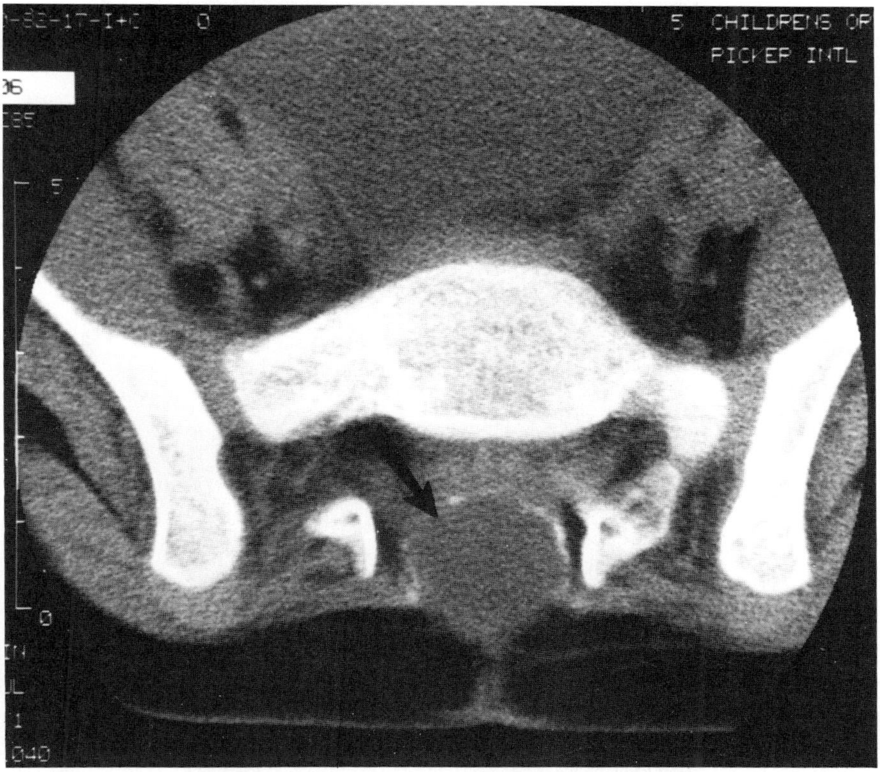

Figure 21-2. Tethered cord due to a dermoid. This shows a computer-assisted tomography scan of the sacral spine demonstrating an open posterior neural arch almost completely filled with a tissue density, which is the almost circular mass outlined by an irregular white border; on slight pressure over this mass the patient screamed in pain. The well-healed scar from previous closure of a meningomyelocele is in the midline directly over the mass and was explored for a neuroma by another group. Our deeper exploration revealed a 2.5-cm dermoid. Complete removal relieved the local tenderness, and the partial paralysis of the lower extremities improved slightly following removal of the dermoid.

episodes of increased pressure or infection.[293] Seizures without overt manifestations cause decreased intellectual performance if not under good control.

Tethered cords from the scar where a spine malformation was repaired or from dermoids (Fig. 21-2), fatty tissue, and herniated disks have been reported in our adolescent and adult population.[1064] These lesions present during rapid growth or increase in weight and during pregnancy. Lipomas (Fig. 21-3) are particularly prone to recur since it is frequently impossible to remove intramedullary fat tissue and to com-

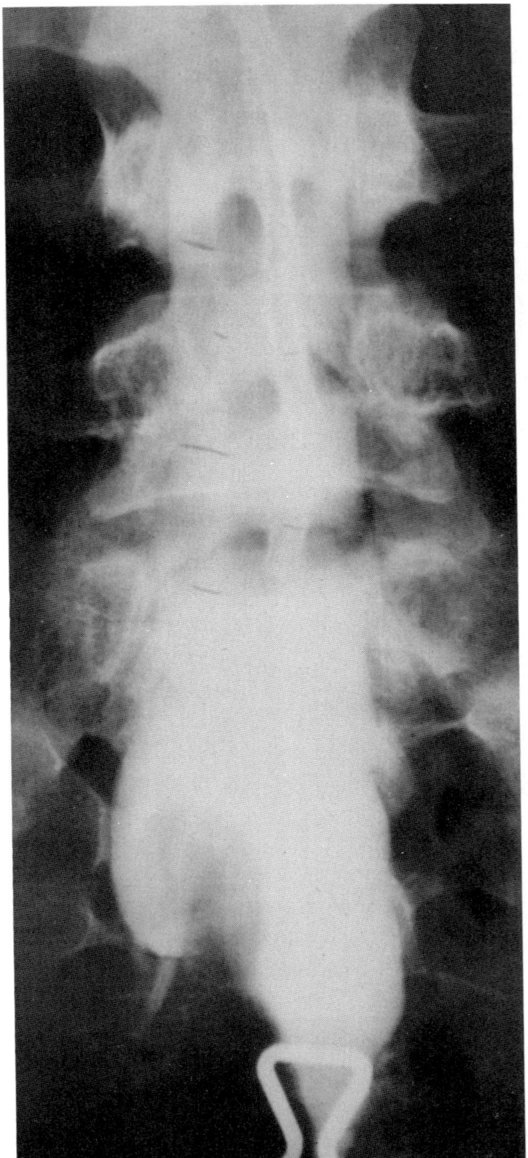

Figure 21-3. Lipoma. This shows a standard myelogram of the lumbosacral spine of a 16-year-old girl with onset of stress incontinence and urinary tract infections. The radiolucent defect in the lower right sacral canal was found to be a lipoma that could be completely removed. Symptoms of urinary sphincter paralysis resolved following surgery.

pletely close the dura (see Chapter 6). Symptoms include local pain and tenderness with or without radiation down the legs, loss of sensation, loss of muscle strength, increasing spasticity, and changes in sphincter or reproductive function. Recently, a middle-aged male with a history of previous spinal surgery for lipomeningomyelocele presented with these symptoms and was successfully operated on with reversal of his symptoms. Two of our older female patients gave us histories of loss of function in their legs during pregnancies many years before. Subsequently, two of our young women became pregnant and developed weakness and pain, symptoms of cord compression (Fig. 21-4). With bed rest they carried to term. Postnatal examinations confirmed the suspicion of herniated discs. Any adolescent or adult with the symptoms listed above should be studied by myelogram.

Renal Function and the Neurogenic Urinary Bladder

Neurogenic impairment of the urinary sphincter and bladder detrusor causes emotional impairment or even death in adolescents and young adults with meningomyelocele. Unfortunately, many individuals in this population today were treated with methods, such as urethrotomy or diversion, that place them at high risk for incontinence and social maladjustment.[285,318,466,613,1057] In the past, many urologists considered obstruction-free drainage of sterile urine more important than adequate, odor-free urine collection. Since the mid-1970s, we have used methods outlined in Chapters 9, 11, and 12 to provide good renal health and socially acceptable methods of urine collection for children with meningomyelocele. Unfortunately, many of today's teenagers and adults have not experienced these more modern and helpful methods of urinary tract management. We have restricted the use of artificial sphincters to older adolescents and adults to avoid complications secondary to growth and possible damage to urinary tracts secondary to teenage rebellion associated with poor self-care, which is a frequent occurrence among our patients.

Forty-nine percent of our adults have ileal conduit surgery, a procedure rarely performed since 1974 (Table 21-2). There are numerous long-term complications such as stomal stenosis, skin ulceration, prolapse, renal failure, infection, hydronephrosis, and stone formation.[753,898,990,1013,1075] Between 10 and 41 percent of renal units, when drained by ileal diversion, are reported to deteriorate by radiographic studies.[753,898,930,990,1075] Although clean intermittent catheterization (CIC) has been recommended by some since 1972,[608] its efficacy has been reported for patients with meningomyelocele only recently.[117,276,603]

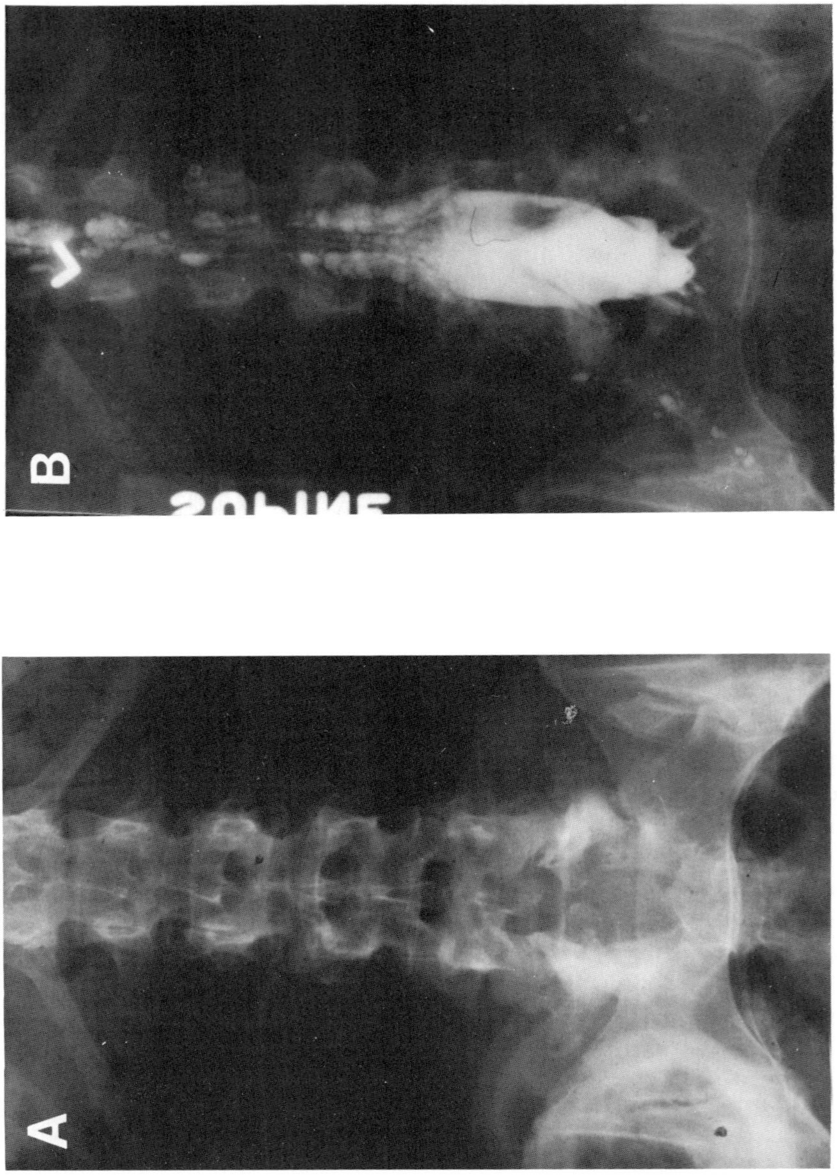
B
A

Table 21-2
Urine and Stool Status

	Urine	Stool	Number	Percentage
No Problem	9 (24%)	15 (41%)		
Odor/leak	14 (38%)[a]	13 (35%)		
Odor/leaking, rare	—	9 (24%)		
Infection/leaking	12 (32%)	—		
Infection/leaking/stone	5 (13%)	—		
Total	40	37		
Urine Collection				
None			9	24%
Ileal Conduit			18	49%
CIC			3	8%
Crede Timed			3	8%
Other			4	11%
Total			37	100%

Data are from Dunne and Shurtleff[292] from an interview survey with 37 adults aged 19–41 years.
[a] Three patients had odor/leaking and infection.

Undiversion has also been recommended, but many patients are either unsuitable candidates or are not willing to undergo the procedure.[411]

Forty-three percent of our population has chronic urinary tract infections (UTIs) (Table 21-2). Previously we reported chronic UTIs and advanced hydronephrosis in 16 percent of adolescent and adult patients; half of these patients had hypertension.[1064] Rickwood and Thomas[930] also reported upper tract abnormalities in 41 percent of 181 adolescents at 16 years of age. During a subsequent follow-up of 43 months (mean), a further 27 percent developed fresh lesions or further deterioration. The risk of upper tract complications was increased with higher lesion levels,

Figure 21-4. Collapse of the intervertebral space with protrusion of the disc: (A) anterior-posterior plain x-ray and (B) myelogram. A 27-year-old white female developed back pain radiating down her left leg with an increased weakness that was originally secondary to a meningomyelocele repaired at her birth. She was 5 months pregnant. Bed rest relieved the pain and stopped the progressive weakness. Because of persistent symptoms after delivery of a normal infant, studies were undertaken. EMG demonstrated membrane instability suggestive of deenervation. The plain A-P film (A) demonstrates missing posterior vertebral arches L4-S2. The myelogram demonstrates a radiolucent filling defect at the L4-S1 interspace found to be a protruding intervertebral disk. Removal of the disk relieved the pain, and the recently lost muscle function returned.

the presence of urinary diversions, and longer periods following diversion.[930]

Little information is available on the degree of renal impairment or the number of patients requiring dialysis or renal transplantation.[318,1057] Rickwood and Thomas[930] stress needless urological deterioration in young adults, primarily due to poor follow-up.

Urinary leakage is a problem for 76 percent of our patients (Table 21-2), and continence problems are reported in 37–45 percent in other series.[318,705] CIC with or without chemical adjuncts or surgery is recommended as the method of choice both to preserve renal health and social acceptability[608] (see Chapter 11). However, little is known about long-term side effects and complications. We have observed complications among males using CIC: six cases of severe epididymitis and one with prostatic calculi. Others report traumatized urethra, urethritis, calculi formation, and epididymitis.[130,277,702] These complications threaten future fertility and are, therefore, real concerns.

Musculoskeletal Kyphosis and Scoliosis

Kyphoscoliosis, a common complication of childhood, increases in 40 percent of lumbar-level patients and 85 percent of patients with high-level lesions during adolescence[566,832,1055] (see Chapter 15). Despite fusion, 60 percent of our young adults have scoliosis or other back problems (Table 21-1).[292] Thirty-five percent of the total group, slightly more than half of those with back problems, have pain, positioning problems, or both. Fifty percent of those with pain are post–spinal-fusion patients. Three of our adult patients have asymptomatic severe kyphotic curves that did not correct with surgery. A fourth is in pulmonary failure in teenage and is expected to live only a short time longer. A fifth developed a decubitus over the gibbus and developed osteomyelitis that took 2 years of bed care and multiple operative procedures to cure. Although instrumentation with various rods and cables has reduced the nonfusion rate and markedly reduced time in the hospital,[832] these procedures have not been used long enough for those affected by them to reach adulthood. Most of our current adult population had fusions without instrumentation and were operated on late, so they were more extensively fused in poor position with residual curves and rigid pelvic obliquity. Fixation of the lumbar spine can prevent the patient with a hip extension or flexion deformity from hyperextending or flexing the lumbar spine as a means of compensation in order to walk or sit. A spine fusion performed elsewhere rendered one of our young adults able to neither sit nor walk. Our orthopedist converted him back to a household walker by performing a girdlestone procedure on both hips. Unless care is taken to

Table 21-3
Ambulatory Status

Motor Level	Wheelchair-Dependent	Wheelchair or Aids	Braces and Crutches	No Aids
L2 and above	75%	25%	—	—
L3-5	8%	38%	38%	16%
Sacral	8%	16%	8%	68%
Overall	30%	27%	16%	27%

Wheelchair-dependent patients cannot ambulate or stand for transfers. Wheelchairs or aids patients can stand with bracing for transfers and limited ambulation in the house or indoors. Patients with brace and crutch ambulatory status are household and community ambulators who may use a wheelchair for more extended periods of mobility. No-aids patients never resort to wheelchair use. Data are from Dunne and Shurtleff[292] from an interview survey of 37 adults aged 19–41 years.

assure an even weight distribution by eliminating pelvic obliquity, the fixed-spine sitting patient will become more prone to decubitus formation, a common problem among our young adults (Table 21-1). Early correction of the collapsing spine to eliminate both sitting and standing imbalance is indicated in order to allow complete correction of the curve and an evenly balanced pelvis.

AMBULATION

During adolescence many patients turn to the use of wheelchairs rather than braces and crutches for many reasons, discussed in Chapter 15. Generally, whether or not an individual will ambulate has been decided by adulthood. Stillwell and Menelaus[1125] reported that 95–100 percent of patients with low-lumbar- and sacral-level lesions are community ambulators, compared with 30–33 percent of those with high-lumbar- and thoracic-level lesions. Our experience is similar: 75 percent with high-lumbar- and thoracic-level lesions and 8 percent with low-lumbar- or sacral-level lesions are wheelchair dependent (Table 21-3).

ARTHRITIS

Another emergent problem is degenerative arthritis severe enough to interfere with ambulation. Thirty-five percent of our patients complained of joint pain (Table 21-1). Seven complained of upper extremity, five of lower extremity, and two of both types of joint pain. Lower extremity degenerative arthritis has been reported by Menelaus[748] and is probably due to a lack both of full sensation and of the ability to cushion the shift of weight during walking by using an active calcaneal fulcrum and anterior leg muscles with a slightly bent knee. The braced patient is unable to bend knee or ankle and loses the protection of these cushioning forces. A jarring force from foot impact, made worse by a swing-through gait, transmits greater forces to the articular surfaces of the joints of the lower extremity and the back.

Unfortunately, the elbow is not built for weightbearing. The radial head develops a classic "tennis elbow" with prolonged arm weightbearing. These painful joints respond to acetylsalicylic acid and nonsteriod inflammatory agents. However, the pain in all joints and the loss of joint stability, particularly at the knee, will force the older patient to rely more frequently on the wheelchair. A surprising number of young and middle-aged adults described these symptoms at Spina Bifida Association of America meetings attended by the primary author, but nothing is written in the medical adult literature about this problem. More needs to be learned, particularly if aggressive ambulatory programs in childhood are antecedents to degenerative joint disease in adulthood. Other orthopedic problems are osteomyelitis with possible amputation of extremities, usually secondary to decubiti, discussed in Chapter 14, and fractures, discussed in Chapter 15.

Decubiti

Decubiti, a major cause of morbidity in the adolescent and young adult, lead to prolonged hospitalization and extensive surgery (see Chapter 14). In our series of young adults, 85 percent have had decubiti requiring inpatient treatment (Table 21-1). An additional 70 percent complained of decubiti as continuing problems.[292] Forty-six percent of these patients reported skin breakdowns only occasionally, 27 percent every 2–5 years, and 27 percent almost persistently. Lonton and associates[664] reported that 26 percent of their patients had had decubiti in the previous year, agreeing with the observation of Okamoto and associates[823] of an annual rate of skin breakdown of 20–25 percent in adolescents. In our adults, decubiti clearly have caused loss of mobility (see Chapter 14) and have led to amputation. Small indolent ulcers of the feet are difficult to heal, probably because of poor skin and other causes (outlined in Chapter 14) as well as poor compliance by adolescents and young adults.

Obesity

Excess body fat is as poorly understood in teenagers and adults as for children with meningomyelocele, as discussed in Chapter 13. Seventy percent of our young adults reported that they were obese, but 52 percent of females and 56 percent of the males were below the 50th percentile for body fat calculated by the weight:arm span^2 $\times$ 100 formula of Roche and associates[942] (see Chapter 13). Although teenage boys were reported to be equivalent to controls for body fat stores estimated by skin-fold thickness, girls with meningomyelocele tended to develop excess fat stores during adolescence.[466,475] Nutritional counseling for teenagers and adults should consider total calorie needs, balance of minimal nutritional requirements, urinary and bowel management, and intrafamily conflicts, all of which are discussed in Chapter 13. At no other time in the life of a patient with meningomyelocele is attainment or maintenance of proper fat stores more important. A fat adolescent or young adult usually becomes a fatter older adult.[272] It is interesting that so few of our patients request counseling from the specialized center for the problem of dietary management, as pointed out in Chapter 22.[824]

Sexual Development

No other problem area for the adolescent and young adult is so laden with myth than sexual development. Although discussed to some extent in Chapters 19 and 20, the biologic problems of sexual development are so unique they deserve comment here as well. Eighty-five percent of our families turn to pediatricians and regional center staff for advice in regard to their children's sexual development and marriage and child-rearing potential.[824] Despite our reported discussions of sexuality, many parents are surprised at the appearance of secondary sexual characteristics in their children who are small and frequently have been infantilized.[466] The most striking finding in Hayden and associates' study[466] of adolescents was a disparity between delayed emotional maturation and early (female) and normal (male) physical sexual development. The authors found that adolescents with meningomyelocele significantly differed from their able-bodied peers in that they experienced increased sedentary life-styles, time alone, and physical problems as well as decreased participation in sports, health, self-esteem, knowledge about sex, and security about their own sex organs and ability to bear children ($p < .01$). In addition, they had fewer dates ($p < 0.05$). We have also reported both the sexual capability and psychosexual problems that impede the normal adjustment of adolescents and adults.[1057,1064]

Gleidman and Roth[403] have described the societal prejudices against physically impaired individuals in education, employment, housing, insurance, and sexuality, as discussed in Chapters 1, 2, and 16–19. In addition, Isaacson and Delgado[529] reported the problem of our American taboo about talking about sex, which inhibits the recovery of spinal cord–injured patients. The latter two authors illustrated this problem by describing the persistence of the myth that spine-injured and chronically disabled patients are incapable of sex despite the Smith papyrus dating from the fourth century B.C. that describes spinal cord–injured males as capable of having erections. Others have also documented that adults with meningomyelocele can perform the sex act, desire sex, satisfy their partners, marry, and have children.[63,212,283,292,318,613,732,1057]

We have reported that women with meningomyelocele are fertile unless they have other anomalies such as cloacal exstrophy.[1057,1064] In Chapter 18, we discussed the sexual potential of patients born with exstrophy. We have also reported increased numbers of UTIs in general during pregnancies of women with meningomyelocele, particularly with ileal diversions.[1064] Above, we commented on back problems associated with these pregnancies, and in Table 21-1 we note that 13 percent of our female patients with meningomyelocele have had prolapse of their uterus and perineal contents postpartum.[292] Of five women with meningomyelocele who became pregnant, three developed prolapse of the uterus or urinary bladder, so 60 percent of mothers with meningomyelocele developed prolapse. Women with any type of myelodysplasia except cloacal exstrophy should be able to experience orgasm, be effective sex partners (potent), and bear children (be fertile), as discussed below. However, societal prejudices and the medical complications listed above may lead to a higher emotional disturbance in females with myelodysplasia, as found by Hayden and associates.[466]

Males with myelodysplasia not only are more concerned about their sexual potential,[466] but each also has the potential for the inability to inseminate a woman (sterility). As we indicated above and in Chapter 8, recurrent UTIs, prostatic calculi, prostatitis, and epididymitis are complications of CIC and an open exstrophic urinary tract. Lower urinary tract infections can also complicate pyocystis with an isolated bladder after ileal diversion. Fertility must be evaluated, therefore, at the end of puberty or when a man with myelodysplasia wishes to either advise, or has been unable to impregnate, his partner. The other three components of the male sex act, however, are more subject to myth and aberrant function.

First, erection may or may not be present, may or may not be coordinated with arousal associated with dreams or thought processes, and may or may not be related to either orgasm or ejaculation.[212] Fortunately, erection and its relationship to the other parts of male sex performance are not necessary for complete performance. Erection has been commonly believed to be necessary for potency and to satisfy the female sex partner. Not true. Several of our older patients with flail penises incapable of erection have described the ability to sexually satisfy and impregnate wives. These accomplishments have been confirmed by their sex partners. In addition, adolescents and adults with flail penises can currently achieve erection with several different types of implantable prosthetic devices.[991] We encourage each of our young patients to look forward to developing erotic erections with pinching the thigh or a flick to the penis or normal erections during puberty if erections are not present during childhood. If not, we assure them that they can obtain penile implants.

Although previously noted to be related to cancer, sickle cell disease, and phenothiazine ingestion, we can add that priapism affects myelodysplastic patients from infancy through teenage. We are unaware of other reports of its association with any form of myelodysplasia.[1202] Although Laurence and Beresford[613] have described one of their 51 married meningocele patients with prolonged episodes of erotic erections, none of which were painful. We have treated three cases of severe, painful, and recurrent episodes of priapism successfully with phenoxybenzamine. Onset of relief is 1–2 hours, and a dose equivalent to an adult dose of 10 mg/day prevents recurrences. We have not had to resort to surgical decompression.[1202]

Since sexuality, fully expressed during puberty and early adulthood, is a combination of self-worth, independence, and sexual identity, we have recommended raising physically impaired children through normal developmental sequences. Those stages include learning about sex and about personal sexual organs. If children are brought up appropriately, they will be capable of orgasm. Orgasm, or the feeling of sexual climax, is described by spinal cord–injured patients as equivalent to their preinjury state.[177,211] Although the genitalia may be totally or partially insensitive, both spinal cord–injured and myelodysplastic patients describe stimulation of other body parts during the love act, leading to orgasm. Comarr[212] has reported details of satisfactory sexual function as well as the use of oral sex by patients with meningomyelocele.

Intellectual and Psychological Performances

During adolescence and young adulthood, patients with myelodysplasia enter into competitive education and work. Subtle hand-eye coordination and neuropsychologic impairment, hygiene problems, obesity, decubiti, and mobility complications (described in Chapters 9–20) add to the depression or "misery" that Dorner[283] describes these individuals experiencing. Some will present with somatic symptoms including headaches, parasthesias, or sensory loss and weakness. Others will present with loss of bowel control and diarrhea. Still others will become silently depressed and drop out. Some will develop sudden weight gain. Others will arrive with decubitus ulcers.

Careful history and physical examination can usually establish the diagnosis of progressive disease or worsening complication. Social, educational, and vocational history, and, when appropriate, neurodiagnostic testing, should be performed with any sudden change in the health of an adolescent or young adult. Most frequently we find a previously adequate program for the child has become an inadequate program for the adolescent or young adult. Therefore, during each yearly evaluation, we explore social and school experiences with the parents and the teenager. With each acceleration in educational requirements, we recommend neuropsychological studies if the patient is having school difficulties or if earlier studies have suggested the older person to be at risk. By detecting neuropsychologic problems of the types discussed in Chapters 16 and 18–20 prior to arriving at a crisis, we can help the high school or college student select appropriate courses and obtain effective vocational counseling.

SUMMARY

Adolescents and young adults with meningomyelocele present all the problems of their childhood as well as the new problems associated with transition to independent adulthood. The multiple problems outlined in this chapter and discussed in detail elsewhere in this text, particularly in Chapters 16 and 20, are managed successfully by a surprising number of those afflicted. It is interesting that many of the more severely impaired have become the least handicapped and best adjusted. The primary author believes we should orient our efforts towards providing timely and efficient medical diagnosis and treatment that allows the child to develop into an effective, independent adult. To do so, we must consider normal developmental phases, particularly the adolescent transition from a latent to an actively practicing, sexual adult.

David Shurtleff

22

Health Care Delivery

The preceding 21 chapters have outlined and discussed an amazingly complex array of medical, social, and educational problems as well as sophisticated and complex treatments. One of the best methods for administering the medical care component has been described by Smith.[1076] His concept was to provide coordination by a generalist who worked with separate clinic staffs in different places within his hospital. The physician coordinator worked with a social worker, the medical specialists, and community resources to assist the family in the care of their child. We have developed our program after that model, but we substituted a pediatrician-nurse specialist for the physician-social worker coordination role.[1048] We have also adopted, in part, the joint clinic meeting time in the same space used by others.[106,144,165,368,779,786,976] We have combined these two approaches for four reasons: (1) 45 percent of our patients who attend our clinics regularly live 3 or more hours away by air, boat, and automobile[824]; (2) the patient's needs and the resources available locally change with time[709]; (3) comprehensive care in one setting is logistically impossible and too costly[709,1048]; and (4) the complexity of care necessitates continuous advocacy on behalf of both family and patient.[1048] These four factors will be discussed in this last chapter prior to an explanation of our own program.

MYELODYSPLASIAS AND EXSTROPHIES: SIGNIFICANCE, PREVENTION, AND TREATMENT
 ISBN 0-8089-1816-8

GEOPOLITICAL CONSIDERATIONS

Health care services for children with severe handicaps vary from single health care providers to multidisciplinary groups of various compositions serving portions of a metropolitan area or all of a population over a broad area. Two or more centers and private practitioners may provide competing care in a small, densely populated area such as Boston, Chicago, Denver, Los Angeles, or Washington, D.C. To some degree, the centers may see patients from outlying areas up to hundreds of miles away. Our single regional center provides primary care or consultation to patients who live locally or up to 2327 miles to the north or 850 miles to the east; these patients are separated from us by mountains, oceans, state borders, and a foreign nation (Fig. 22-1). This area represents 23 percent of the land mass of the United States, but contains only 5.5 million inhabitants. Almost half our patients travel the long distances, and 31 percent of them named the clinic staff as their preferred first contact for most health problems.[824] Seventy-seven percent of those living within 45 minutes of our clinic consider center staff as primary care providers. Reasons for this choice include 24-hour availability of professional staff and longitudinal care, preference of local health care providers to refer all acute illnesses for a comprehensive evaluation due to lack of diagnostic facilities locally, and parental sense of satisfaction with evaluations that distinguish acute common illnesses from complications of existing malformations such as cerebrospinal fluid (CSF) shunt obstructions or infections.[824]

In addition to the logistical problems associated with treating patients from such a vast area, political boundaries confound governmental health care reimbursement schemes. State-based Crippled Children's Services and Medicaid programs vary in their willingness to pay for out-of-state services. Recently, a voluntary health agency reorganized, putting con-

---

Figure 22-1. Seattle regional center catchment area. Scale maps of the (A) New England states with 11 university-associated medical centers providing multidisciplinary care for children with major congenital malformations compared with the (B) WAMI (Washington, Alaska, Montana, and Idaho) and Oregon region served by three independent centers in Seattle, Washington, Portland, Oregon, and Billings, Montana. Circles represent clinics and squares represent medical schools (Seattle and Portland) or combined clinic and teaching sites. (1) ■ WAMI Medical School; (2) ■ University of Oregon Medical School, Portland. Site of collaborative activities; ■ All community sites where medical students and/or resident physicians attend clinics. All but two are WAMI sites; ● Community clinic sites without students or residents; (3) ● Eugene, Oregon, a community clinic site affiliated with the University of Oregon Medical School.

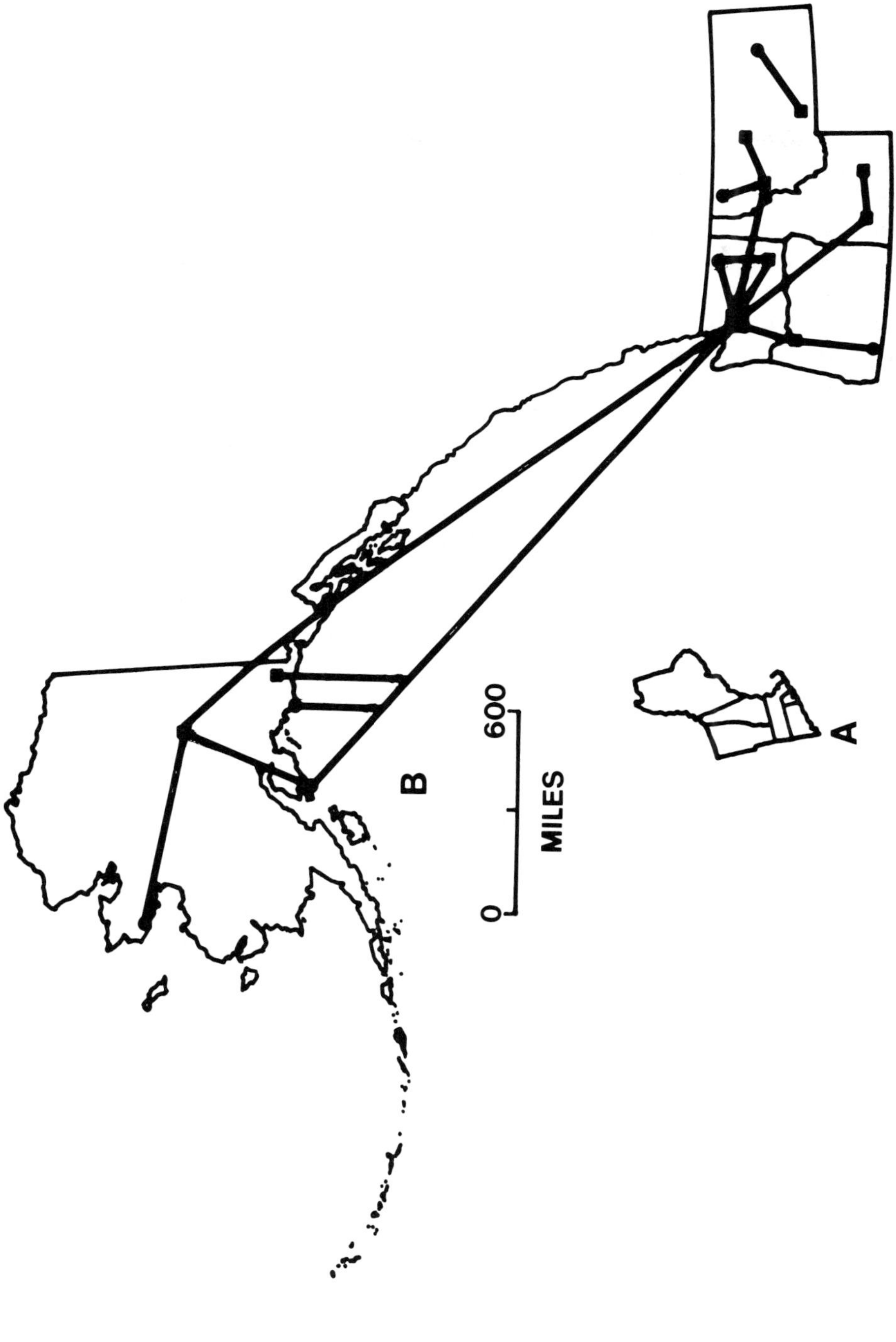
A
B
0
600
MILES

siderable portions of our patient care area outside the region that looks toward Seattle for health care. Previously, these newly excluded areas helped finance our regional patient care center and community clinics. Although care providers and parents still wish to orient toward Seattle, state and voluntary agencies are encouraging them to turn elsewhere for medical consultation.

Due to the complexity of care required and the confusion in regard to who should be providing care, we recommend careful delineation of each patient's status with family and referring physicians. Basically, three types of patients are seen by members of our clinic.

The first group includes patients seen in consultation once or for only one aspect of their multiple problems. We have been contacted by, and have actually seen, patients from throughout the United States, Europe, the Middle East, and the Pacific rim. Most have family or business connections in Seattle; others have arranged special trips to obtain consultation. As with patients from the Pacific Northwest, we attempt to coordinate our consultations with local health and/or education professionals and, whenever possible, encourage local evaluation by experts known to us or obtained from a catalogue of interested specialists and multidisciplinary centers published by the Spina Bifida Association of America.[173]

A second group includes the more common cases referred to us: those we have referred to medical care resources outside the Pacific Northwest and the majority of the 45 percent who live 3 or more hours from our clinic but within the Pacific Northwest. These patients receive some or most of their treatment locally; careful delineation of responsibility for provision of care and clear communication among health care providers and between health care providers and educators are required. Our regional medical school's toll-free line is available to our local physicians throughout the WAMI (Washington, Alaska, Montana, and Idaho) area, providing easier education. As distinct from the first and third groups, the definition of primary care responsibilities frequently varies with changes in both the health care available locally and the patient's needs as well as evolving technology.

We provide primary care for the largest group of patients, most of whom live within 45 minutes of our clinic. This third group, like the second, contains in addition some living in small isolated villages and towns in our vast region and requires careful delineation of primary care responsibilities. We provide emergency care to isolated families through health aides, public health nurses, and family physicians. For example, for these isolated patients we developed an oral agent to relieve the pressure of hydrocephalus subsequent to a CSF shunt obstruction, as described in Chapter 6. This temporary treatment allows time to travel to a neurosurgeon for definitive care. We also instruct primary care physicians in tapping CSF shunts, placing serial casts, and caring for chronic urinary tract infections (UTIs) and decubiti. We develop home care programs as well as encourage our patients from distant areas to obtain as much care locally as possible.

CHANGES IN COMMUNITY RESOURCES AND PATIENT NEEDS

The past 25 years of experience with health care services in the Pacific Northwest has taught us that communities are developing more specialists and that these individuals vary in their ability and willingness to provide services. In Anchorage, Alaska, for example, during two time periods in the past, neurosurgeons have been in practice and willing to operate on children with meningomyelocele and hydrocephalus; for intervals between those two time periods, neurosurgery was not available locally. At present, several neurosurgeons and five perinatologists can treat neonates with open neural tube defects of the spine locally.

Another example of variability occurred in our area's military medical service: the entire neurosurgical staff departed, leaving many families once again dependent on our regional center for these services. Several of our larger cities, previously devoid of any services for the multiply handicapped, have attracted specialists who will individually care for each of every child's problems. Because of the rarity of each problem as well as the rapid evolution of treatments, there is concern that these multiply malformed children with relatively rare disorders will receive care from specialists whose experience is out of date and whose skills are not being used often enough.[709,1145] Our regionalized and local clinics sponsored by state governments and voluntary agencies have been designed in cooperation with a four-state network of medical student and resident physician teaching sites to provide continuous postgraduate teaching and consultation that brings advances in care to the attention of local health care professionals and thereby helps resolve these problems. The University of Washington provides medical student teaching for the WAMI states with assignment of first-, third-, and fourth-year students and resident physicians to learning experiences in local state universities and clinical clerkships in 17 sites in the four states. Our faculty regularly visits these sites and conducts teaching clinics. Other non-WAMI cities have teaching clinics supported by the March of Dimes–Birth Defects Foundation as well as the Alaska and Washington State health departments.

SPECIALTY TEAMS

Although regional center care has been recommended as the model for the care of the children discussed in this text, we believe the complex life course of these children requires a number of individual health

Table 22-1
Specialty Teams in Order of Appearance

Cumulative Number of Team Members	Profession or Person Caring for Patient
Team I: Initial Home Care Team	
1 + ?	Family physician; obstetrician; high-risk perinatologist obstetrician
2 + 3	Mother and father
4	Consulting pediatrician
5 + ?	Extended family
6 + ?	Friends
7	Church or synagogue Leader
	Legal subteam
8	Parent's lawyer
9	Child's advocate
10 + ?	Court social worker
	Judge
	DSHS (Department of Social and Health Services) social worker
	DSHS lawyer
	Foster mother (parents)
Team II: Initial Treatment Team	
11	Neurosurgeon
12	Specialist in developmental pediatrics[a]
13	Plastic surgeon
14	Orthopedic surgeon
15	Urologist
16 + ?	Anesthesiology subteam
17	Pediatric therapist[b]
18 + ?	Neonatal nursing subteam
	Neonatal intensive care
	Intraoperative
	Postoperative
	Infant ward care
19	Social worker
20	Nurse coordinator[b]
21	Neonatologist
22 + ?	Housestaff
Team III: Financial Team	
23	Financial officer of hospital
	Insurance
	Crippled Children's Services

Table 22-1 *Continued*
Specialty Teams in Order of Appearance

Cumulative Number of Team Members	Profession or Person Caring for Patient
24	Admitting office/ER personnel
25 + ?	Voluntary health agencies
	March of Dimes
	Variety club
	Children's hospital
Team IV: Hospital Nursing Team	
26	Birth defects clinic coordinator (or spina bifida clinic coordinator)[b]
27	Public health nurse
28–32	Hospital nurses subteams
	Wards—medical and surgical
	Clinics
	Emergency room
	Intensive care
	Operative
	Postoperative
33 + ?	Specialists
	Bowel and bladder training[b]
	Rehabilitation[b]
	Infant development[b]
Team V: Meningomyelocele or Spina Bifida Clinic (Same as team II)	
	Pediatrician
	Neurosurgeon
	Urologist
	Orthopedist
	Nurse coordinator[b]
	Physical therapist
	Occupational therapist
34	Physiatrist
35	Secretary-scheduler
36	Clerk-receptionist
37	Social worker
38	Psychologist
39	Orthotist-bioengineer
40	Nutritionist
41–43	Technicians
	Radiology
	Isotography

Table 22-1 *Continued*
Specialty Teams in Order of Appearance

Cumulative Number of Team Members	Profession or Person Caring for Patient
	Ultrasound
	Bacteriology
	Biochemistry
Team VI: Specialists	
44–51 +	Otolaryngologist
	Gastroenterology
	Ophthalmologist
	Optometrist
	General surgeon
	Plastic surgeon
	Scoliologist
	Neurologist
	Nuclear medicine
	Bioengineer
	Psychiatrist
	Psychiatric social worker
	Psychologist
Team VII: Home Care Team	
52+	Pediatrician or family physician and staff Spina Bifida
53	Association of America or other peer groups
Team VIII: Preschool Team	
54–55+	Preschool teacher
	Occupational therapist
	Physicial therapist
	Nurse
Team IX: School Team	
56	School teacher
57	Resource or special education teacher
58	Hospital and home teacher
59	Occupational therapist
60	Physical therapist
61	Psychologist
62	Nurse
63	Principal
64	Special education supervisor
65	Social worker or counselor

Table 22-1 *Continued*
Specialty Teams in Order of Appearance

Cumulative Number of Team Members	Profession or Person Caring for Patient
Team X: Vocational Team	
66	Career counselor
67	Welfare assistance worker
68	College counselor
69	Vocational rehabilitation counselor
Team XI: Rest and Recreation (R&R)	
70	R&R or happiness people
71	Day care center
72	Park and play supervisors
73	Summer camp directors
74	Summer camp counselors
75	Special olympics staff
Team XII: Patients Reproductive Team	
76	Family planning conselor or geneticist
77	Perinatologist or developmental pediatrician
78	Obstetrician; family physician and staff
79	Amniocentesiologist; high-risk obstetrician
80	Moralist
81	Ultrasonographer

[a] In our center, physical and occupational therapists cooperate closely in early infant assessment and consultation with the pediatrician and psychologist.
[b] In our clinic, the same person performs these professional responsibilities both in the clinic and while the patient is on the ward. Our nurse is also a consultant to community health workers. At times our nurse provides the only consultation to the physician who works in a community in need of toilet training advice. When necessary, the nurse requests pediatric, urologic, or gastroenterology consultation. Modified from Shurtleff et al.[1048]

professionals and specialty teams. The complex care that requires large numbers of specialists and the widely distributed living situations preclude one team from providing total care.

From the moment, we will set aside the problems of large distances, need for a local physician, professional and interpersonal relationships, and economy in order to restrict our discussion to an ideal patient population managed within the limits of a city or state, as in a metropolitan area. Using such a limited stage for a backdrop, we will introduce, in order of their need, the teams of 81 or more members, as listed in Table 22-1. Rarely do we observe continuity of character for each role. For example, the family physician or referring obstetrician has never in our experience been the same person providing the patient with genetic counseling and obstetric services at the age of the patient's maturity. Our Seattle team uses several specialists—five pediatricians alone—to fill one role of the consulting pediatrician; one of these five is on call at all times. Nevertheless, we will count each role as a single person and assume that a minimum number of personnel will be required to help our patients adjust.

Team I is simultaneously the least knowledgeable about the future for an impaired infant and the most important; basically, it includes baby and family (Figure 22-2).

The local group of friends, possibly church or synagogue members and others, rally around the stricken family to provide immediate and, perhaps, life-long support and help. They are *the* team, as introduced to me by Jullian Joubert, the Bee Keeper from Enumclaw, a septuagenarian born with meningomyelocele and cared for by an innovative pioneer family. This father of three assisted us in developing our approach, which emphasizes family responsibility and independence.

The extended family includes three basic elements: (1) those who help the family with finances, (2) those who provide rest and relaxation (team XI), and (3) those tho provide legal aid. The third group assures our patients the right to life, liberty, and pursuit of happiness. Twenty percent of our severely deformed patients are abandoned and need immediate legal assistance.[470] An average of four, but as many as seven, legal and social service professionals can become involved in a team. We will return to some of these important teams later.

The most dramatic of all teams is the initial treatment team (team II), led by the neurosurgeon who performs critical central nervous system (CNS) surgery. The pediatrician should provide other system diagnoses. Without a smooth functioning subteam of neonatal nurses, most afflicted neonates would not survive. We frequently overlook these individuals who communicate with family and physician and substitute for the mother by providing direct infant care during the first terrible days.

Usually the orthopedic surgeon is needed for an immediate opinion about care of the back or the extremities. The urologist assists with the care of the urinary tract. The plastic surgeon helps close the back in all our cases. Anesthesiology is another much overlooked but critically needed professional team; members talk with parents and become involved in virtually all surgical interventions.

Meanwhile, team III should be alleviating some parental distress—the burden of medical expense. We find a financial helper is needed to guide the family through the complexities of state, federal, and private insurance and voluntary patient care funding agencies. Such a person helps interpret insurance policy fine print and decode government regulations. It literally pays to have a good team III.

Before progressing home from the hospital, the family is aided by nursing groups in team IV. Hospital ward, clinic, specialty, and local community nurses carry the burden of "grandmothering"—helping the mother to mother her child. The clinic coordinator is a nurse and is a true cocaptain with the mother on this critical team. Some of these nurses, the neonatal care specialists, have been mentioned as a part of team II, and others will appear as critical members of other teams.

Team V consists of the specialists providing consultation and care in a multidisciplinary fashion and is usually called the spina bifida or meningomyelocele team, consisting of neurosurgeon, orthopedist, urologist, orthotist, physical and occupational therapists, clinic nurse, and coördinator. Although each contributes significantly to the care of the child, there are no such multidisciplinary teams known to us that meet regularly to discuss coordinated care and set priorities. Frequently, even the supposedly consistent members of the team, who are thought to provide continuity, change. Only three people of our original team remain active: one of the nurses, a pediatrician, and a urologist. The composition, leadership, and method of day-to-day function varies between centers that we have visited. Ideally, the specialty services required of team II and team V will be provided by the same individuals.

Medical and surgical specialty services not usually included in the core multidisciplinary team and used by only a portion of the patients have been listed as team VI. At times these people are needed to provide prolonged and critical care; for example, the otolaryngologist assists us when the Arnold-Chiari malformation causes bulbar palsies and airway obstruction.

The home or primary health care team (team VII) usually, but not always, changes when an impaired child is born. General practitioners will refer to pediatricians for routine care, and primary pediatricians will frequently refer to specialists.[853] One of our most frequent problems is finding a primary care physician with appropriate interests and skills who can afford the time to provide comprehensive primary care for the multiply impaired child.[878] Unfortunately, time for communication, multidisciplinary medical care conferences, and school coordination meetings is not reimbursable time for the private physician. These services are reimbursed by the agencies noted above that also support our community clinics.

Team VIII, including the preschool staff, teacher, occupational therapist, physical therapist, and nurse, is ideal for starting a congenitally malformed child off in life and is assured for our patients in the United States by Public Law 94-142, as discussed in Chapters 2 and 17. This team and teams IX and X (the education and vocational groups) are just as, if not more, important as the spina bifida group, team V. The school teams

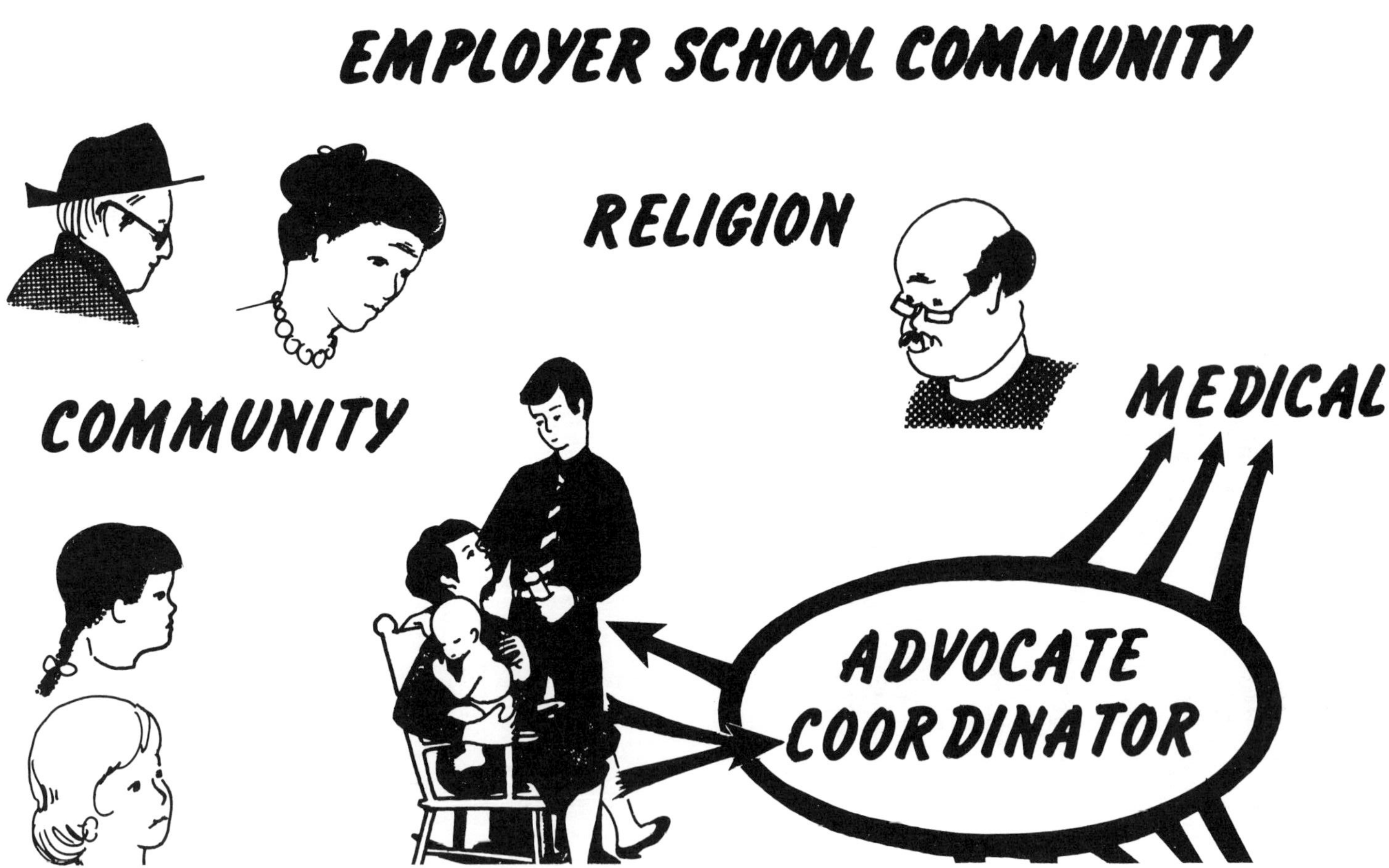
EMPLOYER SCHOOL COMMUNITY
RELIGION
COMMUNITY
MEDICAL
ADVOCATE
COORDINATOR

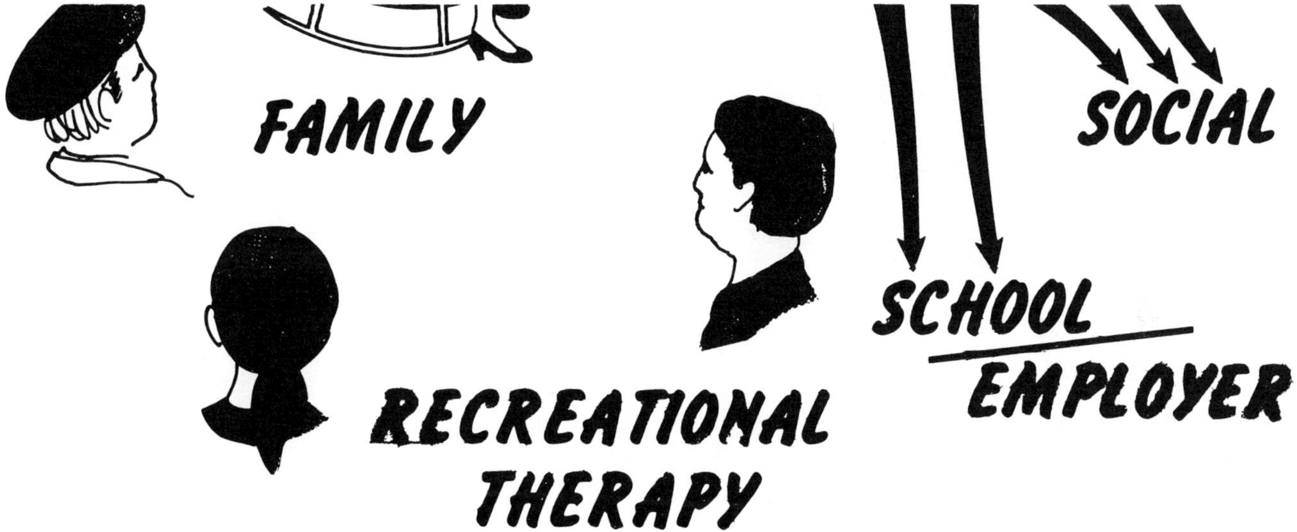

Figure 22-2. Team 1: the family. This illustration has been created to emphasize the important but peripheral relationship the health profession holds in regard to the life and well being of the chronically ill or physically handicapped child. Depending on the family's cultural background, a variety of local community agencies and groups form a support network that allows the child to "individuate," as described in Chapter 19. Prior to that time, some of the same and other social units provide support for the family during the early grieving and adjustment stages (Chapter 18). Throughout the child's life, extended family, school, and eventually employer are critical components of the social network. Someone with medical and social skills can act as both an advocate and coordinator between these social units and the health specialists.

each have a roster with as few as three to four individuals; however, for proper care of the more paralyzed child, special education and regular classroom teachers, occupational and physical therapists, and nurses or aides are required as a minimum. These important educational professionals, second only in importance to the family, team I, provide contact for up to 6 hours a day, 5 days a week, for about 180 days (720–1080 hours) a year for a legally required 15–18 years, or 15,120–18,360 hours during the lifetime of each patient.

The services of team X are usually not available in high school, but are available at age 18 through the Department of Vocational Rehabilitation and Welfare Assistance. For the remainder of the dependent life of the congenitally malformed individual, this team of career counselor, vocational rehabilitation director, and staff is available. Services range from college or graduate school scholarships to skill training and sustenance.

Before closing this section about teams, we would like to return to teams I and XI to reemphasize the family and local teams with particular regard to happiness. Rest and relaxation are too often overlooked. Recreationists and play people, mentioned earlier as team XI, are as important as the schools. Life is terrible without some play. These people in team I are really locally extended family (schools, legal advocates, play people); they enable the congenitally malformed child to enjoy life a little, which is hardly a contribution of the pain-causing and exercise-demanding members of the classic medical-surgical teams II, V, and VI. We try not to, and don't mean to, but we do, unfortunately, hurt little people.[1033]

With the help and guidance of teams I–XI, our patient arrives at independent adulthood and turns to team XII, the family planners—geneticist, amniocentesiologist, and obstetrician. This team helps the patient and spouse either start the cycle anew, or end a new child's life before a new cycle can begin; these two opposite 20th-century sociobiologic phenomena, described by Edgar Wilson,[1224] are discussed in detail in Chapters 1, 2, and 4.

As this review of teams providing services suggests, the patients' needs are too great for any one team to be considered as the sole source of services. To coordinate all these teams through one multidisciplinary setting is both inappropriate and wasteful of the participants' time. Our method of coordinating these services will be discussed below after a further discussion of costs.

COST OF MULTIDISCIPLINARY CARE

As discussed in Chapters 1 and 2, our society has recently passed legislation, and courts have clearly stated the mandates for providing impaired and disabled persons access to the mainstream of society, education, and health services. These laws and mandates have placed enormous financial burdens on state welfare, education, and medical budgets at a time when government has been increasingly reluctant to provide funds for these services. Current private practice reimbursement systems do not adequately compensate the private physican for providing coordinated services. Yet, recent task forces have reported the need for multidisciplinary, coordinated care.[214,709,1145]

Health maintenance organizations and insurance companies are increasingly reluctant to provide coverage for the disabled. In addition, young adults, as noted in Chapter 21, continue to cost our government more on federally mandated subsidies for sustenance and medical care than for medical care only.[65] Our program has been able to demonstrate that modern, early provision of multidisciplinary care provides a more economical program for the third-party payer and graduates a person more likely to be self-sustaining[729,1058,1061] (see Chapters 4 and 5). To provide these services, however, we have been underwritten for coordination and teaching costs by March of Dimes–Birth Defects Foundation, Variety Club, our private hospital's free and partial payment patient care program, and the states of Washington and Alaska. We believe that catastrophic health care coverage should be provided to both the families of disabled infants and children and the disabled themselves from 18 years of age on.[709] Two of our presidents of the United States, Franklin Roosevelt, himself disabled, and John Kennedy, mildly impaired but with a handicapped family member, have demonstrated the ability to initiate private and public programs that have enabled the disabled to succeed. It will only be with concerted effort on behalf of all of us interested in the welfare of the disabled that funds will be available to provide the type of multidisciplinary program that will enable the multihandicapped to become contributing members of society.

THE ADVOCATE-COORDINATOR MODEL FOR CARE OF THE CONGENITALLY MALFORMED

In 1978, we presented our clinic organization to the combined first International Meningomyelocele Seminar and the Spina Bifida Association of America in Cincinnati.[1048] Since that time, our clinic organization and most of our staff have changed. Emphasis has also changed, but the concept of pediatrician or nurse as advocate-coordinator for the patient and family has remained unaltered (Fig. 22-3). Care is taken to have new families and older patients understand that throughout the years either the nurse specialist or pediatrician will be available to help them obtain services locally, through our clinic, or at another national center. We

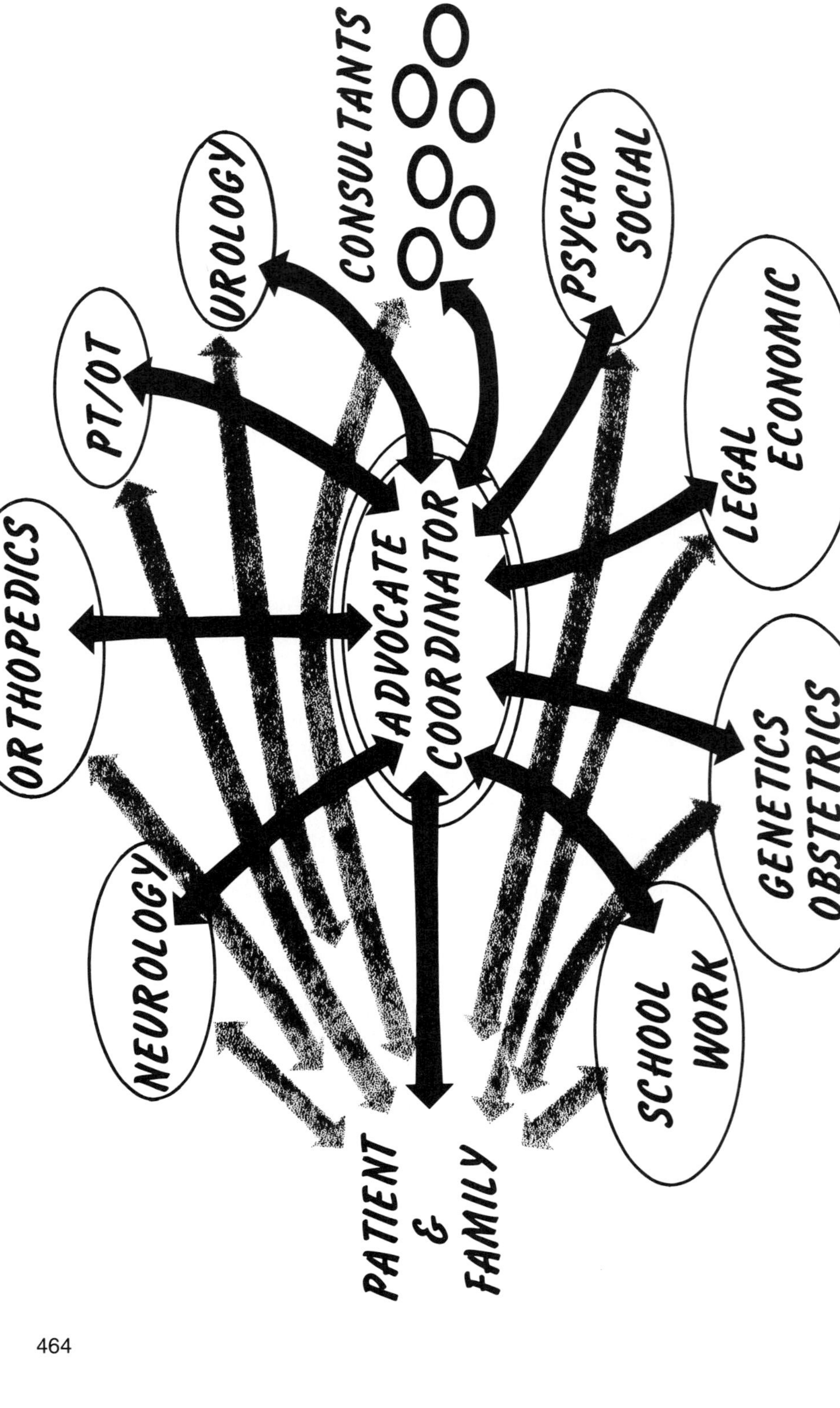
ADVOCATE
COORDINATOR
ORTHOPEDICS
PT/OT
UROLOGY
CONSULTANTS
PSYCHO-
SOCIAL
LEGAL
ECONOMIC
GENETICS
OBSTETRICS
SCHOOL
WORK
PATIENT
&
FAMILY
NEUROLOGY

have exercised our roles as coordinators to provide the latest information from national and international sources to families, health care providers, and educators in the Pacific Northwest. We are also careful as coordinators to assign attending physician responsibilities to our local or regional medical and surgical colleagues when their services are needed by the patient. As advocate-coordinators, we emphasize facilitating communication. For example, Chapters 16 and 17 illustrated how psychosocial evaluations are valuable in timing major surgical procedures and how educators can learn to detect subtle signs of CSF shunt malfunction. The pediatrician and nurse specialist provide interdisciplinary communication, the mortar that holds together the complex of educational, medical, psychological, social, and surgical services needed by our congenitally malformed children.[209] They are also the directors of the clinic staff who schedule patients with various clinic professionals (Table 22-2). The nurses supervise the schedules with one pediatrician of the group. Nurses are the first-line contact for most problems. Both nurse and pediatrician provide primary care to some patients for most health problems and to most patients for a few health problems (Table 22-3).[824]

It is odd that the most sought-after information from the nurse specialist and pediatrician by mothers (85 percent) is about the potential sexual capabilities, marriage, and parenting of their children. The next highest request for information (72 percent) is for medical reports required by schools. Two areas that probably should be more frequently covered include eating and dietary habits, requested by only 40 percent, and emotional problems and growth and development, requested by only 40–48 percent. The complex problems of obesity, behavior, and growth and development, covered in Chapters 13 and 16–20, need to be clarified and distributed among primary care health providers and other local

---

Figure 22-3. Specialist and Advocate Coordinator. Whereas Figure 22-2 emphasizes the important contribution of the local community and social groups, this illustration attempts to emphasize the importance of coordinating the various health specialists' recommendations and treatments. The advocate-coordinator can help explain to families the need for medical and surgical interventions and interpret the patient's needs to the health specialists. Frequently the advocate-coordinator can present the patient's and family's problems and needs to health specialists with a perspective gained from local therapists, school, or other social units. Provision of insight gained from conversations, reports, and conferences can improve the prioritization and type of medical, surgical, and educational treatments. The arrows in this illustration are meant to emphasize the need for an advocate-coordinator to help the family and, eventually, the patient, to communicate between and among different types of specialists.

Table 22-2
Clinical Staff

Person	Percentage of Contact with Patient and Family: Each Visit	Periodic Review	Life Time
Clerk receptionist	100	100	100
Secretary	25	100	100
Pediatrician	80	100	100
Nurse specialist (hygiene) and coordinator	90	100	100
Neurosurgeon	80	100	100
Urologist			
Orthopedic surgeon	80	100	100
Physical therapist	50	100	100
Occupational therapist	50	100	100
Physiatrist	30	100	100
Psychologist	25	100	100
Orthotist	25	80	100
Social worker (medical)	10	25	100
General surgeon	5	—	10
Nutritionist	10	—	20
Plastic surgeon	5	—	10
Scoliogist	—	75	75
Primary care physician	—	100[a]	
Ophthalmologist, optometrist	—	50[a]	80
Psychiatrist, social worker, psychologist	—	10[a]	10
Gastroenterology and biofeedback clinic	—	10	10
Geneticist; high-risk perinatologist	—	—	100[b]
Business agent	—	—	100

[a] Separate regular follow-up programs.
[b] We hope.
Adapted from Shurtleff .[1048]

resources used by parents, or we will have little impact on these complications among our congenitally malformed children.[824]

CLINIC ORGANIZATION

In addition to the primary care and coordination activities discussed above, the nurse specialist and pediatrician provide new case intakes, follow-up, and communication with referral sources and local community

Table 22-3
Perceptions of Mothers for First Contact Care

Reason for Visit	Number of Responses	Child's Local Physician (%)	Other Local Resources (%)	Clinic Staff and Specialists (%)
Immunization update	168	54	32	14
Suspected ear infection	168	80	1	19
Minor accident	169	70	16	14
Suspected urinary tract infection	167	47	6	47
Eyes wander/cross	167	24	39	37
Eating/dietary habits	165	52	8	40
"Lazy" or "stubborn"	162	32	31	37
Unload worries	162	14	50	36
Suspected shunt block	103	22	25	53
Leaky ileal stoma	50	8	40	52
Pressure sore	164	34	4	61
Uncomfortable braces	75	4	28	68
Impaired capacity for play	156	26	6	68
Stool soiling	163	29	3	68
Genetic counseling	161	10	21	69
Literature on spina bifida	167	10	44	46
Growth and development	164	33	19	48
Self-help skills	160	20	12	68
Sex, marriage, parenting	161	10	5	85
Vocational guidance	150	8	40	52
School report	165	27	1	72
Insurance letter	168	31	1	68
Crisis in school	152	18	42	40
Severe emotional problem	167	30	10	60

Adapted from Shurtleff.[1048]

care and service providers. An intake form is used by a trained intake interviewer to obtain information, and the clinic intake staff, clinic chief, and head nurse complete the form for appropriate appointments (Fig. 22-4). New patients are assigned to specialists with relevant skills within our multidisciplinary clinic (Table 22-2) or to other specialty clinics for special diagnostic tests and procedures. The schedule is then prepared for each patient with computer assistance and is (at the time of each clinic visit) transferred to a wall chart for each physician or nurse (Fig. 22-5) so that the patient can be easily tracked and each person in clinic can anticipate the expected sequence of events.

At periods of every 6 months during the first 2 years and at yearly intervals thereafter, a complete review of the central nervous and musculoskeletal systems and urinary tracts takes place along with age-appropriate neuropsychological screening tests (Table 22-4). These tests are routinely performed to determine if further detailed neuropsychological studies, discussed in Chapter 17 (Tables 17-1 and 17-2), are necessary. Following completion of the evaluations, the nurse or pediatrician obtains the consultants' reports, which are discussed at a conference with clinic schedulers, other pediatricians and nurses, students, housestaff, representatives of the occupational and physical therapy staffs, a social worker, and, at times, surgical specialists. These conferences occur after each clinic. A specific attending is assigned for the next period; for example, an orthopedist is designated if an inpatient or outpatient procedure is to be performed. A plan for subsequent follow-up visits is completed (Fig. 22-6). All consultation, patient evaluations, needs for interval planning, or possible therapeutic action, such as obtaining the results of a urine culture, are assigned to the nurse, pediatrician, or another appropriate person. A note is dictated by the pediatrician summarizing all opinions, recommendations, and planned interventions. A copy of this note is sent to the patient's primary care health provider and others involved in the child's care, including local surgical specialists, educators, therapists, and family.

EVALUATION

One important aspect of our multidisciplinary program is ongoing analysis. The data presented in this text have been derived by standardized statistical analysis of patient information recorded on standardized forms (Fig. 22-7). These forms, in whole, in part, or modified, are being used in our community clinics, five other centers in the United States, and the Royal Children's Hospital in Melbourne, Australia. These computer

Figure 22-4. Intake form used for multidisciplinary clinics. This blank form reproduction indicates the types of appointments scheduled prior to seeing the patient in clinic. Actual roentgenographic films or computerized axial tomogram hard copies are necessary, whereas both a copy of the ultrasound and the examiner's report are necessary. Actual operative reports are more helpful than descriptions by name, particularly for orthopedic procedures. The reasons for referral as well as the patient's or family's expectations are clearly delineated. Based on the medical, school, and therapist's reports and the concerns of the person providing referral, the family and patient, nurse coordinator, and pediatrician either obtain more information by telephone or order appropriate tests, special examinations, and consultations.

BIRTH DEFECTS CLINIC

REFERRAL RECD__________
DATE SCH. RECD__________

NEW EVALUATION APPOINTMENT PLAN

Patient Name__________ DX__________
COH# _____ B.D. _____ Age _____ Referred by__________
Funding Source__________ Address__________
Phone__________
Parent/Guardian/Foster__________
Address__________
Phone (home)__________ (work)__________
Time Considerations__________

APPOINTMENTS	TEAM MEMBER(S)	LENGTH OF VISIT	REASON FOR VISIT	SCHEDULED DATE
Clinic Regis.				
Pediatrician				
Orthopedics				
Rehab				
Nurse				
PT				
OT				
Neurosurgery				
Plastic Surgery				
Urology				
Developmental				
Speech				
Audio				
ENT				
Educ. Psych (CONSULT REQD)				
Procedures which require requisition:				
CT SCAN				
EEG				
IVP				
LOOPOGRAM				
RENAL SCAN				
SHUNTOMETRICS				
ULTRASOUND				
URODYNAMICS				
VCUG				
LAB/XRAY				
Other				

Additional Scheduling Instructions__________

DO NOT WRITE BELOW THIS LINE

Birth Defects Clinic Schedule

Time	Patient	Room	Out of Clinic	Attending	Rn	Other Appts.
9:30	Nelson, M	12		Dunne	Kay	
1:30	Wolfe, C	14B	Lunch	Dunne	JoAnne	8:00 PT, 9:00 OT
2:00	Rooks, R		Lunch	Dunne	Mo	11:00 Tapper
2:30	Jurek, A			Dunne	Mo	9:30 VCUG, 11:00 OT
9:30	Roberts, D	10		Hayden	Mo	Suture Removal
10:30	Ogles, D	9		Hayden	Mo	
1:30	Short, P	10		Hayden	Kay	Bath aids, Wheelchair
10:30	Ensley, L	14B		Lemire	Kay	9:00 renogram, 10:00 IVP
11:00	Diaz, R	8		Lemire	Mo	
9:30	Dalton, J	6		McLaughlin		
10:00	Scappini, J	8		McLaughlin	Kay	
10:30	Bishop, J	4		McLaughlin	Mo	
11:00	Rivas, E	5		McLaughlin	Mo	8:30 VCUG, 1:00 OT
1:00	Rosenkranz, G		Lunch	McLaughlin	Kay	8:00 OT
1:30	Banks, R			McLaughlin	Mo	11:45 Dental
2:00	Gleason, S			McLaughlin	Liz	3:00 OT
9:00	Johanson, D	14		Shurtleff	JoAnne	
9:30	Hirschel, R	13		Shurtleff	Mo	
10:30	Baldwin, S	14		Shurtleff	JoAnne	
11:00	Strope, M	14		Shurtleff	JoAnne	
11:30	Carlson, T	13		Shurtleff	JoAnne	10:00 US
1:00	Vandyke, M			Shurtleff	Kiko	10:30 renal US
1:30	Roe, A			Shurtleff	Mo	9:00 VCUG, 1:30 Shunt
2:00	Baldwin, V			Shurtleff	JoAnne	11:00 OT
8:30	Meyers, M	11		Stone	Kiko	8:00 OT, Wheelchair Issues
10:00	Shannon, J	11		Stone		
11:30	Waters, C	16		Stone		11:00 OT, (in clinic)

Figure 22-5. Patient schedule. This reproduction is of a color-coded clinic schedule that is taken from a computer printout and put on a porcelain chalk board with dry ink felt pen. Each physician, surgeon, nurse, and therapist has an individual color. When a patient is in a room, weighed, measured, and ready to be seen, a room number is assigned. On the boards containing the specialists' schedules, the pediatrician and nurse coordinator for the patient are also listed. At a glance, each person in clinic can discover the status of any given patient. When the clinic visit has been completed, a circle is placed around the room number, and the patient released.

Table 22-4
Routine Neuropsychological, Visuomotor, and Developmental Tests

Age[a]	Test	Comments
6 months to adult	Self-care inventory based on Developmental Miles Stories Index	See Chapters 12, 15, and 17[b]
12 and 24 months	Gessell or Bayley	On first and second birthday or until basal levels on Stanford-Binet are achieved
24 and 48 months	Stanford-Binet	On second birthday or when basal levels can be achieved
48 months	DTLA; VMI; McCarthy tapping; Beery Test of Visual-Motor Integration; Motor Free Visual Perception Test	On fourth birthday, or when first seen and a basal level can be achieved, until a maximum score is achieved
4–12 years	Achenbach's Child Behavior Checklist	Each yearly visit
7 years to adult	WISC-R; WISA; DTLA; McCarthy-Tapping; McCarthy-Story; WRAT	Baseline examination when first seen and a basal level can be achieved

Key: DTLA, Detroit Test of Learning Abilities; VMI, Vineland Maturity Index; WISC-R and WISA; WISC-R, Weschler Intelligence Scale for Children and Adults; WRAT, Wide Range Achievement Test.

[a] All tests are used for screening until patient achieves maximum score and are then repeated only when screening for suspected neuropsychological problems (e.g., CSF shunt obstruction, behavior problems, seizure disorder, etc.). Ages are approximate developmental ages and not necessarily chronologic.

[b] Data from Sousa and associates[1095] and Okamoto and associates.[825]

entry forms are also printed out as an abstract of the patient's clinical record (Fig. 22-8). These summaries are particularly useful in a clinic. Computerized medical records have been and are constantly being used to analyze and improve care provided by staff and by University of Washington Health Sciences and School of Education graduate students. The numerous studies from our Division of Congenital Defects as well as the data presented in Chapters 5–7, 12, 13, 15, and 16 are illustrations of our continuous evaluation process. Patients, in turn, derive better care from our combined patient care, teaching, and research activity.

BIRTH DEFECTS FOLLOW-UP PLANNING SHEET

DX__________
RN__________
Attending__________

TODAY'S DATE__________

Appointments	Return Date	Team Member(s)	Length of Visit	Reason	Scheduled Date
Pediatrician					
Orthopedics					
Rehab					
Nurse					
PT					
PT Study					
OT					
Neurosurgery					
Plastic Surgery					
Urology					
Developmental					
B.D. Spine					
Speech					
Audio					
ENT					
Ophthalmology					
Neurodiagnostic Clinic					
Social Services					
CT Scan (requisition)					
EEG (requisition)					
IVP					
Loopogram					
Renal Scan					
Renogram					
Shuntometrics					
Ultrasound					
Urodynamics					
VCUG					
X-ray					
Lab					
Orthotics					
Myelo Study Due					
Other					

Pre-Clinic Needs

Figure 22-6. Clinic schedule chart. The form reproduced in this illustration is used by the nurse coordinator to schedule the patient's next visit. It is filled in during clinic by the various specialists and reviewed with clinic staff at the end of each clinic. The form is then filed in a tickler file according to date of follow-up. Just prior to the anticipated visit, the family is contacted to determine if there are any new concerns or if the visit is necessary.

A

PERMANENT INFORMATION -- Record Type 1 - A

Name ___________________________
(last, first)

Computer Code # ____ Hospital Code __ Date of first contact: __/__/__

General Information

______ Hospital I.D. #

__/__/__ Birthdate

___ Age at first exam

(m = months; d = days)

Sex

1 - male 3 - male-female
2 - female 4 - ?

Labor Information

__ hours of labor

Type of Delivery

1 - vaginal/cephalic 8 - other
2 - vaginal/breech 9 - unknown
3 - C-section

Newborn Information (at birth)

_ . __ kgrams birth weight

__ cm length

__ cm OFC

__ . _ cm lesion length

__ . _ cm lesion width

Initial Surgical Information

Back closure: date __/__/__
age in days __

Shunt: date __/__/__
age in days __

code:

Surgery 00 - not done, improbable
98 - not done, but unknown
99 - unknown whether or when done

Age 00 - not done
98 - not done by 97 days
99 - unknown

Initial Prognosis (at birth)
see criteria for definitions

1 - good c̄ Rx 5 - wait-prog. by reg ctr
2 - good s̄ Rx
4 - poor or hopeless 9 - unknown

Prognosis at First Exam by Center
see criteria for definitions

0 - hopeless 3 - poor
1 - good with Rx 9 - unknown
2 - good without Rx

Primary Diagnosis

01 - meningomyelocele
02 - meningomyelocele with other major anomolies
03 - lumbosacral lipoma or lipomeningocele
06 - extrophy of cloaca with myelocystocele
07 - cord trauma
08 - cord malignancy
09 - sacral anomolies
10 - MM & fetal alcohol syndrome
11 - MM & chromosone disorder
12 - meningocele
97 - combination (list)
98 - other (specify)
99 - unknown

Social Information

__ Education of Father (in years)
12 = high school grad or equiv.
97 - natural father not in home

__ Education of Mother (in years)

Conception of Child

0 - out of wedlock 8 - other
1 - within wedlock 9 - unknown

Marital Status of Parents at Birth

0 - never married 4 - widowed
1 - married 8 - other
2 - separated 9 - unknown
3 - divorced

Occupation of Father at time of Birth

0 - unemployed
1 - professional, technical worker
2 - manager, official, proprietor
3 - clerical, sales
4 - craftsman, foreman, operative
5 - service work, household help, labor
6 - armed forces
7 - student
8 - other (specify)
9 - unknown

Family History of Neural Tube Defects

0 - no
1 - yes
9 - unknown

Patient Follow-up Information

___ Age at Menarche (in months)
998 - male

___ Age at Death (in months)
000 - no death
997 - lost to follow-up
for age in days, see note under Age at First Exam

Cause of Death

0 - no death
1 - urologic (proven by autopsy)
2 - urologic (suspected)
3 - secondary to hydrocephalus
4 - meningitis or other infection
5 - respiratory complications
8 - other (describe)
9 - unknown

Second Hospital Number

__ hospital code

______ hospital ID

Religion

01 - Protestant
02 - Roman Catholic
03 - Greek Orthodox
04 - 7th day Adventist
05 - Mormon
06 - Jehovah's Witness
07 - Other Christian
08 - Jewish
09 - Muslim
10 - Buddist
11 - Other Non-Christian
12 - Athiest
13 - Not Declared
99 - unknown

Gestational Age

__ weeks

Recorded by:

COMMENTS:

3/85

Figure 22-7 *continues*

Figure 22-7. A plan for subsequent follow-up visits. Patient clinical data forms are completed at least every 6 months during the first 2 years of life and yearly thereafter. The first record type is completed only on initial contact, but is reviewed at each visit for accuracy. Each record type can be brought up on the clinic or office computer screen individually or as a table of sequential examinations. An abstract of the patient's record is, therefore, always available even when the patient's hospital chart, many times in more than one volume, is not. Standard definitions of each datum are recorded in a coder's manual and reviewed at least every 6–12 months by representatives from centers involved in an international myelodysplasia study. Not all centers record the same number of observations as on these Seattle forms; some record more, others fewer.

B

SPINAL ALIGNMENT

Curve	Region	Convexity (Primary Curve)	Plumb Alignment
0 - normal 1 - scoliosis 2 - kyphosis 3 - kyphoscoliosis 4 - lordosis 5 - lordoscoliosis 8 - other 9 - unknown	0 - not appl. 1 - cervical 2 - thoracic 3 - lumbar 4 - thoraco-lumbar 8 - other/comb. 9 - unknown	0 - none/not appl. 1 - right 2 - left 9 - unknown	direction/distance _ / _ _ cm sitting (888 if unable to sit or stand) _ / _ _ cm standing 1 - right, 2 - left: codes for direction of displacement from gluteal cleft

HIP	Right			Left			FOOT/ANKLE	Right			Left		
Extension (000)							Dorsiflexion (040) (-) = cc in plantar						
Flexion (135)							Plantarflexion (040) (-) = cc in dorsi						
Test (1)							Heel Position(2)*+						
Abduction (045)							Severity(4)*+						
Adduction (030)							Forefoot Position(3)+						
External Rotation (045) (Lateral)							Severity(4)+						
Internal Rotation (045) (Medial)							Arch (if weight bearing)(5)						
Leg Length (in cm) (888 if indeterminate)							Toes(6)						
Hip Status 1-in socket 2-dislocated 3 - subluxed							Great Toe(6)						
							Thigh-Foot Angle (000-+20) (+) = laterally rotated (-) = medially rotated (888 if indeterminate)						

KNEE	Right			Left			ARTHROGRYPOTIC JOINTS	Right		Left	
Extension (000) (-) = hyperextension							Hip(7)				
Flexion (130)							Knee(7)				
Varus (-08) (code 888 if > 30° v cc)							Ankle(7)				
Valgus (008) (code 888 if > 30° v cc)											
Position while(2) weight bearing											

*measure in weight bearing. +If non-weight bearing, measure fixed deformity only.

(1) Test used	(2) Position	(3) Forefoot position	(4) Severity	(5) Arch	(6) Toes and great toe	(7) Arthrogrypotic
1 - prone ext. 2 - Thomas 3 - other 9 - unknown	0 - neutral 1 - varus 2 - valgus 8 - non-weight bearing 9 - unknown	0 - neutral 1 - adductus 2 - abductus 8 - non-wt. bearing 9 - unknown	0 - 0° - 10° 1 - 10° - 20° 2 - 20° - 30° 3 - > 30° 8 - non-wt. bear. 9 - unknown	0 - neutral 1 - cavus 2 - planus 8 - non-weight bearing 9 - unknown	0 - neutral 1 - hammer 2 - claw 3 - hallux valgus 9 - unknown	0 - none 1 - mild 2 - moderate 3 - severe 9 - unknown

Comments:

Recorded by:

MYELODYSPLASIA STUDY

Lower Extremity Measures: Range of Motion
Record Type 2 - B

Computer Number _ _ _ _   Hospital Code _ _

Date of Evaluation _ _ / _ _ / _ _

Type of Evaluation 1-yearly 2-pre-op 3-post-op 4-follow-up 5-initial

3/85

CASE NUMBER

NAME

BIRTHDATE

C

MUSCLE FUNCTION

codes: 0 - None, 1 - Trace, 2 - Poor, 3 - Fair, 4 - Good, 5 - Normal, 6 - Indeterminant (transferred), 7 - Indeterminant (spastic; contracture), 8 - Indeterminant (abnormal movement), 9 - unknown

Quadratus Lumborum (T_{12} - L_1)
R - 0 1 2 3 4 5 6 7 8 9
L - 0 1 2 3 4 5 6 7 8 9

Abdominals (T_{8-12})
R - 0 1 2 3 4 5 6 7 8 9
L - 0 1 2 3 4 5 6 7 8 9

Iliopsoas (L_{1-2})
R - 0 1 2 3 4 5 6 7 8 9
L - 0 1 2 3 4 5 6 7 8 9

Sartorius (L_{1-3})
R - 0 1 2 3 4 5 6 7 8 9
L - 0 1 2 3 4 5 6 7 8 9

Hip Adductors (L_{2-4})
R - 0 1 2 3 4 5 6 7 8 9
L - 0 1 2 3 4 5 6 7 8 9

Quadriceps (L_{2-4})
R - 0 1 2 3 4 5 6 7 8 9
L - 0 1 2 3 4 5 6 7 8 9

Medial Hamstrings (L_4 - S_2)
R - 0 1 2 3 4 5 6 7 8 9
L - 0 1 2 3 4 5 6 7 8 9

Lateral Hamstrings (L_4 - S_2)
R - 0 1 2 3 4 5 6 7 8 9
L - 0 1 2 3 4 5 6 7 8 9

Extensor Hallicus Longus (L_5 - S_1)
R - 0 1 2 3 4 5 6 7 8 9
L - 0 1 2 3 4 5 6 7 8 9

Flexor Hallicus Longus (S_1 - 2)
R - 0 1 2 3 4 5 6 7 8 9
L - 0 1 2 3 4 5 6 7 8 9

Anterior Tibialis (L_4 - 5)
R - 0 1 2 3 4 5 6 7 8 9
L - 0 1 2 3 4 5 6 7 8 9

Posterior Tibialis (L_4 - 5)
R - 0 1 2 3 4 5 6 7 8 9
L - 0 1 2 3 4 5 6 7 8 9

Peroneus Longus & Brevus (L_5 - S_1)
R - 0 1 2 3 4 5 6 7 8 9
L - 0 1 2 3 4 5 6 7 8 9

Peroneus Teritus (L_5 - S_1)
R - 0 1 2 3 4 5 6 7 8 9
L - 0 1 2 3 4 5 6 7 8 9

Gluteus Medius (L_4 - S_1)
R - 0 1 2 3 4 5 6 7 8 9
L - 0 1 2 3 4 5 6 7 8 9

Gluteus Maximus (L_5 - S_2)
R - 0 1 2 3 4 5 6 7 8 9
L - 0 1 2 3 4 5 6 7 8 9

Gastrocnemius - Soleus (S_1 - 2)
R - 0 1 2 3 4 5 6 7 8 9
L - 0 1 2 3 4 5 6 7 8 9

Toe Extensors (L_5 - S_1)
R - 0 1 2 3 4 5 6 7 8 9
L - 0 1 2 3 4 5 6 7 8 9

Toe Flexors (S_1 - 2)
R - 0 1 2 3 4 5 6 7 8 9
L - 0 1 2 3 4 5 6 7 8 9

Estimated Quality of Muscle Exam

1 - patient cooperative; results accurate
2 - child too young to follow directions or child not cooperative in some positions (please star those muscles not felt to be accurate)
3 - patient uncooperative, crying, etc; results not felt to be accurate.

General Muscle Tone

Upper Ext.	Trunk	Lower Ext.
1-hypotonic	1-hypotonic	1-hypotonic
2-slight hypotonic	2-slight hypotonic	2-slight hypotonic
3-normal	3-normal	3-normal
4-slight hypertonic	4-slight hypertonic	4-slight hypertonic
5-hypertonic	5-hypertonic	5-hypertonic
9-unknown	9-unknown	9-unknown

Motor Level, Right

00 - T10 or above	11 - L1-3
01 - T11	12 - L2-4
02 - T12	13 - L3-4
03 - L1	14 - L4-5
04 - L2	15 - S1-2
05 - L3	16 - S2-3
06 - L4	17 - other; mixed
07 - L5	18 - no loss
08 - S1	19 - L5-S1
09 - S2 or below	99 - Unknown
10 - L1-2	

Motor Level, Left

00 - T10 or above	10 - L1-2
01 - T11	11 - L1-3
02 - T12	12 - L2-4
03 - L1	13 - L3-4
04 - L2	14 - L4-5
05 - L3	15 - S1-2
06 - L4	16 - S2-3
07 - L5	17 - other;mixed
08 - S1	18 - no loss
09 - S2 or below	19 - L5-S1
	99 - Unknown

Sensory Level, Right

00 - T10 or above	05 - S1
01 - T11 or T12	06 - S2
02 - L1-2	07 - S3-4
03 - L3-4	08 - no loss
04 - L5	99 - not recorded

Sensory Level, Left

00 - T10 or above	05 - S1
01 - T11 or T12	06 - S2
02 - L1-2	07 - S3-4
03 - L3-4	08 - no loss
04 - L5	99 - not recorded

Skip, Motor 0 - no 1 - yes 9 - unkn.

Skip, Sensory 0 - no 1 - yes 9 - unk.

Comments:

Recorded by:

MYELODYSPLASIA STUDY

Lower Extremity Measures: Muscle Evaluation
Record Type 3 - C Hospital Code __ __
Computer Case No. __ __ __ __
Date of Eval. __ __/__ __/__ __

Type of Evaluation
1-yearly 3-post-op
2-pre-op 4-followup
5-initial

3/85

CASE No.:

NAME:

B.D.:

Figure 22-7 *continues*

D

Wheelchairs

0 - none
1 - manual
2 - electric
3 - guerney
4 - stroller
8 - other
9 - unknown

Wheelchair Modifications

0 - no 1 - yes(describe):

Wheelchair Cushion

00 - not applicable
01 - none
02 - air, c cells
03 - air, no cells
04 - gel
05 - gel + other
06 - water
07 - light foam
08 - high density foam
09 - laminated foam
10 - hard seat
98 - other
99 - unknown

Wheelchair Transfers

__ t/f bed
__ t/f toilet
__ t/f tub
__ to floor
__ from floor
__ t/f auto

Code: 0 - dependent
1 - max. assist
2 - slight assist
3 - indep. c̄ aids
4 - indep. no aids
9 - unknown

☐ check here if not applicable

Wheeled Devices for Young Children

00 - none
01 - row-car
02 - scooterboard
03 - wheeled cart
04 - kiddie car
05 - trike (foot)
06 - trike (hand)
98 - other
99 - unknown

Braces

00 - none

Long Leg

01 - c̄ thoracic band
02 - c̄ pelvic band
03 - KAFO - metal
04 - KAFO-plastic
05 - KAFO one leg, AFO other leg
06 - other
07 - RGO

Short Leg

25 - metal
26 - plastic
27 - AFO with twisters
28 - twisters only
29 - other
30 - one short leg only
99 - unknown

Other Braces and Splints

00 - none
01 - hip brace
02 - trunk support
03 - Denis Browne
04 - serial casts
05 - night splints foot positioning
06 - UCB insert
98 - other
99 - unknown

Walking Aids (most frequently used)

00 - none

Canes
01 - single point
02 - quad or tripod

Crutches
03 - forearm
04 - axillary

Walkers
05 - pick-up
06 - wheeled
07 - reciprocal
08 - other aid (describe)
09 - joined forearm crutches
99 - unknown

Standing Devices

00 - none
01 - parapodium
02 - hinged parapodium
03 - prone board
04 - verlo
98 - other
99 - unknown

Usual Means of Locomotion

99 - unknown

Non-ambulatory
01 - is carried
02 - scoots/crawls inside, stroller, w.c. outside
03 - dependent in w.c., gurney at home (doesn't wheel self)
04 - partial w.c. indep. at home (pushes self, help for transfers)
05 - indep. in w.c. at home (all mobility and transfers)
06 - w.c. indep. in community (rough ground, ramps, all transfers)

Partially Ambulatory
11 - learning to walk; cruises and/or takes a few steps
12 - scoots/crawls in house, uses aids/braces for amb. away from home
13 - household ambulation, uses w.c. outside

Community Ambulator
21 - ambulates with aids/braces, needs w.c. for long distances
22 - ambulates with aids/braces, no wheel chair needed
23 - complete function without aids/braces

Extend of Independent Mobility

1 - doesn't go out
2 - goes out of house with parent or adult only
3 - out of house indep. to yard
4 - out of yard indep. to neighborhood
5 - out of neighborhood indep.
6 - self-drive auto or public trans. independently
9 - unknown

Type of Gait

00 - no gait
98 - other (describe)
99 - unknown

	Type of Gait	Position of Feet: Neutral	Toeing Out	Toeing In	Windswept Right	Windswept Left
non-functional	standing only	01	02	03	04	05
non-functional	cruises; walks holding on	06	07	08	09	10
with aids	shuffle - rotate (parapodium)	11	12	13	14	15
with aids	swing to (crutches, walker)	16	17	18	19	20
with aids	swing thru (crutches)	21	22	23	24	25
with aids	4-pt. alternating (crutches or 2 canes)	26	27	28	29	30
with aids	2-pt. one aid (crutch or cane)	31	32	33	34	35
with aids	3-pt. feet alternate, arms together (walker)	36	37	38	39	40
no aids	gluteal lurch (feet not dragging)	41	42	43	44	45
no aids	heel walk, poor balance	46	47	48	49	50
no aids	normal	51	52	53	54	55

Comments:

Recorded by:

MYELODYSPLASIA STUDY
Ambulation/Mobility
Record Type 4 - E

Computer Case Number __ __ __ __ Hospital Code __ __

Date of Evaluation __ __/ __ __/ __ __

Type of Evaluation 1-yearly 2-pre-op 3-post-op 4-follow-up 5-initial

3/85

CASE NUMBER:

NAME:

BIRTHDATE:

E

___ ___ ___ Age (m = months; d = days)

___ ___ ___ Height in cm.
(888 = fair measurement not possible)

___ ___ ___ Weight in kg.

___ ___ ___ Arm span in cm.

___ ___. ___ Head size - OFC (in cm)

0 - smaller than -2 SD
1 - within 2 SD + or -
2 - larger than +2 SD
9 - unknown

Blood Pressure

___ ___ ___ systolic

___ ___ ___ dyastolic

Skin Condition

___ ___ description of skin over myelodysplasia site:

Decubitus (since last exam)

00 - none
01 - back-gibbus
02 - sacrum
03 - ischium
04 - penis
05 - perineum
06 - knee
07 - malleoli
08 - heels
09 - dorsum of foot
10 - toes
98 - other or combo: (list)
99 - unknown

Indicate mechanism and describe cause

00 - not applicable
01 - pressure
02 - chemical
03 - shear (friction)
04 - heat
98 - other
99 - unknown

Description of cause:

Shunt Placement

1 - shunt in place
2 - no shunt in place
9 - unknown

Isosorbide Rx (since last exam)

0 - no
1 - yes
9 - unknown

Evidence of Trauma to Brain (since last exam)

0 - none
1 - bloody CSF
2 - subdural hematoma (or subarachnoid)
3 - porencephaly (by x-ray)
4 - meningitis, ventriculitis (gram +)
5 - meningitis, ventriculitis (gram -)
6 - bleeding and infection of CNS
7 - severe shunt obstruction
8 - other (describe):
9 - unknown

Pharyngo-laryngeal Palsy (since last exam)

0 - no 1 - yes 9 - unknown

Difficulty c̄ swallowing

0 - not applicable
1 - none
2 - mild (no Rx)
3 - severe
9 - unknown

Stridor	Apnea
0 - not appl.	0 - not appl.
1 - none	1 - none
2 - mild	2 - mild (no Rx)
3 - severe	3 - severe
9 - unknown	9 - unknown

Other Cranial Nerve Palsies

0 - no
1 - yes
9 - unknown

Other Significant Health Problems or Anomalies

0 - no
1 - yes (describe):
9 - unknown

Seizure Status

00 - none
controlled with:

01 - Dilantin
02 - Phenobarbital
03 - Dilantin and Phenobarbital
04 - Tegretol
05 - other medication (list):
06 - not well controlled c̄ or s̄ meds)
98 - other
99 - unknown

Special Diet

1 - no special diet
2 - for weight control
3 - for bowel management
4 - for bladder management
5 - for allergies
8 - for other or combination (list or describe):

9 - unknown

Occular Abnormalities

Right Eye	Left eye
1 - none	1 - none
2 - esotropia	2 - esotropia
3 - exotropia	3 - exotropia
4 - nystagmus lat gaze	4 - nystagmus lat gaze
5 - nystagmus fixation	5 - nystagmus fixation
8 - other	8 - other
9 - unknown	9 - unknown

General Vision

1 - within normal limits s̄ correction
2 - corrective lenses necessary
3 - indeterminate (too young)
4 - legally blind
8 - other (describe):

9 - unknown

General Hearing

1 - within normal limits
2 - partial hearing loss 1 or both ears)
3 - total hearing loss (1 or both ears)
4 - indeterminate (too young)
8 - other
9 - unknown

Skinfold Thickness ___ ___. ___ cm

Comments:

Recorded by:

MYELODYSPLASIA STUDY

General Health Status
Record Type 5 - **F**

Computer code no. ___ ___ ___ ___ Hospital Code ___ ___

Date of evaluation ___ ___/ ___ ___/ ___ ___

3/85

Hospital No:

Name:

B.D.:

Figure 22-7 *continues*

F

Residual Urine _ _ _ cc

Blood Pressure _ _ _ systolic
_ _ _ diastolic

Tanner Stage
0 1 2 3 4 5 9 - unknown

Urinary Infections
Current infections
0 - no 1 - yes 9 - unknown
Site of current infections (circle 1)
0 - no infec. 4 - pyelonephritis
1 - prostatitis 5 - epididymitis
2 - cystitis 9 - unknown
3 - pyocystis
_ _ Infections since last exam
_ _ Hosp. for infec. since last exam
(99 = unknown)

Urine Collection (circle 2)
01 - diaper 08 - indwell. cath.
02 - incont. pant 09 - valsalva
03 - external col. 10 - crede
04 - timed 11 - art. sphincter
05 - int. cath. 12 - norm c̄ urgency
06 - toilet train. 98 - other (describe
07 - urinary diver. 99 - unknown
00 - no second method
Further description under comments

Program Dates (month/year)
Began _ _ / _ _ Ended _ _ / _ _
(00/00 = program not ended or begun)
(99/99 = date unknown)

Quality of Urine Collection
(check all that apply)
_ good _ rash
_ damp _ decubiti (if due to poor
_ wet peroneal hygiene)
_ odor _ other

Degree of Independence
(use codes under stool indep. for applicable items)
_ emptying bag
_ changing appliance
_ using catheter, diaper, incont. pants, toilet

Stoma Quality
_ not applicable _ crustation
_ stoma good _ herniation
_ bleeding _ stenosis
_ other (describe)

Urinary Bladder Sensation (circle one)
0 - none 3 - fullness
1 - full bladder and passage
2 - passage of urine 9 - unknown

Comments:

Recorded by:

Urine Stream (circle one)
0 - no stream
1 - dribble/no stream
2 - dribble/steam with strain
3 - dribble/stress incontinence
4 - stress incontinence only
5 - normal
8 - not applicable
9 - unknown

Stool Program (circle 3)
00 - no program 07 - colostomy
01 - suppository 08 - high enema
02 - digital stim. 09 - oral med.
03 - timed 10 - reg. controlled
04 - expan. enema 11 - reg. con.- urg.
05 - Fleets bis. 98 - other (describe)
06 - manual remove 99 - unknown
00 - no second program
00 - no third program
Further description under comments

Program Dates (month/year)
Began _ _ / _ _ Ended _ _ / _ _
(00/00 = program not ended or begun)
(99/99 = date unknown)

Quality of Program
_ _ accidents per: 1 - day
2 - week
3 - month
888 - not applicable; no program
999 - unknown

Degree of Independence
1 - dependent 5 - with remind.
2 - takes interest 6 - independent
3 - assists 8 - not applicable
4 - with supervision 9 - unknown

Anal Tone 1 - weak 3 - tight
0 - none 2 - mod 9 - unknown

Anal Squeeze
0 - no 1 - yes 9 - unknown

Anal Sensation
0 - no 1 - yes 9 - unknown

Medications (00 - none, 99 - unknown)

Drug	Dose	began	ended
_ _	_ _ _ mg/day	_ _ / _ _	- _ _ / _ _
_ _	_ _ _ mg/day	_ _ / _ _	- _ _ / _ _
_ _	_ _ _ mg/day	_ _ / _ _	- _ _ / _ _
_ _	_ _ _ mg/day	_ _ / _ _	- _ _ / _ _

Bladder Meds	Antibiotics	Urine Acidification	Stool Regulators
01 - phenoxy	25 - septra	50 - vitamin C	75 - colace
02 - probanth	26 - gantrisin	51 - cranberry j.	76 - senekot
03 - ephedrine	27 - furadantin	52 - acid-ash diet	77 - herbal lax.
04 - ditropan	28 - amoxycillin		78 - metamusil
			79 - diet management
24 - other	49 - other	74 - other	98 - other

MYELODYSPLASIA STUDY
Toilet Training Data
Record Type 6- G

Computer Case No. _ _ _ _ Hospital Code _ _
Date of Evaluation _ _ / _ _ / _ _
Type of Evaluation 1-yearly
4-follow-up
5-initial
7/83

CASE NUMBER:
NAME:
BIRTHDATE:

G

LAB TESTS	BUN	creatinine	creatinine clearance	DMSA renal scan	urine culture
Ordered	__	__	__	__	__
Sent	__	__	__	__	__
Result	__ __	__.__ __	__ __ __	R __ __ __% L __ __ __%	≥10^5 <10^5 9 - unknown

Method of Collection
1 - cath
2 - midstream
3 - double cath
4 - supra pubic
9 - unknown

Testes
0 - undescended
1 - R undesc.
2 - L undesc.
3 - both undesc.
4 - female
9 - unknown

IVP

		none	mild	moderate	severe	cortical scarring and thinning	unknown
Hydronephrosis	R	__	__	__	__	__	__
	L	__	__	__	__	__	__
Nephrolithiasis	R	__	__	__	__		__
	L	__	__	__	__		__
Urinary stones: bladder		__	__	__	__		__
urethra		__	__	__	__		__
prostate		__	__	__	__		__

Anomalies 00 - no __ __ - yes ____________________ (99 = unknown)
If yes, describe & see code book for correct code number)

VCUG ± URODYNAMICS __ __ __ cc residual __ __ __ cc capacity

Trabeculation (bladder outline)
0 - normal
1 - mild
2 - moderate
3 - severe
4 - x-mas tree
5 - smooth
9 - unknown

Bladder Neck (sphincters)
0 - normal
1 - closed
2 - relaxed c̄ funneling
3 - external sphincter spasm (dysynergia)
4 - both relaxed
9 - unknown

Sensation
0 - none
1 - normal
2 - with cath
3 - with filling
4 - at capacity
9 - unknown

Detrusser
0 - normal
1 - reflex
2 - uninhibited (hyperreflexia)
3 - fibrotic
4 - large denervated
5 - areflexic
9 - unknown

		none	WISP	s̄ dilitation	c̄ dilitation	elongation	massive	unknown
Reflux	R	__	__	__	__	__	__	__
	L	__	__	__	__	__	__	__

Comments: (pressures, etc.)

LOOPOGRAM ± DYNAMICS __ __ cc residual __ __ cc capacity
pressure __ __ cm H_2O (mean) __ __ cm H_2O (low) __ __ cm H_2O (high)

		none	Ureteropelvic Junction	ureteroileal	intrinsic to loop	stomal	unknown
Obstruction	R	__	__	__	__	__	__
	L	__	__	__	__	__	__
		none	mild	moderate	severe		unknown
Hydronephrosis	R	__	__	__	__	__	__
	L	__	__	__	__	__	__
Sensation with filling		__	__	__	__	__	__
with contraction		__	__	__	__	__	__

Comments:

RECOMMENDATIONS

MYELODYSPLASIA STUDY
Urology Data
Record Type 7-H

Computer Case No. __ __ __ __ Hospital Code __ __
Date of Evaluation __ __ / __ __ / __ __
7/83

CASE NO.:
NAME:
BIRTHDATE:

Figure 22-7 *continues*

H

State of Residence

01 - Alaska
12 - Idaho
26 - Montana
37 - Oregon
47 - Washington

(see code book for those states not listed)

Size of Community

1 - city (or metropolitan): within 1 hr. of city ≥ 20,000 population
2 - town: within 30 min. of town 5,000 to 19,000 population
3 - small town: within 30 min. of town 1,000 - 5,000 (has shopping)
4 - rural with neighbors: over 30 min. to small town; neighbors with 1 mi.
5 - rural/isolated: neighbors over 1 mi.; over 30 min. to small town (i.e. ranch)
9 - unknown

Years in Current Residence

__ __ years

Living Situation

01 - one or both natural parents
02 - adoptive home
03 - foster home, #1
04 - foster home, #2
05 - foster home, #3 or more
06 - living with relatives
07 - institution or nursing home
08 - emancipated
98 - other (describe)

99 - unknown

Parents (if in natural, adoptive or foster home)

01 - mom and dad
02 - mom only
03 - dad only
04 - mom + stepdad
05 - mom + sig. other
06 - dad + sig. other
07 - dad + stepmom
97 - not applicable
98 - other (describe)
99 - unknown

Single Parents

0 - not applicable
1 - separation
2 - divorce
3 - death of spouse
4 - never married
9 - unknown

Children in Current Home

__ __ children living in current home

Natural Siblings (inlude 1/2 sibs, not step sibs)

__ __ natural siblings (do not include patient)

Legal Status

0 - with natural or adoptive parents
1 - permanent ward of court
2 - temporary ward of court
3 - placed outside natural home, natural parents retain custody
4 - of legal age - no guardian
5 - of legal age - guardian
8 - other (describe)
9 - unknown

Emancipated Patient

0 - not applicable
1 - patient living alone
2 - living with spouse
3 - living with significant other
4 - living with roommate
5 - living with spouse and children
8 - other (describe)

9 - unknown

Father's Occupation (in current home)

00 - unemployment/no income
01 - professional, technical
02 - manager, official, proprietor
03 - clerical, sales
04 - craftsman, foreman, operative
05 - service work, labor
06 - armed forces
07 - AFDC, SSI
08 - student
09 - not in home
98 - other (describe)
99 - unknown

Mother's Occupation (in current home)

00 - homemaker
01 - professional, technical
02 - manager, proprietor
03 - clerical, sales
04 - craftsman, foreman, operative
05 - service work, labor
06 - armed forces
07 - AFDC, SSI fulltime housewife
08 - student
09 - not in home
98 - other (describe)
99 - unknown

Mother's Employment (in current home)

00 - full time homemaker
01 - employment outside of home, F.T.
02 - employment outside of home, P.T.
03 - employment outside of home, irreg.
04 - employment in home, F.T.
05 - employment in home, P.T.
06 - student, F.T.
07 - student, P.T.
08 - wife-farmer
09 - time out from above occupation to raise family
10 - not in home
98 - other (describe)
99 - unknown

▶ **Academic Achievement** (highest grade level achieved)

__ __ 00 - never in school
50 - voc. training completed
51 - nursery or preschool
52 - kindergarten
53 - workshop training completed
96 - ungraded special ed.
99 - unknown

Education/Training (at present)

00 - none
01 - pvt. program for handicapped
02 - pvt. program for "normal"
03 - spec. ed. s̄ contact classes
04 - spec. ed. c̄ contact classes
05 - reg. ed. > 2 grade delay
06 - reg. ed. ± 2 grades
07 - reg. ed. + resource room
08 - higher ed./business or voc. train.
09 - workshop training
10 - developmental center
99 - unknown

Employment (at present)

00 - none
01 - workshop - transitional
02 - workshop - permanent
03 - partial employment
04 - gainful employment
99 - unknown

Therapy Services

__ occupation therapy
__ physical therapy
__ other (describe)

use following codes:
0 - not receiving
1 - sporadic/irregular service
2 - reg. service (≥ 1 time/month)
3 - reg. service (≥ 1 time/week)
4 - reg. service (daily)
5 - reg. but infrequent
9 - unknown

Therapy Services Provided Through:

00 - not applicable
01 - public/private school
02 - Elks
03 - developmental center
04 - medical center (hospital or clinic
98 - other (describe)
99 - unknown

Other Resources (check those applicable

__ none
__ CCS
__ AFDC
__ SSI (include medicaid)
__ Adoption Support
__ MOD
__ Child Support
__ other

MYELODYSPLASIA STUDY
Family and School Data
Record Type 8-I

Computer Case No. __ __ __ __ Hospital Code __ __

Date of Evaluation __ __ / __ __ / __ __

11/82

Case No:

Name:

B.D.:

I

Muscle Function

☐ All uppers grade 5

Shoulder Girdle Elevators
R-0 1 2 3 4 5 6 7 8 9
L-0 1 2 3 4 5 6 7 8 9

Shoulder Girdle Depressors
R-0 1 2 3 4 5 6 7 8 9
L-0 1 2 3 4 5 6 7 8 9

Shoulder Flexors
R-0 1 2 3 4 5 6 7 8 9
L-0 1 2 3 4 5 6 7 8 9

Shoulder Extensors
R-0 1 2 3 4 5 6 7 8 9
L-0 1 2 3 4 5 6 7 8 9

Shoulder Abductors
R-0 1 2 3 4 5 6 7 8 9
L-0 1 2 3 4 5 6 7 8 9

Shoulder Adductors
R-0 1 2 3 4 5 6 7 8 9
L-0 1 2 3 4 5 6 7 8 9

Back Ext. & Scapula Add. (Retraction)
R-0 1 2 3 4 5 6 7 8 9
L-0 1 2 3 4 5 6 7 8 9

Scapula Abductors (Protraction)
R-0 1 2 3 4 5 6 7 8 9
L-0 1 2 3 4 5 6 7 8 9

Elbow Flexors
R-0 1 2 3 4 5 6 7 8 9
L-0 1 2 3 4 5 6 7 8 9

Elbow Extensors
R-0 1 2 3 4 5 6 7 8 9
L-0 1 2 3 4 5 6 7 8 9

Range of Motion
1 - normal
2 - abnormal - Describe
9 - unknown

Upper Extremity Function Test
0 - normal
1 - cogwheeling rigidity
2 - spasticity (waxy)
3 - increased reflexes
4 - clonus (sustained)
5 - 1 + 2
6 - 1 + 3
8 - other (describe)
9 - unknown

* __ **Rapid Alternating Movements**

abnormal:
5-7 years = no pro/supination
7+ years = no or slow pro/supination or elbow excursion

* __ **Intention Tremor**

3-5 years = use finger to finger test, eyes open
6+ years = use finger nose test, eyes closed

* __ **Position Sense**

children 5+ years

Grip Strength

__ __ pounds right
__ __ pounds left

Dominant Hand
1 - right
2 - left
3 - undetermined or both
9 - unknown

Comments:

Recorded by:

*Use codes as follows:
1 - normal
2 - abnormal
3 - unable to determine
9 - unknown

Myelodysplasia Study
Upper Extremity Measures
Record Type 9

Computer Number __ __ __ __ Hosp. No __ __
Evaluation Date __ __ / __ __ / __ __

1/83

Case Number:

Name:

Birthdate:

Figure 22-7 *continues*

J

lesion level __ age (years) __ __ report by __

EATING

Independence Scale** (age in years)

Can	Does	Obs.	Time	Adap.		0 1 2 3 4 5 6 7 8 9 10 11 12 13 14 15 16
			__ __		Finger feed	
			__ __		Drinks from glass	
			__ __		Uses spoon	
			__ __		Uses fork	
			__ __		*Prepares cereal	
			__ __		Cuts with knife	
			__ __		*Makes sandwich	

GROOMING

Independence Scale ** (age in years)

Can	Does	Obs.	Time	Adap.		0 1 2 3 4 5 6 7 8 9 10 11 12 13 14 15 16
			__ __		Washes hands -with help	
			__ __		Washes face -with help	
			__ __		*Washes hands -no help	
			__ __		*Washes face -no help	
			__ __		Dries after bath-no help	
			__ __		Bathes by self	

Report by: (circle one)	Report Code (for Can & Does)	Observation Code	Time	Adaptations/ modifications	**Independence Scale
1-mother 2-father 3-therapist 4-nurse 5-patient 8-other (describe) 9-not recorded	0-fail, child not able or does not do task 1-pass, child does do task 8-not applicable 9-unknown	0-dependent 1-max assist 2-mod assist 3-min assist 4-cues only 5-independent 8-not applicable 9-unknown	Record in seconds (i.e. 1 0 = 10 sec.) or to the nearest minute, preceeded by a (-) (i.e. - 3 = 3 min.) Maximum should be 5 min.	0-none 1-yes, describe in comments 8-not applicable 9-unknown	20% 50%(notch) 80% L2&above(1) L3(2) L4-5(3) S1&below(4)

Comments:

Recorded by:

MYELODYSPLASIA STUDY

Selfcare Skills - Eating and Grooming
Record Type 10a - J

Computer Code Number __ __ __ __ Hospital Code __ __

Date of Evaluation __ __/ __ __/ __ __

11/82

Hospital No:

Name:

B.D.:

lesion level __ age (years) __ __ report by __ **K**

DRESSING (clothing and braces) — Independence Scale ** (age in years) 0 1 2 3 4 5 6 7 8 9 10 11 12 13 14 15 16

Can	Does	Obs.	Time	Adap.	Item	Notes
			__ __		*Socks off	
			__ __		*Pullover shirt - off	
			__ __		*Pants off	
			__ __		*Pullover shirt - on	
			__ __		*Socks on	
			__ __		*Pants on	
			__ __		*Shirt on with buttons	
			__ __		*Shoes on	
			__ __		*Ties shoes	Not achieved by group L2 & above
			__ __		Dresses completely	
			__ __		Choses clothes, gets them	
			__ __		*Removes braces	
			__ __		Braces on - with help	
			__ __		*Braces on - short leg plastic	N.A. L2 & above; N.A. L3
			__ __		*Braces on - short leg metal	N.A. L2 & above; N.A. S1 & below
			__ __		*Braces on - long leg	Not achieved by L2 & above; N.A. L4-5; N.A. S1 & below

Report by:	Report Code	Observation Code	Time	Adaptations/ modifications	**Independence Scale
(circle one) 1-mother 2-father 3-therapist 4-nurse 5-patient 8-other (describe) 9-not recorded	(for Can & Does) 0-fail, child not able or does not do task 1-pass, child does do task 8-not applicable 9-unknown	0-dependent 1-max assist 2-mod assist 3-min assist 4-cues only 5-independent 8-not applicable 9-unknown	Record in seconds (i.e. 1 0 = 10 sec.) or to the nearest minute, preceeded by a (-) (i.e. - 3 = 3 min.) Maximum should be 5 min.	0-none 1-yes, describe in comments 8-not applicable 9-unknown	20% 50%(notch) 80% L2&above(1) L3(2) L4-5(3) S1&below(4)

Comments

Recorded by:

MYELODYSPLASIA STUDY

Selfcare Skills - Dressing
Record Type 10b - K

Computer Code No. __ __ __ __ Hospital Code __ __

Date of Evaluation __ __/ __ __/ __ __

11/82

Hospital No:

Name:

B.D.:

Figure 22-7 *continues*

L

Test Results—RT 11
Developmental Evaluation*—Test Code *0

Test Given	*Test Results*
001 Bayley Scales of Infant Development	__ __ __MDI—Mental Development Index (***49 = below 50***)
	__ __ __PDI—Psychomotor Development Index
	__ __ __Mental-Basal Age (in months)
	__ __ __Mental-Ceiling Age (in months)
	__ __ __Motor-Based Age (in months)
	__ __ __Motor-Ceiling Age (in months)
002 Revised Gesell Developmental Schedules	__ __ __DQ—Developmental Quotient
	__ __ __Fine Motor Age (in months)
Developmental Quotient = (Fine motor age + adaptive age + personal social age + language age) ÷ 4 = developmental age; developmental age ÷ chronological age = DQ	__ __ __Adaptive Age (in months)
	__ __ __Personal Social Age (in months)
	__ __ __Language Age (in months)
	__ __ __Gross Motor Age (in months)
003 Peabody Scales of Fine Motor Development	__ __ __Age Equivalent Score (in months)

M

Test Results—RT 11
Visual Motor/Perceptual Motor Tests—Test Code ***1***

Test Given	*Test Results*
101 Frostig Developmental Test of Visual Perception	__ __ __PQ—Perceptual Quotient __ __ __Eye-Motor (in months) __ __ __Figure-Ground (in months) __ __ __Form Constancy (in months) __ __ __Position in Space (in months) __ __ __Spatial Relations (in months)
102 Motor Free Visual Perception Test (MVPT)	__ __ __PQ—Perceptual Quotient __ __ __Perceptual Age (in months) (110 = greater than 9 years; ***47 = less than 4 years***)
103 Beery Test of Visual Motor Integration (VMI)	__ __ __Visual Motor Age (in months) __ __ __Scale Score
104 Jebsen Taylor Hand Function Test	__ __ __Right Hand % of Mean Score __ __ __Left Hand % of Mean Score __ __ __Dominant Hand 001 = Right 002 = Left 999 = Unknown

Figure 22-7 *continues*

N

Test Results—RT 11
Intelligence Tests—Test Code ***2***

Test Given	*Test Results*
201 Stanford Binet 1961 Revision	__ __ __Mental Age (in months)
	__ __ __IQ
	__ __ __Basal Age (in months)
	__ __ __Ceiling Age (in months)
202 Stanford Binet 1972 Revision	__ __ __Mental Age (in months)
	__ __ __IQ
	__ __ __Basal Age (in months)
	__ __ __Ceiling Age (in months)
203 WISC	__ __ __Verbal IQ
	__ __ __Performance IQ
	__ __ __Full Scale IQ
203 WISC-R	__ __ __Verbal IQ
	__ __ __Performance IQ
	__ __ __Full Scale IQ

O

Test Results—RT 11
Achievement Tests—Test Code ***3***

Test Given	***Test Results***
301 Wide Range Achievement Test (WRAT)	__ __ __Reading (standard score)
	__ __ __Spelling (standard score)
	__ __ __Arithmetic (standard score)

PATIENT'S NAME______________________________BIRTHDATE________

Var.	Col.		
		Computer I.D. Number	__ __ __ __
3	1-2	Hospital Code Number	__ __
5-7	9-14	Date	__ __ __ __ __ __
9-10	17-21	Age (months/days)	__ __ __/__ __
8	15-16	Type of Surgery	__ __
11	22-24	Operation	__ __ __
12	25-27	Operative Indication	__ __ __
13	28-30	Operative Complication	__ __ __
14	31-32	Hospital Where Surgery Performed	__ __
15	33-34	Surgeon	__ __
16	35-37	Late Complications	__ __ __

IND: ____

____

OP: ____

____

M.D.:_________________________Hospital: __________________

Figure 22-7 *continues*

Q

NAME ____________________ Hospital No. ____________________ RECORD TYPE 17

1-4 __ __ __ __ Computer ID

5-10 __ __/__ __/__ __ Birthdate

11-15 __ __ __/__ __ Age of patient in MONTHS/DAYS

16-21 __ __/__ __/__ __ Date of Admission

22-27 __ __/__ __/__ __ Date of Discharge

28-33 __ __/__ __/__ __ Date of Surgery

34-35 __ __ Hospital where surgery performed

36-38 __ __ __ ***Operation*** (__ __ __ __.__ __ __ ICD9CM No.)

39-40 __ __ Revision Number

41-43 __ __ __ ***Indication*** (__ __ __ __.__ __ __ ICD9CM No.)

44-46 __ __ __ Complication

47-48 __ __ Days postop (00-60 = days; 71-79 = 3-12 months; 81-89 = 1-9 years; 99 = unknown)

49-50 __ __ ***Surgeon(s)***

06 = Stuntz	20 = Mulder	37 = Blue	99 = Unknown
19 = Loeser	36 = Kamm	98 = Other	

51-52 __ __ ***Primary symptom complex***

53-54 __ __ ***Secondary symptom complex*** → (Use code below)

01 = sunsetting	05 = change in appetite	09 = decreased schoolwork
02 = bulging fontanelle	06 = lethargy	88 = other (specify below)
03 = vomiting	07 = seizures	99 = unknown
04 = irritability	08 = headaches	

55-56 __ __ ***Observed primary cause of malfunction***

57-58 __ __ ***Observed secondary cause of malfunction*** → (Use code below)

01 = proximal occlusion	04 = shunt too short	07 = no indication
02 = distal occlusion	05 = valve plugged	08 = tube broken
03 = disconnected device	06 = infection present	88 = other (specify below)

59-61 __ __ __ CSF pressure mm H_2O

62-65 __ __ __ __ Protein CSF mg %

66-69 __ __ __ __ Glucose CSF mg %

70-74 __ __ __ __ __ Number red blood cells CSF/mm3

75-79 __ __ __ __ __ Number white blood cells CSF/mm3

80-81 __ __ ***Ventricle size (Degree of Hydrocephalus)***

00 = None	02 = Moderate (1.1–2.0)
01 = Mild (2.1 or greater)	03 = Severe (<1.0 cm)

82-83 __ __ Culture CSF—organism (pre-op + intra-op)

84-85 __ __ Culture CSF—organism (post-op)

Organism
- 00 = None
- 01 = Probable contaminant
- 02 = Staph epi
- 03 = Staph aureus
- 04 = Gram −
- 05 = Gram − Egan +
- 06 = Other

86-88 __ __ __ ***Type of shunting system—reservoir or valve***

201 = Hakim
202 = Hakim (Rickham)
203 = Heyer (Foltz standard to and fro)
204 = Heyer (Omaya)
205 = Heyer (Mishler Double, Lumen)
206 = Heyer (low profile)
207 = Heyer (multipurpose with on-off valve)
208 = Heyer (Foltz reservoir and antisiphon device)
209 = Pudenz-Heyer (Heyer Schulte, standard burr hole)
210 = Pudenz-Heyer (standard, flat bottom)
211 = Holter (Rickham)
212 = Spitz-Holter
213 = Removal; replace with Foltz standard to and fro
214 = Removal prior device; replace with Hakim

89-90 __ __ ***Type of proximal catheter***

00 = None
01 = Standard straight
02 = Standard right angle
03 = Pudenz Flange (Portnoy)
04 = Raimondi, one piece
05 = Pudenz, radio-opaque
06 = "Y" proximal
88 = Other
99 = Unknown

91-93 __ __.__ Length of proximal catheter

84-95 __ __ ***Type of distal catheter***

00 = None
01 = Barium
02 = Silicone
03 = Spring loaded
04 = Raimondi
05 = Pudenz, radio-opaque
06 =
88 = Other
99 = Unknown

96-98 __ __.__ Length of distal catheter
99-100 __ __ Antibiotics #1
101-104 __ __ __.__ mg/kg/day
105-106 __ __ Route
107-108 __ __ Antibiotics #2
109-112 __ __ __.__ mg/kg/day
113-114 __ __ Route
115-116 __ __ Antibiotics #3
117-120 __ __ __.__ mg/kg/day
121-122 __ __ Route

Antibiotics	*Mg/Day*	**Penicillin Dosage*	*Route Codes*
01 = Amikan	15	025 = 25,000 units	01 = PO
02 = Amoxicillin (Ampicillin, 100)	150-200	050 = 50,000 unit	02 = PO + IV
03 = Cetazolin, Cephalothin	40-60	100 = 100,000 units	03 = IM
04 = Chloromphenicol (25)	25-50	150 = 150,000 units	04 = IM + IVent
05 = Gentamycin (2.5)	5-7.5	200 = 200,000 units	05 = IV
06 = Methicillin (50-75)	75-100	250 = 250,000 units	06 = IV + IVent
07 = Nafcillin (40)	60	300 = 300,000 units	07 = IVent
08 = Penicillin	*	350 = 350,000 units	08 = Irrigation
09 = Tobramycin	4-6	400 = 400,000 units	
10 = Vancomycin (30)	45	450 = 450,000 units	
11 = 1/4% Neomycin			
12 = Bacitracin 500,000 u/100cc saline			

123-124 __ __ ***Antibiotics Classification, prophylaxis***

01 = None or inadequate
02 = IV only
03 = IV plus 10 mg IVent methicillin
04 = IV plus 100 mg IVent methicillin
05 = IV plus 100 mg IVent methicillin plus IV plus 2 mg IVent gentamycin

COMMENT: ____________________

9/13/84

Figure 22-7 *continues*

R

Neurology Operations

001 Ventriculo-auricular Shunt Insertion
023 Cysto-ventriculostomy
036 Ventriculo-mastoid Shunt
042 Ventriculo-ureteral Shunt
048 Subarachnoid-ureteral Shunt
054 Subarachnoid-peritoneal Shunt
060 Ventriculostomy
061 Ventriculo-posterior Fossa Shunt
066 Shunt Removal
067 Ventriculo-ventricular Shunt
072 Pneumogram
073 Ventriculogram
074 Pneumo and Ventriculogram
076 Myelogram
078 Implantation of Transnsors
079 Ligation
081 Ventriculo-peritoneal Shunt
088 Thoracic-peritoneal Shunt
091 Lengthening Upper/Lower End of Shunt
092 Open Irrigation of Shunt
093 Craniotomy of Ventriculostomy with Removal of Foreign Body
097 Insertion of Rickham Reservoir
098 Insertion of Omaya Reservoir
129 Ventriculo-pleural Shunt
150 Extraventricular Drainage, External
151 Remove Extraventricular Drainage

Neurology Complications

001 Wound infection
085 Wound dehiscence
082 Shunt Infection (CSF)
025 Blood stream infection
056 Thrombus infection, cardiopulmonary infection
004 CNS infection
052 CNS bloodstream infection
078 Fever NR
060 Wound Infection
002 Shunt non-function
076 Erroneous tube ligation
084 Shunt obstruction, vision loss
090 Disconnected shunt
055 Thrombosis, cardiopulmonary failure
058 Cardiac arrest, procedure complete
059 Cardiac arrest, procedure incomplete
003 CNS Bleed
048 Hyponatremia
049 Dehydration
079 Bradycardia NR
080 Tachycardia NR
046 Seizure NR
047 Motor paralysis
000 None
050 MM sac Full (same as 007)
051 MM Sac full, leaking
053 CNS and Bloodstream infection
054 Pre-op infection persists
057 Death
077 Pre-op indication persists
083 Shunt obstruction
098 Other
099 Unknown/NR
100 Death (same as 057)

Type of Shunting System

201* Hakim
202 Hakim (Rickham)
203* Heyer (Foltz standard to and fro)
204 Heyer (Omaya)
205 Heyer (Mishler Double, Lumen)
206 Heyer (low profile)
207* Heyer (multipurpose with on-off valve)
208 Heyer (Foltz reservoir and antisiphon device)
209* Pudenz-Heyer (Heyer Schulte, standard burr hole)
210* Pudenz-Heyer (standard, flat bottom)
211* Holter (Rickham)
212* Spitz-Holter
213 Torkildsen
214 Codman

Neurology Indications

000 Increased Headsize
001 Increased OFC and vent pressure
002 Increased OFC, vent size/vent pressure
003 Increased ventricular pressure
004 Increased ventricular pressure and size
005 Increased OFC and vent size
006 Papilledema
007 Increased ventricular pressure, acute
008 Broken or dislodged shunt
009 Obstruction proximal/ventricle end
010 Obstruction distal/cardiac/peritoneal end, thrombus
011 Obstruction distal/cardiac/peritoneal end, thrombus
012 Obstruction distal/cardiac/peritoneal end, thrombus
013 Obstruction distal/cardiac/peritoneal end, thrombus
014 Increased shunt transmission pressure
015 CNS infection
016 Bloodstream infection
017 CNS and bloodstream infection
018 Cardiopulmonary emboli with right auriculo thrombus
019 Leaking meningomyelocele
020 Leaking meningocele, increased ventricular size
021 Full meningomyelocele, high transmission pressure
022 Flushing device/valve obstructed
023 Flushing device valve mechanical failure, disconnected
024 Obstruction V.M., proximal, CNS
025 Obstruction V.M., distal, mastoid
026 Social
027 No evidence of dependency "arrested"
028 Both ends of shunt obstructed
029 To decrease size of meningomyelocele
030 Infected tract of shunt and device
031 Sub-galeal fluid collection with obstructed shunt
032 Sub-galeal fluid collection with broken shunt
033 Obstructed ventricle end and broken shunt
034 Obstructed cardiac end and broken shunt
035 Obstruction both ends and broken shunt
036 Prophylactic lengthening of shunt
037 Poor pump filling, no CNS obstruction detected
038 Shunt tube ligated
040 Routine re-evaluation
041 Shunt failure/malfunction/obstruction
042 Flushing valve and bloodstream infection
043 VP shunt distal obstruction
044 For study purposes
045 Replace non-functioning shunt
046 Neurologic loss
047 Subdural hematoma
048 No communication between lateral ventricles (obstruction foramen of Monro)
049 Dural CSF leakage around catheter
050 Enlarging MM without shunt
051 Peritoneal/distal end obstruction
052 Infected shunt with CSF infection
053 Decompression of Arnold-Chiari formation
054 Dislodged, broken shunt with infected CSF
055 Low CSF pressure syndrome
056 Shunt infection resolved
057 Increasing ventricular size (progressive ventriculomegaly)
059 Increasing OFC
060 Sunsetting
061 Bulging fontanelles
062 Vomiting
063 Irritability
064 Appetite change
065 Lethargy
066 Seizures
067 Headaches
068 School work decline
069 Short shunt
070 Plugged valve
998 Other
999 Unknown

*Listed on front

S

NAME ______________________ Hospital No. ______________________ RECORD TYPE 18

1-4 __ __ __ __ Computer ID
5-10 __ __/__ __/__ __ Birthdate
11-15 __ __ __/__ __ Age of patient in Months/Days
16-21 __ __/__ __/__ __ Date of Admission
22-27 __ __/__ __/__ __ Date of Discharge
28-33 __ __/__ __/__ __ Date of Surgery
34-35 __ __ Hospital Where Surgery Performed
36-38 __ __ __ *Operation* (__ __ __ __·__ __ ICD9CM No.)

- 004 = MM Repair—Routine
- 015 = Secondary Closure
- 020 = Removal Lumbar Lipoma, Lipomeningocele or Cystocele (Resection or Excision)
- 024 = Excision of Neurodermal Sinus with Laminectomy
- 027 = Severe Filum Terminale

39-41 __ __ __ *Indication* (__ __ __ __·__ __ ICD9CM No.)

- 006 = Repeat CSF Leakage
- 009 = Increasing neurologic deficit
- 012 = Primary MM removal
- 016 = Breakdown of closure (wound dehiscence)
- 021 = Mass in spinal canal
- 022 = Lipoma or lipomeningocele
- 024 = Neurodermal sinus

42-43 __ __ *Surgeon(s)*

- 06 = Stuntz
- 08 = Gibson
- 11 = Knopp
- 15 = Mulder
- 20 = Loeser
- 26 = Kropp & Stuntz
- 27 = Kropp
- 28 = Blue
- 35 = Kamm
- 36 = Kamm & Kropp
- 98 = Other
- 99 = Unknown

44-45 __ __ *Neural Elements*

- 01 = one-layer pia arachnoid dura
- 02 = neural plaque entubated w/2-layer pia arachnoid
- 03 = myofascial patch; one-layer closure
- 04 = 01 plus neural tissue sacrifice
- 05 = 02 plus neural tissue sacrifice
- 06 = 03 plus neural tissue sacrifice
- 07 = one-layer arachnoid + 2 dura; 2 layer

46-47 __ __ *Myofascial Closure*

- 01 = Midline
- 04 = Four-layer
- 02 = Latissimus dorsi and myofascial
- 05 = One layer lumbodorsal fascial
- 03 = Imbrication ("book")—2 layers of fascia
- 06 = One layer fascia plus free myofascial graft

48-49 __ __ *Skin Closure*

- 01 = Midline (vertical)
- 02 = Midline, right bipedicle graft (side slits)
- 03 = Midline, left bipedicle graft (side slits)
- 04 = Midline, bilateral bipedicle graft (side slits)
- 05 = "T" closure (horizontal and vertical)
- 06 = "Y" or "V" closure
- 07 = Horizontal

50-55 __ __·__/__ __·__cm Width/Length Skin Defect
56-57 __ __ Lesion Level Cephalad (top)
58-59 __ __ Lesion Level Caudad (lower)
60-65 __ __·__/__ __·__cm Width/Length Pedicle
66-71 __ __·__/__ __·__cm Width/Length Mass

Figure 22-7 *continues*

72-74 __ __ __ *Complications*

001 = Wound (not CSF) infection
002 = Skin and myofascial breakdown*
006 = CSF infection
022 = Fluid and electrolyte imbalance
024 = Tachycardia
025 = CSF leak submyofascial
027 = Skin breakdown*
028 = Submyofascial CSF leak plus skin breakdown*
034 = Later next shunt infected
035 = Graft needed for skin breakdown*
* Record size below.

75-80 __ __.__/__ __.__cm Width/Length Skin Slough
81-86 __ __.__/__ __.__cm Width/Length Myofascial Slough
87-91 __ __ __ __ __ White Blood Cells CSF/mm3
92-96 __ __ __ __ __ Red Blood Cells CSF/mm3
97-100 __ __ __ __ Polymorphonuclear cells CSF/mm3
101-104 __ __ __ __ Monocytes (mononuclear) cells CSF/mm3
105-108 __ __ __ __ Glucose CSF mg %
109-112 __ __ __ __ Protein CSF mg %
113-114 __ __ Wound Culture Pre-op/Intra-op
115-116 __ __ CSF Culture Pre-op/Intra-op
117-118 __ __ Wound Culture Post-op
119-120 __ __ CSF Culture Post-op
121-122 __ __ Antibiotics #1
123-126 __ __ __.__ mg/kg/day
127-128 __ __ Route
129-130 __ __ Antibiotics #2
131-134 __ __ __.__ mg/kg/day
135-136 __ __ Route
137-138 __ __ Antibiotics #3
139-142 __ __ __.__ mg/kg/day
143-144 __ __ Route

Organism
00 = None
01 = Probable contaminant
02 = Staph epi
03 = Staph aureus
04 = Gram −
05 = Gram − Egan +
06 = Other

Antibiotics	*Mg/Day*	**Penicillin Dosage*	*Route Codes*
01 = Amikan	15	025 = 25,000 units	01 = PO
02 = Amoxicillin (Ampicillin, 100)	150-200	050 = 50,000 unit	02 = PO + IV
03 = Cetazolin, Cephalothin	40-60	100 = 100,000 units	03 = IM
04 = Chloromphenicol (25)	25-50	150 = 150,000 units	04 = IM + IVent
05 = Gentamycin (2.5)	5-7.5	200 = 200,000 units	05 = IV
06 = Methicillin (50-75)	75-100	250 = 250,000 units	06 = IV + IVent
07 = Nafcillin (40)	60	300 = 300,000 units	07 = IVent
08 = Penicillin	*	350 = 350,000 units	08 = Irrigation
09 = Tobramycin	4-6	400 = 400,000 units	
10 = Vancomycin (30)	45	450 = 450,000 units	
11 = 1/4% Neomycin			
12 = Bacitracin 500,000 u/100 cc saline			

145-146 __ __ *Antibiotics Classification, prophylaxis*

01 = None or inadequate
02 = IV only
03 = IV plus 10 mg IVent methicillin
04 = IV plus 100 IVent methicillin
05 = IV plus 100 mg IVent methicillin plus IV plus 2 mg IVent gentamycin

147-148 __ __ *Delivery*

01 = Labor plus vaginal
02 = Labor plus Caesarean section
03 = Caesarean section 8-9 months (36-40 weeks)
04 = Caesarean section elective "early with prenatal ck" (32-35 weeks)
05 = Vaginal with ventriculostomy

COMMENT: ______________________________

8/1/84

Surgeries

Code	Surgery
000*	Closure, simple
001*	Plastic flap closure
002*	Plastic cover w/resection
003*	Plastic flap w/resection
004**	MM excision—routine
005	Minimal closure
006	Local drain to peritoneum
007	Revision #1
008	Revision #2
009	Revision #3
010	Revision #4
011	Revision #5
012/018	Cord resection
013	Replacement after peeling
014	Replacement of plaque and closure
015**	Secondary closure
016	Exploration
017	Laminectomy w/excision MM or lipoma
018/012	Excision w/cord resection
019	Myelogram
020**	Removal lumbar lipoma, lipomeningocele or cystocele (resection or excision)
021	Excision Rachischis
022*	Opening and drainage w/irrigation and packing of surgical incision
023	Secondary to laminectomy with excision of MM
024**	Excision of neurodermal sinus with laminectomy
025	Debridement or tissue breakdown (necrosis)
026	Removal of meninges w/repair of skin-covered or abdominal meningocele sac with or without nervous element
027**	Sever filum terminale (release of tethered cord)
998	Other
999	Unknown

*Recode and delete
**Listed on front

Indications

Code	Indication
000/001/002/015	Large bulbous sac
003/004/005	Large sac, interfering with development or prostheses
006*	Repeat CSF Leakage
007	Tender
008	Cause for family concern
009*	Increasing neurologic deficit
010	Concern of malignancy
011	Instability of spine, need for fusion
012*	Primary MM repair
013	Full sac post VA shunt
014	Open cord and "neural fid" without sac or membranes
015	Full sac and tender post successful shunt
016*/020	Breakdown of closure (wound dehiscence)
017	MM epithelializing slowly without pressure
018	Exploration
019	Recurrent chemical meningitis
020	Prevent infection in post surgical wound
021*	Mass in spinal canal (suspected)
022*	Lipoma or lipomeningocele
023	Delayed removal of sac with decubitus formation
024*	Neurodermal sinus
998	Other
999	Unknown

*Listed on front

Complications

Code	Complication
000	None
001/004	Local infection
002	Wound breakdown
003/005	CSF leakage
006/007/008/009/018/019	Wound breakdown, CSF infection
014	Blood stream infection
016	Post-op fever, no blood or CNS culture
017	Post-op pneumanitis URI or other
020/023	CSF infection and wound breakdown (meningitis)
024	Tachycardia
077	No change
098	Other
099	Unknown

Figure 22-7 *continues*

101376 999 032 999 999 999 999 75 H002

REPORT NO. MYLIST — MYELODYSPLASIA PATIENT ABSTRACT — RUN DATE 01/11/85

CHART: MY0165599 — CASE: 0087

PERMANENT INFORMATION

BIRTH DATE: 050366 SEX: MALE AGE 1ST EXAM: 3 MONTHS
HOURS OF LABOR: 99 TYPE OF DELIVERY: UNKNOWN
BIRTH WT: 4.40 KG LENGTH: 99 CM OFC: 37 CM LESION LENGTH:99.9 CM WIDTH:99.9 CM
BACK CLOSURE DATE: 999999 AGE: 99 DAYS SHUNT DATE: 999999 AGE: 99 DAYS
PRIMARY DIAGNOSIS: MENINGOMYELOCELE
PROGNOSIS AT BIRTH: UNKNOWN
PROGNOSIS 1ST EXAM: HOPELESS
YEARS EDUCATION OF FATHER: 99 CONCEPTION OF CHILD: CONVEIVED WITHIN WEDLOCK
YEARS EDUCATION OF MOTHER: 99 FAMILY HISTORY OF NEURAL TUBE DEFECTS: UNKNOWN
MARITAL STATUS OF PARENTS AT TIME OF BIRTH: UNKNOWN
OCCUPATION OF FATHER AT TIME OF BIRTH: CRAFTSMAN, FOREMAN, OPERATIVE
AGE AT MENARCHE: 998 MONTHS GESTATIONAL AGE: 99 WEEKS
AGE AT DEATH: 0 MONTHS CAUSE OF DEATH: NO DEATH
RELIGION: UNKNOWN
COMMENTS: RECODED FROM EARLIER DATA COLLECTION FORMS

******************** LOWER EXTREMITY MEASURES: RANGE OF MOTION ********************

SPINAL ALIGNMENT

DATE	CURVE	REGION	CONVEXITY	PLUMB ALIGNMENT	
101566	NORMAL	NOT APPLICABLE	NONE	8/88 CM SITTING	8/88 CM STANDING
061567	NORMAL	NOT APPLICABLE	NONE	0/00 CM SITTING	8/88 CM STANDING
091568	SCOLIOSIS	LUMBAR	RIGHT	9/99 CM SITTING	9/99 CM STANDING
041569	SCOLIOSIS	LUMBAR	RIGHT	9/99 CM SITTING	8/88 CM STANDING
031570	SCOLIOSIS	LUMBAR	RIGHT	9/99 CM SITTING	8/88 CM STANDING
081571	SCOLIOSIS	LUMBAR	RIGHT	9/99 CM SITTING	8/88 CM STANDING
081572	SCOLIOSIS	LUMBAR	RIGHT	9/99 CM SITTING	8/88 CM STANDING
081573	SCOLIOSIS	THORACIC	RIGHT	9/99 CM SITTING	8/88 CM STANDING
103174	SCOLIOSIS	LUMBAR	RIGHT	0/00 CM SITTING	8/88 CM STANDING
091875	SCOLIOSIS	THORACO-LUMBAR	RIGHT	0/00 CM SITTING	8/88 CM STANDING
101277	SCOLIOSIS	THORACO-LUMBAR	RIGHT	0/00 CM SITTING	8/88 CM STANDING
052880	SCOLIOSIS	THORACO-LUMBAR	RIGHT	0/00 CM SITTING	8/88 CM STANDING
010583	SCOLIOSIS	THORACO-LUMBAR	RIGHT	1/02 CM SITTING	8/88 CM STANDING

HIP

	EXTENSION		FLEXION		ABDUCT.		ADDUCT.		EXT ROT		INT ROT		LEG LENGTH	
DATE	R	L	R	L	R	L	R	L	R	L	R	L	R	L
101566	008	008	130	130	033	033	030	030	045	045	045	045	999	999
061567	010	010	130	130	045	045	030	030	045	045	045	045	999	999
091568	010	010	130	130	045	045	030	030	045	045	045	045	999	999
041569	015	015	130	130	045	045	000	000	045	045	000	000	999	999
031570	015	015	130	130	045	045	000	000	045	045	000	000	999	999
081571	015	015	110	110	045	033	000	000	045	045	033	10-	999	999
081572	015	015	100	100	045	045	10-	10-	045	045	010	000	999	999
081573	045	060	130	130	045	045	008	21-	045	045	010	033	999	999
103174	000	888	090	888	030	888	005	888	090	888	000	888	057	888
091875	000	000	100	100	050	050	000	15-	090	090	000	30-	888	888
101277	020	015	095	130	035	035	10-	10-	090	090	000	35-	071	075
052880	000	000	090	090	060	060	000	000	090	090	000	000	071	072
010583	045	045	130	130	045	040	000	-05	090	090	-35	-45	069	072

DATE	TEST USED	HIP STATUS R	HIP STATUS L
101566	UNKNOWN	DISLOCATED	DISLOCATED
061567	UNKNOWN	IN SOCKET	IN SOCKET
091568	UNKNOWN	IN SOCKET	IN SOCKET

A

Figure 22-8 *continues*

Figure 22-8. Computer entry forms used as patient clinical abstracts in clinic. A sample copy of a patient's clinical abstract, which is available during clinic visits in hard copy form. Each screen corresponds to a data collection form in figure 22-7.

041569	UNKNOWN	UNKNOWN	UNKNOWN
031570	UNKNOWN	UNKNOWN	UNKNOWN
081571	UNKNOWN	UNKNOWN	UNKNOWN
081572	UNKNOWN	UNKNOWN	UNKNOWN
081573	UNKNOWN	IN SOCKET	IN SOCKET
103174	UNKNOWN	UNKNOWN	IN SOCKET
091875	UNKNOWN	UNKNOWN	IN SOCKET
101277	UNKNOWN	UNKNOWN	IN SOCKET
052880	UNKNOWN	DISLOCATED	IN SOCKET
010583	THOMAS	DISLOCATED	IN SOCKET

KNEE

	EXTENSION		FLEXION		VARUS		VALGUS		POSITION WHILE	POSITION WHILE
DATE	R	L	R	L	R	L	R	L	WEIGHT BEARING R	WEIGHT BEARING L
101566	000	000	136	136	002	002	002	002	UNKNOWN	UNKNOWN
061567	000	000	112	112	002	002	002	002	N WEIGHT-BEARING	N WEIGHT-BEARING
091568	000	000	112	112	002	002	010	008	UNKNOWN	UNKNOWN
041569	003	003	112	112	002	002	002	002	N WEIGHT-BEARING	N WEIGHT-BEARING
031570	003	003	112	112	002	002	002	002	UNKNOWN	UNKNOWN
081571	030	030	136	112	002	002	010	010	N WEIGHT-BEARING	N WEIGHT-BEARING
081572	060	060	136	136	002	002	010	010	N WEIGHT-BEARING	N WEIGHT-BEARING
081573	030	030	136	136	002	002	010	008	N WEIGHT-BEARING	N WEIGHT-BEARING
103174	047	888	125	888	888	888	888	888	N WEIGHT-BEARING	N WEIGHT-BEARING
091875	050	050	100	090	888	888	888	888	N WEIGHT-BEARING	N WEIGHT-BEARING
101277	040	050	090	090	000	000	000	015	NEUTRAL	VALGUS
052880	030	025	075	080	999	999	999	999	N WEIGHT-BEARING	N WEIGHT-BEARING
010583	030	015	090	090	-10	-10	010	010	N WEIGHT-BEARING	N WEIGHT-BEARING

FOOT/ANKLE

	HEEL POSITION		SEVERITY		FOREFOOT POSITION		SEVERITY	
DATE	R	L	R	L	R	L	R	L
101566	N WEIGHT	N WEIGHT	0 - 10 D	0 - 10 D	NEUTRAL	NEUTRAL	0 - 10 D	0 - 10 D
061567	NEUTRAL	NEUTRAL	0 - 10 D	0 - 10 D	NEUTRAL	NEUTRAL	0 - 10 D	0 - 10 D
091568	N WEIGHT	N WEIGHT	0 - 10 D	0 - 10 D	ADDUCTUS	NEUTRAL	20 - 30	0 - 10 D
041569	VARUS	NEUTRAL	20 - 30	0 - 10 D	ADDUCTUS	NEUTRAL	20 - 30	0 - 10 D
031570	VARUS	NEUTRAL	20 - 30	0 - 10 D	ADDUCTUS	NEUTRAL	20 - 30	0 - 10 D
081571	VARUS	NEUTRAL	> 30 DEG	0 - 10 D	ADDUCTUS	NEUTRAL	> 30 DEG	0 - 10 D
081572	VALGUS	VALGUS	> 30 DEG	> 30 DEG	NEUTRAL	NEUTRAL	0 - 10 D	0 - 10 D
081573	VALGUS	VALGUS	20 - 30	20 - 30	NEUTRAL	NEUTRAL	0 - 10 D	0 - 10 D
103174	VARUS	VARUS	20 - 30	20 - 30	NEUTRAL	ADDUCTUS	0 - 10 D	0 - 10 D
091875	VARUS	VARUS	> 30 DEG	> 30 DEG	ADDUCTUS	NEUTRAL	20 - 30	0 - 10 D
101277	VARUS	VARUS	20 - 30	> 30 DEG	ADDUCTUS	NEUTRAL	20 - 30	0 - 10 D
052880	NEUTRAL	NEUTRAL	0 - 10 D	0 - 10 D	NEUTRAL	NEUTRAL	0 - 10 D	0 - 10 D
010583	N WEIGHT	N WEIGHT	0 - 10 D	0 - 10 D	ADDUCTUS	NEUTRAL	10 - 20	0 - 10 D

	DORSIFLX		PLANTARFLX		ARCH		TOES		GREAT TOE	
DATE	R	L	R	L	R	L	R	L	R	L
101566	020	020	040	040	NEUTRAL	NEUTRAL	UNKNOWN	UNKNOWN	UNKNCWN	UNKNCWN
061567	15-	15-	040	040	NEUTRAL	NEUTRAL	UNKNOWN	UNKNOWN	UNKNCWN	UNKNCWN
091568	000	05-	040	040	PLANUS	NEUTRAL	UNKNOWN	UNKNOWN	UNKNOWN	UNKNOWN
041569	-15	15-	040	040	NEUTRAL	NEUTRAL	UNKNOWN	UNKNOWN	UNKNCWN	UNKNCWN
031570	015	15-	040	040	NEUTRAL	NEUTRAL	UNKNOWN	UNKNOWN	UNKNOWN	UNKNCWN
081571	20-	20-	040	040	NEUTRAL	NEUTRAL	UNKNOWN	UNKNOWN	UNKNOWN	UNKNCWN
081572	000	10-	040	040	PLANUS	PLANUS	UNKNOWN	UNKNOWN	UNKNCWN	UNKNCWN
081573	05-	20-	040	040	NEUTRAL	NEUTRAL	UNKNOWN	UNKNOWN	UNKNOWN	UNKNCWN
103174	005	20-	035	050	CAVUS	PLANUS	NEUTRAL	NEUTRAL	UNKNOWN	UNKNCWN
091875	15-	000	015	015	NEUTRAL	CAVUS	NEUTRAL	NEUTRAL	UNKNOWN	UNKNCWN
101277	10-	000	015	010	NEUTRAL	NEUTRAL	NEUTRAL	NEUTRAL	UNKNCWN	UNKNCWN
052880	05-	000	020	015	NEUTRAL	NEUTRAL	NEUTRAL	NEUTRAL	UNKNOWN	UNKNCWN
010583	000	000	005	005	N WEIGHT	N WEIGHT	NEUTRAL	NEUTRAL	NEUTRAL	NEUTRAL

ARTHROGRYPOTIC JOINTS

	HIP		KNEE		ANKLE		THIGH-FOOT ANGLE	
DATE	R	L	R	L	R	L	R	L
101566	NONE	NONE	NONE	NONE	NONE	NONE	999	999
061567	NONE	NONE	NONE	NONE	NONE	NONE	999	999

B

091568	NONE	NONE	NONE	NONE	NONE	NONE	999 999
041569	NONE	NONE	NONE	NONE	NONE	NONE	999 999
031570	NONE	NONE	NONE	NONE	NONE	NONE	999 999
081571	NONE	NONE	NONE	NONE	NONE	NONE	999 999
081572	NONE	NONE	NONE	NONE	NONE	NONE	999 999
081573	NONE	NONE	NONE	NONE	NONE	NONE	999 999
103174	NONE	NONE	NONE	NONE	NONE	NONE	999 999
091875	NONE	NONE	NONE	NONE	NONE	NONE	999 999
101277	NONE	NONE	NONE	NONE	NONE	NONE	999 999
052880	NONE	NONE	NONE	NONE	NONE	NONE	999 999
010583	NONE	NONE	NONE	NONE	NONE	NONE	000 +25

```
 DATE      COMMENTS
101566     RECODED FROM EARLIER DATA COLLECTION FORMS
           CORRECTIONS MADE 12/31/84

061567     RECODED FROM EARLIER DATA COLLECTION FORMS
           CORRECTIONS MADE 12/31/84

091568     RECODED FROM EARLIER DATA COLLECTION FORMS
           HIP EXTENSION UPDATED AS OF 3/19/84
           MILD RIGHT RIGHT LUMBAR SCOLIOSIS AND LORDOSIS.
           INFO' UPDATED 12/31/84

041569     RECODED FROM EARLIER DATA COLLECTION FORMS
           CORRECTIONS MADE 12/31/84

031570     RECODED FROM EARLIER DATA COLLECTION FORMS
           INFO UPDATED 12/31/84

081571     RECODED FROM EARLIER DATA COLLECTION FORMS
           HIP EXTENSION UPDATED AS OF 3/19/84
           EQUINUS POSITION BOTH FEET.
           INFO UPDATED 12/31/84

081572     RECODED FROM EARLIER DATA COLLECTION FORMS
           INFO UPDATED 12/31/84

081573     RECODED FROM EARLIER DATA COLLECTION FORMS
           CORRECTIONS MADE 12/31/84

103174     RECODED FROM EARLIER DATA COLLECTION FORMS
           LEFT L.E. IN SPLINT.
           INFO UPDATED 12/31/84

091875     RECODED FROM EARLIER DATA COLLECTION FORMS
           INFO UPDATED 12/31/84

101277     RECODED FROM EARLIER DATA COLLECTION FORMS
           HIP EXTENSION UPDATED AS OF 3/19/84
           INFO UPDATED 12/31/84
```

C

Figure 22-8 *continues*

052880 RECODED FROM EARLIER DATA COLLECTION FORMS
INFO UPDATED 12/31/84
RIGHT HIP NOTED TO DISLOCATED AND LEFT HIP IN SOCKET ON L979 AND L980. X-RAY REPORTS.

010583 INFO UPDATED 12/31/84

******************** LOWER EXTREMITY MEASURES: MUSCLE EVALUATION ******************

MUSCLE FUNCTION

```
QUADRATUS LUMBORUM      CODES: 9 - NOT RECORDED
.  ABDOMINALS                    8 - INDETERMINANT (ABNORMAL MOVEMENT)
.  .  ILIOPSOAS                     7 - INDETERMINANT (SPASTIC; CONTR)
.  .  .  SARTORIUS                     6 - INDETERMINANT (TRANSFERRED)
.  .  .  .  HIP ADDUCTORS                 5 - NORMAL
.  .  .  .  .  QUADRICEPS                     4 - GOOD
.  .  .  .  .  .  MEDIAL HAMSTRINGS              3 - FAIR
.  .  .  .  .  .  .  LATERAL HAMSTRINGS             2 - POOR
.  .  .  .  .  .  .  .  EXTENSOR HALLICUS LONGUS       1 - TRACE
.  .  .  .  .  .  .  .  .  FLEXOR HALLICUS LONGUS         0 - NONE
.  .  .  .  .  .  .  .  .  .  ANTERIOR TIBIALIS
.  .  .  .  .  .  .  .  .  .  .  POSTERIOR TIBIALIS
.  .  .  .  .  .  .  .  .  .  .  .  PERONEUS LONGUS & BREVIS
.  .  .  .  .  .  .  .  .  .  .  .  .  PERONEUS TERITUS
.  .  .  .  .  .  .  .  .  .  .  .  .  .  GLUTEUS MEDIUS
.  .  .  .  .  .  .  .  .  .  .  .  .  .  .  GLUTEUS MAXIMUS
.  .  .  .  .  .  .  .  .  .  .  .  .  .  .  .  GASTROCNEMIUS
.  .  .  .  .  .  .  .  .  .  .  .  .  .  .  .  .  TOE EXTENSORS
.  .  .  .  .  .  .  .  .  .  .  .  .  .  .  .  .  .  TOE FLEXORS
```

DATE	RL	RL	RL	RL	RL	RL	RL	RL	RL	RL	RL	RL	RL	RL	RL	RL	RL	RL	RL
101566	99	55	32	00	00	00	00	00	00	00	00	00	00	00	00	00	00	00	00
061567	99	55	32	30	20	30	00	00	00	00	00	00	00	00	00	00	00	11	11
091568	99	33	12	11	00	20	00	00	00	00	00	00	00	00	00	00	00	11	11
041569	99	22	00	00	00	00	00	00	00	00	00	00	00	00	00	00	00	00	00
031570	99	22	00	00	00	00	00	00	00	00	00	00	00	00	00	00	00	00	00
081571	99	11	00	00	00	00	21	00	00	00	00	00	00	00	00	11	00	00	00
081572	99	33	00	00	00	00	00	00	00	00	00	00	00	00	00	00	00	00	00
081573	99	33	00	00	00	00	00	00	00	00	00	00	00	00	00	00	00	00	00
103174	00	11	00	00	11	00	00	00	00	00	00	00	00	00	00	00	01	00	00
091875	99	22	00	00	00	00	00	00	00	00	00	00	00	00	00	00	00	00	00
101277	11	11	00	00	00	00	00	00	00	00	00	00	00	00	00	00	00	00	00
052880	99	22	00	00	00	00	00	00	00	00	00	00	00	00	00	00	00	00	00
010583	99	22	00	00	00	00	00	00	00	00	00	00	00	00	00	00	00	00	00

DATE	ESTIMATED QUALITY OF MUSCLE EXAM
101566	UNKNOWN
061567	UNKNOWN
091568	UNKNOWN
041569	UNKNOWN
031570	UNKNOWN
081571	UNKNOWN
081572	UNKNOWN
081573	UNKNOWN
103174	UNKNOWN
091875	UNKNOWN
101277	UNKNOWN
052880	UNKNOWN
010583	PATIENT COOPERATIVE; RESULTS ACCURATE

D

...............GENERAL MUSCLE TONE..................

DATE	UPPER EXTREM.	TRUNK	LOWER EXTREM.
101566	UNKNOWN	UNKNOWN	UNKNOWN
061567	UNKNOWN	UNKNOWN	UNKNOWN
091568	UNKNOWN	UNKNOWN	UNKNOWN
041569	UNKNOWN	UNKNOWN	UNKNOWN
031570	UNKNOWN	UNKNOWN	UNKNOWN
081571	UNKNOWN	UNKNOWN	UNKNOWN
081572	UNKNOWN	UNKNOWN	UNKNOWN
081573	UNKNOWN	UNKNOWN	UNKNOWN
103174	UNKNOWN	UNKNOWN	UNKNOWN
091875	UNKNOWN	UNKNOWN	UNKNOWN
101277	UNKNOWN	UNKNOWN	UNKNOWN
052880	UNKNOWN	UNKNOWN	UNKNOWN
010583	NORMAL	SLIGHT HYPOTONIC	HYPOTONIC

	MOTOR LEVEL		SENSORY LEVEL		SKIP,	SKIP,
DATE	RIGHT	LEFT	RIGHT	LEFT	MOTOR	SENSORY
101566	L1	L1	L1-2	L1-2	UNKNOWN	UNKNOWN
061567	L1-3	L1	L1-2	L1-2	UNKNOWN	UNKNOWN
091568	L1-3	L1	L1-2	L1-2	UNKNOWN	UNKNOWN
041569	T11	T11	L1-2	L1-2	UNKNOWN	UNKNOWN
031570	T11	T11	L1-2	L1-2	UNKNOWN	UNKNOWN
081571	T11	T11	L1-2	L1-2	UNKNOWN	UNKNOWN
081572	T12	T12	T11 OR T12	T11 OR T12	UNKNOWN	UNKNOWN
081573	T12	T12	T11 OR T12	T11 OR T12	UNKNOWN	UNKNOWN
103174	T11	T11	T11 OR T12	T11 OR T12	UNKNOWN	UNKNOWN
091875	T12	T12	L1-2	L1-2	NO	NO
101277	T12	T12	L1-2	L1-2	NO	NO
052880	T12	T12	L1-2	L1-2	NO	NO
010583	T12	T12	T11 OR T12	T11 OR T12	NO	NO

DATE	COMMENTS
101566	RECODED FROM EARLIER DATA COLLECTION FORMS INFO UPDATED 1/2/85
061567	RECODED FROM EARLIER DATA COLLECTION FORMS INFO UPDATED 1/2/85
091568	RECODED FROM EARLIER DATA COLLECTION FORMS INFO UPDATED 1/2/85
041569	RECODED FROM EARLIER DATA COLLECTION FORMS INFO UPDATED 1/2/85
031570	RECODED FROM EARLIER DATA COLLECTION FORMS INFO UPDATED 1/2/85
081571	RECODED FROM EARLIER DATA COLLECTION FORMS INFO UPDATED 1/2/85
081572	RECODED FROM EARLIER DATA COLLECTION FORMS INFO UPDATED 1/2/85

E

Figure 22-8 *continues*

081573 RECODED FROM EARLIER DATA COLLECTION FORMS
INFO UPDATED 1/2/85

103174 RECODED FROM EARLIER DATA COLLECTION FORMS
INFO UPDATED 1/2/85

091875 RECODED FROM EARLIER DATA COLLECTION FORMS
INFO UPDATED 1/2/85

101277 RECODED FROM EARLIER DATA COLLECTION FORMS
INFO UPDATED 1/2/85

052880 RECODED FROM EARLIER DATA COLLECTION FORMS
INFO UPDATED 1/2/85

010583 INFO UPDATED 1/2/85

******************** UPPER EXTREMITY MEASURES ********************

MUSCLE STRENGTH

DATE	SHOULDER GIRDLE ELEVATORS	SHOULDER GIRDLE DEPRESSORS	SHOULDER FLEXORS	SHOULDER EXTENSORS	SHOULDER ABDUCTORS	SHOULDER ADDUCTORS	BACK EXTENSORS & SCAPULA ADDUCTORS (RETRACTION)	SCAPULA ABDUCTORS (PROTRACTION)	ELBOW FLEXORS	ELBOW EXTENSORS	RANGE OF MOTION	UPPER EXTREMITY FUNCTION TEST
	RL	RL	RL	RL	RL	RL	RL	RL	RL	RL		
101566	99	99	99	99	99	99	55	99	99	99	UNKNOWN	UNKNOWN
061567	99	99	99	99	99	99	55	99	99	99	UNKNOWN	UNKNOWN
091568	99	99	99	99	99	99	33	99	99	99	UNKNOWN	UNKNOWN
041569	99	99	99	99	99	99	55	99	99	99	UNKNOWN	UNKNOWN
031570	99	99	99	99	99	99	55	99	99	99	UNKNOWN	UNKNOWN
081571	99	99	99	99	99	99	00	99	99	99	UNKNOWN	UNKNOWN
081572	99	99	99	99	99	99	55	99	99	99	UNKNOWN	UNKNOWN
081573	99	99	99	99	99	99	55	99	99	99	UNKNOWN	UNKNOWN
103174	55	55	44	44	44	44	44	44	44	44	NORMAL	NORMAL
091875	44	44	44	44	44	44	44	44	44	44	NORMAL	NORMAL
101277	44	44	44	44	44	44	44	44	44	44	ABNORMAL	NORMAL
052880	55	55	55	55	55	55	55	55	55	55	NORMAL	UNKNOWN

DATE	ABNORMAL RAPID ALTERNATING MVMTS	INTENTION TREMOR	ABNORMAL POSITION SENSE	GRIP STRENGTH (POUNDS)	DOMINANT HAND
101566	UNKNOWN	UNKNOWN	UNKNOWN	R:99 L:99	UNDETERM
061567	UNKNOWN	UNKNOWN	UNKNOWN	R:99 L:99	UNDETERM
091568	UNKNOWN	UNKNOWN	UNKNOWN	R:99 L:99	UNDETERM
041569	UNKNOWN	UNKNOWN	UNKNOWN	R:99 L:99	UNDETERM

F

031570	UNKNOWN	UNKNOWN	UNKNOWN	R:99 L:99	UNKNOWN
081571	UNKNOWN	UNKNOWN	UNKNOWN	R:99 L:99	UNKNOWN
081572	UNKNOWN	UNKNOWN	UNKNOWN	R:99 L:99	LEFT
081573	UNKNOWN	UNKNOWN	UNKNOWN	R:99 L:99	UNKNOWN
103174	ABNORMAL	ABNORMAL	NORMAL	R:99 L:99	RIGHT
091875	NORMAL	ABNORMAL	NORMAL	R:99 L:99	RIGHT
101277	ABNORMAL	ABNORMAL	NORMAL	R:99 L:99	RIGHT
052880	ABNORMAL	ABNORMAL	NORMAL	R:99 L:99	RIGHT

```
 DATE     COMMENTS
101566    RECODED FROM EARLIER DATA COLLECTION FORMS
          INFO UPDATED 1/2/85________________________________________
          -----------------------------------------------------------
          -----------------------------------------------------------
          -----------------------------------------------------------
061567    RECODED FROM EARLIER DATA COLLECTION FORMS
          INFO UPDATED 1/2/85________________________________________
          -----------------------------------------------------------
          -----------------------------------------------------------
          -----------------------------------------------------------
091568    RECODED FROM EARLIER DATA COLLECTION FORMS
          INFO UPDATED 1/2/85________________________________________
          -----------------------------------------------------------
          -----------------------------------------------------------
          -----------------------------------------------------------
041569    RECODED FROM EARLIER DATA COLLECTION FORMS
          INFO UPDATED 1/2/85________________________________________
          -----------------------------------------------------------
          -----------------------------------------------------------
          -----------------------------------------------------------
031570    RECODED FROM EARLIER DATA COLLECTION FORMS
081571    RECODED FROM EARLIER DATA COLLECTION FORMS
081572    RECODED FROM EARLIER DATA COLLECTION FORMS
081573    RECODED FROM EARLIER DATA COLLECTION FORMS
103174    RECODED FROM EARLIER DATA COLLECTION FORMS
091875    RECODED FROM EARLIER DATA COLLECTION FORMS
101277    RECODED FROM EARLIER DATA COLLECTION FORMS
052880    RECODED FROM EARLIER DATA COLLECTION FORMS
          INFO UPDATED 1/2/85________________________________________
          -----------------------------------------------------------
          -----------------------------------------------------------
          -----------------------------------------------------------
```

******************** AMBULATION/MOBILITY **

DATE	WHEELCHAIRS	MOD	CUSHION	WHEELED DEVICE
101566	STROLLER	UNK	UNKNOWN	NONE
061567	STROLLER	UNK	UNKNOWN	UNKNOWN
091568	UNKNOWN	UNK	UNKNOWN	UNKNOWN
041569	STROLLER	UNK	UNKNOWN	UNKNOWN
031570	MANUAL	UNK	UNKNOWN	NONE
081571	MANUAL	UNK	UNKNOWN	NONE
081572	MANUAL	UNK	UNKNOWN	NONE
081573	MANUAL	UNK	UNKNOWN	NONE
103174	MANUAL	UNK	UNKNOWN	NONE
091875	MANUAL	UNK	UNKNOWN	NONE
101277	MANUAL	UNK	UNKNOWN	NONE
052880	MANUAL	UNK	UNKNOWN	NONE
010583	MANUAL	NO	NONE	NONE

WHEELCHAIR TRANSFERS

DATE	T/F BED	T/F TOILET	T/F TUB	TO FLOOR	FROM FLOOR	T/F AUTO
101566	NOT APPLIC	NOT APPLIC	NOT APPLIC	NOT APPLIC	NOT APPLIC	NOT APPLIC
061567	NOT APPLIC	NOT APPLIC	NOT APPLIC	NOT APPLIC	NOT APPLIC	NOT APPLIC
091568	NOT APPLIC	NOT APPLIC	NOT APPLIC	NOT APPLIC	NOT APPLIC	NOT APPLIC
041569	NOT APPLIC	NOT APPLIC	NOT APPLIC	NOT APPLIC	NOT APPLIC	NOT APPLIC

G

Figure 22-8 *continues*

031570	MAX HELP	MAX HELP	MAX HELP	UNKNOWN	UNKNOWN	UNKNOWN
081571	MAX HELP	MAX HELP	MAX HELP	UNKNOWN	UNKNOWN	UNKNOWN
081572	MAX HELP	MAX HELP	MAX HELP	UNKNOWN	UNKNOWN	UNKNOWN
081573	MAX HELP	MAX HELP	MAX HELP	UNKNOWN	UNKNOWN	UNKNOWN
103174	MAX HELP	DEPENDENT	DEPENDENT	DEPENDENT	DEPENDENT	DEPENDENT
091875	IND NO AID	DEPENDENT	DEPENDENT	DEPENDENT	DEPENDENT	SLIGHT HEL
101277	MAX HELP	MAX HELP	MAX HELP	DEPENDENT	DEPENDENT	SLIGHT HEL
052880	INDEP W/AI	INDEP W/AI	DEPENDENT	DEPENDENT	DEPENDENT	INDEP W/AI
010583	INDEP W/AI	MAX HELP	MAX HELP	DEPENDENT	DEPENDENT	SLIGHT HEL

DATE	TYPE OF GAIT	BRACES
101566	NO GAIT	NONE
061567	NO GAIT	NONE
091568	NO GAIT	NONE
041569	NO GAIT	NONE
031570	STANDING ONLY; NEUTRAL	LONG LEG WITH PELVIC BAND
081571	NO GAIT	NONE
081572	NO GAIT	NONE
081573	NO GAIT	NONE
103174	NO GAIT	NONE
091875	NO GAIT	NONE
101277	NO GAIT	NONE
052880	NO GAIT	NONE
010583	NO GAIT	NONE

DATE	OTHER BRACES AND SPLINTS	WALKING AIDS	STANDING DEVICES
101566	NONE	NONE	UNKNOWN
061567	NONE	NONE	UNKNOWN
091568	DENIS BROWNE	UNKNOWN	UNKNOWN
041569	NONE	UNKNOWN	UNKNOWN
031570	NONE	NONE	UNKNOWN
081571	NONE	NONE	UNKNOWN
081572	NONE	NONE	UNKNOWN
081573	NONE	NONE	UNKNOWN
103174	NONE	NONE	UNKNOWN
091875	NONE	NONE	UNKNOWN
101277	NONE	NONE	UNKNOWN
052880	NONE	NONE	UNKNOWN
010583	NONE	NONE	NONE

DATE	USUAL MEANS OF LOCOMOTION	EXTENT OF INDEPENDENT MOBILITY
101566	IS CARRIED	GOES OUT OF HOUSE WITH ADULT ONL
061567	DEPENDENT IN W.C. GURNEY AT HOME	UNKNOWN
091568	DEPENDENT IN W.C. GURNEY AT HOME	UNKNOWN
041569	DEPENDENT IN W.C. GURNEY AT HOME	UNKNOWN
031570	DEPENDENT IN W.C. GURNEY AT HOME	UNKNOWN
081571	SCOOTS/CRAWLS INSIDE, STROLLER, W.C. OUT	UNKNOWN
081572	PARTIAL W.C. INDEPENDENT AT HOME	UNKNOWN
081573	PARTIAL W.C. INDEPENDENT AT HOME	UNKNOWN
103174	PARTIAL W.C. INDEPENDENT AT HOME	UNKNOWN
091875	INDEPENDENT IN W.C. AT HOME	UNKNOWN
101277	W.C. INDEPENDENT IN COMMUNITY	UNKNOWN
052880	W.C. INDEPENDENT IN COMMUNITY	UNKNOWN
010583	W.C. INDEPENDENT IN COMMUNITY	OUT OF YARD INDEP. TO NEIGHBORHO

DATE	COMMENTS
101566	RECODED FROM EARLIER DATA COLLECTION FORMS INFO UPDATED 1/2/85
061567	RECODED FROM EARLIER DATA COLLECTION FORMS INFO UPDATED 1/2/85

H

091568 RECODED FROM EARLIER DATA COLLECTION FORMS
INFO UPDATED 1/2/85

041569 RECODED FROM EARLIER DATA COLLECTION FORMS
INFO UPDATED 1/2/85

031570 RECODED FROM EARLIER DATA COLLECTION FORMS
INFO UPDATED 1/2/85

031571 RECODED FROM EARLIER DATA COLLECTION FORMS
INFO UPDATED 1/2/85

081572 RECODED FROM EARLIER DATA COLLECTION FORMS
INFO UPDATED 1/2/85

081573 RECODED FROM EARLIER DATA COLLECTION FORMS
INFO UPDATED 1/2/85

103174 RECODED FROM EARLIER DATA COLLECTION FORMS
INFO UPDATED 1/2/85

091875 RECODED FROM EARLIER DATA COLLECTION FORMS
INFO UPDATED 1/2/85

101277 RECODED FROM EARLIER DATA COLLECTION FORMS
CAPABLE OF DOING FLOOR TRANSFERS BUT DOES NOT DO THEM AT HOME (DEPENDENT).

052880
010583 RECODED FROM EARLIER DATA COLLECTION FORMS

******************** GENERAL HEALTH STATUS ********************

DATE	AGE MTHS	HEIGHT (CM)	WEIGHT (KG)	ARM SPAN	HEAD SIZE	BLOOD PRES SYST	BLOOD PRES DYAST	SKIN FOLD
101566	5	99	999	999	99.9	999	999	99.9
061567	14	99	999	999	99.9	777	777	99.9
071567	999	99	999	999	99.9	777	777	99.9
091568	28	99	999	999	99.9	777	777	99.9
041569	35	99	999	999	99.9	777	777	99.9
031570	46	99	999	999	99.9	999	999	99.9
031571	63	99	999	999	99.9	999	999	99.9
081072	999	99	999	999	99.9	999	999	99.9
081572	75	99	999	999	99.9	999	999	99.9
081573	88	99	999	999	99.9	777	777	99.9

Figure 22-8 *continues*

103174	102	10	40	127	53.6	98	80	99.9
091875	96	23	42	135	54.0	999	999	99.9
101277	137	32	55	150	57.0	100	70	99.9
052880	168	49	71	163	57.5	100	70	99.9
010583	199	84	74	174	57.9	110	82	99.9

DATE	DECUBITIS	MECHANISM
101566	UNKNOWN	UNKNOWN
061567	UNKNOWN	UNKNOWN
071567	NONE	NOT APPLICABLE
091568	UNKNOWN	UNKNOWN
041569	UNKNOWN	UNKNOWN
031570	BACK - GIBBUS	PRESSURE
081571	UNKNOWN	UNKNOWN
081072	NONE	NOT APPLICABLE
091572	NONE	NOT APPLICABLE
081573	NONE	NOT APPLICABLE
103174	NONE	NOT APPLICABLE
091875	NONE	NOT APPLICABLE
101277	PENIS	PRESSURE
052880	NONE	NOT APPLICABLE
010583	NONE	NOT APPLICABLE

DATE	SKIN CONDITION OVER MYELODYSPLASIA SITE	SHUNT PLACEMENT	ISOSORBIDE TREATMENT
101566	EPITHELIZATION; NOT LEAKING OR TENDER	NO SHUNT IN PLACE	NO
061567	EPITHELIZATION; NOT LEAKING OR TENDER	SHUNT IN PLACE	NO
071567	UNKNOWN	SHUNT IN PLACE	UNKNOWN
091568	EPITHELIZATION; NOT LEAKING OR TENDER	SHUNT IN PLACE	NO
041569	EPITHELIZATION; NOT LEAKING OR TENDER	SHUNT IN PLACE	NO
031570	EPITHELIZATION; NOT LEAKING OR TENDER	SHUNT IN PLACE	NO
081571	EPITHELIZATION; NOT LEAKING OR TENDER	SHUNT IN PLACE	NO
081072	UNKNOWN	SHUNT IN PLACE	UNKNOWN
091572	EPITHELIZATION; NOT LEAKING OR TENDER	SHUNT IN PLACE	NO
081573	EPITHELIZATION; NOT LEAKING OR TENDER	SHUNT IN PLACE	NO
103174	EPITHELIZATION; NOT LEAKING OR TENDER	SHUNT IN PLACE	NO
091875	EPITHELIZATION; NOT LEAKING OR TENDER	SHUNT IN PLACE	NO
101277	EPITHELIZATION; NOT LEAKING OR TENDER	SHUNT IN PLACE	NO
052880	WELL-HEALED SCAR; NOT LEAKING OR TENDER	SHUNT IN PLACE	NO
010583	WELL-HEALED SCAR; NOT LEAKING OR TENDER	NO SHUNT IN PLACE	NO

DATE	EVIDENCE OF TRAUMA TO BRAIN	SEIZURE STATUS	SPECIAL DIET
101566	MENINGITIS, VENTRICULITIS (GR	UNKNOWN	UNKNOWN
061567	MENINGITIS, VENTRICULITIS (GR	UNKNOWN	UNKNOWN
071567	UNKNOWN	UNKNOWN	UNKNOWN
091568	MENINGITIS, VENTRICULITIS (GR	UNKNOWN	UNKNOWN
041569	MENINGITIS, VENTRICULITIS (GR	UNKNOWN	UNKNOWN
031570	MENINGITIS, VENTRICULITIS (GR	UNKNOWN	UNKNOWN
081571	MENINGITIS, VENTRICULITIS (GR	UNKNOWN	UNKNOWN
081072	UNKNOWN	UNKNOWN	UNKNOWN
091572	MENINGITIS, VENTRICULITIS (GR	UNKNOWN	UNKNOWN
081573	MENINGITIS, VENTRICULITIS (GR	UNKNOWN	UNKNOWN
103174	NONE	CONTROLLED WITH DILANTOIN, P	UNKNOWN
091875	NONE	CONTROLLED WITH DILANTOIN, P	UNKNOWN
101277	NONE	CONTROLLED WITH PHENOBARBITO	UNKNOWN
052880	NONE	CONTROLLED WITH DILANTOIN, P	UNKNOWN
010583	NONE	NONE	NO SPECIAL DIET

DATE	PHARYNGO-LARYNGEAL PALSY	DIFFICULTY SWALLOWING	STRIDOR	APNEA	OTHER CRANIAL PALSIES	OTHER HEALTH PROBLEMS
101566	YES	INFO AVAIL	INFO AVAIL	INFO AVAIL	UNKNOWN	INFO AVAIL
061567	YES	INFO AVAIL	INFO AVAIL	INFO AVAIL	UNKNOWN	INFO AVAIL
071567	UNKNOWN	INFO AVAIL	INFO AVAIL	INFO AVAIL	UNKNOWN	INFO A
091568	NO	INFO AVAIL	INFO AVAIL	INFO AVAIL	UNKNOWN	INFO A
041569	UNKNOWN	INFO AVAIL	INFO AVAIL	INFO AVAIL	UNKNOWN	INFO A

031570	UNKNOWN	INFO AVAIL	INFO AVAIL	INFO AVAIL	UNKNOWN	INFO AVAIL
081571	UNKNOWN	INFO AVAIL	INFO AVAIL	INFO AVAIL	UNKNOWN	INFO AVAIL
081072	UNKNOWN	INFO AVAIL	INFO AVAIL	INFO AVAIL	UNKNOWN	INFO AVAIL
081572	UNKNOWN	INFO AVAIL	INFO AVAIL	INFO AVAIL	UNKNOWN	INFO AVAIL
081573	UNKNOWN	INFO AVAIL	INFO AVAIL	INFO AVAIL	UNKNOWN	INFO AVAIL
103174	NO	INFO AVAIL	INFO AVAIL	INFO AVAIL	NO	INFO AVAIL
091875	NO	INFO AVAIL	INFO AVAIL	INFO AVAIL	NO	INFO AVAIL
101277	NO	INFO AVAIL	INFO AVAIL	INFO AVAIL	NO	INFO AVAIL
052880	NO	INFO AVAIL	INFO AVAIL	INFO AVAIL	NO	INFO AVAIL
010583	NO	NOT APPLICABLE	NOT APPLICABLE	NOT APPLICABLE	NO	NO

OCULAR ABNORMALITIES

DATE	RIGHT EYE	LEFT EYE	GENERAL VISION	GENERAL HEARING
101566	NONE	NONE	UNKNOWN	UNKNOWN
061567	NONE	NONE	UNKNOWN	UNKNOWN
071567	UNKNOWN	UNKNOWN	UNKNOWN	UNKNOWN
091568	ESOTROPIA	NONE	UNKNOWN	UNKNOWN
041569	ESOTROPIA	NONE	UNKNOWN	UNKNOWN
031570	ESOTROPIA	NONE	UNKNOWN	UNKNOWN
081571	ESOTROPIA	NONE	UNKNOWN	UNKNOWN
081072	UNKNOWN	UNKNOWN	UNKNOWN	UNKNOWN
081572	ESOTROPIA	NONE	UNKNOWN	UNKNOWN
081573	ESOTROPIA	NONE	UNKNOWN	UNKNOWN
103174	NONE	NONE	UNKNOWN	UNKNOWN
091875	NONE	NONE	UNKNOWN	UNKNOWN
101277	NONE	NONE	UNKNOWN	UNKNOWN
052880	NONE	NONE	UNKNOWN	UNKNOWN
010583	OTHER	OTHER	WITHIN NORMAL LIMITS	WITHIN NORMAL LIMITS

```
DATE     COMMENTS
101566   RECODED FROM EARLIER DATA COLLECTION FORMS
061567   RECODED FROM EARLIER DATA COLLECTION FORMS
071567   RECODED FROM EARLIER DATA COLLECTION FORMS
         INFO UPDATED 1/2/85________________________________________
         ___________________________________________________________
         ___________________________________________________________
         ___________________________________________________________
091568   RECODED FROM EARLIER DATA COLLECTION FORMS
041569   RECODED FROM EARLIER DATA COLLECTION FORMS
031570   RECODED FROM EARLIER DATA COLLECTION FORMS
081571   RECODED FROM EARLIER DATA COLLECTION FORMS
081072   RECODED FROM EARLIER DATA COLLECTION FORMS
         INFO UPDATED 1/2/85________________________________________
         ___________________________________________________________
         ___________________________________________________________
         ___________________________________________________________
081572   RECODED FROM EARLIER DATA COLLECTION FORMS
081573   RECODED FROM EARLIER DATA COLLECTION FORMS
103174   RECODED FROM EARLIER DATA COLLECTION FORMS
091875   RECODED FROM EARLIER DATA COLLECTION FORMS
101277   RECODED FROM EARLIER DATA COLLECTION FORMS
052880   RECODED FROM EARLIER DATA COLLECTION FORMS
010583   ___________________________________________________________
         ___________________________________________________________
         ___________________________________________________________
         ___________________________________________________________
         ___________________________________________________________
```

******************** TOILET TRAINING DATA **

	BLOOD PRES		RESID	CURRENT	SITE OF	......SINCE LAST EXAM......	
DATE	SYST	DYAST	URINE	INFECT.	INFECT.	# OF INFECT.	# TIMES HOSP.
101566	999	999	999	UNKNOWN	UNKNOWN	99	99
061567	777	777	40	YES	UNKNOWN	99	99
071567	777	777	40	YES	UNKNOWN	99	99

K

Figure 22-8 *continues*

091568	777	777	30	YES	UNKNOWN	99	99
041569	777	777	20	NO	UNKNOWN	99	99
031570	999	999	999	UNKNOWN	UNKNOWN	99	99
081571	999	999	15	UNKNOWN	UNKNOWN	99	99
081072	999	999	70	YES	UNKNOWN	99	99
081572	999	999	70	YES	UNKNOWN	99	99
081573	777	777	30	YES	UNKNOWN	99	99
103174	98	80	40	YES	UNKNOWN	99	99
091875	999	999	30	YES	UNKNOWN	99	99
101277	100	72	50	YES	UNKNOWN	99	99
052880	100	70	200	UNKNOWN	UNKNOWN	99	99
010583	110	82	999	UNKNOWN	UNKNOWN	3	0

			URINE PROGRAM		QUALITY OF
DATE	URINE COLLECTION METHODS		BEGAN	ENDED	URINE COLLECTION
101566	DIAPER	UNKNOWN	99/99	99/99	RASH
061567	DIAPER	UNKNOWN	99/99	99/99	GOOD
071567	DIAPER	UNKNOWN	99/99	99/99	GOOD
091568	DIAPER	UNKNOWN	99/99	99/99	RASH
041569	DIAPER	UNKNOWN	99/99	99/99	GOOD
031570	DIAPER	UNKNOWN	99/99	99/99	GOOD
081571	DIAPER	UNKNOWN	99/99	99/99	GOOD
081072	DIAPER	UNKNOWN	99/99	99/99	WET
081572	DIAPER	UNKNOWN	99/99	99/99	WET
081573	DIAPER	UNKNOWN	99/99	99/99	GOOD
103174	DIAPER	UNKNOWN	99/99	99/99	GOOD
091875	DIAPER	UNKNOWN	99/99	99/99	GOOD
101277	EXTERNAL COLLECT	UNKNOWN	99/99	99/99	GOOD
052880	EXTERNAL COLLECT	UNKNOWN	99/99	99/99	GOOD
010583	EXTERNAL COLLECT	INTERMITTENT CAT	06/74	00/00	GOOD

DEGREE OF INDEPENDENCE			
DATE	EMPTYING BAG	CHANGING APPLIANCE	USING CATHETER, DIAPER, ETC
101566	UNKNOWN	UNKNOWN	NOT APPLICABLE
061567	UNKNOWN	UNKNOWN	NOT APPLICABLE
071567	UNKNOWN	UNKNOWN	NOT APPLICABLE
091568	UNKNOWN	UNKNOWN	TOTALLY DEPENDENT
041569	UNKNOWN	UNKNOWN	TOTALLY DEPENDENT
031570	UNKNOWN	UNKNOWN	NOT APPLICABLE
081571	UNKNOWN	UNKNOWN	NOT APPLICABLE
081072	UNKNOWN	UNKNOWN	NOT APPLICABLE
081572	UNKNOWN	UNKNOWN	NOT APPLICABLE
081573	UNKNOWN	UNKNOWN	NOT APPLICABLE
103174	UNKNOWN	UNKNOWN	NOT APPLICABLE
091875	UNKNOWN	UNKNOWN	NOT APPLICABLE
101277	TOTALLY INDEPENDENT	TOTALLY DEPENDENT	UNKNOWN
052880	CARRIES OUT W/REMIND	TOTALLY DEPENDENT	UNKNOWN
010583	TOTALLY INDEPENDENT	TOTALLY DEPENDENT	TOTALLY INDEPENDENT

DATE	URINARY BLADDER SENSATION	TANNER STAGE	URINE STREAM	STOMA
101566	UNKNOWN	6	DRIBBLE/NO STREAM	
061567	UNKNOWN	6	DRIBBLE/NO STREAM	
071567	UNKNOWN	6	DRIBBLE/NO STREAM	
091568	UNKNOWN	6	DRIBBLE/NO STREAM	
041569	UNKNOWN	6	DRIBBLE/NO STREAM	
031570	UNKNOWN	6	DRIBBLE/NO STREAM	
081571	UNKNOWN	6	DRIBBLE/NO STREAM	
081072	UNKNOWN	6	DRIBBLE/NO STREAM	
081572	UNKNOWN	6	DRIBBLE/NO STREAM	
081573	UNKNOWN	6	DRIBBLE/NO STREAM	
103174	UNKNOWN	6	NO STREAM	
091875	UNKNOWN	6	DRIBBLE/NO STREAM	
101277	UNKNOWN	6	NOT APPLICABLE	
052880	UNKNOWN	6	DRIBBLE/NO STREAM	
010583	NONE	6	DRIBBLE/STREAM WITH STRAIN	NOT APPLIC.

DATE	STOOL PROGRAM(S)			PROGRAM DATES BEGAN	ENDED
101566	NO PROGRAM	UNKNOWN	UNKNOWN	99/99	99/99
061567	SUPPOSITORY	UNKNOWN	UNKNOWN	99/99	99/99
071567	SUPPOSITORY	UNKNOWN	UNKNOWN	99/99	99/99
091568	SUPPOSITORY	UNKNOWN	UNKNOWN	99/99	99/99
041569	SUPPOSITORY	UNKNOWN	UNKNOWN	99/99	99/99
031570	NO PROGRAM	UNKNOWN	UNKNOWN	99/99	99/99
031571	NO PROGRAM	UNKNOWN	UNKNOWN	99/99	99/99
081072	SUPPOSITORY	UNKNOWN	UNKNOWN	99/99	99/99
081572	SUPPOSITORY	UNKNOWN	UNKNOWN	99/99	99/99
081573	SUPPOSITORY	UNKNOWN	UNKNOWN	99/99	99/99
103174	SUPPOSITORY	UNKNOWN	UNKNOWN	99/99	99/99
091875	SUPPOSITORY	UNKNOWN	UNKNOWN	99/99	99/99
101277	SUPPOSITORY	UNKNOWN	UNKNOWN	99/99	99/99
052880	OTHER	UNKNOWN	UNKNOWN	99/99	99/99
010583	EXPANSION ENEMA	ORAL MEDICATION	NO PROGRAM	00/77	00/00

DATE	QUALITY OF PROGRAM	DEGREE OF INDEPENDENCE	ANAL TONE	ANAL SQUEEZE	ANAL SENSAT.
101566	NOT APPLICABLE	UNKNOWN	NONE	NO	NO
061567	NOT APPLICABLE	UNKNOWN	TIGHT	NO	NO
071567	NOT APPLICABLE	TOTALLY DEPENDENT	UNKNOWN	UNKNOWN	UNKNOWN
091568	NOT APPLICABLE	UNKNOWN	TIGHT	NO	NO
041569	6 ACCIDENTS PER WEEK	UNKNOWN	NONE	NO	NO
031570	99 ACCIDENTS PER UNKNOWN	UNKNOWN	NONE	NO	NO
031571	99 ACCIDENTS PER UNKNOWN	UNKNOWN	NONE	NO	NO
081072	2 ACCIDENTS PER WEEK	TOTALLY DEPENDENT	UNKNOWN	UNKNOWN	UNKNOWN
081572	2 ACCIDENTS PER WEEK	TOTALLY DEPENDENT	NONE	NO	NO
081573	2 ACCIDENTS PER WEEK	TOTALLY DEPENDENT	NONE	NO	NO
103174	2 ACCIDENTS PER WEEK	TOTALLY DEPENDENT	NONE	NO	NO
091875	2 ACCIDENTS PER WEEK	ASSISTS WITH PROGRAM	NONE	NO	NO
101277	2 ACCIDENTS PER WEEK	ASSISTS WITH PROGRAM	NONE	NO	NO
052880	6 ACCIDENTS PER WEEK	TOTALLY DEPENDENT	UNKNOWN	UNKNOWN	UNKNOWN
010583	0 ACCIDENTS PER MONTH	TOTALLY DEPENDENT	UNKNOWN	UNKNOWN	UNKNOWN

MEDICATIONS

DATE	DRUG	DOSAGE MG-DAY	DATES BEGAN	ENDED
010583		500	06/68	00/00
010583		999	06/68	00/00
010583		010	06/79	00/00
010583		999	06/79	00/00

DATE	COMMENTS
101566	RECODED FROM EARLIER DATA COLLECTION FORMS
061567	RECODED FROM EARLIER DATA COLLECTION FORMS
071567	RECODED FROM EARLIER DATA COLLECTION FORMS
091568	RECODED FROM EARLIER DATA COLLECTION FORMS
041569	RECODED FROM EARLIER DATA COLLECTION FORMS
031570	RECODED FROM EARLIER DATA COLLECTION FORMS
031571	RECODED FROM EARLIER DATA COLLECTION FORMS
081072	RECODED FROM EARLIER DATA COLLECTION FORMS
081572	RECODED FROM EARLIER DATA COLLECTION FORMS
081573	RECODED FROM EARLIER DATA COLLECTION FORMS
103174	RECODED FROM EARLIER DATA COLLECTION FORMS
091875	RECODED FROM EARLIER DATA COLLECTION FORMS
101277	RECODED FROM EARLIER DATA COLLECTION FORMS
052880	RECODED FROM EARLIER DATA COLLECTION FORMS
010583	BID CIC BID URO SHEATH. --

-- **M**

******************** UROLOGY DATA ***

Figure 22-8 *continues*

LAB TEST RESULTS

DATE	BUN	CREAT-ININE	CREATININE CLEARANCE	DMSA RENAL SCAN RIGHT %	DMSA RENAL SCAN LEFT %	URINE CULTURE	METHOD OF COLLECTION
101566	99	999	999	999	999	UNKNOWN	UNKNOWN
061567	99	999	999	999	999	100,000 OR MORE	CATHETER
071567	99	999	999	999	999	100,000 OR MORE	CATHETER
091568	99	999	999	999	999	100,000 OR MORE	CATHETER
041569	99	999	999	999	999	LESS THAN 100,000	CATHETER
031570	99	999	999	999	999	UNKNOWN	UNKNOWN
081571	99	999	999	999	999	UNKNOWN	UNKNOWN
081072	99	999	999	999	999	100,000 OR MORE	CATHETER
081572	99	999	999	999	999	100,000 OR MORE	CATHETER
081573	99	999	999	999	999	100,000 OR MORE	CATHETER
103174	99	999	999	999	999	100,000 OR MORE	CATHETER
091875	99	999	999	999	999	100,000 OR MORE	CATHETER
101277	99	999	999	999	999	100,000 OR MORE	CATHETER
052880	99	999	999	999	999	UNKNOWN	UNKNOWN
061484	0	999	999	999	999	UNKNOWN	UNKNOWN

IVP

CODES: 0 - NONE, 1 - MILD, 2 - MODERATE, 3 - SEVERE, 4 - CORTICAL SCARRING, 9 - UNKNOWN

DATE	HYDRONEPHROSIS R	HYDRONEPHROSIS L	NEPHROLITHIASIS R	NEPHROLITHIASIS L	URINARY STONES: BLADDER	URINARY STONES: URETHRA	URINARY STONES: PROSTATE	ANOMALIES	TESTES
101566	0	2	0	0	0	0	0	6	0
061567	0	0	0	0	0	0	0	6	0
071567	0	0	0	0	0	0	0	6	0
091568	0	0	0	0	0	0	0	6	0
041569	0	0	0	0	0	0	0	6	0
031570	9	9	0	0	0	0	0	6	0
081571	9	9	0	0	0	0	0	6	0
081072	9	9	0	0	0	0	0	6	0
081572	9	9	0	0	0	0	0	6	0
081573	0	0	0	0	0	0	0	5	9
103174	0	0	0	0	0	0	0	0	0
091875	9	9	0	0	0	0	0	0	0
101277	9	9	0	0	0	0	0	0	0
052880	9	9	0	0	0	0	0	0	0
061484	9	9	9	9	9	9	9	9	9

VCUG +- URODYNAMICS

DATE	RESIDUAL	CAPACITY	TRABECULATION	BLADDER NECK	SENSATION
101566	999	999		EXTERNAL SPHINCTER SPASM	UNKNOWN
061567	40	125		RELAXED WITH FUNNELING	UNKNOWN
071567	40	125		RELAXED WITH FUNNELING	UNKNOWN
091568	30	75		RELAXED WITH FUNNELING	UNKNOWN
041569	20	100		RELAXED WITH FUNNELING	UNKNOWN
031570	999	999		UNKNOWN	UNKNOWN
081571	15	75		RELAXED WITH FUNNELING	UNKNOWN
081072	70	125		RELAXED WITH FUNNELING	UNKNOWN
081572	70	125		RELAXED WITH FUNNELING	UNKNOWN
081573	30	998		RELAXED WITH FUNNELING	UNKNOWN
103174	40	70		RELAXED WITH FUNNELING	UNKNOWN
091875	30	100		EXTERNAL SPHINCTER SPASM	UNKNOWN
101277	50	200		EXTERNAL SPHINCTER SPASM	UNKNOWN
052880	200	300		EXTERNAL SPHINCTER SPASM	UNKNOWN
061484	430	450		RELAXED WITH FUNNELING	UNKNOWN

DATE	DETRUSSER	REFLUX RIGHT	REFLUX LEFT
101566	UNKNOWN	NONE	WITHOUT DILITATION
061567	UNKNOWN	NONE	NONE
071567	UNKNOWN	NONE	NONE
091568	UNKNOWN	NONE	NONE
041569	UNKNOWN	NONE	NONE

N

031570	UNKNOWN	NONE	NONE
081571	UNKNOWN	NONE	NONE
081072	UNKNOWN	NONE	NONE
081572	UNKNOWN	NONE	NONE
081573	UNKNOWN	NONE	NONE
103174	UNKNOWN	NONE	NONE
091875	UNKNOWN	NONE	NONE
101277	UNKNOWN	NONE	NONE
052880	UNKNOWN	NONE	NONE
061484	UNKNOWN	NONE	NONE

LOOPOGRAM +- DYNAMICS

DATE	RESIDUAL	CAPACITY	PRESSURE (CM WATER) MEAN	LOW	HIGH	OBSTRUCTION RIGHT	LEFT
101566	99	99	99	99	99	UNKNOWN	UNKNOWN
061567	99	99	99	99	99	UNKNOWN	UNKNOWN
071567	99	99	99	99	99	UNKNOWN	UNKNOWN
091568	99	99	99	99	99	UNKNOWN	UNKNOWN
041569	99	99	99	99	99	UNKNOWN	UNKNOWN
031570	99	99	99	99	99	UNKNOWN	UNKNOWN
081571	99	99	99	99	99	UNKNOWN	UNKNOWN
081072	99	99	99	99	99	UNKNOWN	UNKNOWN
081572	99	99	99	99	99	UNKNOWN	UNKNOWN
081573	99	99	99	99	99	UNKNOWN	UNKNOWN
103174	99	99	99	99	99	UNKNOWN	UNKNOWN
091875	99	99	99	99	99	UNKNOWN	UNKNOWN
101277	99	99	99	99	99	UNKNOWN	UNKNOWN
052880	99	99	99	99	99	UNKNOWN	UNKNOWN
061484	0	0	0	0	0	UNKNOWN	UNKNOWN

DATE	HYDRONEPHROSIS RIGHT	LEFT	SENSATION WITH FILLING	SENSATION WITH CONTRACTION
101566	UNKNOWN	UNKNOWN	UNKNOWN	UNKNOWN
061567	UNKNOWN	UNKNOWN	UNKNOWN	UNKNOWN
071567	UNKNOWN	UNKNOWN	UNKNOWN	UNKNOWN
091568	UNKNOWN	UNKNOWN	UNKNOWN	UNKNOWN
041569	UNKNOWN	UNKNOWN	UNKNOWN	UNKNOWN
031570	UNKNOWN	UNKNOWN	UNKNOWN	UNKNOWN
081571	UNKNOWN	UNKNOWN	UNKNOWN	UNKNOWN
081072	UNKNOWN	UNKNOWN	UNKNOWN	UNKNOWN
081572	UNKNOWN	UNKNOWN	UNKNOWN	UNKNOWN
081573	UNKNOWN	UNKNOWN	UNKNOWN	UNKNOWN
103174	UNKNOWN	UNKNOWN	UNKNOWN	UNKNOWN
091875	UNKNOWN	UNKNOWN	UNKNOWN	UNKNOWN
101277	UNKNOWN	UNKNOWN	UNKNOWN	UNKNOWN
052880	UNKNOWN	UNKNOWN	UNKNOWN	UNKNOWN
061484	UNKNOWN	UNKNOWN	UNKNOWN	UNKNOWN

DATE	COMMENTS
101566	RECODED FROM EARLIER DATA COLLECTION FORMS
061567	RECODED FROM EARLIER DATA COLLECTION FORMS
071567	RECODED FROM EARLIER DATA COLLECTION FORMS
091568	RECODED FROM EARLIER DATA COLLECTION FORMS
041569	RECODED FROM EARLIER DATA COLLECTION FORMS
031570	RECODED FROM EARLIER DATA COLLECTION FORMS
081571	RECODED FROM EARLIER DATA COLLECTION FORMS
081072	RECODED FROM EARLIER DATA COLLECTION FORMS
081572	RECODED FROM EARLIER DATA COLLECTION FORMS
081573	RECODED FROM EARLIER DATA COLLECTION FORMS
103174	RECODED FROM EARLIER DATA COLLECTION FORMS
091875	RECODED FROM EARLIER DATA COLLECTION FORMS
101277	RECODED FROM EARLIER DATA COLLECTION FORMS
052880	RECODED FROM EARLIER DATA COLLECTION FORMS
061484	--

O

Figure 22-8 *continues*

******************** FAMILY AND SCHOOL DATA **

DATE	STATE OF RESIDENCE	SIZE OF COMMUNITY	YEARS IN CURR. RESIDENCE
101566	UNKNOWN	FURTHER INFO AVAILABLE IN DIFFERENT FMT	99
061567	UNKNOWN	FURTHER INFO AVAILABLE IN DIFFERENT FMT	99
071567	UNKNOWN	FURTHER INFO AVAILABLE IN DIFFERENT FMT	99
091568	WASHINGTON	FURTHER INFO AVAILABLE IN DIFFERENT FMT	99
041569	UNKNOWN	FURTHER INFO AVAILABLE IN DIFFERENT FMT	99
031570	UNKNOWN	FURTHER INFO AVAILABLE IN DIFFERENT FMT	99
081571	UNKNOWN	FURTHER INFO AVAILABLE IN DIFFERENT FMT	99
081072	UNKNOWN	FURTHER INFO AVAILABLE IN DIFFERENT FMT	99
081572	UNKNOWN	FURTHER INFO AVAILABLE IN DIFFERENT FMT	99
081573	UNKNOWN	FURTHER INFO AVAILABLE IN DIFFERENT FMT	99
031174	WASHINGTON	FURTHER INFO AVAILABLE IN DIFFERENT FMT	99
103174	UNKNOWN	FURTHER INFO AVAILABLE IN DIFFERENT FMT	99
091875	WASHINGTON	FURTHER INFO AVAILABLE IN DIFFERENT FMT	99
101277	WASHINGTON	FURTHER INFO AVAILABLE IN DIFFERENT FMT	99
052880	WASHINGTON	FURTHER INFO AVAILABLE IN DIFFERENT FMT	99
010583	WASHINGTON	CITY: WITHIN 1 HOUR OF CITY OF 20,000 +	8

DATE	LIVING SITUATION	PARENTS	SINGLE PARENTS	CHLDRN IN HOME	NAT. SIB.
101566	UNKNOWN	FURTHER INFO AVAIL	FURTHER INFO AVAIL	99	99
061567	UNKNOWN	FURTHER INFO AVAIL	FURTHER INFO AVAIL	99	99
071567	UNKNOWN	FURTHER INFO AVAIL	FURTHER INFO AVAIL	99	99
091568	ONE OR BOTH NATURAL	FURTHER INFO AVAIL	FURTHER INFO AVAIL	99	4
041569	UNKNOWN	FURTHER INFO AVAIL	FURTHER INFO AVAIL	99	99
031570	UNKNOWN	FURTHER INFO AVAIL	FURTHER INFO AVAIL	99	99
081571	UNKNOWN	FURTHER INFO AVAIL	FURTHER INFO AVAIL	99	99
081072	UNKNOWN	FURTHER INFO AVAIL	FURTHER INFO AVAIL	99	99
081572	UNKNOWN	FURTHER INFO AVAIL	FURTHER INFO AVAIL	99	99
081573	UNKNOWN	FURTHER INFO AVAIL	FURTHER INFO AVAIL	99	99
031174	ONE OR BOTH NATURAL	FURTHER INFO AVAIL	FURTHER INFO AVAIL	2	4
103174	UNKNOWN	FURTHER INFO AVAIL	FURTHER INFO AVAIL	99	99
091875	ONE OR BOTH NATURAL	FURTHER INFO AVAIL	FURTHER INFO AVAIL	1	4
101277	ONE OR BOTH NATURAL	FURTHER INFO AVAIL	FURTHER INFO AVAIL	2	1
052880	ONE OR BOTH NATURAL	FURTHER INFO AVAIL	FURTHER INFO AVAIL	1	4
010583	ONE OR BOTH NATURAL	MOM AND DAD	NOT APPLICABLE	1	4

DATE	LEGAL STATUS	EMANCIPATED PATIENT	FATHERS OCCUPATION
101566	UNKNOWN	UNKNOWN	UNKNOWN
061567	UNKNOWN	UNKNOWN	UNKNOWN
071567	UNKNOWN	UNKNOWN	UNKNOWN
091568	UNKNOWN	UNKNOWN	SERVICE WORK, LABOR
041569	UNKNOWN	UNKNOWN	UNKNOWN
031570	UNKNOWN	UNKNOWN	UNKNOWN
081571	UNKNOWN	UNKNOWN	UNKNOWN
081072	UNKNOWN	UNKNOWN	UNKNOWN
081572	UNKNOWN	UNKNOWN	UNKNOWN
081573	UNKNOWN	UNKNOWN	UNKNOWN
031174	W/NAT OR ADOPT PARENTS	UNKNOWN	CRAFTSMAN, FOREMAN, OPER
103174	UNKNOWN	UNKNOWN	UNKNOWN
091875	W/NAT OR ADOPT PARENTS	UNKNOWN	SERVICE WORK, LABOR
101277	W/NAT OR ADOPT PARENTS	UNKNOWN	MANAGER, OFFICIAL, PROPR
052880	W/NAT OR ADOPT PARENTS	UNKNOWN	CRAFTSMAN, FOREMAN, OPER
010583	W/NAT OR ADOPT PARENTS	NOT APPLICABLE	MANAGER, OFFICIAL, PROPR

DATE	MOTHERS OCCUPATION	MOTHERS EMPLOYMENT	ACADEMIC ACHIEVEMENT
101566	UNKNOWN	UNKNOWN	NEVER IN SCHOOL
061567	UNKNOWN	UNKNOWN	NEVER IN SCHOOL
071567	UNKNOWN	UNKNOWN	NEVER IN SCHOOL
091568	UNKNOWN	UNKNOWN	NEVER IN SCHOOL
041569	UNKNOWN	UNKNOWN	NEVER IN SCHOOL

P

031570	UNKNOWN	UNKNOWN	NEVER IN SCHOOL
081571	UNKNOWN	UNKNOWN	NEVER IN SCHOOL
081072	UNKNOWN	UNKNOWN	UNGRADED SPECIAL EDUCATIO
081572	UNKNOWN	UNKNOWN	UNGRADED SPECIAL EDUCATIO
081573	UNKNOWN	UNKNOWN	UNGRADED SPECIAL EDUCATIO
031174	UNKNOWN	FULL TIME HOMEMAKER	UNGRADED SPECIAL EDUCATIO
103174	UNKNOWN	UNKNOWN	UNGRADED SPECIAL EDUCATIO
091875	UNKNOWN	FULL TIME HOMEMAKER	UNGRADED SPECIAL EDUCATIO
101277	UNKNOWN	FULL TIME HOMEMAKER	UNGRADED SPECIAL EDUCATIO
052880	UNEMPLOYED OUTSIDE HOME	FULL TIME HOMEMAKER	UNGRADED SPECIAL EDUCATIO
010583	UNEMPLOYED OUTSIDE HOME	FULL TIME HOMEMAKER	UNGRADED SPECIAL EDUCATIO

DATE	EDUCATION/TRAINING	EMPLOYMENT
101566	NONE	NONE
061567	NONE	NONE
071567	NONE	NONE
091568	NONE	NONE
041569	NONE	NONE
031570	NONE	NONE
081571	NONE	NONE
081072	SPECIAL EDUC WITHOUT CONTACT CLASS	NONE
081572	SPECIAL EDUC WITHOUT CONTACT CLASS	NONE
081573	SPECIAL EDUC WITHOUT CONTACT CLASS	NONE
031174	SPECIAL EDUC WITHOUT CONTACT CLASS	NONE
103174	SPECIAL EDUC WITH CONTACT CLASSES	NONE
091875	SPECIAL EDUC WITHOUT CONTACT CLASS	NONE
101277	SPECIAL EDUC WITH CONTACT CLASSES	NONE
052880	SPECIAL EDUC WITHOUT CONTACT CLASS	NONE
010583	SPECIAL EDUC WITH CONTACT CLASSES	NONE

DATE	OCCUPATION THERAPY	PHYSICAL THERAPY	OTHER THERAPY
101566	FURTHER INFO AVAILABLE	FURTHER INFO AVAILABLE	FURTHER INFO AVAILABLE
061567	FURTHER INFO AVAILABLE	FURTHER INFO AVAILABLE	FURTHER INFO AVAILABLE
071567	FURTHER INFO AVAILABLE	FURTHER INFO AVAILABLE	FURTHER INFO AVAILABLE
091568	FURTHER INFO AVAILABLE	FURTHER INFO AVAILABLE	FURTHER INFO AVAILABLE
041569	FURTHER INFO AVAILABLE	FURTHER INFO AVAILABLE	FURTHER INFO AVAILABLE
031570	FURTHER INFO AVAILABLE	FURTHER INFO AVAILABLE	FURTHER INFO AVAILABLE
081571	FURTHER INFO AVAILABLE	FURTHER INFO AVAILABLE	FURTHER INFO AVAILABLE
081072	FURTHER INFO AVAILABLE	FURTHER INFO AVAILABLE	FURTHER INFO AVAILABLE
081572	FURTHER INFO AVAILABLE	FURTHER INFO AVAILABLE	FURTHER INFO AVAILABLE
081573	FURTHER INFO AVAILABLE	FURTHER INFO AVAILABLE	FURTHER INFO AVAILABLE
031174	FURTHER INFO AVAILABLE	FURTHER INFO AVAILABLE	FURTHER INFO AVAILABLE
103174	FURTHER INFO AVAILABLE	FURTHER INFO AVAILABLE	FURTHER INFO AVAILABLE
091875	FURTHER INFO AVAILABLE	FURTHER INFO AVAILABLE	FURTHER INFO AVAILABLE
101277	FURTHER INFO AVAILABLE	FURTHER INFO AVAILABLE	FURTHER INFO AVAILABLE
052880	FURTHER INFO AVAILABLE	FURTHER INFO AVAILABLE	FURTHER INFO AVAILABLE
010583	NOT RECEIVING	NOT RECEIVING	NOT RECEIVING

DATE	THERAPY SERVICES PROVIDED THROUGH	OTHER RESOURCES
101566	FURTHER INFO AVAILABLE	
061567	FURTHER INFO AVAILABLE	
071567	FURTHER INFO AVAILABLE	
091568	FURTHER INFO AVAILABLE	
041569	FURTHER INFO AVAILABLE	
031570	FURTHER INFO AVAILABLE	
081571	FURTHER INFO AVAILABLE	
081072	FURTHER INFO AVAILABLE	
081572	FURTHER INFO AVAILABLE	
081573	FURTHER INFO AVAILABLE	
031174	FURTHER INFO AVAILABLE	
103174	FURTHER INFO AVAILABLE	
091875	FURTHER INFO AVAILABLE	CCS
101277	FURTHER INFO AVAILABLE	CCS
052880	FURTHER INFO AVAILABLE	CCS
010583	NOT APPLICABLE	CCS

Q

Figure 22-8 *continues*

DATE	COMMENTS
101566	RECODED FROM EARLIER DATA COLLECTION FORMS INFO UPDATED 1/2/85
061567	RECODED FROM EARLIER DATA COLLECTION FORMS INFO UPDATED 1/2/85
071567	RECODED FROM EARLIER DATA COLLECTION FORMS INFO UPDATED 1/2/85
091568	RECODED FROM EARLIER DATA COLLECTION FORMS INFO UPDATED 1/2/85
041569	RECODED FROM EARLIER DATA COLLECTION FORMS INFO UPDATED 1/2/85
031570	RECODED FROM EARLIER DATA COLLECTION FORMS INFO UPDATED 1/2/85
081571	RECODED FROM EARLIER DATA COLLECTION FORMS INFO UPDATED 1/2/85
081072	RECODED FROM EARLIER DATA COLLECTION FORMS INFO UPDATED 1/2/85
081572	RECODED FROM EARLIER DATA COLLECTION FORMS INFO UPDATED 1/2/85
081573	RECODED FROM EARLIER DATA COLLECTION FORMS INFO UPDATED 1/2/85
031174	RECODED FROM EARLIER DATA COLLECTION FORMS INFO UPDATED 1/2/85
103174	RECODED FROM EARLIER DATA COLLECTION FORMS INFO UPDATED 1/2/85
091875	RECODED FROM EARLIER DATA COLLECTION FORMS INFO UPDATED 1/2/85

R

```
101277   RECODED FROM EARLIER DATA COLLECTION FORMS
         INFO UPDATED 1/2/85

052880   RECODED FROM EARLIER DATA COLLECTION FORMS
         INFO UPDATED 1/2/85

010583

******************** TEST RESULTS - FROSTIG                          **************

        TC01
 DATE    .                                    AGE  TEST LOCATION
103174  997  999  999  999  999  999          102  H002
091875  240  999  999  999  999  999           96  H002
101277  251  999  999  999  999  999          137  H002

******************** TEST RESULTS - JEBSON TAYLOR HAND FUNCTION      **************

        TF01
 DATE    .                                    AGE  TEST LOCATION
081572  997  033  002  999  999  999           75  H002
091875  064  044  002  999  999  999           96  H002
101277  046  033  002  999  999  999          137  H002

******************** TEST RESULTS - WISC                             **************

        TH01
         .    .    FULL SCALE IQ
 DATE    .         .                          AGE  TEST LOCATION
022874  063  055  056  999  999  999           93  H002
031174  063  055  056  999  999  999          999  H002

******************** TEST RESULTS - WRAT                             **************

        READING (STANDARD SCORE)
         .    SPELLING (STANDARD SCORE)
         .    .    ARITHMETIC (STANDARD SCORE)
 DATE    .    .    .                          AGE  TEST LOCATION
022874  059  056  057  999  999  999           93  H002
```

S

SUMMARY

We recommend a multidisciplinary program that provides the patient's family with a professional advocate pair of a physician or surgeon and a nurse or social worker. The advocates should help the family obtain complex medical services from a vast array of health providers and integrate this care with the patient's education and social life. Every program, regardless of modifications necessary to accommodate local differences, should focus on helping the patient and family achieve as near normal growth and development as possible. There are no clear-cut distinctions among medical, educational, and social factors that contribute to the normalized growth and final outcome for a patient born with any of the severe congenital malformations discussed in this text. Carefully standardized records of patients' medical problems and interventions should, therefore, be analyzed to measure progress toward the final outcome and provide insight into better methods of care. Maximum self-sufficiency should remain the goal for all patients. Keep in mind that the patient and his or her world, present and future, should be the central focus of the health care program.

REFERENCES

1. Aadalen RJ, O'Phelan EH, Chisholm TC, et al: Exstrophy of the bladder: Long-term results of bilateral posterior iliac osteotomies and two-stage anatomic repair. Clin Orthop 151:193–200, 1980
2. Abrams N, Buckner MD: Medical Ethics: A Clinical Textbook and Reference for the Health Care Professions. Cambridge, MIT Press, 1983
3. Abramson M, Ash MJ, Nash WR: Handicapped adolescents—A time for reflection. Adolescence 14(55):557–565, 1979
4. Abt AF: Abt-Garrison History of Pediatrics. Philadelphia, WB Saunders, 1965
5. Adams B: Like It Is: Fact and Feelings About Handicaps From Kids Who Know. New York, Walker, 1979
6. Adams CF: Nutritive Value of American Foods in Common Units. Agriculture Handbook No. 456. Washington, D.C., 1975, AR5-USDA
7. Adams GR: The effects of physical attractiveness on the socialization process, in Lucker GW, Ribbens KA, McNamara JA (eds): Psychological Aspects of Facial Form. Ann Arbor, Center for Human Growth and Development, 1980, pp 25–47
8. Adams GR, Cohen AS: Children's physical and interpersonal characteristics that affect student–teacher interactions. J Exp Educ 43:1–5, 1974
9. Adams GR, Crane P: An assessment of parents' and teachers' expectations of preschool children's social preference for attractive or unattractive children and adults. Child Dev 51(1):224–237, 1980
10. Adams GR, Crossman SM: Physical Attractiveness: A Cultural Imperative. New York, Libra, 1978
11. Adams GR, Huston TL: Social perception of middle-aged persons varying in physical attractiveness. Dev Psychobiol 11:656–658, 1975
12. Adams GR, LaVoie JC: The effects of sex of child, conduct and facial attractiveness on teacher expectancy. Education 95:76–83, 1974
13. Adams GR, LaVoie JC: Parental expectations of educational and personal-social performance and childrearing patterns as a function of attractiveness, sex and conduct of the child. Child Study J 5:125–142, 1975
14. Adams GR, LaVoie JC: Teacher expectations: A review of the student characteristics used in expectancy formation. J Instruct Psych Mono 4:1–28, 1977
15. Adams MM, Finley S, Hansen H, et al: Utilization of prenatal genetic diagnosis in women 35 years of age and older in the United States, 1977 to 1978. Am J Obstet Gynecol 139(16):673–677, 1981
16. Adoption Assistance and Child Welfare Act, PL 96-272, 1980
17. Agarwal H, Lee BY, Corcoran L, et al: Energy expenditure in quadriplegic patients. JPEN 8:99, 1984
18. Agness PJ: Learning disabilities need assessment. Spina Bifida Insights 11(1):2, 1983
19. Ajir F, Levin AB, Duff TA: Effect of prophylactic methicillin on cerebrospinal fluid shunt infections in children. Neurosurgery 9:6–8, 1981
20. Akins C, Davidson R, Hopkins T: The child with myelodysplasia, in

Scheiner AP, Abroms IF (eds): The Practical Management of the Developmentally Disabled Child. St. Louis, CV Mosby, 1980, pp 116–144

21. Aldrich RA: Human life-span development: A life science for Epoch B, in Hess HO (ed): The Nature of a Human Society: A Symposium on the Bicentennial of the United States of America. Philadelphia, Fortress Press, 1977, pp 171–185
22. Alexander SW, Altemeier WA: Penicillin prophylaxis of experimental staphylococcal wound infections. Surg Gynecol Obstet 120:243–254, 1954
23. Alland A: Adoption in Cultural Evolution: An Approach for Medical Anthropology. New York, Columbia University Press, 1970
24. Allen TD, Spence HM, Salyer KF: Reconstruction of the external genitalia in exstrophy of the bladder: Preliminary communication. J Urol 111:830–834, 1974
25. Allison L: Blood and Guts (A Working Guide to Your Own Insides). Boston, Little, Brown, 1976
26. Alpern GD, Boll TJ: Developmental Profile. Indianapolis, Indiana Psychology Developmental Publications, 1972
27. Altshuler A, Meyer J, Butz MC: Even children can learn to do clean self-catheterization. Am J Nurs 77(1):97–101, 1977
28. AMA Council on Scientific Affairs: Genetic counseling and prevention of birth defects. JAMA 248:221–224, 1981
29. AMA Council on Scientific Affairs: Maternal serum alpha-fetoprotein monitoring. JAMA 247:1478–1481, 1982
30. Ambrose SS: The repair of genital defects associated with persistent cloaca. J Urol 111:256–259, 1974
31. Ambrose SS, O'Brien DP III: Surgical embryology of the exstrophy-epispadias complex. Surg Clin North Am 54(6):1379–1390, 1974
32. American Academy of Pediatrics: Symposium on Myelomeningocele. St. Louis, CV Mosby, 1972, p 157
33. American Academy of Pediatrics: Doe compromise passed by senate. News Comments 35(9):3–4, 1984
34. American Academy of Pediatrics: Joint policy statement. Principles of treatment of disabled infants. Pediatrics 73(4):559–560, 1984
35. American Academy of Pediatrics, Committee on Bioethics: Treatment of critically ill newborns. Pediatrics 72:565–566, 1983
36. Ames MD, Schut L: Results of treatment of 171 consecutive myelomeningoceles—1963 to 1968. Pediatrics 50:466–470, 1972
37. Amuso SJ, Mankin HJ: Hereditary spondylolisthesis and spina bifida. Report of a family in which the lesion is transmitted as an autosomal dominant through three generations. J Bone Joint Surg [Am] 49:507–513, 1967
38. Anderl H, Jakse Q, Marberger H: Reconstruction of abdominal wall and mons pubis in females with bladder exstrophy. Urology 22:247–250, 1983
39. Anderson EM: Handwriting and spina bifida. Spec Educ Forward Trends 3(2):17–20, 1976

40. Anderson EM, Clarke L: Disability in Adolescence. London, Methuen, 1982
41. Anderson EM, Plewis I: Impairment of motor skill in children with spina bifida cystica and hydrocephalus: An exploratory study. Br J Psychol 68:61–70, 1977
42. Anderson EM, Spain B: The Child with Spina Bifida. London, Methuen, 1977
43. Anderson FM: Occult spinal dysraphism: A series of 73 cases. Pediatrics 55(6):826–835, 1975
44. Anderson FM: Ventriculocardic shunts. J Pediatr 82:222–227, 1973
45. Andrews RJ, Elkins J: The Management and Education of Children with Spina Bifida and Hydrocephalus. ERDC Report No. 32. Canberra, Australian Government Publishing Service, 1981
46. Ansell JS: Surgical treatment of exstrophy of the bladder with emphasis on neonatal primary closure. J Urol 121:650–653, 1979
47. Apley J: The infant with stridor: A follow-up survey of 80 cases. Arch Dis Child 28:423–435, 1953
48. Appelgarth DA, Kirby LI, Lowry RB: Screening for neural tube defects. Can Med Assoc J 21:116–117, 1978
49. Asch A: The experience of disability: A challenge for psychology. Am Psychol 39(5):529–536, 1984
50. Asher M, Olson J: Factors affecting the ambulatory status of patients with spina bifida cystica. J Bone Joint Surg [Am] 65(3):350–356, 1983
51. Atimed S: Management of neurogenic bladder. Spina Bifida Mag March:3–5, 1980
52. Ayme S, Mattei JF: Brief clinical report: HARD (+/−E) syndrome: Report of a sixth family with support for autosomal-recessive inheritance. Am J Med Genet 14:759–766, 1983
53. Aziz IA: Neural tube defects in the Sudan. J R Coll Surg Edinb 28(3):151–153, 1983
54. Bachman DS, Hodges IJ, Freeman JM: Computerized axial tomography in neurologic disorders in children. Pediatrics 59:352–363, 1977
55. Badell-Ribera A, Shulman K, Paddock N: The relationship of nonprogressive hydrocephalus to intellectual functioning in children with spina bifida cystica. Pediatrics 37(5):787–793, 1966
56. Bailey BH: Bedsores. London, E Arnold, 1967
57. Bailey SK: Ethics and the public service. Public Admin Rev 24(4):234–243, 1964
58. Bajaj PS, Welsh F, Shadid EA: Versatility of lumbar transposition flaps in the closure of meningomyelocele skin defects. Ann Plast Surg 2(2):103–108, 1979
59. Bakan D: Slaughter of the Innocents. San Francisco, Jossey-Bass Press, 1979
60. Baker EM: Vitamin C requirements in stress. Am J Clin Nutr 20:583, 1967
61. Banta JV, Casey JM, Bedell L, et al: Long term ambulation in spina bifida. Dev Med Child Neurol 25:110, 1983

62. Banta JV, Whiteman S, Dyck PM, et al: Fifteen year review of myelodysplasia. J Bone Joint Surg [Am] 58:726, 1976
63. Barden BA, Meyer DC, Stelling FH: Myelodysplasia—Fate of those followed for twenty years or more. J Bone Joint Surg [Am] 57(5):643–647, 1975
64. Barsel G, Pueschel SM, Hall AH, et al: Experience with prenatal diagnosis in Rhode Island. RI Med J 61(7):273–278, 1978
65. Bartlett S: Employment Opportunities for Disabled Americans Act. H.R. 2030. Congressional Record: Proceedings and Debates of the 99th Congress, First Session. Washington, D.C., 131:43, April 15, 1985
66. Bartlett MD, Wolf LS, Shurtleff DB, et al: The assessment of hip flexion contraction. Arch Phys Med Rehabil 66:620–625, 1985
67. Barton V: Nutritional support of the spinal cord injury patient. Perspect Nutr Supp 2:1–4, 1985
68. Bartoshesky LE: Genetics and the child with developmental disabilities, in Scheiner AP, Abroms IF (eds): The Practical Management of the Developmentally Disabled Child. St. Louis, CV Mosby, 1980, pp 221–249
69. Bartoshesky LE, Haller J, Scott RM, et al: Seizures in children with meningomyelocele. Am J Dis Child 139:400–416, 1985
70. Battle CU: The role of the primary care physician, in Scheiner AP, Abroms IF (eds): The Prenatal Management of the Developmentally Disabled Child. St. Louis, CV Mosby, 1980, pp 1–20
71. Bayer C: Zur technik der operation der spina bifida and encephalocele. Prog Med Wochenschr 17:317, 332, 345, 1892
72. Bayer C: Ztchr f Heilk Berl. Vor der Operation der Spina Bifida and Encephalocoele. Zeitzchrift fur Heilkronen Berlin 18:405, 1897
73. Bayles M: Ethics and Population. Cambridge, Schenkman, 1976, pp ix–xiii
74. Bayley N: Constancy and variability in growth of intelligence from birth to eighteen years. J Genet Psychol 75:165–196, 1949
75. Bayston R: Antiobiotic prophylaxis in shunt surgery. Dev Med Child Neurol 35(suppl):99–103, 1975
76. Bayston R, Lari J: A study of the sources of infection in colonised shunts. Dev Med Child Neurol 16(suppl 32):16–22, 1975
77. Beal VA: Nutritional intake, in McCammon R (ed): Human Growth and Development. Springfield, IL, Charles C Thomas, 1970, p 63
78. Beals RK: Spastic paraplegic and dyplegia, and evaluation of nonsurgical and surgical factors influencing the prognosis for ambulation. J Bone Joint Surg [Am] 48:827–846, 1966
79. Beck AT: Cognitive Therapy and the Emotional Disorders. New York, New American Library, 1976
80. Becker RD: Recent developments in child psychiatry (I). The restrictive emotional and cognitive environment reconsidered: A redefinition of the concept of therapeutic restraint. Isr Ann Psychiatr Rel Disc 13:239–258, 1975
81. Beckwith JB: The congenitally malformed. VII. Exstrophy of the bladder and cloacal exstrophy. Northwest Med 65:407–410, 1966

82. Beckwith L: Relations between attributes of mothers and their infant's I.Q. scores. Child Dev 42:1083–1097, 1971
83. Beckwith L, Cohen SE, Kopp CB, et al: Caregiver–infant interactions and early cognitive development in preterm infants. Child Dev 47:579–587, 1976
84. Beery KE, Buktenica NA: Developmental Test of Visual Motor Integration Manual. Chicago, Follett, 1976
85. Bell DC, Bell LB: Parental validation and support in the development of adolescent daughters, in Grotevant HD, Cooper LR (eds): Adolescent Development in the Family. San Francisco, Jossey-Bass, 1983
86. Belsky J, Lerner RM, Spainer GB: The Child in the Family. Reading, MA, Addison-Wesley, 1984
87. Bennett KA: Lumbo-sacral malformations and spina bifida occulta in a group of proto-historic Modoc Indians. Am J Phys Anthropol 36:435–440, 1972
88. Bentovim A: Emotional disturbances of handicapped preschool children and their families: Attitudes to the child. Br Med J 3:579–581, 1972
89. Berg K, Isaksson B: Body composition and nutrition of school children with cerebral palsy. Acta Paediatr Scand 204:41–52, 1970
90. Berger G: Physical Disabilities. New York, Franklin Watts, 1979
91. Bergsma D (ed): Conference on the Clinical Delineation of Birth Defects. Baltimore, The National Foundation, 1974, p 97
92. Berman P: Letter: Congenital abnormalities associated with maternal clomiphene ingestion. Lancet 2(7940):878, 1975
93. Bernstein RA: Two expert deceivers. Seattle Times, January 28, 1985, pp A4
94. Berscheid E: An overview of the psychological effects of physical attractiveness, in Lucker GW, Ribbens KA, McNamara JA (eds): Psychological Aspects of Facial Form. Ann Arbor, Center for Human Growth and Development, 1980, pp 1–23
95. Berscheid E, Walster E: Physical attractiveness, in Berkowitz L (ed): Advances in Experimental Social Psychology, vol. 7. New York, Academic Press, 1974
96. Bettelheim B: The Uses of Enchantment: The Meaning and Importance of Fairy Tales. New York, Alfred A. Knopf, 1976
97. Beirig JR, Linn JE: The Baby Doe Law and Regulations as They Affect Infants Born with Spina Bifida. Chicago, Sidley and Austin, 1985
98. Binder HJ: Absorption and secretion of water and electrolytes by small and large intestine, in Slesenger MH, Fordtran JS (eds): Gastrointestinal Disease Pathophysiology Diagnosis Management (ed 3), vol. 1. Philadelphia, WB Saunders, 1983, pp 811–829
99. Birkel P: Cognitive development and measurement of intelligence in physically handicapped children. Prax Kinderpsychol Kinderpsychiatr 29(7):264–268, 1980
100. Black P: Selective treatment of infants with myelomeningocele. Neurosurgery 5:334–338, 1979

101. Black RB, Furlong R: Prenatal diagnosis: The experience in families who have children. Am J Med Genet 19:729–739, 1984
102. Blackburn G, Bistridh B, Maini B, et al: Nutritional and metabolic assessment of the hospitalized patient. JPEN 1:11–22, 1977
103. Blaiklock CR, Demetriou EL, Rayner CR: The use of a latissimus dorsi myocutaneous flap in the repair of spinal defects in spina bifida. Br J Plast Surg 34(3):356–361, 1981
104. Blakeley CR, Mills WG: The obstetric and gynaecological complications of bladder exstrophy and epispadius. Br J Obstet Gynaecol 88:167–173, 1981
105. Bleck EE: Low motor prognosis in cerebral palsy. Dev Med Child Neurol 17:18–24, 1975
106. Bleck EE, Nagel DA: Physically Handicapped Children—A Medical Atlas for Teachers. Orlando, FL, Grune & Stratton, 1982
107. Bloom S: The Doctor and His Patient—A Sociological Interpretation. New York, Russell Sage Foundation, 1963
108. Blos P, Finch SM: Sexuality and the handicapped adolescent, in Downey JA, Low NL (eds): The Child with Disabling Illness. Philadelphia, WB Saunders, 1974, p 538
109. Blum RH: The Management of the Doctor–Patient Relationship. New York, McGraw-Hill, 1960
110. Blum RW: The adolescent with spina bifida. Clin Pediatr (Phila) 22:331–334, 1983
111. Bobroff M: Discussion of Edgerton MT (ed): Plastic reconstruction of congenital defects associated with spina bifida and cranium bifidum. Surg Clin North Am 32:1327, 1952
112. Boles ET: Discussion of principles of management of exstrophy of the cloaca. Am J Surg 119:98, 1970
113. Boning H: Specific Skill Builders. Rockville Center, Baldwin, NY, Barnellhoft, 1970
114. Booth BE, Gates J, Morris RC: Grocery store baking soda: A source of sodium bicarbonate in the management of metabolic acidosis. Clin Pediatr (Phila) 23(2):94–96, 1984
115. Borberg A: Clinical and genetic investigations into sclerosis and Recklinghausen's neurofibromatosis. Acta Psychiatr Neurol 71:239, 1951
116. Borzyskowski M: Management of the neuropathic bladder in childhood. Dev Med Child Neurol 26:401–404, 1984
117. Borzyskowski M, Mundy AR, Neville BGR, et al: Neuropathic vesicourethral dysfunction in children. A trial comparing clean intermittent catheterization with expression combined with drug treatment. Br J Urol 54:641–644, 1982
118. Boston VE, Wilkinson AJ: A retrospective analysis of conservative versus active management in severe open myelomeningocele. Z Kinderchir 28:340–347, 1979
119. Bower TGR: Development in Infancy. San Francisco, WH Freeman, 1974
120. Bradley RH, Caldwell BM: Early home environment and changes in

mental test performance in children from 6–36 months. Dev Psychobiol 12(2):93–97, 1976

121. Braham J, Front D, Sarova-Pinhas I, et al: Brain atrophy, hydrocephalus and dementia in adults. Isr J Med Sci 5:1213–1218, 1969
122. Braine MDS, Heimer CB, Wortis H, et al: Factors associated with impairment of the early development of prematures. Monogr Soc Res Child Dev 30:4, 1966
123. Breed AL, Ibler I: The motorized wheelchair: New freedom, new responsibility and new problems. Dev Med Child Neurol 24:366–371, 1982
124. Breslau N, Staruch KS, Mortimer EA Jr: Psychological distress in mothers of disabled children. Am J Dis Child 136(8):682–686, 1982
125. Breslow N: A generalized Kruskal-Wallis test for comparing K samples subject to unequal patterns of censorship. Biometrika 57:579–594, 1970
126. Bricker D, Bailey E, Bruder MB: The efficacy of early intervention and the handicapped infant: A wise or wasted resource, in Wolraich M, Routh DK (eds): Advances in Developmental and Behavioral Pediatrics, vol. 5. Greenwich, CT, JAI Press, 1984, pp 373–423
127. Bricker D, Carlson L, Schwarz R: A discussion of early intervention for infants with Down syndrome. Pediatrics 67(1):45–46, 1981
128. British Medical Journal: Perspectives in spina bifida (editorial). 2:909–910, 1978
129. Brock DJH, Barron L, Van Heyningen V: Prenatal diagnosis of neural-tube defects with a monoclonal antibody specific for acetylcholinesterase. Lancet 1(8419):5–8, 1985
130. Brock WA, Eddie PS, Harback LB, et al: Intermittent catheterization in the management of neurogenic vesical dysfunction in childhood. J Urol 125:391, 1981
131. Brocklehurst G: Spina Bifida for the Clinician. Philadelphia, JB Lippincott, 1976
132. Brocklehurst G, Gleave JRW, Lewin W: Early closure of myelomeningocele with special reference to leg movement. Br Med J 1:666–669, 1967
133. Bronfenbrenner U: The Ecology of Human Development: Experiments by Nature and Design. Cambridge, MA, Harvard University Press, 1979
134. Brothwell DR, Powers R: Congenital malformations of the skeleton in earlier man, in Brothwell DR (ed): The Skeletal Biology of Earlier Human Populations, vol. VIII. Oxford, Pergamon Press, 1968, p 173
135. Browder JA: The pediatrician's orientation to infant stimulation programs. Pediatrics 67(1):42–44, 1981
136. Brown B: Personal communication, 1985
137. Brown et al *v*. Board of Education of Topeka, Shawnea Country, Kansas et al. 347 US 483, 1954
138. Bruce AMB, Lorber J, Sheddon WIH, et al: Persistent bacteraemia following ventriculo-caudal shunt operations for hydrocephalus in infants: Dev Med Child Neurol 5:461–470, 1963
139. Bruch H: Eating Disorders. New York, Basic Books, 1973

140. Brunt D: Characteristics of upper limb movements in a sample of meningomyelocele children. Percept Mot Skills 51:431–437, 1980
141. Buck Bell 274 US 200, 1927
142. Budoff M: Implementing due process safeguards: Its application to special educational and its implications for teacher training. Cambridge, MA, Research Institute for Educational Problems, 1976
143. Bunch WH: Treatment protocols, tentative and personal, still evolving, in Lovell WW, Winter RB (eds): Pediatric Orthopedics. Philadelphia, JB Lippincott, 1978, pp 381–426
144. Bunch WH, Cass AS, Bensman AS, et al: Modern Management of Myelomeningocele. St. Louis, Warren H Green, 1972
145. Bureau of Education for the Handicapped: A summary of the evaluation of the Handicapped Children's Early Education Program (HCEEP). Report prepared by the planning staff of official child development. Washington, D.C., Bureau of Education for the Handicapped, 1976
146. Burke JF: The effective period of preventive antiobiotic action in experimental incisions and dermal lesions. Surgery 50:161–168, 1961
147. Burkitt D: Don't Forget Fiber in Your Diet. New York, Arco, 1984
148. Burlingham D: Notes on problems of motor restraint during illness, in Lowenstein RM (ed): Drives, Affects, Behavior. New York, International Universities Press, 1953
149. Burnett C: Giant Steps for Steven. Berlin, NJ: Spina Bifida Foundation, 1980
150. Butler C: Effects of powered mobility on self-initiative behavior of very young, locomotor-disabled children. Unpublished Doctor of Education Dissertation, University of Washington, 1983
151. Butler C: Personal communication, 1985
152. Butler C, Okamoto GA, McKay TM: Motorized wheelchair driving by disabled children. Arch Phys Med Rehabil 65:95–97, 1984
153. Callaghan RP, Cohen SJ, Stewart GT: Septicemia due to colonization of Spitz-Holter valves by *Staphylococci*: Five cases treated with methicillan. Br Med J 1:860–866, 1961
154. Calussen C: Computerized axial tomography of the spine. Neurol Pediatr 8:405, 1977
155. Campbell M: Clinical Pediatric Urology. Philadelphia, WB Saunders, 1951
156. Campbell MM, Hayden PW, Davenport S: Psychological adjustment of adolescents with myelodysplasia. J Youth Adoles 6(4):397–407, 1977
157. Campbell S: Early prenatal diagnosis of neural tube defects by ultrasound. Clin Obstet Gynecol 20:351–359, 1977
158. Candia A, Zegel HG: The occurrence of Wilms tumor in two patients with exstrophy of the bladder. J Urol 128(3):589–590, 1982
159. Cappanari SC, Rau B, Abram HS, et al: Voodoo in the general hospital. JAMA 232:938–940, 1975
160. Capute AJ, Biehl RF: Functional developmental evaluation, a prerequisite to habilitation: Symposium on habilitation of the handicapped child. Pediatr Clin North Am 20:3–24, 1973

161. Carey JC, Greenbaum B, Hall BD: The OEIS complex (omphalocele, exstrophy, imperforate anus, spinal defects). Birth Defects OAS 14(6B): 253–263, 1978
162. Carr J: Helping Your Handicapped Child: A Step-by-Step Guide to Everyday Problems. Harmondsworth, England, Penguin Books, 1980
163. Carr J, Halliwell MD, Pearson AM: Educational attainments of spina bifida children attending ordinary or special schools. Z Kinderchir 34(4):364–370, 1981
164. Carratello P: My Body. Rachelle Cracchiolo/Mary Dupuy Smith Publications, 1980
165. Carroll N: The orthopedic and orthotic management of the spina bifida child, in Weiss M (ed): Clinical Neurosurgery. Baltimore, Williams & Wilkins, 1982, pp 413–435
166. Carroll N: The orthotic management of the spina bifida child. Clin Orthop 102:108–114, 1974
167. Carroll NC, Sharrard WJW: Long-term follow up posterior ileopsoas transplantation for paralytic dislocation of the hip. J Bone Joint Surg [Am] 54:551–560, 1972
168. Carter CO, David PA, Laurence KM: A family study of major central nervous system malformations in South Wales. J Med Genet 5:81–106, 1968
169. Carter CO, Evans K: Spina bifida and anencephalus in Greater London. J Med Genet 10:209–234, 1973
170. Carter CO, Evans KA, Till K: Spinal dysmorphism: Genetic relation to neural tube malformations. J Med Genet 13(5):343–350, 1976
171. Carter EA, McGoldrick M: The Family Life Cycle. New York, Gardner, 1980
172. Casey Youngwirth *v.* the State of Washington, a Dependency Hearing, Superior Court of Pierce County, 1977
173. Catalogue: Health Specialists and Multiple Disciplinary Clinics Caring for Patients with Meningomyelocele (Spina Bifida). Chicago, Spina Bifida Association of America, 1985
174. Caudal BF, Brazier MAB: Prevention of Neural Tube Defects: The Role of Alpha-Fetoprotein. New York, Academic Press, 1978
175. Chance PF, Smith DW: Hyperthermia and meningomyelocele and anencephaly (letter). Lancet 1:769–770, 1978
176. Chandler LS, Andrews MS, Swanson MW: Movement Assessment of Infants: A Manual. Rolling Bay, WA, Published by the Authors, 1980
177. Chapman W, Hill M, Shurtleff DB: Management of the Neurogenic Bowel and Bladder. Oakbrook, IL, Eterna Press, 1979
178. Charlip R, Charlip MB: Handtalk. New York, Scholastic/Four Winds, 1974
179. Charney EB, Rosenblum M, Finegold D: Linear growth in a population of children with myelomeningocele. Z Kinderchir 34:415–419, 1981
180. Charney EB, Weller SC, Sutton LH, et al: Management of the newborn

with myelomeningocele: Time for a decision-making process. Pediatrics 75:58–64, 1985

181. Charron J, Delisle R: Carcinoma of the sigmoid: A complication of ureterosigmoidostomy. Can J Surg 25(3):253–257, 1982
182. Chedd G: Who shall be born? Science 81:33–40, 1981
183. Cheek WR, Laurent JP, Cech DA: Operative repair of lumbosacral myelomeningocele. Technical note. J Neurosurg 59(4):718–722, 1983
184. Chemke J, Czernobilsky B, Mundel G, et al: A familial syndrome of central nervous system and ocular malformations. Clin Genet 7:1–17, 1975
185. Chen H, Wooley PV: A developmental assessment chart for noninstitutionalized Down Syndrome children. Growth 42:157–165, 1978
186. Chervenak FA, Berkowitz RL, Tortora M, et al: The management of fetal hydrocephalus. Am J Obstet Gynecol 151:933–942, 1985
187. Chervenak FA, Berkowitz RL, Romero R, et al: The diagnosis of fetal hydrocephalus. Am J Obstet Gynecol 147(6):703–716, 1983
188. Chervenak FA, Duncan L, Ment LR, et al: Perinatal management of meningomyelocele. Obstet Gynecol 63(3):376–380, 1984
189. Chiari H: Uber Verandesungen des Kleinhirns, des pons und der medulla oblongata in folge von congenitaler hydrocephalie des Grosshirns. Denksher Akad Wiss Wein 63:71–116, 1896
190. Child Abuse Amendment of 1984, PL 98-457, 98 stat 1749
191. Chodak GW, Plaut ME: Use of systemic antibiotics for prophylaxis in surgery: A critical review. Arch Surg 112:326–334, 1977
192. Christianson RE, van den Berg BJ, Milkorich L, et al: Incidence of congenital anomalies among white and black live births with long-term follow-up. Am J Public Health 71(12):1333–1341, 1981
193. Christie DL, O'Grady LR, Mack DV: Incompetent lower esophageal sphincter and gastroesophageal reflux in recurrent acute pulmonary disease of infancy and childhood. J Pediatr 93(1):23–27, 1978
194. Cicarelli V, Granger R: The Impact of Head Start: An Evaluation of the Effects of Head Start on Children's Cognition and Affective Development. Athens, OH, Westinghouse Learning Corporation, 1969
195. Clark DH, Walsh JW, Luce EA: Closure of myelorachischisis defects with reverse latissimus dorsi myocutaneous flaps. Neurosurgery 11(3):423–425, 1982
196. Clarke A, Clarke A: Early Experiences: Myth and Evidence. New York, Free Press, 1976
197. Clarren SK, Smith DW, Harvey MAS, et al: Hyperthermia—A prospective evaluation of a possible teratogenic agent in man. J Pediatr 95:81–83, 1979
198. Clarren SK, Smith DW: The fetal alcohol syndrome. N Engl J Med 298(19):1063–1067, 1978
199. Claussen CO, Lohkamp FW, Von Bazan VB: The diagnosis of congenital spinal disorders in computed tomography (CT). Neuropaediatrie 8(4):405–417, 1977

200. Clean Intermittent Catheterization for Boys (pamphlet). Oakbrook, IL, Eterna Press, 1982
201. Clean Intermittent Catheterization for Girls (pamphlet). Oakbrook, IL, Eterna Press, 1982
202. Cleland J: Contribution to the study of spina bifida, encephalocele and anencephalus. J Anat 17:257, 1883
203. Clewell WH, Johnson ML, Meier PR, et al: A surgical approach to the treatment of fetal hydrocephalus. N Engl J Med 306(22):1320–1325, 1982
204. Clifford M, Walster E: The effect of physical attractiveness on teacher expectations. Sociol Educ 46:248–258, 1973
205. Cobb LS, Hancock KA: Development of the child with a physical disability, in Wolraich M, Routh DK (eds): Advances in Developmental and Behavioral Pediatrics, vol. 5. Greenwich, CT, JAI Press, 1984, pp 75–107
206. Cochrane DD, Myles ST: Management of intrauterine hydrocephalus. J Neurosurg 57:590–596, 1982
207. Cockran JH Jr, Edstrom LE, Dibbell DG: Usefulness of the innervated tensor fascia lata flap in paraplegic patients. Ann Plast Surg 7:286–288, 1981
208. Cohen MA, Gross PJ: The Developmental Resource: Behavioral Sequences for Assessment and Program Planning, vol. I and II. Orlando, FL, Grune & Stratton, 1979
209. Colgan MT: The child with spina bifida. Am J Dis Child 135:854–858, 1981
210. Collis VR: The effects of selective treatment of myelomeningocele on a neonatal unit. Dev Med Child Neurol 14(Suppl 27):34–37, 1972
211. Comarr AE: Marriage and divorce among patients with spinal cord injury. I-IV, in Proceedings of the Eleventh Annual Clinical Spinal Cord Injury Conference. Bronx, NY, Veterans Administration Hospital, 1962, pp 163–215
212. Comarr AE: Neurological disturbances of sexual function among patients with myelodysplasia, in McLaurin RL (ed): Myelomeningocele. Orlando, FL, Grune & Stratton, 1977, pp 797–808
213. Committee on Nutrition: Obesity in childhood. Pediatrics 66:772, 1967
214. Conference Report: Critical Needs of the Child with Long-Term Orthopedic Impairment. Chicago, American Academy of Orthopedics, 1985
215. Congenital Malformations Surveillance. Atlanta, Centers for Disease Control, 1975
216. Connell HM, McConnel TS: Psychiatric sequelae in children treated operatively for hydrocephalus in infancy. Dev Med Child Neurol 23:505–517, 1981
217. Codman and Shurtleff, Control of hydrocephalus using the Holter ventriculoatrial shunt system. Extracorporal Medical Specialities, Billerica, MA, 1968
218. Cook RC, Zachary RB: Operative management of the neurogenic bladder in children: Diversion through intestinal conduits. Surgery 63:825–831, 1968

219. Coon V, Donato G, Horeser C, et al: Normal ranges of hip motion in infants six weeks, three months, and six months of age. Clin Orthop 110:256–260, 1975
220. Cooper I, Rynearson E, MacCarty C, et al: Consequences of spinal cord injury. J Clin Endocrinol Metab 10:858–870, 1950
221. Cooperman GM: Meningomyelocele: To treat or not to treat. Can Med Assoc J 116:1339–1340, 1977
222. The Cordis-Hakim Valve System for Ventricular Shunting (ed 4). Cordis Neurological Corp, Miami, FL, 1972
223. Coren S, Porac C: Fifty centuries of righthandedness: The historic record. Science 198:631–632, 1977
224. Corter C, Trehub S, Boukydis C, et al: Nurses' judgements of the attractiveness of premature infants. Infant Behav Dev 1:373–380, 1978
225. Council for Exceptional Children: Editor's note. Except Child 47:492–493, 1981
226. Cox S, Posanick P, Worthington P, et al: Energy expenditure after spinal cord injury. JPEN 8:99, 1984
227. Craig TJ, Van Natta PA: Disability and depressive symptoms in two communities. Am J Psychiatry 140(5):598–601, 1982
228. Crandall BF, Brazier MAB (eds): Prevention of Neural Tube Defects: The Role of Alpha-Fetoprotein. Orlando, FL, Academic Press, 1978
229. Crandall BF, Lebherz TB, Freihube R: Neural tube defects: Maternal serum screening and prenatal diagnosis. Pediatr Clin North Am 25:619–629, 1978
230. Creasy MR, Alberman ED: Congenital malformations of the central nervous system in spontaneous abortions. J Med Genet 13:9–16, 1976
231. Creating Your Kids: A Look at the Puppet Workshop, in Caputo L (ed): Keeping Up With the Kids (pamphlet). Fall 1983
232. Crnic KA, Friedrich WN, Greenberg MT: Adaptation of families with mentally retarded children: A model of stress, coping, and family ecology. Am J Ment Defic 88(2):125–138, 1983
234. Crowell RM, Tew JM Jr, Mark VH: Aggressive dementia associated with normal pressure hydrocephalus. Report of two unusual cases. Neurology (Minneap) 23:461–464, 1973
235. Cruse PJE, Foord R: A five-year prospective study of 23,649 surgical wounds. Arch Surg 107:206–210, 1973
236. Cull C, Wyke MA: Memory function of children with spina bifida and shunted hydrocephalus. Dev Med Child Neurol 26(2):177–183, 1984
237. Culley WJ, Middleton TO: Calorie requirements of mentally retarded children with and without motor dysfunction. J Pediatr 75:380–384, 1969
238. Curtis BH: Principles of orthopedic management in myelomeningocele, in American Academy of Orthopedic Surgeons Symposium on Myelomeningocele. St. Louis, CV Mosby, 1972, p 157
239. Curtis BH, Butler JE, Emerson CE: Follow up study of 100 patients over the age of 12 with meningomyelocele, in American Association of Ortho-

pedic Surgeons Symposium on Myelomeningocele. St. Louis, CV Mosby, 1972

240. Dalens B, Raynaud EJ, Gaulme J: Teratogenicity of valproic acid (letter). J Pediatr 97(2):332–333, 1980

241a. Dallaire L, Melancon SB, Pottier M, et al: Date of conception and prevention of neural tube defects. Clin Genet 26:304–307, 1984

241b. Dandy WE: Diagnosis and treatment of hydrocephalus due to occlusions of the foramina of Magendie and Luschka. Surg Gynecol Obstet 32:112, 1921

242a. Daniel RK, Priest DC, Wheatley DC: Etiologic factors in pressure sores: An experimental model. Arch Phys Med Rehabil 62:492–498, 1981

242b. Dardour JC, Vilain R, Castro D: Evaluation of 10 years surgical treatment for decubitus ulcer. Sem Hop Paris 60:1051–1056, 1984

243a. Darling R: Parents, Physicians, and Spina Bifida. Institute of Society, Ethics and the Life Sciences. Hastings Center Report, Hudson, NY, 1977

243b. Darling RB: Families Against Society: A Study of Reactions to Children with Birth Defects. Beverly Hills, Sage, 1979

244a. Darling RB: The birth defective child and the crisis of parenthood, in Callahan E, McCluskey K (eds): Life-Span Developmental Psychology: Nonnormative Life Events. Orlando, FL, Academic Press, 1983, pp 115–147

244b. Darling RB: Parent-professional interaction: The roots of misunderstanding, in Seligman M (ed): The Family with a Handicapped Child: Understanding and Treatment. Orlando, FL, Grune & Stratton, 1983, pp 95–121

245a. Darling RB, Darling J: Children Who are Different: Meeting the Challenges of Birth Defects in Society. St. Louis, CV Mosby, 1982

245b. Darling RB, Darling J: Helping Techniques I: Counseling: Children Who Are Different. St. Louis, CV Mosby, 1982, pp 192–218

246a. Darwin C: The Origin of Species and the Descent of Man. New York, Modern Library, 1836, p 429

246b. Davies D, Adendorff D: A large rotation flap raised across the midline to close lumbo-sacral meningomyeloceles. Br J Plast Surg 30(2):166–168, 1977

247a. Davis F: Deviance disavowal: The management of strained interaction by the visibly handicapped. Soc Prob 9:120–132, 1961

247b. Davol IH, Hastings ML: Effects of sex, age, reading ability, SES, and display position on measures of spatial relations in children. Percept Mot Skills 24:375–387, 1967

248a. Davson H: Dynamic aspects of the cerebrospinal fluid. Dev Med Child Neurol 14(suppl 27):1–16, 1972

248b. Death drugs for some spina bifida babies? (editorial). Med News Trib 19(18), 1978

249a. Dekaban AS, Bartelmez GW: Complete disraphism in 14 somite human embryo. Am J Anat 115:27–42, 1964

249b. DeKlerk DJJ, DeVilliers JC: Frontal encephaloceles. S Afr Med J 47:1350–1355, 1973

250. DeKlotz RL: Care of infants with myelomeningocele. Pediatrics 74:162, 1984
251. DeLange SA: Selection for treatment of patients with spina bifida operta. Dev Med Child Neurol 16(suppl 32):27–30, 1974
252. DeLuca P, Torella M, Festa B: Pregnancy complicated by ISO-Rh in patient born with bladder exstrophy and operated on by sigmoidal implantation of the ureters. Arch Obstet Gynecol 87(5–6):203–213, 1982
253. DeMaria JE, Alton DJ, Krueger RP, et al: Renal function in continent patients after surgical closure of bladder exstrophy. J Urol 124(1):85–88, 1980
254. Dember CP: Motivation and the cognitive revolution. Am Psychol 29:161–178, 1974
255. Demenais F, LeMerrier M, Briard ML, et al: Neural tube defects in France: Segregation analysis. Am J Med Genet 11:287–298, 1982
256. deMol J: Psychic disturbance in normal pressure hydrocephalus. Acta Neurol Belg 78(6):321–340, 1978
257. Demographic Aspects of Aging and the Older Population in the United States. Current Population Reports, Special Studies Series Bureau of the Census, U.S. Superintendent of Public Documents Washington, DC, 59, May 1976, p 23
258. DeMyer W: The median cleft face syndrome: Differential diagnosis of cranium bifidum occultum, hypertelorism and median cleft nose, lip and palate. Neurology (Minneap) 17:961–971, 1967
259. Denhoff E: Current status of infant stimulation or enrichment programs for children with developmental disabilities. Pediatrics 67(1):32–37, 1981
260. DeSouza LJ, Carroll M: Ambulation of the braced myelomeningocele patient. J Bone Joint Surg 58(AM):1112–1118, 1976
261. Desprez JD, Kiehn CL, Eckstein W: Closure of large meningomyelocele defects by composite skin-muscle flaps. Plast Reconstr Surg 47:234–238, 1971
262. DeVoogt HJ, VanderSluis C: Preliminary evaluation of alpha-adrenergic blocking agents in children with neurogenic bladder due to myelomeningocele. Dev Med Child Neurol 37(Suppl):82–88, 1976
263. DeVroede G: Constipation mechanisms and management, in Sleisenger MH, Fordtran JS (eds): Gastrointestinal Disease Pathophysiology Diagnosis Management (ed 3), vol. 1. Philadelphia, WB Saunders, 1983, p 288
264. Dewhurst J, Toplis PJ, Shepherd JH: Ivalon sponge hysterosacropexy for genital prolapse in patients with bladder exstrophy. Br J Obstet Gynaecol 87(1):67–69, 1980
265. Dias L: Personal communication, 1985
266. Dias L: Use of computers in the International Myelodysplasia Study. Presented at the American Academy of Cerebral Palsy and Developmental Medicine Meeting, Seattle, WA, September 2–5, 1985
267. Dias L, Mazur J: Personal communication, 1985
268. Dibbell DG, McGraw JB, Edstrom LE: Providing useful and protective

sensibility to the sitting area in patients with meningomyelocele. Plast Reconstr Surg 64:796–799, 1979

269. Dibbell DG: Use of a Long Island flap to bring sensation to the sacral area in young paraplegics. Plast Reconstr Surg 54:200, 1974
270. Dickens C: Oliver Twist. New York, New American Library, 1961
271. Dietrich S, Okamoto G: Bowel training for children with neurogenic dysfunction: A follow up. Arch Phys Med Rehabil 63(4):166–170, 1982
272. Dietz WH: Childhood obesity: Susceptibility, cause and management. J Pediatr 103:676–686, 1983
273. Diller L, Gordon WA, Swinyard C, et al: Psychological and educational studies with spina bifida children. ERDC Document EDO 34347, US DHEW. Washington, D.C., US Office of Education, 1969
274. Diller L, Swinyard CA, Epstein FJ: Cognitive function in children. in Swinyard CA (ed): Decision Making and the Defective Newborn: Proceedings of a conference on Spina Bifida and Ethics. Springfield, IL, Charles C Thomas, 1978
275. Dinno WD, Shearer L, Weisskopf B: Chondrodysplastic dwarfism, cleft palate and micrognathia in a neonate, a new syndrome? Eur J Pediatr 123(1):39–42, 1976
276. Diokno AC, Kass E, Lapides J: A new approach to myelodysplasia. J Urol 116:771–772, 1976
277. Diokno AC, Sonda PL, Hollander JB, et al: The fate of patients started on clean intermittent self-catheterization therapy 10 years ago. J Urol 129:1120, 1983
278. Dion KK: Young children's stereotyping of facial attractiveness. Dev Psychobiol 9:183–188, 1973
279. Dion KK, Berscheid E: Physical attractiveness and peer perception among children. Sociometry 37:1–12, 1974
280. Doctors face new rules on "Baby Doe" treatment. Seattle Times, December 8, 1984, p A1
281. Donn SM: Fetal hydrocephalus: A perinatal dilemma. J Reprod Med 27(9):589–592, 1982
282. Doran PA, Guthkelch AM: Studies in spina bifida. J Neurol Neurosurg Psychiatry 24:331–343, 1961
283. Dorner S: Adolescents with spina bifida: How they see their situation. Arch Dis Child 51:539–544, 1976
284. Dorner S: The relationship of physical handicap to stress in families with an adolescent with spina bifida. Dev Med Child Neurol 17:765–776, 1975
285. Dorner S: Sexual interest and activity in adolescents with spina bifida. J Child Psychol Psychiatry 18(3):229–237, 1977
286. Drago JR, Wellner L, Sanford EJ, et al: Role of intermittent catheterization in the management of children with myelomeningocele. J Urol 118:92–94, 1977
287. Drotar D: Psychological perspective in chronic childhood illness. J Pediatr Psychol 6:211–228, 1981
288. Drotar D, Baskiewicz A, Irvin N, et al: The adaptation of parents to the

birth of an infant with a congenital malformation: A hypothetical model. Pediatrics 56(5):710–717, 1975

289. Drummond DS, Harechania RG, Rosenthal AM, et al: A study of pressure distributions measured during balanced and unbalanced sitting. J Bone Joint Surg 64:1034–1039, 1982
290. Dudgeon B, Jaffe KM, Shurtleff DB: Variations in mid lumbar meningomyelocele: Implications for ambulation. Arch Phys Med Rehab 66:553, 1985.
291. Duff RS, Campbell AGM: Moral and ethical dilemmas in the special care nursery. N Engl J Med 289:890–894, 1973
292. Dunne KB, Shurtleff DB: The adult with meningomyelocele: A preliminary report, in McLaurin R, Oppenheimer S (eds): Myelomeningocele: A Multidisciplinary Approach. New York, Praeger (in press)
293. Dunne KB, Shurtleff DB: Epilepsy in myelomeningocele. Presented at the Society for Research into Hydrocephalus and Spina Bifida. 29th Annual Scientific Meeting. Manchester, England, July 3–6, 1985
294. Dyson JL, Kohler HG: Anencephaly and ovulation stimulation (letter). Lancet 1:1256–1257, 1973
295. Eastman NJ: Induced abortion and contraception: A consideration of ethical philosophy in obstetrics. Obstet Gynecol Surv 22:3–11, 1967
296. Edgerton MT: Symposium on pediatric surgery: Plastic repair of congenital defects associated with spina bifida and cranium bifidum. Surg Clin North Am 32:933–950, 1952
297. Education for All Handicapped Children Act of 1975, PL 94-142, 89 Stat 773 (1975)
298. Eisenberg L: Reading retardation: I. Psychiatric and sociologic aspects. Pediatrics 37:352–365, 1966
299. Elkind D: Cognitive development and psychopathology: Observations on egocentrism and ego defense, in Schapler E (ed): New Developments in Child Psychopathology. New York, Plenum, 1976
300. Elkind D, Larson M, Van Doorninck W: Perceptual decentration in learning and performance in slow and average readers. J Educ Psychol 56:50–56, 1965
301. Elwood JM, Elwood JH: Epidemiology of anencephalus and spina bifida. New York, Oxford University Press, 1980
302. Emery AE: Folates and fetal central-nervous-system malformations (letter). Lancet 1:703, 1977
303. Emery JL: Fibrin and thrombosis in the central nervous system in children with particular reference to congenital hydrocephalus. J Clin Pathol 17:348–352, 1964
304. Emery JL: Infanticide, filicide, and cot death. Arch Dis Child 60:505–507, 1985
305. Emery JL, Lendon RG: Clinical implications of cord lesions in neurospinal dysraphism. Dev Med Child Neurol 14(suppl 27):45–51, 1972
306. Eng CC: The relationship between the eye-hand coordination and visual

perception test scores of children with myelomeningocele. Masters Thesis, University of Washington, 1981
307. Englebach W: Endocrine Medicine, vol. 1. Springfield, IL, Charles C Thomas, 1932, pp 261–292
308. Englehardt HT: Euthanasia and children: The injury of continued existence. J Pediatr 83:170–171, 1983
309. Englemann S: Corrective Reading Program. Chicago, Science Research Associates, 1975
310. Englemann S, Osborn G: DISTAR. Language 1: An Instruction System (ed 2). Chicago, Science Research Associates, 1976
311. Engstrom FM, Roche AF, Mukherjee D: Differences between arm span and stature in white children. J Adolesc Health Care 2:19–22, 1981
312. Ericson C, Lidgren L, Lindberg L: Cloxacillin in prophylaxis of postoperative infections of the hip. J Bone Joint Surg [Am] 55:808–1073, 1973
313. Erickson MT: MMPI profiles of parents of young retarded children. Am J Ment Defic 73:728–732, 1969
314. Erikson EH: Childhood and Society. New York, Norton, 1950
315. Erikson M, Larsson G, Windbladh B, et al: The influence of amphetamine addiction on pregnancy and the newborn infant. Acta Pediatr Scand 67(1):95–99, 1978
316. Erikson ML: Assessment: A Basis for Management, in Marcene L Powell (ed): Assessment and Management of Developmental Changes in Children (ed 2). St. Louis, CV Mosby, 1976
317. Evans EP, Tew B: The energy expenditure of spina bifida children during walking and wheelchair ambulation. Z Kinderchir 34:425–427, 1981
318. Evans K, Hickman V, Carter CO: Handicap and social status of adults with spina bifida cystica. Br J Prev Soc Med 28:85–92, 1974
319. Evans RC, Thomas MD, Williams LA: Shunt blockage in hydrocephalic children: The use of the valvogram. Clin Radiol 27:489–495, 1976
320. Everett ED, Strausbaugh LJ: Antimicrobial agents and the central nervous system. Neurosurgery 6(6):691–714, 1980
321. Fabrega H: The study of disease in relation to culture. Behav Sci 17:183–203, 1972
322. Farber B: Notes on sociological knowledge about families with mentally retarded children, in Schreiber M (ed): Social Work and Mental Retardation. New York, John Day, 1970
323. Fassler J: One Little Girl. New York, Human Sciences Press, 1969
324. Fay G: Personal communication, 1985
325. Feetham SL, Tweed H, Perrin JS: Practical problems in selection of spina bifida infants for treatment in the USA. Z Kinderchir 28(4):301–306, 1979
326. Feifel H: Perception of death. Ann Acad Sci 164:669–677, 1969
327. Feiwell E, Sakai D, Blatt T: The effect of hip reduction on function in patients with myelomeningocele. J Bone Joint Surg [Am] 60:169–173, 1978
328. Feldman KW, Schaller RT, Feldman JA, et al: Tap water scald burns in children. Pediatrics 62(1):1–7, 1978
329. Fellous M, Boue J, Malbrunot C, et al: A five-generation family with

sacral agenesis and spina bifida: Possible similarities with the mouse T-locus. Am J Med Genet 12:465–487, 1982

330. Feremback D: Frequency of spina bifida occulta in prehistoric human skeletons. Nature 199:100, 1963
331. Fernandez-Serrats AA, Guthkelch AH, Parker SA: The prognosis of open myelocele with a note on a trial of Laurence's operation. Dev Med Child Neurol 13(Suppl):65–74, 1967
332. Ferris: Considerations Generales et Observations Particulaires sur le Spina Bifida. J Gen Med Chir Pharm Franc Etrang 27:162–176, 1806
333. Ferry PC: On growing new neurons: Are early intervention programs effective? Pediatrics 67(1):38–41, 1981
334. Field TM, Vega-Lahr N: Early interactions between infants with craniofacial anomalies and their mothers. Infant Behav Dev 7:527–530, 1984
335. Filshov B, Boll TJ: Handbook of Clinical Neuropsychology. New York, John Wiley, 1981
336. Fineman RM, Jorde LB, Martin RA, et al: Spinal dysraphia as an autosomal dominant defect in four families. Am J Med Genet 12:457–464, 1982
337. Finnie NR: Handling the Young Cerebral Palsied Child at Home (ed 2). New York, DP Dutton, 1975
338. Firooznia H, Rafii M, Golimbu C, et al: Computed tomography of pressure sores, pelvic abscess and osteomyelitis in patients with spinal cord injury. Arch Phys Med Rehabil 63:545–548, 1982
339. Fishler K, Graliker BV, Koch R: The predictability of intelligence with Gesell developmental scales in mentally retarded infants and young children. Am J Ment Defic 69:515–525, 1965
340. Fishman MA, Palkes HS: The validity of psychometric testing in children with congenital malformations of the central nervous system. Dev Med Child Neurol 16:180–185, 1974
341. Fishman MA, Palkes HS, Shackelford GD, et al: Lacunar-skull deformity and intelligence. Pediatrics 59(2):296–299, 1977
342. Fitzsimmons JS: Laryngeal stridor and respiratory obstruction associated with myelodysplasia. Dev Med Child Neurol 15:533–536, 1973
343. Flanigan RC, Casale AJ, McRoberts JW: Cloacal exstrophy. Urology 23:227–233, 1984
344. Flatz G, Sukthomya L: Fronto-enthmoidal encephalomeningoceles in the population of Northern Thailand. Humangenetik 11:1–8, 1970
345. Fleisher DR: Diagnosis and treatment of disorders of defecation in children. Pediatr Ann 5:70–101, 1976
346. Fletcher J: Ethics and euthanasia, in Weir RF (ed): Ethical Issues in Death and Dying. New York, Columbia University Press, 1977, p 348
347. Fletcher J: Morals and Medicine. Princeton, NJ, Princeton University Press, 1954
348. Fletcher J: The morality and ethics of prenatal diagnosis, in Abrams N, Buckner MD (eds): Medical Ethics: A Clinical Textbook and Reference

for the Health Care Professions. Cambridge, MA, The MIT Press, 1983, pp 443–451

349. Fletcher J: Spina bifida with myelomeningocele: A case study in attitudes towards defective newborns, in Swinyard CB (ed): Decision-making and the Defective Newborn. Springfield, IL, Charles C Thomas, 1978, pp 281–303
350. Folkman S, Schaefer C, Lazarus RS: Cognitive processes as mediators of stress and coping, in Hamilton V, Warburton DW (eds): Human Stress and Cognition. New York, John Wiley, 1979
351. Foltz EL, DeFeo DR: Double compartment hydrocephalus—A new clinical entity. Neurosurgery 7:551–559, 1980
352. Foltz EL, Shurtleff DB: Five-year comparative study of hydrocephalus in operated and non-operated children (113 cases). J Neurosurg 20:1064–1079, 1963
353. Foltz EL, Shurtleff DB: Conversion of communicating hydrocephalus to stenosis or occlusion of the aqueduct during ventricular shunting. J Neurosurg 24:520–529, 1966
354. Foltz EL, Shurtleff DB: Myelomeningocele: To treat or not to treat. A neurosurgeon's perspective. Clin Neurosurg 20:147–163, 1973
355. Fonkalsrud EW, Linde LM: Successful management of vesicointestinal fistula: Reports of two cases. J Pediatr Surg 5:309–314, 1970
356. Forbes GB: Lean body mass and fat in obese children. Pediatrics 34:308, 1964
357. Forrest DM: Spina bifida: Some problems in management. Proc R Soc Med 70:233–239, 1977
358. Forrester RM: Ethical and social aspects of treatment of spina bifida. Lancet 2:1033, 1968
359. Fost N: Counseling families who have a child with a severe congenital anomaly. Pediatrics 67(3):321–324, 1981
360. Fraiberg S: Insights From the Blind. New York, Basic Books, 1977
361. Frame PT, Watankunakorn C, McLaurin RL, et al: Penetration of nafcillin, methicillin, and cefazolin into human brain tissue. Neurosurgery 12:142–147, 1983
362. Francis V, Korsch BM, Morris MJ: Gaps in doctor-patient communications: Patients' response to medical advice. N Engl J Med 280(10): 535–540, 1969
363. Frankel B: Childbirth in the Ghetto: Folk Beliefs of Negro Women in a North Philadelphia Hospital Ward. San Francisco, R & E Research Associates, 1977
364. Frankenburg WK, Dodds JB, Fandal AW, et al: Denver Developmental Screening Test Reference Manual. Revised 1975 Edition. Boulder, University of Colorado Medical Center, 1975
365. Fraumeni JF Jr, Li FP, Dalager N: Teratomas in children: Epidemiological features. J Nat Cancer Inst 51:1425–1430, 1973
366. Frazier CH: Surgery of the Spine and Spinal Cord. New York, Appleton, 1918

367. Freeman JM: Early management and decision making for the treatment of myelomeningocele: A critique (letter). Pediatrics 73(4):564–566, 1984

368. Freeman JM: Practical Management of Meningomyelocele. Baltimore, University Park Press, 1974

369. Freeman MVR, Williams DW, Schimke RN, et al: The Robert's syndrome. Clin Genet 5:1–16, 1974

370. Freeston MB: An inquiry into the effect of the spina bifida child on family life. Dev Med Child Neurol 13:456–461, 1971

371. Fried K, Liban E, Lurie M, et al: Polycystic kidneys associated with malformations of the brain, polydactyly and other birth defects in newborn sibs. A lethal syndrome showing autosomal-recessive pattern of inheritance. J Med Genet 8:285–290, 1971

372. Friedrich WN: Ameliorating the psychological impact of chronic physical disease on the child and family. J Pediatr Psychol 2:26–31, 1977

373. Friedrich WN: Unpublished data, 1985

374. Friedrich WN, Friedrich W: Comparison of psychosocial assets of parents with a handicapped child and their normal controls. Am J Ment Defic 85:551–553, 1981

375. Friedrich WN, Wilturner LT, Cohen DS: Coping resources and parenting the retarded child. Am J Ment Defic 90(2):130–139, 1985

376. Frostig M: Developmental Test of Visual Perception. Palo Alto, CA, Consulting Psychologists Press, 1966

377. Frostig M, Horne D: The Frostig Program for the Development of Visual Perception: Teacher's Guide. Chicago, Follett, 1964

378. Fry I, McKinna JA, Simon G, et al: Some observations on the lower urinary tract in infants with spina bifida cystica. Proc R Soc Med 59:420–421, 1966

379. Frykberg T, Olsen L: Infection as a cause of peritoneal catheter dysfunction in ventriculo-peritoneal shunting in children. Z Kinderchir 38(Suppl 11):84–86, 1983

380. Fuchs VR: Who Shall Live? Health, Economics, and Social Choice. New York: Basic Books, 1974

381. Fulford GE, Cairns TP: The problems associated with flail feet in children and their treatment with orthoses. J Bone Joint Surg [Br] 60:93–95, 1978

382. Gallo A: Spina bifida: The state of the art of medical management, in C Levine (ed.) The Hastings Center Report. Hastings-on-Hudson, NY, 1984, 14(2):10–13

383. Garber SL, Krouskop TA: Wheelchair cushion modification and its effect on pressure. Arch Phys Med Rehabil 65:579–583, 1984

384. Gardner E, O'Rahilly R, Prolo D: The Dandy-Walker and Arnold-Chiari malformations. Arch Neurol 32:393–406, 1975

385. Gardner WJ: Myelomeningocele, the result of rupture of the embryonic neural tube. Cleve Clin Q 27:88, 1960

386. Garland MJ: Rescue, unless . . . A review of the ethics of infant euthanasia, in Wolraich M, Routh DK (eds): Advances in Developmental and Behavioral Pediatrics, vol. 4. Greenwich, CT, JAI Press, 1983, pp 181–203

387. Gartel B, Haddow JE, Fletcher JL, et al. (eds): Maternal Serum Alpha-Fetoprotein: Issues in the Prenatal Screening and Diagnosis of Neural Tube Defects. National Center for Health Care Technology Conference Proceedings. Washington, D.C., U.S. Government Printing Office, 1980
388. Garwood SG: Educating young handicapped children: A developmental approach. Germantown, Aspen Systems, 1979
389. Gath A: The effect of mental subnormality on the family. Br J Hosp Med 8:147–150, 1972
390. Geiger RC: Sexuality of people with cerebral palsy. Med Asp Human Sex 9:70–83, 1975.
391. George R, Leibrock L, Epstein M: Long-term analysis of CSF shunt infections. A 25-year experience. J Neurosurg 51:804–811, 1979
392. Geraghty J, Feely M: Antibiotic prophylaxis in neurosurgery: A randomized controlled trial. J Neurosurg 60:724–726, 1984
393. Getman GN, Kane ER, Halgren MR, et al: The Physiology of Readiness, an Action Program for the Development of Perception for Children. Minneapolis, Program to Accelerate School Success, 1964
394. Gibson EJ: Learning to read. Science 148:1066–1072, 1965
395. Gibson EJ: Principles of Perceptual Learning and Development. New York, Meredith Corporation, 1969
396. Gibson EJ, Levin H: The Psychology of Reading. Cambridge, MA, The MIT Press, 1972
397. Gierup J: Micturition studies in infants and children. Scand J Urol Nephrol 4:191–207, 1970
398. Giesy JD, Barry JM, Fuchs EF, et al: Initial experience with the Rosen Incontinence Device. J Urol 125:794–795, 1981
399. Gilsanz V, Cleveland RH, Reid BS: Duplication of the mullerian ducts and genitourinary malformations. Part II: Analysis of malformations. Radiology 144(4):797–801, 1982
400. Glancy J: A dynamic orthotic system for young myelomeningoceles. Orthot Prosthet 30:3–15, 1976
401. Glancy J, Lindseth RE: The polypropylene solid-ankle orthosis. Orthot Prosthet 26:14–26, 1972
402. Glick PL, Harrison MR, Nakayama DK, et al: Management of ventriculomegaly in the fetus. J Pediatr 105(1):97–105, 1984
403. Gliedman J, Roth W: The Unexpected Minority. Handicapped Children in America. Orlando, FL, Harcourt, Brace, Janovich, 1980
404. Gluckman S, Barling J: Effects of a remedial program on visual motor perception in spina bifida children. J Genet Psychol 136:195–202, 1980
405. Gluthkelch AN, Pang D, Vries JK: Influence of closure technique on results in myelomeningocele. Childs Brain 8(5):350–355, 1981
406. Go KG, Melchoir HJ, Lakke JPWF: A thermosensitive device for the evaluation of the patency of ventriculo-atrial shunts in hydrocephalus. Acta Neurochir (Wien) 19:209–216, 1968
407. Goffman E: Stigma: Notes on the Management of Spoiled Identity. Englewood Cliffs, NJ, Prentice-Hall, 1963

408. Goldfarb W: Infant rearing and problem behavior. Am J Orthopsychiatry 13:249–265, 1943
409. Goldman AS, Lash JW, Dayton D, et al: Congenital Defects. Child Health and Human Development: An Evaluation and Assessment of the State of the Science (Pub #82-2304). Washington, D.C, U.S. Department of Health and Human Services, 1981, p V-3
410. Goldstein G, Arulanantham K: Neural tube defect and renal anomalies in a child with fetal alcohol syndrome. J Pediatr 93(4):636–637, 1978
411. Goldstein HR, Hensle TW: Urinary undiversion in adults. J Urol 128:143–150, 1982
412. Gorlin RV, Jens JP, Cohen MM Jr: Syndromes of the Head and Neck (ed 2). New York, McGraw-Hill, 1976
413. Gosden C, Brock DJ: Prenatal diagnosis of exstrophy of the cloaca. Am J Med Genet 8(1):95–109, 1981
414. Gottfried AW, Brody M: Interrelationships between and correlations of psychometric and Piagetian scales of sensorimotor intelligence. Dev Psychobiol 2(3):379–387, 1975
415. Gouin-Decaurie T: Quelques symptomes de'efants atyiques en regard des theories de Jean Piaget. Contributions a l'etude des science de'l homme. 2:87–93, 1953
416. Graham P, Howman-Giles R: Evaluations of CSF shunt patency by means of technetium-99M DTPA. J Neurosurg 57:262–266, 1982
417. Graivier L: Exstrophy of the cloaca. Am Surg 34(5):387–390, 1968
418. Gray SW, Skandalakis JE: Embryology for surgeons. London, WB Saunders, 1972, p 422
419. Greenacre P: Infant reactions to restraint: Problems in the fate of infantile aggression. Am J Orthopsychiatry 14:204–218, 1944
420. Gressang JD: Perceptual processes of children with myelomeningocele and hydrocephalus. Am J Occup Ther 28(4):226–230, 1974
421. Grimm RA: Hand function and tactile perception in a sample of children with myelomeningocele. Am J Occup Ther 30(4):234–240, 1976
422. Groden G: Mental ability, reaction time, perceptual motor and motor abilities in handicapped children. Percept Mot Skills 28:27–30, 1969
423. Groden G: Simple and complex motor proficiency. Am J Ment Defic 74:373–375, 1969
424. Grogan C, Ekvall S: Body composition of spina bifida patients as determined by K_{40} urinary creatinine and anthropometric measurements in international union of nutritional science. Proceedings of Tenth International Congress of Nutrition, Kyoto, Japan, 1975
425. Grogan C, Ekvall S: The effect of nutrient intake and physical activity on the body composition of meningomyelocele patients as determined by K_{40} urinary creatinine and anthropometric measurements, in Federal Proceedings Abstracts. Chicago, Federation of American Societies for Experimental Biology, 1977
426. Gross RH: Newborns with myelodysplasia—The rest of the story. N Engl J Med 312(25):1632–1634, 1985

427. Gross RH, Cox A, Tatyrek R, et al: Early management and decision making for the treatment of myelomeningocele. Pediatrics 72:450–458, 1983
428. Gross RH, Cox AD, Tatyrek R, et al: Letter to the editor. Pediatrics 74(1):166–167, 1984
429. Grundy DJ, Silva JR: Major amputation in paraplegic and tetraplegic patients. Int Rehabil Med 6:162–165, 1984
430. Grundy M, Tosh P, McLeish RD, et al: An investigation of the centers of pressure under the foot while walking. J Bone Joint Surg [Br] 57:98–103, 1975
431. Guidotti TL: American Indian anthropology and medicine. JAMA 240(4):348, 1978
432. Guiney EJ, Fitzgerald RJ, Mehigan D, et al: Surgical closure of myelomeningocele: Problems and consequences of the introduction of a policy of selection. Ir J Med Sci 146(8):260–262, 1977
433. Guiney EJ, MacCarthy P: Implications of a selective policy in the management of spina bifida. J Pediatr Surg 16(2):136–138, 1981
434. Guralnik MJ, Richardson HB, Jr, Heiser KE: A curriculum in handicapping conditions for pediatric residents. Except Child 48:338–346, 1982
435. Gurdjian ES, Thomas LM: Cerebral vasospasm. Surg Gynecol Obstet 129:931–948, 1969
436. Gustafson JM: Mongolism, parental desires, and the right to life, in Weir RF (ed): Ethical Issues in Death and Dying. New York, Columbia University Press, 1977, p 145
437. Gustafson L, Hagberg B: Recovery in hydrocephalic dementia after shunt operation. J Neurol Neurosurg Psychiatry 41:940–947, 1978
438. Guthkelch AN, Pang D, Vries JK: Influence of closure technique on results in myelomeningocele. Childs Brain 8(5):350–355, 1981
439. Guthrie JT: Models of reading and reading disability. J Educ Psychol 65:9–18, 1973
440. Guttmann L: Problem of treatment of pressure sores in spinal paraplegics. Br J Plast Surg 8:196–213, 1955
441. Haas S, Epps CH Jr, Adams JP: Normal ranges of hip motion in the newborn. Clin Orthop 91:114–118, 1973
442. Habal MB, Vries JK: Tension free closure of large meningomyelocele defects. Surg Neurol 8:177–180, 1977
443. Haddad HM, Wilkins L: Congenital anomalies associated with gonadal aplasia: Review of 55 cases. Pediatrics 23:885–902, 1959
444. Hagard S, Carter F, Milne RG: Screening for spina bifida cystica—A cost-benefit analysis. Br J Prev Soc Med 30:45–53, 1976
445. Hagberg B: The sequelae of spontaneously arrested infantile hydrocephalus. Dev Med Child Neurol 4:583–587, 1962
446. Haines SJ: Systemic antibiotic prophylaxis in neurological surgery. Neurosurgery 6:355–361, 1980
447. Hakim S, Duran de la Roche F, Burton JD: A critical analysis of valve

shunts used in the treatment of hydrocephalus. Dev Med Child Neurol 15:230–255, 1973

448. Hald T, Bradley WE: The Urinary Bladder Neurology and Dynamics. Baltimore, Williams & Wilkins, 1982

449. Hall JC, O'Quigley J, Giles GR, et al: Upper limb anthropometry: The value of measurement variance studies. Am J Clin Nutr 33(8):1846–1851, 1980

450. Halliwell MD, Carr JG, Pearson AM: The intellectual and educational functioning of children with neural tube defects. Z Kinderchir 31(4):375–381, 1980

451. Hammill D, Larsen S: Test of Written Language. Austin, TX, Pro-Ed, 1983

452. Hamill PVV, Drizd TA, Johnson CL, et al: Physical growth: National Center for Health Statistics percentiles. Am J Clin Nutr 32:607–629, 1979

453. Hammock MK, Milhoray TN, Baron IS: Normal pressure hydrocephalus in patients with myelomeningocele. Dev Med Child Neurol 18(suppl 37):55–68, 1976

454. Hanna MK, Williams DI: Genital function in males with vesical exstrophy and epispadias. Br J Urol 44:169–174, 1972

455. Hannigan KF: Teaching intermittent self-catheterization to young children with myelodysplasia. Dev Med Child Neurol 21:365–368, 1979

456. Hara M, Kadowaki C: A new method for measuring cerebrospinal fluid flow in shunts. J Neurosurg 58:557–561, 1983

457. Harbart J, Haddad D, McCullough D: Quantitation of cerebrospinal fluid shunt flow. Radiology 112:379, 1974

458. Harber JR: Perception and perceptual motor integration: There is a difference. Percept Mot Skills 49:919–924, 1979

459. Hare EH, Laurence KM, Payne H, et al: Spina bifida cystica and family stress. Br Med J 2:757–760, 1966

460. Harkins E: Effects of the empty nest transition: A self report of psychological well being. J Marriage Fam 40(3):549–556, 1978

461. Harrison MR, Golbus MS, Filly RA: The Unborn Patient: Prenatal Diagnosis and Treatment. Orlando, FL, Grune & Stratton, 1984

462. Harrison MR, Gobus MS, Filly RA: Management of the fetus with a correctible congenital defect. JAMA 246(7):774–777, 1981

463. Haskins J, Stifle M: Quiet Revolution. New York, Thomas Crowell, 1979

464. Hayden PW: Adolescents with meningomyelocele. Pediatr Rev 6(8):245–252, 1985

465. Hayden PW, Chapman WH, Stevenson JK: Exstrophy of the cloaca. Am J Dis Child 125:879–883, 1973

466. Hayden PW, Davenport LH, Campbell MM: Adolescents with myelodysplasia: Impact of physical disability on emotional maturation. Pediatrics 64(1):53–59, 1979

467. Hayden PW, Foltz EL, Shurtleff DB: Effect of an oral osmotic agent on ventricular fluid pressure of hydrocephalic children. Pediatrics 41:955–967, 1968

468. Hayden PW, Lemire JR, Scott CR, et al: Children with congenital defects (multiple approaches to neural tube defects). Washington State Medical Association Annual Meeting, Spokane, 1974
469. Hayden PW, Rudd TG, Dizmang D: Evaluation of surgically treated hydrocephalus by radionuclide clearance studies of the cerebrospinal fluid shunt. Dev Med Child Neurol 16(suppl 32):72–78, 1974
470. Hayden PW, Shurtleff DB, Broy AB: Custody of the myelodysplastic child: Implications for selection for early treatment. Pediatrics 53(2):253–256, 1974
471. Hayden PW, Shurtleff DB, Stuntz TJ: A longitudinal study of shunt function in 360 patients with hydrocephalus. Dev Med Child Neurol 25:334–337, 1983
472. Hayes JT, Gross HP: Orthopedic implications of myelodysplasia. JAMA 184:762–767, 1963
473. Hayes JT, Gross HP, Dow S: Surgery for paralytic defects secondary to myelomeningocele and myelodysplasia. J Bone Joint Surg [Am] 46:1577–1597, 1964
474. Hayes-Allen, MC: Obesity and short stature in children with myelomeningocele. Dev Med Child Neurol 14(suppl 22):59–64, 1972
475. Hayes-Allen MC, Tring FL: Obesity: Another hazard for spina bifida children. Br J Prev Soc Med 27:192–196, 1972
476. Haygood VP, Wahbeh CJ: Prospects for the prenatal diagnosis and obstetric management of cloacal exstrophy: A report of two cases. J Reprod Med 28:807–810, 1983
477. Haynes BF, Check WR, Mintz AA: Treatment of meningomyelocele in infants and nonindigent patients. Am J Dis Child 127:182–186, 1974
478. Haynes SG, Gibson JB, Kurland LT: Epidemiology of neural-tube defects and Down's syndrome in Rochester, Minnesota, 1935–1971. Neurology (Minneap) 24:691–700, 1974
479. Heimburger RF: Early repair of myelomeningocele (spina bifida cystica). J Neurosurg 37:594–600, 1974
480. Hemmer R: Postoperative causes of death in hydrocephalic children. Analysis and conclusions about therapy. Acta Neurochir (Wien) 48:95–103, 1979
481. Hentoff N: The awful privacy of Baby Doe. Atlantic Monthly 55:54–62, January 1985
482. Hepper NG, Black LF, Fowler WS: Relationships of lung volume to height and arm span in normal subject and in patients with spinal deformity. Am Rev Respir Dis 91:356–362, 1965
483. Hewitt D: Geographical variations in the mortality attributed to spina bifida and other congenital malformations. Br J Prev Soc Med 17:13–22, 1963
484. Heyer-Schulte Systems for the Treatment of Hydrocephalus. American Heyer-Schulte Corp, Goleta, Calif
485. Hibbard ED, Smithells RW: Folic acid metabolism and human embryopathy. Lancet 1:1254, 1965

486. Hide DW, Williams HP, Ellis HL: The outlook for the child with a myelomeningocele for whom early surgery was considered inadvisable. Dev Med Child Neurol 14:304–307, 1972
487. Hillesmaa VK, Bardy AH, Grunstrom ML, et al: Valproic acid during pregnancy. Lancet 1:883, 1980
488. Hindse-Nielsen S: Spina bifida-prognose: Erblichkeit ein klinische studie. Acta Chir Scand 80:525–578, 1938
489. Hobson DA, Legal J: Stand up wheelchair for severely handicapped children. Interclin Info Bull 12:15–17, 1972
490. Hoffer MD: Joint motion limitation in newborns. Clin Orthop 148:94–96, 1980
491. Hoffer MM, Feiwell E, Perry R, et al: Functional ambulation in patients with myelomeningocele. J Bone Joint Surg 55AM:137–148, 1973
492. Hoffman HJ, Henrick EB, Humphreys RP: Management of hydrocephalus. Monogr Neural Sci 8:21–25, 1982
493. Hoffman HJ, Taecholarn C, Hendrick EB, et al: Lipomyelomeningoceles and their management. Neurosurgery 5:107–117, 1985
494. Hoffman L: Foundations of Family Therapy. New York, Basic Books, 1981
495. Hoffmaster B: Would you want to be normalized? Westminster Inst Rev 1(4):3–6, 1982
496. Holder AR: The duty to prolong life, in Abrams N, Buckner MD (eds): Medical Ethics: A Clinical Textbook and Reference for the Health Care Professions. Cambridge, MA, MIT Press, 1983, p 378
497. Holinger PC, Holinger LD, Reichert TJ, et al: Respiratory obstruction and apnea in infants with bilateral abductor vocal cord paralysis, meningomyelocele, hydrocephalus and Arnold-Chiari syndrome. J Pediatr 92(3):368–373, 1978
498. Holm B: Personal communication, 1985
499. Holmes LB, Driscoll SG, Atkins LA: Etiologic heterogeneity of neural tube defects. N Engl J Med 294(7):365–369, 1976
500. Holmes TH, Rahe RH: The social readjustment rating scale. J Psychosom Res 11:213–218, 1967
501. Holroyd J: The questionnaire on resources and stress: An instrument to measure family response to a handicapped family member. J Community Psychol 2:92–94, 1974
502. Holroyd J, McArthur D: Mental retardation and stress on the parents: A contrast between Down's syndrome and childhood autism. Am J Ment Defic 80:431–436, 1976
503. Hook EB: Incidence and prevalence as measures of the frequency of birth defects. Am J Epidemiol 116:743–747, 1982
504. Hook EB, Schrinemachers DB, Cross PK: Use of prenatal cytogenetic diagnosis in New York State. N Engl J Med 305:1410–1412, 1981
505. Horai J, Naccari N, Fatoullah E: The effects of expertise and physical attractiveness upon opinion agreement and liking. Sociometry 37:601–606, 1974

506. Horoszowski H, Israeli A, Heim M, et al: A new orthopedic fixation method in the treatment of bladder exstrophy. Clin Orthop 165:200–203, 1982
507. Hosking GP: Fits in hydrocephalic children. Arch Dis Child 49:633–635, 1974
508. Hourcade J, Pautte HP: A review of the therapeutic intervention research on gross and fine motor progress in young children with cerebral palsy. Am J Occup Ther 38:462–468, 1984
509. Howell C, Caldamone A, Snyder H, et al: Optimal management of cloacal exstrophy. J Pediatr Surg 18(4):365–369, 1983
510. Hsia YE, Bratu M, Herbordt A: Genetics of the Meckel syndrome (dysencephalia splanchnocystica). Pediatrics 48:237–247, 1971
511. Huff CW, Ramsey PL: Myelodysplasia: The influence of the quadriceps and hip abductor muscles on ambulatory function and stability of the hip. J Bone Joint Surg [Am] 60:432–443, 1978
512. Hunt GM: Spina bifida: Implications for 100 children at school. Dev Med Child Neurol 23(2):160–172, 1981
513. Hunt GM, Holmes AG: Factors relating to intelligence in treated cases of spina bifida cystica. Am J Dis Child 130:823–827, 1976
514. Hunt G, Lewin W, Gleave J, et al: Predictive factors in open myelomeningocele with special reference to sensory level. Br Med J 4:197–201, 1973
515. Hunter AGW: Neural tube defects in Eastern Ontario and Western Quebec: Demography and family data. Am J Med Genet 19:45–63, 1984
516. Hurd RW, Wilder BJ, Van Rinsvelt HA: Valproate, birth defects, and zinc (letter). Lancet 1(8317):181, 1983
517. Hutchinson DH: Has Chapter 766 accomplished its goals? The views of parents of children with special needs (Doctoral dissertation, University of Massachusetts, 1978). Dissertation Abstracts International (University Microfilms #ISSN0419-4209), 39(2180A), 1978
518. Ignelzi RJ, Kirsch WM: Follow-up analysis of ventriculoperitoneal and ventriculoatrial shunts for hydrocephalus. J Neurosurg 42:679–682, 1975
519. Ikeme AC: Pregnancy in women after repair of bladder exstrophy. Two case reports. Br J Obstet Gynecol 88(3):327–328, 1981
520. Illingworth RS: The predictive value of developmental assessment in infancy. Dev Med Child Neurol 13:721, 1971
521. In the Matter of the Guardianship of Joseph Hamlin, An Incompetent Person, November 1, 1984. 689 Pacific 2nd 372
522. In the Matter of the Guardianship of Joseph Hamlin, An Incompetent Person, November 1, 1984. 102 Wash 2nd 810
523. Ingraham FD, Hamlin H: Spina bifida and cranium bifidum. II. Surgical treatment. New Engl J Med 228:631–641, 1943
524. Ingraham FD, Matson DD: Neurosurgery of Infancy and Childhood (ed 2). Springfield, IL, Charles C Thomas, 1969
525. Ingraham FD, Swan H: Spina bifida and cranium bifidum. I. A survey of five hundred and forty-six cases. New Engl J Med 228(18):559–563, 1943

526. Ingram TTS, Naughton JA: Pediatric and psychological aspects of cerebral palsy associated with hydrocephalus. Dev Med Child Neurol 4:287–291, 1961
527. International Clearinghouse for Birth Defects Monitoring Systems: 1980 Report. Stockholm, Swedish National Board of Health and Welfare, 1982
528. Irving Independent School District *v*. Tatro, 104 SC 3371 (1984)
529. Isaacson J, Delgado HE: Sex counseling for those with spinal cord injuries. Soc Casework 55:622–627, 1974
530. Ivemark BI: Implications of agenesis of the spleen on the pathogenesis of conotruncus anomalies in childhood. Acta Paediatr Scand 44(Suppl): 1–100, 1958
531. Ives E, Coffey R, Carter CO: A family study of bladder exstrophy. J Med Genet 17:139–141, 1980
532. Jackson JBS: Peculiar form of spina bifida with imperforation of the duodenum and rectum. Boston Med Surg J 59:355, 1858
533. Jackson PH, Lorber J: Brain and ventricular volume in hydrocephalus. Z Kinderchir 39(suppl II):91–93, 1984
534. Jacobs LJ: Hidden dangers, hidden costs. Amicus 4(2):86–88, 1979
535. Jacobsen CB, Berlin CM: Possible reproductive detriment in LSD users. JAMA 222(11):1367–1373, 1972
536. James CM, Lassman LP: Spinal Dysraphism: Spina Bifida Occulta. London, Butterworth, 1972
537. James HE: Intrinsically dervied deformational defects secondary to dysraphism. Semin Perinatol 7:253–256, 1983
538. James HE: Radical removal of conus and cauda equina lipomas: It can be done safely. Section of Pediatric Neurological Surgery of the American Association of Neurological Surgeons, 12th Annual Meeting, Toronto, Canada, November 1983
539. James HE, Walsh JW, Wilson HD, et al: Prospective randomized study of therapy of CSF shunt infection. Neurosurgery 7:459–463, 1980
540. James HE, Williams J, Brock W, et al: Radical removal of lipomas of the conus and cauda equina with laser microneurosurgery. Neurosurgery 15(3):340–343, 1984
541. James HE, Wilson HD, Connor JD, et al: Intraventricular cerebrospinal fluid antibiotic concentrations in patients with intraventricular infections. Neurosurgery 10:50–54, 1982
542. James N, Laurence KM, Miller M: Diet as a factor in aetiology of neural tube defects. Z Kinderchir 31(4):302–307, 1980
543. James WH: Clomiphene, anencephaly and spina bifida (letter). Lancet 1:603, 1977
544. James WH: Hyperthermia and meningomyelocele and anencephaly (letter). Lancet 1:770, 1978
545. Janerich DT, Piper J: Shifting genetic patterns in anencephaly and spina bifida. J Med Genet 15:101–105, 1978
546. Jastak JF, Jastak SR: The Wide Range Achievement Test. Wilmington, DE, Guidance Associates, 1965

547. Jebsen RH, Taylor N, Trieschmann RB, et al: An objective and standardized test of hand function. Arch Phys Med Rehabil 50:311–319, 1969
548. Jefcoate RV: Electronic technology for disabled people. Rehabilitation 38:110–115, 1977
549. Jeffs RD: Complications of exstrophy surgery. Urol Clin North Am 10(3):509–518, 1983
550. Jeffs RD: Exstrophy and cloacal exstrophy. Urol Clin North Am 5(1):127–140, 1978
551. Jennings MT, Clarren SK, Kokich VG, et al: Neuroanatomic examination of spina bifida aperta and the Arnold-Chiari malformation in a 130-day human fetus. J Neurol Sci 54:325–338, 1982
552. Johnson BE, Westgate HO: Methods of predicting vital capacity in patients with thoracic scoliosis. J Bone Joint Surg [Am] 52:1433, 1970
553. Johnson DG, Herbst JJ, Oliveros MA, et al: Evaluation of gastroesophageal reflux surgery in children. Pediatrics 59:62–68, 1977
554. Johnson FE, Hamill PVV, Lameshow S: Skinfold thickness of children 6–11 years. United States Center for Health Statistics, Vital and Health Statistics—Series 11, No. 120, DEHEW Publications No. (HSU)73-1602. Washington, D.C., U.S. Government Printing Office, 1972
555. Johnson FE, Hamill PVV, Lamesho S: Skinfold thickness of youths 12–17 years, United States. National Center for Health Statistics, Vital and Health Statistics—Series 11, No. 132, DHEW Publications No. (HRA) 74-1614. Washington, D.C., U.S. Government Printing Office, 1974
556. Johnson MK, Zuck FN, Wingate K: The motor age test: Measurement of motor handicaps with neuromuscular disorders such as cerebral palsy. J Bone Joint Surg [Am] 33:698–705, 1951
557. Johnson PR: Selective nontreatment of spina bifida: A case study in ethical theory and application. Bioethics Quarterly 3(2):91–111, 1981
558. Johnston JH, Kogan SJ: The exstrophic anomalies and their surgical reconstruction. Curr Probl Surg 1:39, 1974
559. Jones KL, Smith DW, Hall BD, et al: A pattern of craniofacial and limb defects secondary to aberrant tissue bands. J Pediatr 84:90–95, 1974
560. Jones R: The Acorn People. Nashville, Abingdon Press, 1976
561. Jones R, Sisk D: Early perceptions of orthopedic disability: A developmental study. Rehabil Lit 34:42–43, 1967
562. Joosten J: Accounting for changes in family life of families with spina bifida children. Z Kinderchir 28(4):412–417, 1979
563. Jordan R, McLauglin J, Nickel R, et al: Laryngeal dysfunction in infants with neural tube defects. Dev Med Child Neurol 26(2):245, 1984
564. Juul KD: Special education in Europe, in Kaufman JM, Hallahan DP (eds): Handbook of Special Education. Englewood Cliffs, NJ, Prentice-Hall, 1981
565. Kagan J, Sontag LW, Baker CT, et al: Personality and IQ change. J Abnorm Soc Psychol 56:261–266, 1958
566. Kahanovitz N, Duncan JW: The role of scoliosis and pelvic obliquity on functional disability in myelomeningocele. Spine 6:494–497, 1981

567. Kahn H, Panariello V, Saeli J, et al: Effect of cranberry juice on urine. J of Am Diet Asso 51:251–254, 1967
568. Kalnins IV, Churchill MP, Terry GE: Concurrent stresses in families with a leukemic child. J Pediatr Psychol 5:81–92, 1980
569. Kane J: Mental and personality correlates of motor ability, in Wall WD, Varma VP (eds): Advances in Educational Psychology, I. New York, Barnes and Noble, 1972
570. Kapit W, Elson LM: The Anatomy Coloring Book. New York, Harper & Row, 1977
571. Kaplan L, Powell BR, Grynbaum BB, et al: Comprehensive follow-up study of cord dysfunction and its result in disabilities. National Advisory Council on Vocational Rehabilitation, Vocational Rehabilitation Administration, Department of Health, Education and Welfare, RD 548, 1966
572. Kapp-Simon K: Psychological adaptation of patients with craniofacial malformations, in Lucker GW, Ribbens KA, McNamara JA (eds): Psychological Aspects of Facial Form. Ann Arbor, MI, Center for Human Growth and Development, 1980, pp 143–160
573. Kaufman AS: Intelligent Testing with the WISC-R. New York, Wiley, 1979
574. Kaufman J: How We Are Born, How We Grow, How Our Bodies Work and How We Learn. New York, Golden Press, 1975
575. Kaufman JJ: Ammoniagenic coma following ureterosigmoidostomy. J Urol 131(4):743–745, 1984
576. Kazarian G, Goldstein P: Ankyloblepharon filiforme adnatum with hydrocephalus, meningomyelocele and imperforate anus. Am J Ophthalmol 84:355–357, 1977
577. Kegan R: The Evolving Self. Cambridge, MA, Harvard University Press, 1982
578. Kellerman J, Zeltzer L, Ellenberg L, et al: Psychologic effects of illness in adolescents. I. Anxiety, self esteem, and perception of control. J Pediatr 97:126–131, 1980
579. Kendall IIO, Kendall FP, Wadworth GE: Muscles, Testing and Function (ed 3). Baltimore, Williams & Wilkens, 1971
580. Kephart N: The Slow Learner in the Classroom. Columbus, OH, Charles E Merrill, 1960
581. Keucher TR, Mealey J: Long-term results after ventriculoatrial and ventriculoperitoneal shunting for infantile hydrocephalus. J Neurosurg 50:179–186, 1979
582. Khoury MJ, Erickson JD, James LM: Etiologic heterogeneity of neural tube defects, II. Clues from family studies. Am J Hum Genet 34:980–987, 1982
583. The Kids on the Block (pamphlet). Washington, D.C., The Kids on the Block, Fall 1983
584. Kilfoyle RM, Foley JJ: The hip in myelomeningocele. J Bone Joint Surg [Am] 52:827, 1970

585. Kirk S: Early education of the mentally retarded. Urbana, IL, University of Illinois Press, 1958
586. Kleak RE, Richardson SA, Ronald L: Physical appearance cues and interpersonal attraction in children. Child Dev 45:305–310, 1974
587. Klein RM, Fowler RS Jr: Pressure relief training device: The microcalculator. Arch Phys Med Rehabil 62:500–501, 1981
588. Knobloch H, Pasamanick B: Developmental Diagnosis. Hagerstown, NY, Harper & Row, 1974
589. Knobloch WH, Layer JM: Retinal detachment and encephalocele. J Pediatr Ophthalmol 8:181–184, 1971
590. Knox EG: Anencephaly and dietary intake. Br J Prev Soc Med 26:219–223, 1972
591. Knox EG: Fetus–fetus interaction—A model aetiology for anencephalus. Dev Med Child Neurol 12:167–177, 1970
592. Knox EG: Twins and neural tube defects. Br J Soc Med 28:73–80, 1974
593. Kohn M, Rosman BL: A social competence scale and symptom checklist for the preschool child. Dev Psychobiol 6:430–444, 1972
594. Kolodny A: Results of surgery in spina bifida. JAMA 101:1626–1630, 1933
595. Kopits SE: Orthopedic aspects, in Freeman JM (ed), Practical Management of Meningomyelocele. Baltimore, University Park Press, 1974
596. Korsch BM, Gozzi EK, Francis V: Gaps in doctor–patient communication. I. Doctor–patient interaction and patient satisfaction. Pediatrics 42:855–870, 1968
597. Krane RJ, Siroky MB: Clinical Neuro-Urology. Boston, Little, Brown, 1979
598. Krause MV, Mahan LK: Food, Nutrition, and Diet Therapy. Philadelphia, WB Saunders, 1984
599. Kretchmer N: Whither birth defects. Perspect Biol Med 8:15–29, 1964
600. Kropp R, Stuntz T: Full thickness pedicle graft for closure of meningomyelocele sac. Presentation to the American Association of Plastic and Reconstructive Surgeons, San Francisco, 1976
601. Krupp S, Kuhn W, Zaed GA: The use of innervated flaps for the closure of ischial pressure sores. Paraplegia 21:119–126, 1983
602. Kutner L: Due process of euthanasia: The living will, a proposal. Indiana Law J 44:539–554, 1969
603. Kyker J, Gregory JG, Shah J, et al: Comparison of intermittent catheterization and supravesical diversion in children with meningomyelocele. J Urol 118:90, 1977
604. Lamid S, El Ghatit AZ: Smoking, spasticity and pressure sores in spinal cord injured patients. Am J Phys Med 62:300–306, 1983
605. Land LC: Study of the sensory integration of children with myelomeningocele, in McLaurin RL (ed): Myelomeningocele. Orlando, FL, Grune & Stratton, 1977
606. Langlois JH, Downs C: Peer relations as a function of physical attractiveness: The eye of the beholder or behavioral reality? Child Dev 50:409–418, 1979

607. Langlois JH, Stephen C: The effects of physical attractiveness and ethnicity on children's behavioral attributions and peer preferences. Child Dev 48:1694–1698, 1977

608. Lapides J, Diokno C, Silber SJ, et al: Clean, intermittent self-catheterization in the treatment of urinary tract disease. J Urol 107:458, 1972

609. Lappe M: Can eugenic policy be just? in Milunsky A (ed): The Prevention of Genetic Disease and Mental Retardation. Philadelphia, WB Saunders, 1975, pp 456

610. Lasagna L: Life, Death and the Doctor. New York, Knopf, 1968

611. Laurence KM: Effect of early surgery for spina bifida on survival and quality of life. Lancet 1:301–304, 1974

612. Laurence KM: The survival of untreated spina bifida cystica. Dev Med Child Neurol 11(suppl):10–19, 1966

613. Laurence KM, Beresford A: Continence, friends, marriage, and children in 51 adults with spina bifida. Dev Med Child Neurol 17(suppl 35):123–128, 1975

614. Laurence KM, Bligh AS, Evans KT, et al: Vertebral abnormalities in parents and sibs of cases of spina bifida cystica, encephalocele and anencephaly. Proceedings of the International Congress for Padiatrie, Wien, Osterrsich, August 29 to September 4, 1971, pp 415–421

615. Laurence KM, Coates S: Spontaneously arrested hydrocephalus: Results of re-examination of 82 survivors from a series of 182 unoperated cases. Dev Med Child Neurol 13(suppl):4, 1967

616. Laurence KM, Evans RC, Weeks RD, et al: The reliability of prediction of outcome of spina bifida. Dev Med Child Neurol 18(suppl 37):150–156, 1976

617. Laurence KM, James N, Miller MH, et al: Double-blind randomized controlled trial of folate treatment before conception to prevent recurrence of neural tube defects. Br Med J 282:1509–1511, 1981

618. Laurence KM, Tew BJ: The natural history of spina bifida cystica and cranium bifidum cysticum: Major central nervous system malformations in South Wales. Arch Dis Child 46(245):127–138, 1971

619. LaVielle CJ, Campbell DA: Neurofibromatosis and intrathoracic meningocele. Radiology 70:62–66, 1958

620. LaVoie JC, Adams GR: Teacher expectancy and its relation to physical and interpersonal characteristics of the child. Alberta J Educ Res 22:122–132, 1974

621. Laws ER: Neurosurgical Management. Practical Management of Myelomeningocele. Baltimore, University Park Press, 1974

622. Layde PM, Erickson JD, Falek H, et al: Congenital malformations in twins. Am J Hum Genet 32:69–78, 1980

623. Layde PM, Von Allmen SD, Oakley GP: Maternal serum alpha-fetoprotein screening: A cost benefit analysis. Am J Public Health 69:566–572, 1979

624. Lazarus RS, Folkman S: Stress, Appraisal, and Coping. New York, Springer, 1984

625. Leck I: Changes in the incidence of neural tube defects. Lancet 2:791–793, 1966
626. Leck I: The geographical distribution of neural tube defects and oral clefts. Br Med J 40:309–395, 1984
627. Leck I, Iles CA, Sharman IM, et al: Proceedings: A study of the extent to which maternal nutrition after delivery reflects the situation in early pregnancy. Br J Prev Soc Med 28:66, 1974
628. Leck I, Millar ELM: Short-term changes in the incidence of malformations. Br J Prev Soc Med 17:1–5, 1963
629. Leck J: Epidemiological clues to the causation of neural tube defects, in Dobbing J (ed): Prevention of Spina Bifida and Other Neural Tube Defects. London, Academic Press, 1983, pp 155–182
630. Leichty E: Teratological omens. Unpublished Ph.D. dissertation, University of Chicago, 1960
631. Lejeune J: The William Allen memorial award lecture: On the nature of man. Am J Hum Genet 22:121–128, 1970
632. Lemire RJ: Neural tube defects: Clinical correlations. Clin Neurosurg 30:165–177, 1983
633. Lemire RJ, Beckwith JB, Warkany J: Anencephaly. New York, Raven Press, 1978
634. Lemire RJ, Graham CB, Beckwith JB: Skin-covered sacrococcygeal masses in infants and children. J Pediatr 79(6):948–954, 1971
635. Lemire RJ, Loeser JD, Leach RW, et al: Normal and Abnormal Development of the Human Nervous System. Hagerstown, NY, Harper & Row, 1975
636. Lemire RJ, Shephard TH, Alvord ED Jr: Caudal myeloschisis (lumbosacral spina bifida cystica) in a five millimeter (horizon XIV) human embryo. Anat Rec 152:9–16, 1965
637. Leonard CO, Freeman JM: Spina bifida: A new disease. Pediatrics 68:136–137, 1981
638. Lepor H, Shapiro E, Jeffs RD: Urethral reconstruction in boys with classical bladder exstrophy. J Urol 131:512–515, 1984
639. Letters to the Editor: Care of infants with myelomeningocele. Pediatrics 74(1):162–166, 1984
640. Letts RM, Fulford R, Hobson DA: Mobility aids for the paraplegic child. J Bone Joint Surg [Am] 58:38–41, 1976
641. Levin GW: Functional evaluation of eighteen myelomeningocele patients. Clin Orthop 100:101–107, 1974
642. Levin HS, Benton AL, Grossman RG: Neurobehavioral Consequences of Closed Head Injury. New York and Oxford, Oxford University Press, 1982
643. Levinson RM: Family crisis and adaptation: Coping with a mentally retarded child. Dissertation Abstracts International 36:8336A–8337A, 1976 (University Microfilms No. 76-8221)
644. Lewis M, Fox N: Predicting cognitive development from assessments in

infancy, in Camp BW (ed): Advances in Behavioral Pediatrics, vol. 1. Greenwich, CT, JAI Press, 1980, pp 53–67

645. Lewis M, McGurck H: Evaluation of infant intelligence. Science 178:1174, 1972

646. Lichtenstein BW: Distant neuroanatomic complications of spina bifida. Arch Neurol Psychiatry 47:195–214, 1942

647. Light JK, Scott FB: Treatment of the epispadius exstrophy complex with the AS792 artificial urinary sphincter. J Urol 129:738–740, 1983

648. Lightowler CD: Meningomyelocele: The price of treatment. Br Med J 2:385–387, 1971

649. Lilly S: Children With Exceptional Needs. New York, Holt, Rinehart & Winston, 1979

650. Lima SV, Noroes JA, Carvalheira F, et al: Bladder exstrophy primary reconstruction with human dura mater. Monogr Paediatr 12:50–54, 1981

651. Lindseth RE: Posterior iliac osteotomy for fixed pelvic obliquity. J Bone Joint Surg [Am] 60:17–22, 1978

652. Lindseth RE, Glancy J: Polypropylene lower-extermity braces for paraplegia due to myelomeningocele. J Bone Joint Surg [Am] 56:556–563, 1974

653. Lippman-Hand A, Piper M: Prenatal diagnosis for the detection of Down Syndrome: Why are so few eligible women tested? Prenat Diagn 1:249–257, 1981

654. Lister, JB: The Collected Papers of Joseph B. Lister. Oxford, Clarendon Press, 1909

655. Little JR, Rhoton AL Jr, Mellinger JF: Comparison of ventriculoperitoneal and ventriculoatrial shunts for hydrocephalus in children. Mayo Clin Proc 47:396–401, 1972

656. Llenado M, Grogan C: Myelomeningocele, in Palmer S, Etevall S (eds): Pediatric Nutrition in Developmental Disorders. Springfield, IL, Charles C Thomas, 1978, p 55

657. Loeser JD, Sells CJ, Shurtleff DB: The management of patients with cerebrospinal fluid shunts. J Fam Pract 6:285–289, 1978

658. Lohkamp F, Calussen C: Computertomographische diagnostik des Gehirns: Erganzung der transversalen standardschicten durch frontale und clivoparallele schichten. Fortschr Neurol Psychiatry 45(6):372–380, 1977

659. Longfellow HW: The Song of Hiawatha. Mount Vernon, NY, Peter Pauper Press, 1942

660. Lonton AP: Hand preference in children with meningomyelocele and hydrocephalus. Dev Med Child Neurol 18(suppl 37):143–149, 1976

661. Lonton AP: The relationship between intellectual skills and the computerised axial tomograms of children with spina bifida and hydrocephalus. Z Kinderchir 28(4):368–374, 1979

662. Lonton AP, Barrington MA, Lorber J: Lacunar skull deformity related to intelligence in children with myelomeningocele and hydrocpehalus. Dev Med Child Neurol 17(suppl 35):58–64, 1975

663. Lonton AP, Loughlin AM, O'Sullivan AM: The employment of adults with spina bifida. Z Kinderchir 39(suppl II):132–134, 1984
664. Lonton AP, O'Sullivan AM, Loughlin AM: Spina bifida adults. Z Kinderchir 38(suppl II):110–112, 1983
665. Lorber J: Ethical problems in the management of myelomeningocele and hydrocephalus, in Abrams N, Buckner MD (eds): Medical Ethics: A Clinical Textbook and Reference for the Health Care Professions. Cambridge, MA, MIT Press, 1983, pp 373–378
666. Lorber J: Results of treatment of myelomeningocele: An analysis of 524 unselected cases with special reference to possible selection for treatment. Dev Med Child Neurol 13:279–303, 1971
667. Lorber J: The family history of spina bifida cystica. Pediatrics 35(41):589–595, 1965
668. Lorber J: Selective treatment of myelomeningocele: To treat or not to treat? Pediatrics 53:307–308, 1974
669. Lorber J: Spina bifida cystica: Results of treatment of 270 consecutive cases with criteria for selection for the future. Arch Dis Child 47:854–873, 1972
670. Lorber J, Pucholt V: When is a shunt no longer necessary? An investigation of 300 patients with hydrocephalus and myelomeningocele: 11–22 year follow-up. Z Kinderchir 34:327–329, 1984
671. Lorber J, Salfield SA: Results of selective treatment of spina bifida cystica. Arch Dis Child 56(11):822–830, 1981
672. Lorber J, Salfield S, Lorton T: Isosorbide in the management of infantile hydrocephalus. Dev Med Child Neurol 25:502–511, 1983
673. Lorber J, Schloss AL: The adolescent with myelomeningocele. Dev Med Child Neurol 15(suppl 29):113–114, 1973
674. Lotimer LE: Pregnancy and delivery following bilateral uterosigmoid transplant for exstrophy of the bladder. Am J Obstet Gynecol 67:281–285, 1954
675. Lucker GW: Esthetics and a quantitative analysis of facial appearance, in Lucker GW, Ribbens KA, McNamara JA (eds): Psychological Aspects of Facial Form. Ann Arbor, MI, Center for Human Growth and Development, 1980, pp 49–79
676. Lucker GW, Ribbens KA, McNamara JA (eds): Psychological Aspects of Facial Form. Ann Arbor, MI, Center for Human Growth and Development, 1980
677. Ludlow J, Allen L: The effects of early intervention and preschool stimulus on the development of the Down's Syndrome child. J Ment Defic Res 23:29–44, 1979
678. Lundstrom R: Rubella during pregnancy. A follow-up study of children born after an epidemic of rubella in Sweden, 1951, with additional investigations on prophylaxis and treatment of maternal rubella. Acta Pediatr 51(suppl 133):1–110, 1962
679. Luthart T: Bacterial infections in ventriculo-auricular shunt systems. Dev Med Child Neurol 12(suppl 23):105–109, 1970

680. Lynch JJ: The Broken Heart: The Medical Consequences of Loneliness. New York, Basic Books, 1977
681. Lynn AM, Stuntz JT, Ward BH: Pneumocephalus: An unusual presentation of a persistent neurenteric fistula. J Pediatr 93(5):818–820, 1978
682. Lyons AS, Petrucelli RJ: Medicine: An Illustrated History. New York, Harry W. Abrams, 1978
683. Macias R, Tena L: Myelomeningocele: New technique for skin repair. Childs Brain 10(2):73–78, 1983
684. Mackel JC, Lindseth RE: Scoliosis in myelodysplasia. J Bone Joint Surg [Am] 57:1031, 1975
685. "Madison Avenue and the Handicapped." National Public Radio, 7:50 AM, June 27, 1985
686. Maguire D: Deciding for yourself: The objective, in Weir RF (ed): Ethical Issues in Death and Dying. New York, Columbia University Press, 1972, pp 320–347
687. Malis LI: Prevention of neurosurgical infection by intraoperative antibiotics. Neurosurgery 5:339–343, 1979
688. Maloley A, Weber S, Smith DR: Patterns of strabismus in meningomyelocele. Am Orthop J 27:115–118, 1977
689. Maloney MP, Ward MP: Mental Retardation and Modern Society. New York, Oxford University Press, 1979
690. Malthus TR: An Essay on Population, vol. 1. London, J.M. Dent, 1958
691. Manenica K: Identification of factors related to obesity in children with myelomeningocele. Masters Thesis, University of Washington, 1982
692. Mansson HH: Justifying the final solution, in Weir RF (ed): Ethical Issues in Death and Dying. New York, Columbia University Press, 1977, pp 308–319
693. Marion JP, Kassman G, Farnhoff PM, et al: Acceptance of amniocentesis by low-income patients in an urban hospital. Am J Obstet Gynecol 138:11–15, 1980
694. Marsh N, Gould AP, Clutton HH, et al: Report of a committee of the society nominated November 10, 1882 to investigate spina bifida and its treatment by the injection of Dr. Morton's iodoglycerine solution. Clin Soc Trans 18:339, 1885
695. Marshall R, Newnham RE, Rawstron JR, et al: Features of 13–15 trisomy syndrome with normal karotype (letter). Lancet 1:556, 1964
696. Marshall VF, Muecke EL: Variations in exstrophy of the bladder. J Urol 88:766–796, 1962
697. Martin PM: Marital breakdown in families of patients with spina bifida cystica. Dev Med Child Neurol 17:757–763, 1975
698. Masters JC, Cerreto MC, Mendlowitz DR: The role of the family in coping with childhood chronic illness, in Barish TG, Bradley LA (eds): Coping with Chronic Disease. Orlando, FL, Academic Press, 1983
699. Mather G, Humphries L: Anthropometric changes in spinal cord injury. Annual Meeting of the American Spinal Cord Injury Association, Houston, TX, 1984

700. Matson DD: Surgical treatment of myelomeningocele. Editorial in Pediatrics 42:225–227, 1968
701. Mawdsley T, Rickham PP: Improvement in the postoperative mortality following operation for open myelomeningocele. Dev Med Child Neurol 13(suppl 25):68–70, 1971
702. Maynard FM, Dioknow AL: Clean intermittent catheterization for spinal cord injury patient. J Urol 128:447–480, 1982
703. Mazur J: Personal communication, 1985
704. Mazur JM, Stillwell A, Menelaus M: Significance of spasticity in the upper and lower limbs in myelomeningocele. Presented at the American Academy of Cerebral Palsy and Developmental Medicine meetings, Seattle, Washington, September 2–5, 1985
705. McAndrew I: Adolescents and young people with spina bifida. Dev Med Child Neurol 21:619–629, 1979
706. McAndrew I: Children with a handicap and their families. Child Care Health Dev 2:213–237, 1976
707. McBride ML: Sib risks of anencephaly in spina bifida in British Columbia. Am J Med Genet 3(4):377–387, 1979
708. McCarthy MF Jr, Wenzel RP: Postoperative spinal fluid infections after neurosurgical shunting procedures. Pediatrics 59:793, 1977
709. McCollough NC, Clark MW, MacEwen GD, et al: Conference Report: Critical Needs of the Child with Long Term Impairment. Chicago, American Academy of Orthopaedic Surgeons, 1985
710. McCollum AT: The Chronically Ill Child: A Guide for Parents and Professionals. New Haven, CT, Yale University Press, 1975
711. McCormick RA: To save or let die. JAMA 229:172–176, 1974
712. McCormick RA: To save or let die: The dilemma of modern medicine, in Weir RF (ed): Ethical Issues in Death and Dying. New York, Columbia University Press, 1977, pp 173–184
713. McCormick WF: Is anencephaly a single entity? A brief note on the morphologic heterogeneity of anencephaly. Birth Defects 3(1):94–96, 1971
714. McCracken GH Jr, Mize SG, Threlkeld N: Intraventricular gentamicin therapy in gram-negative bacillary meningitis of infancy. Report of the Second Neonatal Meningitis Cooperative Study Group. Lancet 1(8172): 787–791, 1980
715. McCullough DC: Personal communication, 1983
716. McCullough DC, Balzier-Martin LA: Current prognosis in overt neonatal hydrocephalus. J Neurosurg 57:378–383, 1982
717. McCullough DC, Kane JG, Presper JH, et al: Antibiotic prophylaxis in ventricular shunt surgery: I. Reduction of operative infection rates with methicillin. Childs Brain 7:182–189, 1980
718. McCullough DC, Kufta C, Axelbaum SP, et al: Computerized axial tomography in clinical pediatrics. Pediatrics 59:173–181, 1977
719. McCullough P: Launching children and moving on, in Carter EA, McGoldrick M (eds): The Family Life Cycle: A Framework for Family Therapy. New York, Gardner Press, 1980

720. McDonald CM, Jaffe KM, Shurtleff DB: Clinical assessment of muscle strength in children with meningomyelocele: Accuracy and stability of measurements over time. Arch Phys Med Rehabil (in press)
721. McGuire EJ: Clinical Evaluation and Treatment of Neurogenic Vesical Dysfunction. Baltimore, Williams & Wilkins, 1984
722. McKay D: Personal communication, 1985
723. McKay DA: McKay hip stabilization in meningomyelocele. Orthop Trans 1:87–88, 1977
724. McKay DA: The McKay plate for kyphosis of the spine. Presented at the Scoliosis Research Society, Louisville, KY, September 1975
725. McKibbon B, Porter RW: The incidence of vitamin C deficiency in meningomyelocele. Dev Med Child Neurol 9:338, 1967
726. McLaughlin JF: Unpublished data, 1985
727. McLaughlin JF, Marks WM, Jones G: Prospective management of exstrophy of the cloaca and myelocystocele following prenatal ultrasound recognition of neural tube defects in identical twins. Am J Med Genet 19(4):721–727, 1984
728. McLaughlin JF, Shurtleff DB: Management of the newborn with myelodysplasia. Clin Pediatr (Phila) 18(8):463–476, 1979
729. McLaughlin JF, Shurtleff DB, Lamers JY, et al: Influence of prognosis on decisions regarding the care of newborns with myelodysplasia. N Engl J Med 312(25):1589–1634, 1985
730. McLaughlin JF, Shurtleff DB, Lemire RJ, et al: A process for care selection in myelodysplasia. Z Kinderchir 37:161–164, 1982
731. McLaurin RL: Infected cerebrospinal fluid shunts. Surg Neurol 1:191–195, 1973
732. McLaurin RL: Myelomeningocele. Orlando, FL, Grune & Stratton, 1977
733. McLaurin RL: Myelomeningocele repair. Contemp Neurosurg 6(17):1–6, 1984
734. McLaurin RL: Treatment of infected ventricular shunts, in O' Brien MS (ed): Pediatric Neurological Surgery. New York, Raven Press, 1978, pp 125–133
735. McLaurin RL, Dodson D: Infected ventriculo-atrial shunt: Some principles of treatment. Dev Med Child Neurol 13(suppl 25):71, 1971
736. McLone DG: An Introduction to Hydrocephalus. Pittsburgh, Children's Memorial Hospital, 1982
737. McLone DG: Long-term follow-up of patients with myelomeningocele. Proceedings of the Congress of Neurological Surgeons, 32nd Annual Meeting, Toronto, Canada, October 3–8, 1982
738. McLone DG: Results of treatment of children born with myelomeningocele. Clin Neurosurg 30:407–412, 1983
739. McLone DG: Technique for closure of myelomeningocele. Childs Brain 6(2):65–73, 1980
740. McLone DG, Czyzewski D, Raimondi AJ, et al: Central nervous system infections as a limiting factor in the intelligence of children with myelomeningocele. Pediatrics 70:338–342, 1982

741. McLone DG, Dias L, Kaplan WE, et al: Concepts in the management of spina bifida. Concepts Pediatr Neurosurg 5:97–106, 1985

742. McLone DG, Mutlner S, Naidich TP: Lipomeningoceles of the conus medullaris, in American Society for Pediatric Neurosurgery (ed): Concepts in Pediatric Neurosurgery 3. Basil, S. Karger, 1983, pp 170–171

743. McNair P: Curator of Ethnology. British Columbia Provincial Museum, Victoria, B.C., Canada, personal communication, July 8, 1985

744. Mealey J, Gilmore RL, Bubb MP: The prognosis of hydrocephalus overt at birth. J Neurosurg 39:348–355, 1973

745. Meckel JF: Beschreibung zweier durch sehr ahnliche Bildungsabweichung entstellter Geschwister. Deutsch Arch Physiol 7:99–172, 1822

746. Meleis AI, Jonsen AR: Ethical crises and cultural differences. West J Med 138(6):889–895, 1983

747. Menashi M, Ornoy A, Cohen MM: Anencephaly in trisomy 18: Related or unrelated? Teratology 15:325–328, 1977

748. Menelaus MB: Orthopedic Management of Spina Bifida Cystica (ed 2). New York, Churchill Livingstone, 1980, pp 57–60

749. Menelaus MB: Orthopedic management of children with myelomeningocele: A plea for realistic goals. Dev Med Child Neurol 18(suppl 37):3–11, 1976

750. Meyer BC: Truth and the physician, in Weir RF (ed): Ethical Issues in Death and Dying. New York, Columbia University Press, 1977, p 42

751. Michejda M: The fetal neural tube: Is intervention progress? Casey Holter Memorial Lecture. Z Kinderchir 39(suppl II):85, 1985

752. Mickle JP, McLennen JE: Malignant teratoma arising within a lipomeningocele. Case report. J Neurosurg 43(6):761–763, 1975

753. Middleton AW Jr, Hendren WH: Ileal conduits in children at the Massachusetts General Hospital from 1955 to 1970. J Urol 115:591, 1976

754. Miezio PM: Parenting Children with Disabilities: A Professional Source for Physicians and Guide for Parents. New York, Marcel Dekker, 1983

755. Milgram S: Behavioral study of obedience. J Abnorm Soc Psychol 67:371–378, 1963

756. Miller E, Sethi L: The effect of hydrocephalus on perception. Dev Med Child Neurol 13(suppl 25):77–81, 1971

757. Miller J: The Human Body. New York, Viking Press, 1983

758. Miller JQ, Selden RF: Arhinencephaly, encephalocele and 13–15 trisomy syndrome with normal chromosomes. Neurology 17:1087–1091, 1967

759. Miller P, Smith DW, Shepard TH: Maternal hyperthermia as a possible cause of anencephaly. Lancet 1:519–521, 1978

760. Milunsky A (ed): The Prevention of Genetic Disease and Mental Retardation. Philadelphia, WB Saunders, 1975

761. Milunsky A: Alpha-fetaprotein and the prenatal detection of neural tube defects. Am J Public Health 69:552–553, 1979

762. Milunsky A, Atkins L: Prenatal diagnosis of genetic disease, in Milunsky A (ed): The Prevention of Genetic Disease and Mental Retardation. Philadelphia, WB Saunders, 1975, p 221

763. Milunsky A, Graef JW, Gaynor MF, et al: Methotrexate-induced congenital malformations. Pediatrics 72:790–795, 1968
764. Minuchin S: Families and Family Therapy. Cambridge, MA, Harvard University Press, 1974
765. Mitchell CO, Lipschitz DA: Arm length measurement as an alternative to height in nutritional assessment of the elderly. Journal of Parenteral and Enteral Nutrition 6(3):226–229, 1982
766. Mitchell ME: Urinary tract diversion and undiversion in the pediatric age group. Surg Clin North Am 61(5):1147–1164, 1981
767. Mitchell ME: Undiversion. AMA Update Series 3(6):1984
768. Moe JH, Winter RB, Bradford DS, et al: Scoliosis and Other Spinal Deformities. Philadelphia, WB Saunders, 1978, pp 239–287
769. Mollard P: Bladder reconstruction in exstrophy. J Urol 124:525, 1980
770. Monson D, Shurtleff C: Altering attitudes toward the physically handicapped through print and nonprint media. Lang Arts 56(2):163–170, 1979
771. Montagnani CA: One stage functional reconstruction of exstrophied bladder: Report of two cases with six-year follow-up. Z Kinderchir 30(1):23–27, 1982
772. Moore JE: Spina bifida, with a report of three hundred and eighty-five cases treated by excision. Surg Gynecol Obstet 1(2):137–140, 1905
773. Moore LG, Van Arsdale PW, Glittenberg JE, et al: The Biocultural Basis of Health: Expanding Views of Medical Anthropology. St. Louis, CV Mosby, 1980
774. Moos R: Family Environment Scale, Palo Alto, CA, Consulting Psychologists Press, 1974
775. Mordock JB: The separation-individuation process and developmental disabilities. Except Child 40:176–184, 1979
776. Morgagni GB: The Seats and Causes of Disease Investigated by Anatomy. London, R Miller and J Cadell, 1769
777. Morison JE: Congenital malformations in one of monozygotic twins. Arch Dis Child 24:214, 1949
778. Morton M: Spina bifida operta, treatment by injection. Br Med J 1:381, 1875
779. Motloch W: Orthotic philosophies of treatment. Clin Prosthet Orthot 8:9–11, 1984
780. Motloch W: Parapodium: Orthotic device for neuromuscular disorders. Artif Limb 15:36–47, 1971
781. Motulsky AG: Brave new world: Ethical issues in prevention, treatment and research of human defects, in Motulsky A, Powledge TM (eds): Birth Defects. Amsterdam, Excerpta Medica, 1974, p 311
782. Munro IR: The psychological effects of surgical treatment of facial deformity, in Lucker GW, Ribbens KA, McNamara JA (eds): Psychological Aspects of Facial Form. Ann Arbor, MI, Center for Human Growth and Development, 1980, pp 171–199
783. Murdock A: How much value in muscle charting? A study of the relation

between neonatal assessment of muscle power and later mobility in children with spina bifida defects. Physiotherapy 66:221–223, 1980

784. Murphree AH: A functional analysis of southern folk beliefs concerning birth. Am J Obstet Gynecol 102:125–134, 1968
785. Mustarde JC: Reconstruction of the spinal canal in severe spina bifida. Plast Reconstr Surg 42:109–114, 1968
786. Myers GJ, Cerone SB, Olson AL: A Guide for Helping the Child with Spina Bifida. Springfield, IL, Charles C Thomas, 1981
787. Myers MG, Shoenbaum SC: Shunt fluid aspiration. An adjunct in the diagnosis of CSF shunt infection. Am J Dis Child 129:220–222, 1975
788. Myrick RD, Bowman R: Becoming a Friendly Helper: Handbook for Student Facilitator. Minneapolis, Educational Media Corporation, 1981
789. Myrick RD, Bowman RP: Children Helping Children: Teaching Students to Become Friendly Helpers. Minneapolis, Educational Media Corporation, 1981
790. Myrick RD, Bowman R: Children Helping Children—Becoming a Friendly Helper. Minneapolis, Educational Media Corporation, 1982 (film)
791. Naggon L, MacMahon: Ethnic differences in the prevalence of anencephaly and spina bifida in Boston, Massachusetts. N Engl J Med 227:1119–1123, 1967
792. Naglo AS, Hellstrom B: Results of treatment of myelomeningocele. Acta Pediatr Scand 65:565–569, 1976
793. Naidich TP, McLone DG, Mutlner S: A new understanding of dorsal disraphism with lipoma (lipomyeloschisis): Radiologic evaluation and surgical correction. AJR 140(6):1065–1078, 1983
794. Naito H, Toya S, Shizawa H, et al: High incidence of acute postoperative meningitis and septicemia in patients undergoing craniotomy with ventriculoatrial shunt. Surg Gynecol Obstet 137:810–812, 1973

794a. Nance WC: Anencephaly and Spina Bifida: An Etiologic Hypothesis in Birth Defects Original Article Series: The Second Conference on the Clinical Delineation of Birth Defects: Part VI, D. Bergoina (ed), The Williams and Wilkens Co (Publisher) Baltimore, MD, 1971

795. Nash DFE: Congenital spinal palsey. Br Med J 5005:1333–1337, 1956
796. Nash DFE: Spina bifida and allied disorders. Hosp Med 4:439–448, 1968
797. Nash DF: Ellison. Br Med J 5005:1333–1337, 1956
798. Nathanson RB, Lambert J: Integrating disabled employees into the work place. Personnel J 60(2):109–113, 1981
799. Neel JV: Notes on the effects of measles and measles vaccine in a virgin-soil population of South American Indians. Am J Epidemiol 91:418–429, 1970
800. Nellhaus S: Head circumference from birth to eighteen years. Composite international and interracial graphs. Pediatrics 41:106–114, 1968
801. Nelson GD, Kendall TE, Shaw RC, et al: Meningomyelocele repair. Use of bipedicle flaps. J Kans Med Soc 78(9):382–384, 1977
802. Nevin NC, Harley JMG: Clomiphene and neural tube defects. Ulster Med J 45:59–64, 1976

803. Nevin RS, McCubbin HI, Birkebak RC: Stress and Coping with Spina Bifida: A Family Perspective. Oakbrook, Eterna Press, 1984
804. Newacheck PW, Bendetti PP, McManus P: Trends in childhood disability. Am J Public Health 74(3):232–236, 1984
805. Newman J: Handicapped persons and their families: Philosophical, historical and legislative perspectives, in Seligman M (ed): The Family with a Handicapped Child: Understanding and Treatment. Orlando, FL, Grune & Stratton, 1983, pp 3–25
806. News Release: Crippled daughter sues parents for abandoning her. Seattle Times, February 11, 1979, p A2
807. Nichols MM: Fetal anomalies following maternal trimethadione ingestion (letter). J Pediatr 82(5):885–886, 1973
808. Nielsen HH: A longitudinal study of the psychological aspects of myelomeningocele. Scand J Psychol 21:45–54, 1980
809. Nielson K, Nielson KK: Adenocarcinoma in exstrophy of the bladder—The last case in Scandinavia? A case report and review of the literature. J Urol 130(6):1180–1182, 1983
810. Nihira K, Meyers CE, Mink IT: Home environment, family adjustment, and the development of mentally retarded children. Appl Res Ment Retard 1:5–24, 1980
811. Nio NH, Hull CH, Jenkins JG, et al: SPSS: Statistical Package for the Social Sciences (ed 2). New York, McGraw-Hill, 1982
812. Nishimura H, Takano K, Tanimura T, et al: High incidence of several malformations in the early human embryos as compared with infants. Biol Neonate 10:93–107, 1966
813. Nishimura H, Takano K, Tanimura T, et al: Normal and abnormal development of human embryos: First report of the analysis of 1,213 intact embryos. Teratology 1:281–290, 1968
814. Norwood C: Terata: Only 88 out of 100 American babies are born without defects. If the birth defect crisis continues, "Terata" will become a household word. Mother Jones, January 15–21, 1985
815. Nosik WA: Repair of lumbar and cranial meningocele with tantalum gauze. J Neurosurg 8:498–503, 1951
816. Nulsen FE, Spitz EB: Treatment of hydrocephalus by direct shunt from ventricle to jugular vein. Surg Forum 2:399–403, 1952
817. Oakland JA, Sherman WE: An examination of Erickson's theory from the perspective of a study of congenitally paraplegic children in Proceedings of 46th Annual Meeting of American Orthopsychiatric Association, New York, April 8, 1969
818. O'Brien M, Parent A, Davis B: Management of ventricular shunt infections. Childs Brain 5(3):304–309, 1979
819. O'Brien WS, McLanahan CS: Review of the neurosurgical management of myelomeningocele at a regional pediatric medical center. Proceedings of Concepts of Pediatric Neurosurgery I, American Society for Pediatric Neurosurgery. Basil, S. Karger, 1981

820. O'Connell F, Gardner WJ: Metabolism in paraplegia. JAMA 153:706–711, 1953
821. Oesch I, Jeffs R: Staged functional closure of bladder exstrophy (author's translation). Z Kinderchir 33(1):74–83, 1981
822. Offer D: The Psychological World of the Teenager. New York, Basic Books, 1969
823. Okamoto GA, Lamers JV, Shurtleff DB: Skin breakdown in patients with myelomeningocele. Arch Phys Med Rehabil 64:20–23, 1983
824. Okamoto GA, Shurtleff DB: Perceived first contact care for disabled children. Pediatrics 67:530–535, 1981
825. Okamoto GA, Sousa J, Telzrow RW, et al: Toileting skills in children with meningomyelocele: Rates of learning. Arch Phys Med Rehabil 65:182–185, 1984
826. Olness K, McPharland FA, Piper J: Biofeedback: A new modality in the management of children with fecal soiling. J Pediatr 96(3):505–509, 1980
827. Olshansky S: Chronic sorrow: A response to having a mentally defective child. Soc Casework 43:190–193, 1962
828. O'Neill JA, Grosfeld JL, Bolest ET, et al: Surgical treatment of meconium ileus. Am J Surg 119:99–105, 1970
829. Opitz JM, Gilbert EF: Editorial comment: CNS anomalies and the midline as a "developmental field." Am J Med Genet 12:443–455, 1982
830. Opitz JM, Howe JJ: The Meckel syndrome (dysencephalia splanchocystica, the Gruber syndrome). Birth Defects 5:167–179, 1969
831. Orenstein A: Organizational issues in implementing special education legislation. Paper presented at the Annual Meeting of the Society for the Study of Social Problems, Boston, 1979, p 22
832. Osebold WR, Mayfield JK, Winter RB, et al: Surgical treatment of paralytic scoliosis associated with myelomeningocele. J Bone Joint Surg [Am] 64(6):841–856, 1982
833. Padget DH: Spina bifida and embryonic neuroschisis: A causal relationship. Johns Hopkins Med J 123:233–252, 1968
834. Pagon RA, Chandler JW, Collie WR et al: Hydrocephalus, agyria, retinal dysplasia, encephalocele (Hard ± E) syndrome: An autosomal recessive condition. Birth Defects 14(6B):233–241, 1978
835. Pallister P: Personal communication, 1985
836. Pallister P, Opitz J: Personal communication, 1985
837. Pang D, Casey K: Use of an anal sphincter pressure monitor during operations on the sacral spinal cord and nerve roots. Neurosurgery 13(5):562–568, 1983
838. Park TS, Hoffman HJ, Hendrick EB, et al: Experience with surgical decompression of the Arnold-Chiari malformation in young infants with myelomeningocele. Neurosurgery 13:147–152, 1983
839. Parkash S, Bhander M: Rectus abdominis myocutaneous island flap for bridging defect after cystectomy for bladder exstrophy. Urology 20(5):536–537, 1982

840. Parkes CM, Stevenson-Hinde J: The Place of Attachment in Human Behavior. New York, Basic Books, 1982
841. Parsons JG: Assessments of aptitudes in young people of school-leaving age handicapped by hydrocephalus or spina bifida cystica. Dev Med Child Neurol 14(suppl 27):101–107, 1972
842. Parsons JG: Short-term verbal memory in hydrocephalic children. Dev Med Child Neurol 20(suppl):75–77, 1969
843. Parsons T: The Social System. New York, Free Press, 1951
844. Passarge E, True CW, Sneoka WT, et al: Malformations of the central nervous system in trisomy 18 syndrome. J Pediatr 69:771–778, 1966
845. Patten BM: Embryological stages in the establishing of myeloschisis with spina bifida. Am J Anat 93:365–396, 1953
846. Patten BM, Barry A: The genesis of exstrophy of the bladder and epispadius. Am J Anat 90:35–57, 1952
847. Patterson JM, McCubbin HI: Chronic illness: Family stress and coping, in Figley CR, McCubbin HI (eds): Stress and the Family, vol. II. New York, Brunner/Mazel, 1983, pp 21–36
848. Patterson TJ, Till K: The use of rotational flaps following excision of lumbar myelomeningoceles: An aid to closure of large defects. Br J Surg 46:605–608, 1959
849. Patzold U, Pfingst E, Trostdorf E: Der "normal pressure hydrocephalus." Fortschr Neurol Psychiatry 42:281–290, 1974
850. Paulozzi LJ: Personal communication, 1984
851. Peach B: The Arnold-Chiari malformation: Morphogenesis. Arch Neurol 12:527–535, 1965
852. Pearson PH: The results of treatment: The hours of our dilemma. Dev Med Child Neurol 24:417–418, 1982
853. Pediatric Manpower Committee: Projecting pediatric practice patterns. Pediatrics 62:646, 1978
854. Morse T: The agonizing decision of Joanne and Roger Pell. Good Housekeeping 174:76–77, 1972
855. Pemberton M, Gastineau CF: Mayo Clinic Diet Manual: A Handbook of Dietary Practices. Philadelphia, WB Saunders, 1981
856. Penfield W, Cone W: Spina bifida and cranium bifidum. JAMA 98:454–460, 1932
857. Pennsylvania Association for Retarded Children, Nancy Beth Bowman et al. *v*. Commonwealth of Pennsylvania, NIA, David H. Kurtzman et al. 334 F. Supp. 1257, 1971
858. Pennsylvania Association for Retarded Children et al., Plaintiffs *v*. Commonwealth of Pennsylvania, NIA et al., Defendants, 343 F. Supp. 279, 1972
859. People You'd Like to Meet: A K-6 Birth Defects Curriculum Project. Seattle, Washington, Comprehensive Health Education Foundation, 1981
860. Perkash I: Management of neurogenic dysfunction of the bladder and bowel, in Kottke FJ, Stillwell GK, Lehman JF (eds): Krusen's Handbook

of Physical Medicine and Rehabilitation (ed 3). Philadelphia, WB Saunders, 1982, pp 724–745

861. Perrin JC, McLaurin RL: Infected ventriculoatrial shunts. A method of treatment. J Neurosurg 27:21–26, 1967
862. Perry J, Antonelli D, Ford W: Analysis of knee-joint forces during flexed knee stance. J Bone Joint Surg [Am] 57:961–967, 1975
863. Peter Mills et al. *v*. Board of Education of the District of Columbia et al. 348 F. Suppl 866 (1972)
864. Peters CR, Dinner MI, Wacksman J: Escutcheon and external genitalia reconstruction following childhood correction of urinary bladder exstrophy. Ann Plast Surg 6(2):117–120, 1981
865. Phillips SF: Megacolon: Congenital and acquired, in Sleisenger MH, Fordtran JS (eds): Gastrointestinal Disease Pathophysiology Diagnosis Management (ed 3), vol. 1. Philadelphia, WB Saunders, 1983, p 912
866. Piaget J: The Child's Conception of the World. New York, Harcourt Brace, 1929
867. Piaget J: The Principles of Genetic Epistomology. New York, Basic Books, 1972
868. Pickering LK, Ericsson LD, Ruiz-Palacios, et al: Intraventricular and parental gentamicin therapy for ventriculitis in children. Am J Dis Child 132(5):480–483, 1978
869. Pieper B: The Teacher and the Child with Spina Bifida. Chicago, IL, Spina Bifida Association of America, 1977
870. Pieper E: Sticks and Stones: The Story of Loving a Child. Syracuse, NY, Human Policy Press, 1976
871. Piercy SL, Gregory JG, Young PH: Ventriculo-peritoneal shunt pseudocyst causing ureteropelvic junction obstruction in child with myelomeningocele and retrocaval ureter. J Urol 132:345–348, 1984
872. Pietsch P, Lober R, Wurfel S: Gynecologic and obstetric problems in patients with ureterointestinal anastomosis in bladder exstrophy. Zentralbl Gynakol 105(22):1450–1456, 1983
873. Piotrowski M: Functioning of normal and neurogenic bladder. Association of Rehabilitation of Nursing J 5:13–30, 1980
874. Piotrow PT: World population: The present and future crisis, in Headline Series 251. New York, Foreign Policy Association, 1980, p. 32
875. Piper MC, Pless IB: Early intervention for Down syndrome: A controlled trial. Pediatrics 65:463–468, 1980
876. Pipes PL: Nutrition in Infancy and Childhood (ed 2). St. Louis, CV Mosby, 1981
877. Pless BI: Practical problems and their management, in Scheiner AP, Abroms IF (eds): The Prenatal Management of the Developmentally Disabled Child. St. Louis, CV Mosby, 1980, pp 116–144
878. Pless BI, Satterwhite B, VanVechten D: Chronic illness in childhood: A regional survey of care. Pediatrics 58:37, 1976
879. Powers JT, Healey A: Inservice training for physicians serving handicapped children. Except Child 48:332–336, 1982

880. Powledge TM, Fletcher J: Guidelines for the ethical, social and legal issues in prenatal diagnosis: A report from the Genetic Research Group of the Hastings Center, Institute of the Society of Ethics and the Life Sciences. N Engl J Med 300:168–172, 1979
881. President's Commission for the Study of Ethical Problems in Medicine and Biomedical and Behavioral Research: Deciding to Forego Life-Sustaining Treatment. Washington, D.C., U.S. Government Printing Office, 1983
882. Prince B: Myelomeningocele. Part IV: Psychosocial problems and social work interventions. West J Med 12(4):297–298, 1974
883. Provis HS, Ellis RWB: An anthropometric study of Edinburgh school children. Part 1 Methods. Data and assessment of maturity. Arch Dis Child 30:328–337, 1955
884. Puckell CL, Reinisch JF, Montie JE: Free flap phalloplasty. J Urol 128:294–297, 1982
885. Pudenz RH, Russell FE, Hurd AH, et al: Ventriculo-auriculotomy. A technique for shunting cerebrospinal fluid into the right auricle. Preliminary report. J Neurosurg 14:171–179, 1957
886. Puppets: Principles and Politics, in Caputo L (ed): Keeping Up With the Kids (pamphlet). U.S. Government Printing Office, Washington, D.C. Spring 1984
887. Purpura DP, Gallagher JJ, Tjossem TD: Mental Retardation. U.S. Department of Health and Human Services. Child Health and Human Development U.S. Government Printing Office: Washington, D.C.: An Evaluation and Assessment of the State of the Science. (Pub No. 82-2304), 1981, pp VI1–VI42
888. Raimondi AJ, Soare P: Intellectual development in shunted hydrocehalic children. Am J Dis Child 127:664–671, 1974
889. Ralis ZA: The role of mechanical intrauterine pressure in the pathogenesis of paralytic limb deformities. J Bone Joint Surg [Br] 56:383, 1974
890. Ralis ZA: Traumatizing effect of breech delivery on infants with spina bifida. J Pediatr 87(4):613–616, 1975
891. Rapaport D, Gill MD, Schafer R: Diagnostic Psychological Testing. New York, International Universities Press, 1968
892. Rapier J, Adelson R, Carey R, et al: Changes in children's attitudes toward the physically handicapped. Except Child 39:219–223, 1972
893. Record RG: Anencephalus in Scotland. Br J Prev Soc Med 15:93-105, 1961
894. Record RG: Congenital malformations of the central nervous system. II—Maternal reproductive history and familial incidence. Br J Soc Med 4:26–50, 1950
895. Redman JF, Seibert JJ, Page BC: Cloacal exstrophy in identical twins. Urology 17(1):73–74, 1981
896. Rehabilitation Act of 1973, 29 USC Section 701 et. seq. enacted Sept. 26, 1973. Public Law 93–12, 87 Stat. 355
897. Reid R: Spina bifida: The fate of the untreated. Hastings Center Rep 7(4):16–19, 1977

898. Reid-Pitts W Jr, Muecke EC: A 20-year experience with ileal conduits: The fate of the kidneys. J Urol 122:154, 1979
899. Reigel D: Personal Communication, 1983
900. Reigel D: Kyphectomy and myelomeningocele repair. Modern techniques in surgery. Neurosurgery 13:1–9, 1979
901. Reigel D: Spina bifida, in McLaurin RL, Shulman K, Hendrick EB, et al (eds): Pediatric Neurosurgery. Surgery of the Developing Nervous System. Orlando, FL, Grune & Stratton, 1982, pp 23–43
902. Reigel D: Spina Bifida. Section of Pediatric Neurosurgery of the American Association of Neurological Surgeons. Orlando, FL, Grune & Stratton, 1978, pp 23–43
903. Reigel D: Tethered spinal cord. Concept Pediatr Neurosurg 4:142–164, 1983
904. Reigel DH, Dallman DE, Scarff TB, et al: Intra-operative evoked potential studies of newborn infants with meningomyelocele. Dev Med Child Neurol 37(suppl):42–49, 1976
905. Reigel DH, Dallman DE, Scarff TB, et al: Transcephalic impedance measurement during infancy. Dev Med Child Neurol 19(3):295–304, 1977
906. Reilly P: The role of law in the prevention of genetic disease, in Milunsky A (ed): The Prevention of Genetic Disease and Mental Retardation. Philadelphia, WB Saunders, 1975, p 422
907. Reitan RM, Davidson LA (eds): Clinical Neuropsychology: Current Status and Application. Washington, D.C., V.H. Winston, 1974
908. Rekate HL, Ruch T, Nulsen FE: Diphtheroid infections of cerebrospinal fluid shunts. A changing pattern of shunt infection in Cleveland. J Neurosurg 52:553–556, 1980
909. Relman AS: The Saikewiez decision: A medical viewpoint. Am J Law Med 4(3):233–242, 1977
910. Remigailo RV, Woodward JR, Andrews HG, et al: Cloacal exstrophy: 18-year survival of untreated case. J Urol 116:811–813, 1976
911. Rennels MS, Wald ER: Treatment of *Haemophilus influenzae* type b meningitis in children with cerebrospinal fluid shunts. J Pediatr 97:424–426, 1980
912. Repasky D, Rickard K, Lindseth R: Ascorbic acid and fractures in children with myelomeningocele. J Am Diet Assoc 69:511–513, 1976
913. Report by a working-party: Ethics of selective treatment of spina bifida. Lancet 1:85–88, 1975
914. Richards IDG, McIntosh HT: Spina bifida survivors and their parents: A study of problems and services. Dev Med Child Neurol 15:292–304, 1973
915. Richardson AB, Guralnick MJ, Tupper DB: Training pediatricians for effective involvement with preschool handicapped children and their families. Ment Retard 16:3–7, 1978
916. Richardson JT: Memory and intelligence following spontaneously arrested congenital hydrocephalus. Br J Soc Clin Psychol 17(3):261–267, 1978
917. Richardson S: Some social consequences of handicapping. Pediatrics 32:291–297, 1963

918. Richardson SA: Age and sex differences in values toward physical handicaps. Health Soc Behav 11:207–214, 1970
919. Richardson SA: Attitudes and behavior toward the physically handicapped. Birth Defects 7(4):15–34, 1976
920. Richardson SA: Attitudes and behavior toward the physically handicapped, in Bergsma D, Pulver AE (eds): Developmental Disabilities: Psychologic and Social Implications. New York, Alan R. Liss, 1976, pp 15–34
921. Richardson SA: Children's values in regard to disabilities: A reply to Yuker. Rehabil Psych 28(3):131–140, 1983
922. Richardson SA: Handicap, appearance and stigma. Soc Sci Med 5:621–628, 1971
923. Richardson SA, Green A: When is black beautiful? Coloured and white chidren's reactions to skin colour. Br J Educ Psych 41(part I):61–69, 1971
924. Richardson SA, Hastorf AH, Goodman N, et al: Cultural uniformity in reaction to physical disabilities. Am Soc Rev 26:241–247, 1961
925. Rickard K, Brady MS, Gresham EL: Nutritional management of the chronically ill child. Congenital heart disease and myelomeningocele. Pediatr Clin North Am 24(1):157–175, 1977
926. Rickey G: Kids on the Block. Good News America. Washington, D.C., The Kids on the Block, 1983
927. Rickham PP: The swing of the pendulum: The indications for operating on myelomeningocele. Med J Aust 2(20):743–746, 1976
928. Rickham PP: Vesico-intestinal fissure. Arch Dis Child 35:97–102, 1960
929. Rickham PP, Penn IA: The place of the ventriculostomy reservoir in the treatment of myelomeningocele and hydrocephalus. Dev Med Child Neurol 7:296–301, 1965
930. Rickwood AMK, Thomas DG: The upper urinary tract in adolescents and young adults with myelomeningocele. Z Kinderchir 39(suppl II):104–106, 1984
931. Ring JC, Cates KL, Belani KK, et al: Rifampin for CSF shunt infections caused by coagulase-negative staphylococcis. J Pediatr 95(2):317–320, 1979
932. Robards MF, Thomas GG, Rosenbloom L: Survival of infants with unoperated myeloceles. Br Med J 4:12–13, 1975
933. Robert E, Robert JM, Lapors C: Is valproic acid teratogenic? Rev Neurol (Paris) 139(6–7):445–447, 1983
934. Roberts CJ, Evans KT, Hibbard BM, et al: Diagnostic effectiveness of ultrasound in detection of neural tube defects. Lancet 2(8358):1068–1069, 1983
935. Roberts JB: A child with double cleft of lip and palate, protrusion of the intermaxillary portion of the upper jaw and imperfect development of the bones of the four extremities. Ann Surg 70:252–253, 1919
936. Robertson JA: The right to procreate and in utero fetal therapy. J Legal Med 3(3):333–366, 1982

937. Robertson JA: Involuntary euthanasia of defective newborns: Legal analysis. Stanford Law Rev 27:214–269, 1975
938. Robertson JA, Frost N: Passive euthanasia of defective newborn infants: Legal considerations, in Abrams N, Buckner MD (eds): Medical Ethics: A Clinical Textbook and Reference for the Health Care Professions. Cambridge, MA, MIT Press, 1983, pp 382–389
939. Robinson JM, Hewson JE, Parker PM: The walking ability of fourteen to seventeen year old teenagers with spina bifida—A physiotherapy study. Z Kinderchir 31:421–427, 1980
940. Robinson V: David in Silence. Philadelphia, JB Lippincott, 1966
941. Rocereto LR: Root work and the root doctor. Nurs Forum 12:414–427, 1973
942. Roche AF, Siervogel RM, Chumelea WC, et al: Grading body fatness from limited anthropometric data. Am J Clin Nutr 34:2831–2838, 1981
943. Roney H: Obesity and Leanness. Philadelphia, Lea & Febiger, 1940
944. Roos P: Normalization, de-humanization, and conditioning—Conflict of harmony. Ment Retard 8:12–14, 1970
945. Rose GK: Splint age for severe spina bifida cystica. J Bone Joint Surg [Br] 52:178–179, 1970
946. Rose GK, Henshaw JT: A swivel walker for paraplegia: Medical and technical considerations. Biomech Engineer 7:420–425, 1972
947. Rosenbaum P, Barmitt R, Brand HL: A developmental intervention programme designed to overcome the effects of impaired movement in spina bifida infants. Clin Dev Med 55:145–156, 1975
948. Rosenkrantz JG, Bailey WC, Dumars KW: Incomplete exstrophy of the cloaca. J Urol 91:540–542, 1964
949. Rosenstein BD, Greene WB, Herrington RT, et al: Effect of ambulatory status on bone density in myelomeningocele. Presented at the American Academy of Cerebral Palsy and Developmental Medicine Meetings, Seattle, Washington, September 2–5, 1985
950. Roth JA: The treatment of tuberculosis as a bargaining process, in Rose A (ed): Human Behavior and Social Processes. Boston, Houghton-Mifflin, 1962
951. Rubovitz FE, Arnkoff M: Pregnancy associated with exstrophy of the bladder. J Urol 62:52–57, 1949
952. Ruderman R, Francis R, Mosca VS, et al: The ambulatory management of foot ulceration in myelodysplasia. Z Kinderchir 37:123, 1982
953. Rueda J, Carroll NC: Hip instability in patients with myelomeningocele. J Bone Joint Surg [Br] 54:422–431, 1972
954. Rummelhardt S, Donner G: Long-term observations following urinary drainage into the intact large intestine. Z Urol Nephrol 76(9):561–565, 1983
955. Rutter M: The long-term effects of early experience. Dev Med Child Neurol 22:800–815, 1980
956. Rutter M: Scientific Foundations of Developmental Psychiatry. London, William Heinemann Medical Books, 1980
957. Ruysch F: Observationum anatomico-chirurgicarum centuria. Amster-

dam: H & T Boom, 1691 (Cited in Stark GD (ed): Spina Bifida: Problems and Management. Oxford, Blackwell Scientific Publications, 1977)

958. Ryan P: Widening their horizons: A model career development program for severely physically disabled youth. Rehabil Lit 40(3):72–74, 1979
959. Sabbeth BF, Leventhal JM: Marital adjustment to chronic childhood illness: A critique of the literature. Pediatrics 73:762–768, 1984
960. Sadovnick AD, Baird PA: A cost-benefit analysis of prenatal diagnosis for neural tube defects selectively offered to relatives of index cases. Am J Med Genet 12:63–73, 1982
961. Safford PL, Arbitman DC, Townsend WB: Developmental Intervention with Young Physically Handicapped Children. Springfield, IL, Charles C Thomas, 1975
962. Saint-Hilaire LG: Description d'un monstre humain re avant l'ere chretienne, compare a an pareil monstre de l'epoque actuelle; et considerations zootomiques et physiologiques sur le caractere de ces monstruosltes, dites ancephales; sur l'independance de deformation de chique sexe; et sur l'existence de deux noyauxdan l'os basilaire. Ann Sci Natl 7:357, 1826
963. Salk JE: Limits to growth, in Hess HO (ed): The Nature of Human Society: A Symposium on the Bicentennial of the United States of America. Philadelphia, Fortress Press, 1977, pp 162–171
964. Salk JE: The Survival of the Wisest. New York, Harper & Row, 1973, pp 100–105
965. Salmon JH: Adult hydrocephalus: Evaluation of shunt therapy in 80 patients. J Neurosurg 37:423–428, 1972
966. Salmon JH: Isolated unilateral hydrocephalus following ventriculoatrial shunt. J Neurosurg 32:219–226, 1970
967. Salmon JH: The collapsed ventricle: Management and prevention. Surg Neurol 9(16):349–352, 1978
968. Sand PL, Taylor N, Hill M, et al: Hand function in children with myelomeningocele. Am J Occup Ther 28(2):87–90, 1974
969. Sand PL, Taylor N, Rawlings M, et al: Performance of children with spina bifida manifesta on the Frostig Developmental Test of Visual Perception. Percept Mot Skills 37:539–546, 1973
970. Sandusky WR: Post-operative infections and anti-microbial prophylaxis for surgical infections, in Mandell GL, Douglas RG Jr, Bennet JE (eds): Principles and Practice of Infectious Diseases. New York, John Wiley and Sons, 1979, pp 2248–2256
971. Sarason IG, Johnson JH, Siegel JM: Assessing the impact of life changes: Development of the life experiences survey. J Consult Clin Psychol 45:932–946, 1978
972. Savitz MH, Katz SS: Rationale for prophylactic antibiotics in neurosurgery. Neurosurgery 9:142–144, 1981
973. Savitz MH, Malis LI, Meyers BR: Prophylactic antibiotics in neurosurgery. Surg Neurol 2:95–100, 1974
974. Say B, Coldwell JG: Hereditary defect of the sacrum. Humangenetik 27:231–234, 1975

975. Scarff JE: Treatment of hydrocephalus: An historical and critical review of methods and results. J Neurol Neurosurg Psychiatry 26:1–26, 1963
976. Schafer MF, Dias LS: Myelomeningocele: Orthopedic Treatment. Baltimore, Williams & Wilkins, 1983
977. Schardein JL: Drugs as Teratogens. Cleveland, CRC Press, 1976
978. Scheiner AP, Abroms IF (eds): The Practical Management of the Developmentally Disabled Child. St. Louis, CV Mosby, 1980
979. Scherzer AL, Gardner GG: Studies of the school-age child with meningomyelocele: I. Physical and intellectual development. Pediatrics 47(2):424–430, 1971
980. Schilling M, Siepp J, Patterson EG, et al: The First Three Years: Programming for Atypical Infants and Their Families. A United Cerebral Palsy Nationally-Organized Collaborative Project to Provide Comprehensive Services. New York, United Cerebral Palsy Associations, 1974
981. Schimke RT, Black PH, Mark VH, et al: Indolent Staphylococcus albus or aureus bacteremia after ventriculoatriostomy. N Engl J Med 264:264–270, 1961
982. Schinzel A, Smith DW, Miller JR: Monozygotic twinning and structural defects. J Pediatr 95:921–930, 1979
983. Schmid W, Muhletzaler JP, Briner J, et al: Ring chromosome 13 in a polymalformed anencephalic. Humangenetik 27:63–66, 1975
984. Schoenbaum SC, Gardner P, Shillite J: Infections of CSF shunts: Epidemiology, chemical manifestations and therapy. J Infect Dis 131:543–552, 1975
985. Schultz TL, Sorenson LM: The Organic Puppet Theater: Children's Activities in Health Awareness. St. Paul, Night Owl Press, 1983
986. Schut L, Bruce DA: The Arnold-Chiari malformation. Orthop Clin North Am 9(4):913–921, 1978
987. Schut L, Bruce DA, Sutton LN: The management of the child with a lipomyelomeningocele, in Carmel PW (ed): Clinical Neurosurgery, vol. 28. Baltimore, Williams & Wilkins, 1981, p 464
988. Schut L, Groff RA: Redundant nerve roots as a cause of complete myelographic block. A case report. J Neurosurg 28:394–395, 1968
989. Schwalbe E: Die Morphologie der Missbildugen der Menschen und der Tiere Jena. Ergebn & Wissenschmed Leipz, pp 45–46, 1909
990. Schwarz GR, Jeffs RD: Ileal conduit diversion in children: Computer analysis of follow up from 2 to 16 years. J Urol 114:285, 1975
991. Scott FB, Bradley WE, Timm GW: Management of erectile impotence: Use of implantable inflatable prosthesis. Urology 11(1):80–82, 1973
992. Scott FB, Light JK, Fishman I, et al: Implantation of an artifical sphincter for urinary incontinence. Contemp Surg 18:11–16, 25–27, 30–31, 34, 1981
993. Scott JA: Report of the Heights and Weights (and Other Measurements) of School Pupils in the County of London in 1959. London, London County Council, 1961
994. Scragg RKD, Dorsch MM, McMichael AJ, et al: Birth defects and

household water supply. Epidemiological studies in the Mount Gambier region of South Australia. Med J Aust 2:577–579, 1982

995. Seegmiller BR, King WL: Relations between behavioral characteristics of infants, their mothers' behaviors, and performance on the Bayley Mental and Motor Scales. J Psychology 90:99–111, 1975
996. Seiferth J: Types of neurogenic bladder in children with spina bifida, and response to treatment with phenoxybenzamine. Dev Med Child Neurol 37(suppl):94–96, 1976
997. Sella A, Foltz EL, Shurtleff DB: A three-year developmental study of treated and untreated hydrocephalic children. J Pediatr 69:887–891, 1966
998. Seller MJ, Nevin NC: Periconceptual vitamin supplementation and the prevention of neural tube defects in south-east England and Northern Ireland. J Med Genet 21:325–330, 1984
999. Sells CJ, Shurtleff DB: Cerebrospinal fluid shunt systems. West J Med 127:93–98, 1977
1000. Sells CJ, Shurtleff DB, Loeser JD: Gram negative cerebrospinal fluid shunt-associated infections. Pediatrics 59:613–618, 1977
1001. Sensenig EC: The early development of the meninges of the spinal cord in human embryos. Contrib Embryol 34:145–157, 1951
1002. Sever LE: A case of meningomyelocele in a kindred with multiple cases of spondylolisthesis and spina bifida occulta. J Med Genet 11(1):94–96, 1974
1003. Sever LE: Incidence and prevalence as measures of the frequency of birth defects (letter). Am J Epidemiol 118(4):608–609, 1983
1004. Sever LE: An epidemiologic study of neural tube defects in Los Angeles County II. Etiologic factors in an area with low prevalence at birth. Teratology 25(3):323–334, 1982
1005. Sever LE: Zinc and human development: A review. Hum Ecol 3(1):43–57, 1957
1006. Sever LE, Sanders M, Monsen R: An epidemiologic study of neural tube defects in Los Angeles County I. Prevalence at birth based on multiple sources of case ascertainment. Teratology 25(3):315–321, 1982
1007. Sever LE: Zinc deficiency in man. Lancet 1:887, 1973
1008. Shaffer J: Personal communication, 1984
1009. Shaffer J, Friedrich WN, Shurtleff DB, et al: Cognitive and achievement status of children with meningomyelocele. Pediatr Psychol 10(3):325–336, 1985
1010. Shane Lemel *v*. the State of Washington, a Show Cause Hearing, Superior Court of Wakiakum, Cowlitz County, 1976
1011. Shapiro E, Lepor H, Jeffs RD: The inheritance of the exstrophy/epispadias complex. J Urol 132:308–310, 1984
1012. Shapiro K, Fried A: Childhood spinal dysraphism. Contemp Neurosurg 6:1–7, 1985
1013. Shapiro SR, Lebowitz R, Colodny AH: Fate of 90 children with ileal conduit urinary diversion a decade later: Analysis of complications, pyelography, renal function and bacteriology. J Urol 114:289, 1975

1014. Sharrard WJW: Congenital paralytic dislocation of the hip in children with myelomeningocele. J Bone Joint Surg [Br] 41:622, 1959

1015. Sharrard WJW: Paediatric Orthopaedics and Fractures. Oxford and Edinburgh, Blackwell Scientific Publications, 1971

1016. Sharrard WJW: Posterior ileopsoas transplantation in the treatment of paralytic dislocation of the hip. J Bone Joint Surg [Br] 46:426–444, 1964

1017. Sharrard WJW: The segmental innervation of the lower limb muscles in man. Ann R Coll Surg Engl 35:106–112, 1964

1018. Sharrard WJW: Specific orthopaedic problems, in Brocklehurst G (ed): Spina Bifida for the Clinician. Philadelphia, JB Lippincott, 1976, pp 116–118

1019. Sharrard WJW, Drennan JC: Osteotmy excision of the spine for lumbar kyphosis in older children with meningomyelocele. J Bone Joint Surg [Br] 54:50, 1972

1020. Sharrard WJ, Zachary RB, Lorber J: The long-term evaluation of a trial of immediate and delayed closure of spina bifida cystica. Clin Orthop 50:197–201, 1967

1021. Sharrard WJW, Zachary RB, Lorber J: Survival and paralysis in open myelomeningocele with special reference to the time of repair of the spinal lesion. Dev Med Child Neurol 13:35–50, 1967

1022. Sharrard WJ, Zachary RB, Lorber J, et al: A controlled trial of immediate and delayed closure of spina bifida cystica. Arch Dis Child 38:18–22, 1963

1023. Shaw A: Dilemmas of "informed consent" in children. N Engl J Med 289:885–890, 1973

1024. Shaw A: The ethics of proxy consent, in Swinyard C (ed): Decision Making and the Defective Newborn. Springfield, IL, Charles C Thomas, 1978, pp 589–597

1025. Sheldon CA, McKinley CR, Hartig PR, et al: Carcinoma at the site of ureterosigmoidostomy. Dis Colon Rectum 26(1):55–58, 1983

1026. Shelley M: Frankenstein. New York, Regents Publishers, 1981

1027. Shepherd K, Hickstein R, Shepherd R: Neurogenic faecal incontinence in children with spina bifida: Rectosphincteric responses and evaluation of a physiological rationale for management, including biofeedback conditioning. Aust Paediatr J 19:97–99, 1983

1028. Shiota K: Neural tube defects and maternal hyperthermia in early pregnancy. Am J Med Genet 12:281–288, 1982

1029. Shively RE, Schafer ME, Kernalian DA: The spread of sensibility into previously anaesthetic skin following intercostal flap transfer in a paraplegic. Ann Plast Surg 5:396–400, 1980

1030. Shkolnik A, McLone DG: Intraoperative real-time ultrasonic guidance of intracranial shunt tube placement in infants. Radiology 141(2):515–517, 1981

1031. Shkolnik A, McLone DG: Intraoperative real-time ultrasonic guidance of intracranial shunt tube placement in infants. Radiology 144(3):573–576, 1982

1032. Shoeing HA, Iversen IA: Numerical scoring of self-care status: A study of the Kenny Self Card Evaluation. Arch Phys Med Rehabil 49:199, 1968

1033. Shore MF: Red is the color of hurting. National Institute of Mental Health, National Institute of Health, Bethesda, MD 20014. Copy in care of Superintendent of Documents. Washington, D.C., U.S. Government Printing Office, 1965

1034. Shrybman J, Matsonkas G: The principal and the special education hearing. Nat Element Princ 58(1):30–33, 1978

1035. Shulman K: Use of outcome predictors in severe myelodysplasia. Clin Pediatr (Phila) 18(8):476–480, 1979

1036. Shurtleff CF: Bibliography of Children's Books About Disabilities. Seattle, Children's Orthopedic Hospital and Medical Center, 1985

1037. Shurtleff CF: Personal communication, 1985

1038. Shurtleff DB: Central nervous system infection with hydrocephalus and myelodysplasia. Clin Pediatr (Phila) 12:310–314, 1973

1039. Shurtleff DB: Characteristics of the various CSF shunt systems. Clinic Pediatr (Phila) 17(2):154–160, 1978

1040. Shurtleff DB: Ethics of fetoscopy, in Rocker I, Laurence KM (eds): Fetoscopy. Elsevier, North-Holland Biomedical Press, 1981, pp 313–324

1041. Shurtleff DB: Independence achievement of congenitally handicapped children. Pediatr Digest 19:15–22, 1977

1042. Shurtleff DB: Management of birth defects. University of Washington Medicine, 1976

1043. Shurtleff DB: Management of myelodysplasia: A decision for abortion, involuntary euthanasia or treatment. Contin Educ Fam Phys 6(6):36–54, 1977

1044. Shurtleff DB: Meningomyelocele: The price of treatment, in Gellis SS (ed): Yearbook of Pediatrics. Chicago, Yearbook Medical Publishers, 1973, pp 333–336

1045. Shurtleff DB: Myelodysplasia: Management and treatment, in Gluck L (ed): Current Problems in Pediatrics, vol. X. Chicago, Yearbook Medical, 1980, pp 1–90

1046. Shurtleff DB: Myelodysplasia: Problems of long term survival and social function. West J Med 122:199–205, 1975

1047. Shurtleff DB: Prognosis of meningomyelocele. South Med J 68(1):2–3, 1975

1048. Shurtleff DB: The team approach: Multidisciplinary, interdisciplinary: Is it real? Spina Bifida Ther 2(1):57–70, 1979

1049. Shurtleff DB: Timing of learning: Meningomyelocele patients. J Am Phys Ther Assoc 46:135–148, 1965

1050. Shurtleff DB: Transillumination of the skull in infants and children. Am J Dis Child 107:14–24, 1964

1051. Shurtleff DB, Christie D, Foltz EL: Ventriculo-auriculostomy associated infection. A 12-year study. J Neurosurg 35:686–699, 1971

1052. Shurtleff DB, Foltz EL: Comparative study of meningomyelocele repair of cerebrospinal fluid shunt as primary treatment in spina bifida. Dev Med Child Neurol 13(suppl):57–64, 1967

1053. Shurtleff DB, Foltz EL, Loeser JD: Hydrocephalus: A definition of its progression and relationship to intellectual functions, diagnosis and complications. Am J Dis Child 125:688–693, 1973

1054. Shurtleff DB, Foltz EL, Weeks, RD, et al: Therapy of staphylococcus epidermidis: Infections associated with cerebrospinal fluid shunts. Pediatrics 53:55–62, 1974

1055. Shurtleff DB, Gordon LH, Goiney R, et al: Myelodysplasia: The natural history of kyphosis and scoliosis—A preliminary report. Dev Med Child Neurol 18(suppl 37):126–133, 1976

1056. Shurtleff DB, Hayden PW: The treatment of hydrocephalus with isosorbide, an oral hyperosmotic agent. J Clin Pharmacol 12:108–114, 1972

1057. Shurtleff DB, Hayden PW, Chapman WH, et al: Myelodysplasia: Problems of long-term survival and social function. West J Med 122:199–205, 1975

1058. Shurtleff DB, Hayden PW, Loeser JD, et al: Myelodysplasia: Decision for death or disability. N Engl J Med 291:1005–1011, 1974

1059. Shurtleff DB, Hayden PW, Weeks R, et al: Temporary treatment of hydrocephalus and myelodysplasia with isosorbide. Preliminary report. J Pediatr 83:651–657, 1973

1060. Shurtleff DB, Kronmal R, Foltz EL: Follow-up comparison of hydrocephalus with and without myelomeningocele. J Neurosurg 42:61–68, 1975

1061. Shurtleff DB, Lamers J: Clinical considerations in the treatment of myelodysplasia, in Crandall DB, Brazier MAB (eds): The Prevention of Neural Tube Defects: The Role of Alpha-Fetoprotein. Orlando, FL, Academic Press, p 103–122, 1978

1062. Shurtleff DB, Lamers J, Goiney T, et al: Are myelodysplastic children fat? Anthropometric measures: A preliminary report. Spina Bifida Ther 4(1): 1–21, 1982

1063. Shurtleff DB, Menelaus MB, Staheli LT et al: The natural history of flexion deformity of the hip in myelodysplasia. In Press J. Pediat Orthop 1985

1064. Shurtleff DB, Sousa JC: The adolescent with myelodysplasia: Development, achievement, sex, and deterioration. Del Med J 49(11):631–638, 1977

1065. Shurtleff DB, Stuntz JT, Hayden PW: Experience with 1201 cerebrospinal fluid shunt procedures. Pediatr Neurosci 12:49–57, 1985–6

1066. Simon G: Causes of late death due to hydrocephalus and myelomeningocele. Prog Pediatr Surg 13:105–108, 1979

1067. Simpson JL, Dische R, Morillo-Cucci G: Triploidy (69, XXY) in a liveborn infant. Ann Genet (Paris) 15:103–106, 1972

1068. Sinclair JG: Intestinal hernia with eversion and exstrophic bladder. J Pediatr 26:78–81, 1945

1069. Singer P: Predicting the quality of their lives. The New York Times Book Review. September 30, 1984, pp 14–15: on Weir RF: Selective Nontreatment of Handicapped Newborns: Moral Dilemmas in Neonatal Medicine. New York, Oxford University Press, 1984

1070. Singh M, Singh S: Possible relationship between clomiphene and neural tube defects (case report). J Pediatr 93(5):152, 1978

1071. Siris IE: Spina bifida: Treatment and analysis of 84 cases. Ann Surg 103:97–123, 1936

1072. Skef Z, Bellinger MF, Blomain EW, et al: Use of inferior rectus myocutaneous flap for coverage of bladder exstrophy defect. J Pediatr Surg 17(6):718–720, 1982

1073. Smith AD: Adult spina bifida survey in Scotland: Educational attainment and employment. Z Kinderchir 38(suppl II):107–109, 1983

1074. Smith DW, Clarren SK, Harvey MAS: Hyperthermia as a possible teratogenic agent. J Pediatr 92:878–883, 1978

1075. Smith ED: Follow up studies on 150 ileal conduits in children. J Pediatr Surg 7:1, 1972

1076. Smith ED: Spina bifida and the total care of spinal myelomeningocele. Springfield, IL, Charles C Thomas, 1965

1077. Smith GK, Smith ED: Selection for treatment in spina bifida. Br Med J 4:189–197, 1973

1078. Smith K: Parents need to stay smart on education. Spina Bifida Insights 11(1):2, 1983

1079. Smithells RW, Nevin NC, Seller MJ, et al: Further experience of vitamin supplementation for prevention of neural tube defect recurrences. Lancet 1(8332):1027–1031, 1983

1080. Smyth BT, Piggot J, Forsythe WI, et al: A controlled trial of immediate and delayed closure of myelomeningocele. J Bone Joint Surg [Br] 56:297–304, 1974

1081. Snow LF: Traditional health beliefs and practices among lower class black Americans. West J Med 139(6):820–828, 1983

1082. Snow LF, Johnson SM, Mayhew HE: The behavioral implications of some old wives' tales. Obstet Gynecol 51:727–732, 1978

1083. Snyder CC: A new therapeutic concept of the exstrophied bladder. Plast Reconstr Surg 22:1–10, 1958

1084. Snyder M, Tanke ED, Berschied E: Social perception and interpersonal behavior: On the self-fulfilling nature of social stereotypes. J Pers Soc Psychol 35:656–666, 1977

1085. Snyder RT, Freud SL: Reading readiness and its relationship to maturational unreadiness as measured by the spiral after-effect and visual perceptual techniques. Percept Mot Skills 25:841–854, 1967

1086. Soare PL, Raimondi AJ: Intellectual and perceptual motor characteristics of treated myelomeningocele children. Am J Dis Child 131:199–204, 1977

1087. Sobol H: My Brother Steven is Retarded. New York, Macmillan, 1977

1088. Soboloff HR: Early intervention—Fact or fiction? Dev Med Child Neurol 23:261–266, 1981

1089. Sokal DL, Byrd JR, Chen ATL, et al: Prenatal diagnosis: Racial and geographic variation for older women in Georgia. JAMA 244:1355–1357, 1980

1090. Soler NG, Walsh CH, Malins JM: Congenital malformations in infants of diabetic mothers. Q J Med 45:303–313, 1976

1091. Soper RT, Kilger K: Vesico-intestinal fissure. J Urol 92(5):490–501, 1961

1092. Sory B, Coldwell JG: Hereditary defect of the sacrum. Humangenetik 27:231–234, 1975

1093. Soskin RM: Handicapped advocacy: A last hurrah? Amicus 5:69–71, 1980

1094. Sousa JC, Gordon LH, Shurtleff DB: Assessing the development of independence of daily living skills in patients with spina bifida. Dev Med Child Neurol 18(suppl 37):134–142, 1976

1095. Sousa JC, Telzrow RW, Holm RA, et al: Developmental guidelines for children with myelodysplasia. J Am Phys Ther Assoc 63(1):21–29, 1983

1096. Spain B: Verbal and performance ability in pre-school children with spina bifida. Dev Med Child Neurol 16:773–780, 1974

1097. Speer JB: Baby Doe from a Seattle perspective. Grand Rounds, Children's Orthopedic Hospital, December 8, 1984

1098. Spencer R: Exstrophia splanchica (exstrophy of the cloaca). Surgery 57:751–756, 1965

1099. Spina Bifida Association of America, 343 South Dearborn Street, Suite 319, Chicago, IL, (312) 663-1562

1100. Spitz RA: Hospitalism: An inquiry into the genesis of psychiatric conditions in early children, in Fenichel O, Greenacre P, Hartmann H, et al (eds): Psychoanalytic Study of the Child. New York, International Press, 1945

1101. Stacey M: Charisma, power and altruism: A discussion of research in a child development center. Soc Health Ill 2:64–90, 1980

1102. Staheli L: Personal communication, 1985

1103. Stark E: Disabilities, Puppets, and Play. Psychol Today 17(9):14–15, 1983

1104. Stark G: The nature and cause of paraplegia in myelomeningocele. Paraplegia 9:219–223, 1972

1105. Stark G (ed): Spina Bifida: Problems and Management. London, Blackwell Scientific Publications, 1977

1106. Stark G, Drummond M: Results of selective early operation in myelomeningocele. Arch Dis Child 48:676–682, 1973

1107. Stark G, Drummond M: Spina bifida as an obstetric problem. Dev Med Child Neurol 12(suppl 12):157–160, 1970

1108. State Adoption Support of 1971, RCW 74.13.100

1109. Stedman DJ, Amastasion PR, Gordon IJ: How can effective early intervention programs be delivered to potentially retarded children? Office of the Secretary of the US Department of Health, Education, and Welfare. Washington, D.C., Bureau of Education for the Handicapped, 1972

1110. Stein RE, Jessop DJ: Relationship between health status and psychological adjustment among children with chronic conditions. Pediatrics 73:169–174, 1984

1111. Stein SB: About Handicaps. New York, Walker, 1974

1112. Stein SC, Feldman JG, Friedlander M, et al: Is myelomeningocele a disappearing disease? Pediatrics 69(5):511–514, 1982
1113. Stein SC, Schut LA: Hydrocephalus in myelomeningocele. Childs Brain 5:413–419, 1979
1114. Stein SC, Schut LA: Selection for early treatment in myelomeningocele: A retrospective analysis of various selection procedures. Pediatrics 54(5):553–557, 1974
1115. Stein SC, Schut L, Ames MD: Selection for early treatment in myelomeningocele: A retrospective analysis of various selection procedures. Pediatrics 54:553–557, 1974
1116. Stein SC, Schut LA, Borns P: Lacunar skull deformity (Luckenschadel) and intelligence in myelomeningocele. J Neurosurg 41:10–13, 1974
1117. Steinbock B: Baby Jane Doe in the Courts. Hastings Center Rep Hastings-on-Hudson, NY, 14(2):13–19, 1984
1118. Stephens S: Learning difficulties and children born with neural tube defects. Spina Bifida Ther 4:63–76, 1982
1119. Stern J, Linke R: Assessment of weight in spinal cord injury patients. The America Dietetic Association 66th Annual Meeting, San Antonio, Texas, 1983
1120. Stewart JM, Stoll S: Familial caudal regression anomalad and maternal diabetes. J Med Genet 16(1):17–20, 1979
1121. Stewart TD: Incidence of separate neural-arch defects in the lumbar vertebrae of Eskimos. Am J Phys Anthropol 16:51–62, 1931
1122. Stewart TD: The age incidence of neural-arch defects in Alaskan natives, considered from the standpoint of etiology. J Bone Joint Surg [Am] 35:937–950, 1953
1123. Stillman PL, Sabers DL, Redfield DL: Use of trained mothers to teach interviewing skills to first-year medical students: A follow-up study. Pediatrics 60:165–169, 1977
1124. Stillman R: Collier Azusa Scale. Dallas, Collier Center for Communication Disorders, 1974
1125. Stillwell A, Menelaus MB: Walking ability in mature patients with spina bifida. J Pediatr Orthop 3:184–190, 1983
1126. Stover S, Fleming W: Recurrent bactiuria in complete spinal cord injury. Patients on external condom drainage. Arch Phys Med Rehabil 61:178–181, 1980
1127. Strach EH: Methods of bracing in the rehabilitation of the paraplegic child. Paraplegia 11:137–143, 1973
1128. Strassburg MA, Greenland S, Portigal LD, et al: A population-based case-control study of anencephalus and spina bifida in a low-risk area. Dev Med Child Neurol 25:632–641, 1983
1129. Strauss RP: Surgery activism and aesthetics: A sociological perspective on treating facial disfigurement, in Lucker GW, Ribbens KA, McNamara JA (eds): Psychological Aspects of Facial Form. Ann Arbor, MI, Center for Human Growth and Development, 1980
1130. Strickland B: Legal issues that affect parents, in Seligman M (ed): The

Family with a Handicapped Child: Understanding and Treatment. Orlando, FL, Grune & Stratton, 1983, pp 27–59

1131. Strom R, Rees R, Slaughter H, et al: Child-rearing expectations of families with atypical children. Am J Orthopsychiatry 51:285–296, 1981
1132. Stuart RB: Helping Couples Change. New York, Guilford, 1980
1133. Sudnow D: Passing On. Englewood Cliffs, NJ, Prentice-Hall, 1967
1134. Sugarman B: Infection and pressure sores. Arch Phys Med Rehabil 66:177–179, 1985
1135. Sullivan-Bolyai S, Swanson M, Shurtleff DB: Toilet training the child with neurogenic impairment of bowel and bladder function. Issues Comprehen Pediatr Nurs 7:33–43, 1984
1136. Sunburst Communications, Pleasantville, NY 10570
1137. Sutow WW, Pryde AW: Incidence of spina bifida occulta in relation to age. Am J Dis Child 91:211–217, 1956
1138. Sutton LN, Bruce DA, Schut L: Hydranecephaly versus maximal hydrocephalus: An important clinical distinction. Neurosurgery 6(1):35–38, 1980
1139. Swift J: A modest proposal for preventing the children of Ireland from being a burden to their parents and country, in Eddy WA (ed): Satires and Personal Writings. London, Oxford University Press, 1973, p 21
1140. Swinyard CA (ed): Decision Making and the Defective Newborn: Proceedings of a Conference on Spina Bifida and Ethics. Springfield, IL, Charles C Thomas, 1978
1141. Tachdjian MO: Pediatric Orthopedics. Philadelphia, WB Saunders, 1972, pp 887–944
1142. Taggart JR, Walker AE: Congential atresia of the foraminia of luschka and magendie. Arch Neurol Psychiatr 48:583–612, 1942
1143. Tank ES, Lindenauer SM: Principles of management of exstrophy of the cloaca. Am J Surg 119:95–98, 1970
1144. Tanner JM, Whitehorse RH: Revised standards for triceps and subscapular skinfolds in British children. Arch Dis Child 50:142–143, 1975
1145. The Task Force on Pediatric Education: The Future of Pediatric Education, A Report. Evanston, IL, American Academy of Pediatrics, 1978, pp 24–25
1146. Taussig HB: A study of the German outbreak of phocomelia. The thalidomide syndrome. JAMA 180:1106–1114, 1962
1147. Taylor AI: Autosomal trisomy syndromes: A detailed study of 27 cases of Patau's syndrome. J Med Genet 5:227–252, 1968
1148. Taylor N, Pemberton DR: Verlo: Orthosis for children with severe motor handicaps. Arch Phys Med Rehabil 53:534–535, 1972
1149. Taylor N, Sand PL: Verlo orthosis: Experience with different developmental levels in normal children. Arch Phys Med Rehabil 56:120–122, 1975
1150. Taylor N, Sand PL, Jebsen RH: Evaluation of hand function in children. Arch Phys Med Rehabil 54:129–135, 1973
1151. Tew B: The psychological and educational consequences of spina bifida and its complications. Dev Med Child Neurol 20:240, 1978

1152. Tew BJ, Laurence KM: Mothers, brothers, and sisters of patients with spina bifida. Dev Med Child Neurol 29(suppl):69–76, 1973
1153. Tew BJ, Laurence KM: The relationship between spina bifida children's intelligence test scores on school entry and school leaving: A preliminary report. Child Care Health Dev 9:13–17, 1983
1154. Tew BJ, Laurence KM: Some sources of stress found in mothers of spina bifida children. Br J Prev Soc Med 29:27–30, 1975
1155. Tew B, Laurence KM: The ability and attainments of spina bifida patients born in South Wales between 1956–1962. Dev Med Child Neurol 14(suppl 27):124–131, 1972
1156. Tew B, Laurence KM: The effects of hydrocephalus on intelligence, visual perception, and school attainments. Dev Med Child Neurol 17(6)(suppl 35):129–134, 1975
1157. Tew B, Laurence KM: The validity of psychometric studies on children with spina bifida. Dev Med Child Neurol 16:186–188, 1974
1158. Tew BJ, Laurence KM, Payne H, et al: Marital stability following the birth of a child with spina bifida. Br J Psychiatry 131:79–82, 1977
1159. Tew BJ, Payne H, Laurence KM: Must a family with a handicapped child be a handicapped family? Dev Med Child Neurol 16:(suppl 32):95–98, 1974
1160. The Task Force on Pediatric Education: The Future of Pediatric Education, A Report. Elk Grove Village, IL, American Academy of Pediatrics, 1978, pp 24–25
1161. Theilgard A, Lundsteen C, Parring H, et al: Trisomy 8 syndrome. A psychological and somatic study of a mentally non-retarded male with 46 XY/47 XY, +8 chromosome constitution. Clin Genet 12:227–232, 1977
1162. Thomas LI, Thompson TC, Straub LR: Transplantation of the external oblique muscle for abductor paralysis. J Bone Joint Surg [Am] 32:207–219, 1950
1163. Thompson A: Prenatal advances pose ethics problems. The Seattle Times, October 7, 1984, p E2
1164. Thornton PA: Influence of exogenous ascorbic acid on calcium and phosphorous metabolis in the chick. J Nutr 100:1479, 1970
1165. Timson J: A study of the first degree relatives of the parents of spina bifida children. Clin Genet 3:99–102, 1972
1166. Tobiasen JM: Psychosocial correlates of congenital facial clefts: A conceptualization model. Cleft Palate J 21(3):131–139, 1984
1167. Todres DT, Krane D, Howell MC, et al: Pediatricians' attitudes affecting decision making in defective newborns. Pediatrics 60:197–201, 1977
1168. Trieschmann RB: The psychological, social, and vocational adjustment to spinal cord injury, in Pan EL, Backer TE, Vash CL (eds): Annual Review of Rehabilitation, vol. I. New York, Springer, 1980
1169. Trowbridge A: Three cases of spina bifida, successfully treated. Boston Med Surg J 1:753, 1828
1170. Tsignoglon S, Forrest DM: A technique for insertion of Holter ventriculoatrial shunts for infantile hydrocephalus. Br J Surg 58:367–372, 1971

1171. Tulpius N: Obs Med Lib. III Cap. XXIX, XXX, p 229, 1641
1172. 2,4,5-T spina bifida and after. NZ Med J 86(592):99–100, 1977
1173. Tyrrel S: Some problems of incontinent children attending ordinary school. Public Health 89:77–80, 1975
1174. Umlauf R: Personal communication, 1985
1175. United States of America *v.* University Hospital, 729 S.2d 144 (2nd cir. 1984)
1176. U.S. Department of Health, Education and Welfare/Public Health Service: Surveillance Summary. Temporal trends in the incidence of birth defects—United States. MMWR 28(34):401–402, 1979
1177. U.S. Department of Health, Education and Welfare/Public Health Service: International notes. Dengue-Mexico. MMWR 28(34):402–404, 1979
1178. Van den Berg BJ: Personal communication, 1982
1179. Van Went JJ, Van Went GF, Delleman JW, et al: Spina bifida and so-called asphenia syndrome occurring separately in sibs. Teratology 15:195–198, 1977
1180. Vanderhof KD: Euthanasia: Fetal-neonatal-infanticide. Northwest Inst Ethics Life Sci Bull 1:4–5, 1976
1181. Varni JW and Wallander JL: Adherence health-related regimens in pediatric chronic disorders. Clinical Psych Rev (in press)
1182. Varni JW, Wallander JL: Pediatric chronic orthopaedic disabilities: Hemophilia and spina bifida as exemplary disorders, in Routh DK (ed): Handbook of Pediatric Psychology. New York, Guilford Press, (in press)
1183. Veatch RM: Severe handicaps raise major issues of medical ethics. The Seattle Times. Sunday, August 22, 1982, pp A-19
1184. Veatch RM: The technical criteria fallacy. Hastings Center Rep 7(4): 15–16, 1977
1185. Venes JL: Control of shunt infection: Report of 150 consecutive cases. Neurosurgery 45:311–314, 1976
1186. Venes JL: Letter to the editor. Pediatrics 74(1):162–163, 1984
1187. Venes JL: Mental retardation in children with myelomeningocele: An acquired disease? Presented at the Annual Meeting of the American Association of Neurological Surgeons, Pediatric Section, New York, December 1980
1188. Venes JL, Stevens EA: Surgical findings in tethered cord secondary to myelomeningocele repair. Concepts Pediatr Neurosurg 4:165–185, 1983
1189. Vernon MD: Perception Through Experience. London, Methuen, 1970
1190. Vogel FS: The anatomic character of the vascular anomalies associated with anencephaly: With consideration of the role of abnormal angiogenesis in the pathogenesis of the cerebral malformation. Am J Pathol 39:163–169, 1961
1191. Votsey M: A Constant Burden: The Reconstitution of Family Life. London, Routledge and Kegan Paul, 1975
1192. Waechter EH: Congenital anomalies. Nurs Forum 16(3,4):299–318, 1977
1193. Wald SL, McLaurin L: Cerebrospinal fluid antibiotic levels during treatment of shunt infections. J Neurosurg 52:41–46, 1980

1194. Walker JH, Thomas M, Russell IT: Spina bifida and the parents. Dev Med Child Neurol 13:462–476, 1971
1195. Wallace SJ: The effect of upper-limb function on mobility of children with myelomeningocele. Dev Med Child Neurol 15(suppl 29):84–91, 1973
1196. Walsh JW: Management of wounds in anaesthetic tissue. Surg Clin North Am 64:809–819, 1984
1197. Walters BC, Hoffman HJ, Hendrick EB, et al: Cerebrospinal fluid shunt infection: Influences on initial management and subsequent outcome. J Neurosurg 60:1014–1021, 1984
1198. Warkany J: Congenital Malformations. Notes and Comments. Chicago, Yearbook Medical Publishers, 1971
1199. Warkany J, Beandry PHP, Hornstein S: Attempted abortion with aminopterin (4-aminopteroylglutamie acid). Am J Dis Child 97:274–281, 1959
1200. Warkany J, Passarge E, Smith LB: Congenital malformations in autosomal trisomy syndromes. Am J Dis Child 112:502–517, 1966
1201. Warren RB, Warner TF, Hafez GR: Late development of colonic adenocarcinoma 49 years after ureterosigmoidostomy for exstrophy of the bladder. J Urol 124(4):550–551, 1980
1202. Wasmer JM, Carrion HM, Mekras G, et al: Evaluation and treatment of priapism. J Urol 125(2):204–207, 1981
1203. Waters EG: Cloacal dysgenesis: Related anomalies and pregnancies. Obstet Gynecol 59(3):398–402, 1982
1204. Wechsler D: WISC-R Manual. New York, Psychological Corporation, 1974
1205. Weicker L Jr: Defining liberty for handicapped Americans. Am Psychol 39(5):518–523, 1984
1206. Wein AJ, Raezer D: Physiology of Micturition, in Krane RJ, Siroky MB (eds): Clinical Neuro-Urology. Boston, Little, Brown, 1979, pp 1–35
1207. Weir RF (ed): Ethical Issues in Death and Dying. New York, Columbia University Press, 1977
1208. Weiss SR, Raskind R: Further experience with the ventriculoperitoneal shunt: Prophylactic antibiotics. Int Surg 53:300–303, 1970
1209. Wertham F: A Sign for Cain: An Exploration of Human Violence. New York, Macmillan, 1962, p 153
1210. Wertham F: The geranium in the window: The "euthanasia" murders, in Horan DT, Mull D (ed): Death, Dying, and Euthanasia. Washington, D.C., University Publications of America, 1977, pp 602–641
1211. Whang CJ, Cauthen JC, Garcia-Bengochea F: Successful treatment of ventriculitis by continuous intraventricular irrigation with gentamicin solution. Surg Neurol 2:91–94, 1974
1212. White BL, Kaban BT, Attanucci JS: The Origins of Human Competence. Lexington, MA, Lexington Books, 1979
1213. White OR, Haring NG: Exceptional teaching. Columbus, OH, Charles E Merrill, 1976
1214. Wikler L, Wasow M, Hatfield E: Chronic sorrow revisited: Parent vs. professional depiction of the adjustment of parents of mentally retarded children. Am J Orthopsychiatry 51:63–70, 1981
1215. Wilkins J: Nutrition and wound healing. Perspect Nutr Supp 1:1–3, 1984

1216. Williams B: The March of Dimes and abortion. Homiletic Pastoral Rev 74:48–58, 1973
1217. Williams G: The Sanctity of Life and the Criminal Law. New York, Alfred A. Knopf, 1957, p 146
1218. Williams LO, Anderion AD, Campbell J, et al: Energy code of walking and of wheelchair propulsion by children with myelodysplasia: Comparison with normal children. Dev Med Child Neurol 25:617–624, 1983
1219. Williams RH: Our role in the generation, modification and termination of life. Arch Intern Med 124:215–237, 1969
1220. Williams SR: Nutrition and Diet Therapy (ed 2). St. Louis, CV Mosby, 1973
1221. Williamson RA, Schauberger CW, Varner MW, et al: Heterogeneity of prenatal onset hydrocephalus: Management and counseling implications. Am J Med Genet 17:497–508, 1984
1222. Willner AE: Abstraction, associative focusing, and similarities tests: Towards more clinically sensitive and better understood tests. Psychol Rep 29:688–731, 1971
1223. Wilner IA: Familial repetition of myelomeningocele. J Mich Med Soc 48:727, 1949
1224. Wilson E: Sociobiology. Cambridge, MA, Harvard University Press, 1975
1225. Wilson RW, Drury TF: Factors affecting the use of limitations of activity as a health status measure, in National Center for Health Statistics, Silver Anniversary of the National Health Survey Act. Baltimore, MD, NCHS, 1981
1226. Windham GC, Edmonds LD: Current trends in the incidence of neural tube defects. Pediatrics 70(3):333–337, 1982
1227. Winston KR, Schuster SR, Mickle P: Management of large skin defects in newborn children with myelodysplasia: A new method. J Pediatr Surg 13:303–306, 1978
1228. Wolf B: Anna's Silent World. New York, JB, Lippincott, 1977
1229. Wolf LS, McLaughlin JF: Early motor development in infants with meningomyelocele. Presented at the American Academy of Cerebral Palsy and Developmental Medicine, Washington, D.C., October 1984
1230. Wolfensberger W: The Principle of Normalization in Human Services. Toronto, National Institute on Mental Retardation, 1972
1231. Wolraich ML: Medical, ethical, and legal issues in selective use of rehabilitative care in the management of children with spina bifida. Spina Bifida Ther 2:213–222, 1980
1232. Wolraich ML: Pediatric training in developmental disabilities. Ment Retard 17:133–136, 1979
1233. Woodhouse CR, Ransley PG, Williams DI: The patient with exstrophy in adult life. Br J Urol 55:632–635, 1983
1234. Woodhouse CRJ, Kellet MJ: Anatomy of the penis and its deformities in exstrophy and epispadias. J Urol 132(6):1122–1124, 1984
1235. Woolf CM: A genetic study of spina bifida in Utah. Soc Biol 22(3):216–220, 1975
1236. World Health Organization: International Classification of Impairments, Disabilities, and Handicaps. Geneva, World Health Organization, 1980

1237. Wright BA: Changes in attitudes toward people with handicaps. Rehabil Lit 34(2):354–357, 1973
1238. Wright J, Wright B: Personal communication, 1985
1239. Wright PF, Kaiser AB, Bowman CM, et al: The pharmacokinetics and efficacy of an aminoglycoside administered into the cerebral ventricles in neonates: Implications for further evaluation of this route of therapy in meningitis. J Infect Dis 143:141–147, 1981
1240. Wright YM, Clark WE, Breg WR: Cranio-rachischisis in a partially trisomic 11 fetus in a family with reproductive failure and a reciprocal translocation, t (6p+; 11q−). J Med Genet 11:69–75, 1974
1241. Yamanaka M: Myelodysplasia, pathogenesis of hip flexion contracture and its influence on ambulation. Unpublished paper, 1981
1242. Yashon D: Prognosis in infantile hydrocephalus: Past and present. J Neurosurg 20:105–111, 1963
1243. Yates G: Moulded plastics in bracing. Clin Orthop 102:46–57, 1974
1244. Yen S, MacMahon B: Genetics of anencephaly and spina bifida? Lancet 2:623–626, 1968
1245. Yngve DA, Douglas R, Roberts JM: The cable-type reciprocating gait orthosis in myelomeningocele. Dev Med Child Neurol 25:116–117, 1983
1246. Yngve DA, Lindseth RE: Effectiveness of muscle transfer in meningomyelocele hips measured by radiographic indices. J Pediatr Orthop 2:121–125, 1982
1247. Yogev R, Davis AT: Neurosurgical shunt infections. A review. Childs Brain 6:74–81, 1980
1248. Young HF, Nulsen FE, Weiss MH, et al: The relationship of intelligence and cerebral mantle in treated infantile hydrocephalus. Pediatrics 52(37):38–44, 1973
1249. Young MH: Cognitive development in cerebral palsy children. Ph.D. Dissertation, State University of New York, 1977
1250. Yu HC, Patterson RH, Jr.: Prophylactic antimicrobial agents after ventriculoatriostomy for hydrocephalus. J Pediatr Surg 8:881–884, 1973
1251. Yuker HE, Block JR, Young JH: The measurement of attitudes toward disabled persons. Alberson, NY, Human Resources Center, 1966
1252. Zachary RB: Ethical and social aspects of treatment of spina bifida. Lancet 2:457, 1968
1253. Zansmer E, Tower G: A quotient for the evaluation of motor development. Phys Ther 46:725–731, 1966
1254. Zaporozhets AV: The development of perception in the preschool child. Eur Res Soc Res Cogn Dev 2(100):82–107, 1965
1255. Zook EG, Dzenitis AJ, Bennett JE: Repair of large myelomeningoceles. Arch Surg 98:41–43, 1969
1256. Zwiren GT, Patterson JH: Exstrophy of the cloaca: Report of a case treated surgically. Pediatrics 35:687–692, 1965

Index

Page numbers in *italics* refer to figures; page numbers followed by t refer to tables.